Somatic Patterning

Somatic Patterning

How to Improve Posture and Movement and Ease Pain

Mary Ann Foster

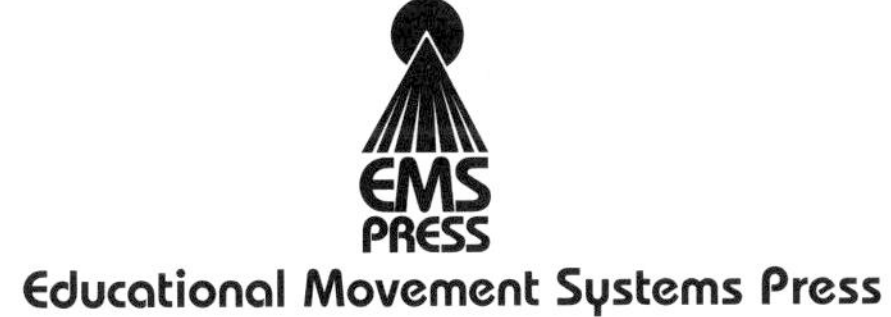

Editor: Mary Anne Maier
Designer: Teresa Bennett
Computer Consultant and Designer: Scott Harmon
Illustrator, Photographer, and Compositor: Mary Ann Foster

Published by EMS Press, Longmont, Colorado.
First Edition, 2nd printing

Printed in the United States.

Library of Congress Cataloging-in-Publication Data

Foster, Mary Ann
Somatic Patterning: How to improve posture and movement and ease pain.
A sourcebook for massage, bodywork, and somatic practitioners.
Includes bibliographical references.
Includes index.

ISBN 978-0-9713700-0-5
Library of Congress Control Number: 2003115443
1. Massage. 2. Health. 3. Exercise. 4. Self-help. 5. Somatics. 6. Alternative health care.

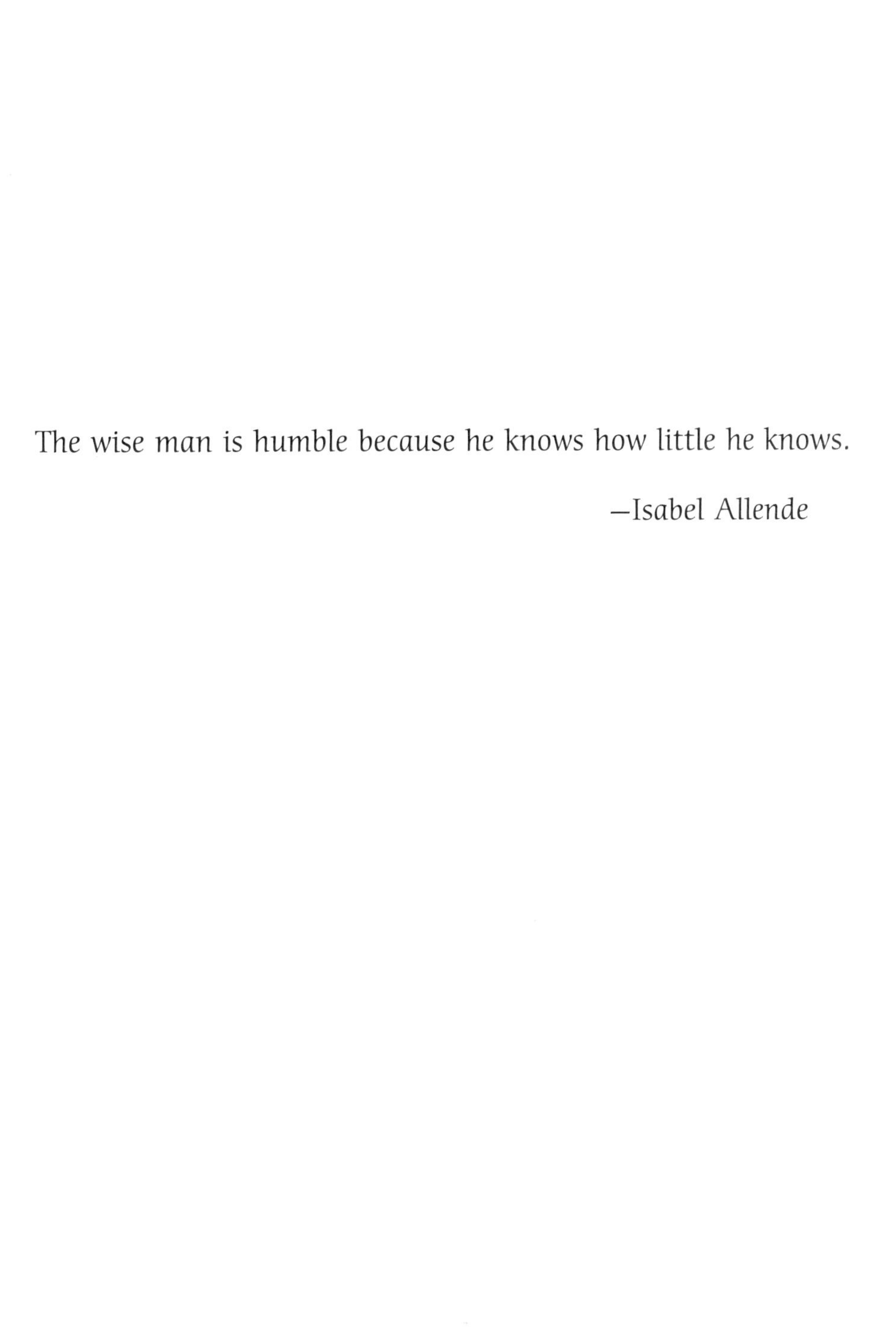

The wise man is humble because he knows how little he knows.

—Isabel Allende

Contents

PART 2: PRACTICE

PART 3: HISTORY

HOW TO USE THIS BOOK

This text will enhance whatever personal or professional posture and movement applications to which you may wish to apply it. It can be read and studied as a whole or used in sections. Use this sourcebook as:

- a personal guide to change your posture and movement.
- a sourcebook if you are a massage therapist or teacher, bodyworker, somatic practitioner and educator, dance or yoga teacher, or healthcare practitioner.
- a textbook if you are a massage school teacher or somatic educator.
- an exercise guide for you and your clients and/or students.

Glossary terms are in bold; anatomical terms as well as words or points of emphasis are in italics. Although I have attempted to explain anatomical or medical terms as they arise, you may need to consult a medical dictionary or anatomy book on occasion.

There are a number of special features in the book to help you integrate the material. They are designed to provide you with experiential studies so that this material can be learned through personal experience. The words *exercise* and *exploration* are used interchangeably throughout the text because somatic patterning exercises are more than a mechanical body-building technique—they are a deliberate yet fluid exploration of body movement.

The special features used in the book can be identified by the icons shown in the following list. These features include:

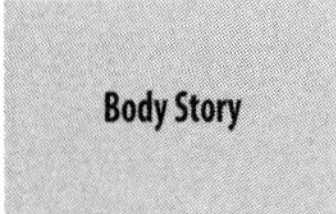

Body Stories: Case studies and historical stories provided for their educational value. To maintain the confidentiality of clients, the names and settings of the case histories are fictitious.

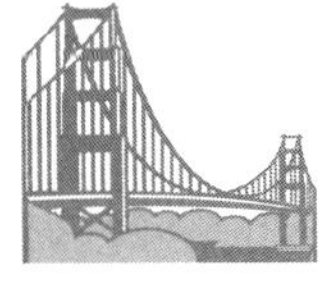

Bridge to Practice: Practical application for practitioners such as massage therapists or somatic educators to apply the material to work with clients.

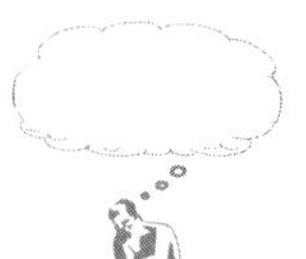

Critical Thinking Questions: Sprinkled throughout the text to spur problem-solving thought processes to develop creative ways of thinking on your feet and applying somatic patterning to therapeutic sessions.

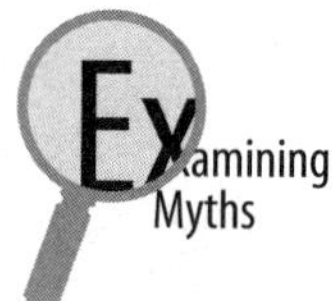

Examining Myths: Short pieces that look at the logic (and missing logic) behind popular myths about posture and movement.

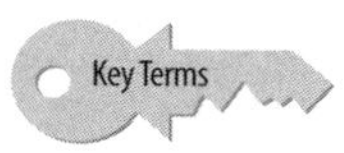

Key Terms: The general terms commonly used in somatic studies, some conventional and some not, provided to clarify the somatic vernacular. A list of key terms is provided at the end of each chapter as a review of the main points covered in that chapter.

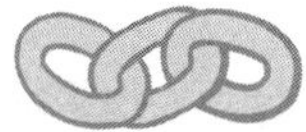

Links to Application: Short tips and practical ways to apply somatic patterning to daily living activities.

Patterning Exercise

The patterning exercises are the meat of the somatic patterning practice.

1. They are simple movement exercises and visualizations that correlate to the text. All the patterning exercises can be done alone or in a classroom setting.
2. Some are designed to practice with a partner to integrate touch with movement. Although the patterning exercises in Part 2 relate to the text, they are not meant to represent the techniques of any one school unless specifically stated.

Patterning Exercises: The patterning exercises are the meat of the somatic patterning practice. They are simple movement exercises and visualizations that correlate to the text. All the patterning exercises can be done alone or in a classroom setting. Some are designed to practice with a partner to integrate touch with movement. Although the patterning exercises in Part 2 relate to the text, they are not meant to represent the techniques of any one school unless specifically stated. A list of all the patterning exercises can be found on pps. 412-413.

To make this book user friendly as an educational guide, you have my permission to copy up to 10 exercises for each client or student with whom you want to share the patterning exercises.

It is my hope that you will enjoy this book, that it will inspire a new perspective, that it will provide you with a background to understand whatever intuitive patterning you may already be doing, and that it will help you feel better and move with more ease.

In fact, just reading this book will help you, whether you actually do the exercises or just start thinking about your posture. Many of the people who read it prior to publication commented that after reading it, they found themselves sitting straighter, practicing the exercises while at their jobs or in their cars, and becoming more aware of their posture and body-use habits in all aspects of their lives. Just the fact that you have read this far indicates you are interested in change, so it is highly likely that this information will seep into your awareness whether you actively apply it or not.

You may be thinking that this is beginning to sound like a pep talk. Well, it is—one specifically designed to motivate you to take charge of your body and free yourself from the clutches of faulty body-use habit and poor posture. I guarantee that if you begin reading this book your awareness of your posture and movement will change. Also, you may improve your body patterns, you may feel better and look better, your body may last longer, and you might even have a better quality of life. You only get one body, so let this book help you make it work well for you. Why wait? Begin now!

PREFACE

This writing project got its start nearly 20 years ago when I began to notice that there was tremendous overlap in the principles and methods of the various somatic modalities. Different schools were often teaching exactly the same concepts and methods but using different terms. Although they claimed that their approaches were unique, it often seemed to me that they were unable to explain clearly why or how.

Despite the confusions within the field, I found what I identified as the somatic patterning modalities to be incredibly effective, both personally and professionally, and wanted to know why. To this end, I often found myself studying 20 or 30 books at the same time, and lugging a bag of books to refer to in movement classes I taught to bodyworkers, which was just too hard on my body! Finally, I decided to distill the most useful information I compiled on somatic patterning into one book, and here is that book.

The prolific anatomist John Basmajian mentions in the preface of one of his texts that "writing a book compares to minor marital infidelity." Now I know what he means. With this in mind, I want to acknowledge the unconditional patience and support my husband, Gary, has given even when I have abandoned him to this project. I appreciate the volumes of feedback Gary has given me, the research he has helped me with, and the many hours he has spent with me discussing and ironing out theoretical conflicts. Also, many thanks to Mary Anne, my editor, whose patience and humor kept me going when I ran out of gas; to Teresa and Scott for their design and technical support; to Ed for computer help; to readers who gave me feedback; and to my many family members, colleagues, students, and clients for their undying enthusiasm about this project.

Lastly, one huge issue I had in creating this book was in producing the images of the many types of body patterns. In my opinion, many of the books about posture and movement today emphasize unflattering and posed pictures of what goes wrong with posture, or show incredibly beautiful shots of professional athletes and dancers who are able to move in a range far beyond the average person. In looking for a middle ground, I used a lot of unposed images of children, workers, or pedestrians to illustrate natural, spontaneous movement patterns. Also, I tried to keep the images of what is healthy more abundant than those of what goes wrong with the body. To this end, I want to extend a huge amount of gratitude to all the people who let me use their pictures, to those who generously let me raid their family albums (Lorraine, Kate, Deborah, Doug, Mary Lou and others), and to my beautiful models, especially Ashley, Michelle, Deborah, Mary, and Stephanie, whose images bring the patterning exercises to life.

INTRODUCTION

This book is about posture and movement. As such, it is an excellent sourcebook for somatic practitioners and movement teachers, particularly for teachers who integrate postural education into their classes, including dance, yoga, exercise, and massage training classes. But it was written first and foremost with the massage therapist and bodyworker in mind. Why?

Because this is my area of expertise. I have been a massage therapist and bodyworker since 1981, specializing in a patterning-style bodywork where I combine posture and movement education with hands-on work to help clients change the patterns that cause their pain and dysfunction. In addition, I have been teaching movement classes to massage therapists and somatic educators in both private training programs and massage schools since 1987. When I began teaching movement at massage schools, there were actually students who could not understand why it was important. Now, most massage therapists know how important it is for them to use good body mechanics while working to avoid pain and burnout. Massage magazines today are full of stories about how to recover from carpal tunnel syndrome and from shoulder, neck, and back pain, and how to avoid these problems in our work. *This sourcebook offers the first comprehensive look at posture and movement for massage therapists, bodyworkers, movement educators, and somatic practitioners, as well as for their clients and students.*

Most massage schools now offer some type of ergonomic training in Swedish classes, and may even have a separate class devoted specifically to this type of education. Most schools also have classes that address somatic, or body-mind patterns, i.e., how emotional patterns and traumas show up in the body problems that many massage clients and practitioners deal with daily. This book was written to be a practitioner's sourcebook as well as a text for both of these types of classes.

With books popping up left and right for massage therapists these days, you might be asking how this book is different and how it can help you. *Somatic Patterning* is unique in that it pulls together a broad body of information about body-mind patterns that until now you would have needed to study at least 40 books, many of them obscure, to understand.

Somatic Patterning **is a practical and comprehensive sourcebook that can help you in three ways:**

- **It gives you concrete tools to improve your own posture and movement so that you can have a long and prosperous career without burnout.**

To have a successful career in this field, a practitioner must use effective body mechanics, have a strong and healthy body, and practice attentive self-care. One of the primary sources of the repetitive-stress injuries that many of us experience may be ergonomics, but all ergonomic problems are rooted in poor posture and faulty body-use habits. This book goes far beyond the typical posture studies taught to massage therapists. It draws on a broad array of somatics and biomechanical approaches to provide theoretical information and simple exercises for you to improve your posture and movement not just on the job, but in all aspects of your life.

- **It gives you simple, logical, and easy-to-teach exercises for your clients.**

If you're like most massage therapists, you probably teach your clients stretches and relaxation exercises to help them with the problems for which they come to you for relief. Most of the problems that clients need help with are rooted in poor posture and faulty movement habits, and this book is chock-full of exercises that you can share with your clients to help solve these problems. *To make this text more user friendly, I encourage you to photocopy the exercises right out of the book and share them with your clients. (See the copyright page for photocopying parameters.)*

- **It gives you a template for understanding body-mind patterns in such a way that you can apply your new understanding directly to your table work with clients, which will boost your skill level and help you get better results.**

Most massage practitioners learn a lot of hands-on techniques. But understanding which technique to use when on whom for the best results is another kind of knowledge altogether. I know from my own practice and my experience supervising massage therapists over the years that we all struggle with this issue. It is important because whenever we practice hands-on work, we are continuously stretching, moving, and repositioning the client's body. Whatever the choices we make about these movements of our client's body will help to shape a pattern in the muscles, joints, and nerves involved—a pattern that may stem from an ideal the practitioner holds, but is more often random.

Somatic Patterning addresses this issue by giving you a detailed template from which to understand the body-mind patterns that promote alignment, health, and well-being. With this information, you can make informed choices about how you touch your clients, and not only improve your skill level, but get better results.

This text is the result of an intense study of the broad and diverse fields that work to change body-mind patterns. I coined the term "somatic patterning" as an umbrella for these approaches to wed two distinct approaches, the field of somatics with the generic process of patterning. Somatic approaches excel at working with the body-mind connection, particularly in cultivating body awareness. By making us aware of the continual flow of sensations through the body, particularly those sensations generated by movement, somatics teaches us to use awareness as a guide to improving mental, physical, and emotional health.

But a guide may be of little use without a map.

Awareness through movement is a first step in changing body-mind patterns; patterning gives the somatic process direction. Patterning is a generic term to describe any method of intentionally changing body patterns to improve posture and movement. Some of the most widely recognized systems of patterning are muscle conditioning used in physical therapy for rehabilitation, ergonomic education for reducing repetitive stress injuries taught to office workers, and biofeedback for reducing the ill effects of stress. I believe that patterning systems such as these provide the direction and content needed for comprehensive somatic education, which *Somatic Patterning* was written to describe.

Whenever massage therapists integrate movement education into hands-on work, they are practicing somatic patterning. It is my hope that somatic patterning as a paradigm and a comprehensive body of work will become a standard study in massage schools. As a paradigm, somatic patterning can make massage more effective and refined, offering an array of practical approaches for working *with* rather than *on* the client's body-mind patterns in a comprehensive and holistic manner.

Massage therapists and movement educators, it is my hope that this sourcebook will give you more tools to improve your own posture and movement so that you can have a long and productive career. Also, if you are the type of massage therapist who likes to teach your clients stretches and relaxation skills in order to give them the tools with which to help themselves, this sourcebook will provide you with many new tools in postural education. And lastly, it is my hope that you can more fully integrate somatic patterning skills into your massage or bodywork practice or classes to boost your skill level as well as the effectiveness of your work. In support of this, I welcome all questions and comments about this work that you may have. To contact me, please send me an e-mail through **www.EMSPress.com.**

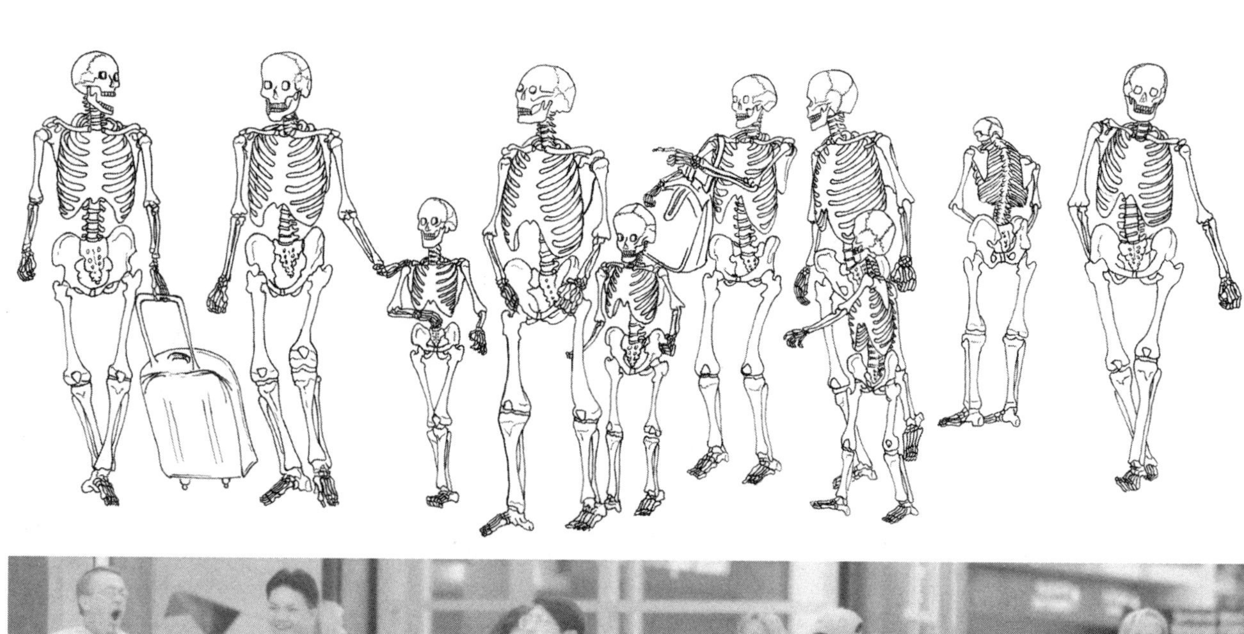

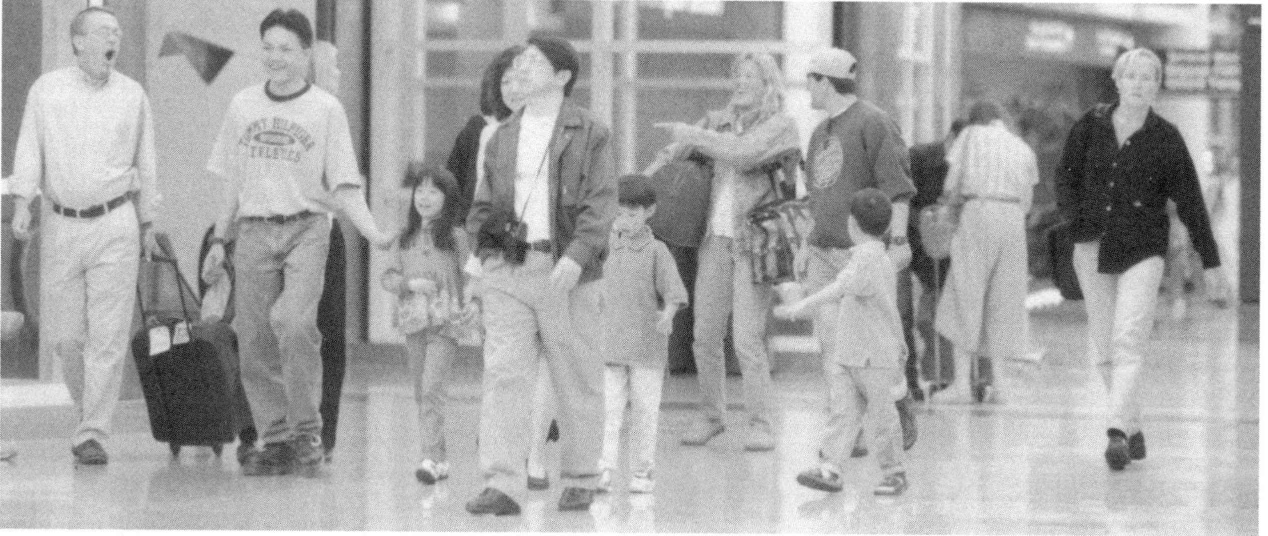

Part 1: Theory

Somatic patterning is so broad a field that its essence is often obscured by the diverse approaches it encompasses. Simply put, *somatic* refers to anything involving the "body-mind" relationship, and *patterning* refers to the process of intentionally changing body-mind patterns to improve posture and movement. Part 1 introduces the eclectic field of somatic patterning to the reader by presenting its theoretical underpinnings.

Chapter 1 begins with an introduction to the influences that shape body-mind patterns of posture and movement, with an emphasis on the sensorimotor learning processes of early motor development. This chapter explains that our patterns of posture and movement are not only molded and conditioned by early emotions and environmental conditions, but also remain an outward manifestation of our deepest thoughts and feelings throughout our lifetimes. This body-mind congruency is stressed throughout the text.

Many somatic patterning methods grew out of the need to address dysfunctional body-mind patterns that show up as general discomfort and ill-health, and can lead to pain and injury. Chapter 2 addresses this issue of dysfunctional patterns, discussing what occurs in the body that leads to patterns of pain and tension, and how to work with dysfunctional patterns.

Because there are so many different somatic schools and methods, knowing how to choose which technique to use when and to apply where can be confusing. To attempt to clear up this confusion, Chapter 3 presents the primary concepts and principles of somatic patterning that have been compiled from an extensive survey of the field. Chapter 4 categorizes the primary approaches and their application to specific types of body-mind issues.

This first part introduces simple patterning exercises for readers to build somatic awareness, learn relaxation techniques, deal with patterns of pain, work with breathing, and begin sensing the body both at rest and in movement. It concludes with a look at the steps of the patterning process in Chapter 5 to launch the reader into the many patterning exercises presented in Part 2.

OVERVIEW OF CHAPTER 1

SOMATIC PATTERNING
- A Historical Perspective
- Posture and Attitude
- The Human Movement Crisis

SOMATIC PATTERNING APPROACHES AND PATTERN RECOGNITION

FORCES THAT SHAPE MOVEMENT
- Biological and Behavioral Foundations of Movement
  - *Upright Posture*
  - *Opposable Thumbs*
  - *Neoteny*
  - *The Cerebral Cortex*
- Sensorimotor Learning
  - *Movement Precedes Sensation and Perception*
  - *Imprinting and Family Patterns*
  - *Body Awareness and Self-Image*
  - *Movement Initiated by Input from Sense Organs*
- Defense Mechanisms
  - *Fight, Flight, Freeze Responses*
  - *Muscular Armor and Bracing*
  - *Habituation and Holding Patterns*
  - *The Startle "Reflex"*
  - *Emotional Tone*
- Parallels between Human and Other Animal Movements
  - *Prevertebral Patterns*
  - *Vertebral Patterns*

INTEGRATED MOVEMENT AND POSTURE
- Body-Mind Integration
- Postural Integration
- Models of Somatic Integration

Fundamentals of Somatic Patterns and Movement

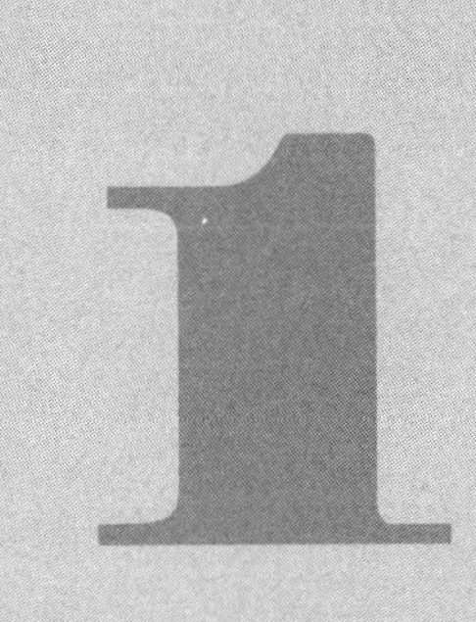

"In its simplest and most basic form . . . the problem is this: man is a self-conscious and therefore a self-controlling organism; but how is he to control the aspect of himself which does the controlling? . . . There is a point in which control becomes self-paralysis—as if I want simultaneously to throw a ball and hold it to its course with my hand." —Alan Watts

In its simplest and most basic form . . . the problem is this: man is a self-conscious and therefore a self-controlling organism; but how is he to control the aspect of himself which does the controlling?. . . There is a point in which control becomes self-paralysis—as if I want simultaneously to throw a ball and hold it to its course with my hand.

—Alan Watts

The predicament to which Watts refers in this eloquent summary of the human quandary is a direct outgrowth of our most recent physical adaptation: the human brain. The feature that renders our highly sophisticated brain unique, setting man and woman apart from all other animals, is our unique *cerebral cortex*. Although small in mass (the cerebral cortex is made up of a thin layer of tissue that covers the brain like a glove), the range of function made possible by the human cortex is immense. Unlike the cerebral cortex of other animals, the sophisticated circuitry of the human cortex gives rise to powers of reasoning and to an innate ability to think creatively. This capacity distinguishes Homo sapiens from all other animals. The cerebral cortex in humans also carries with it the mental powers to analyze, plan, reflect, and visualize, which have spawned advanced feats of human accomplishment that range from medicine and electronics to economics and politics. How and what humans think have led to our dominion over the planet. Yet while our technologies may have liberated us from the wild lifestyle of the animal kingdom, we shall see that they have not liberated us from the needs of the animal body.

Although the anatomical features and biological functions of humans are similar to those of other animals, our cerebral cortex marks human behavior with a feature not found in quadrupeds. We are self-conscious, possessing a unique capacity for reflective thinking, *an ability to be aware of awareness*. This unique trait has brought with it no shortage of political, environmental, and medical advances and problems, the most obvious being that by the very act of self-awareness, a person tends to stop action to observe it, literally interrupting the flow of a movement sequence. The natural movement of an animal is characterized by the creature's reflexive grace, economy of form, and balanced coordination, all marked by the absence of self-awareness. All too often, stiffness, pain, and effort characterize the normal movement of a human being. To understand why this is so, and what we can do about it, this text examines how somatic patterns form, what we can do to change faulty patterns, and most importantly, what we can do to cultivate healthy patterns. Let's begin with a look at what a fleeting thought about movement triggers in the body.

Thoughts have a strong effect on posture and movement. Take, for instance, the single thought of rising from a seated position. The mere image of standing up sets a flood of physiological processes into motion. These processes occur subconsciously with such precision and speed that they are largely imperceptible. First the brain, in preparation for coordinating the pending motion, initiates a chain of barely perceptible biological responses. Reflexive neurological circuits in the brain scan the memory banks in search of the exact program for "standing up." Once the memory is retrieved, the program is implemented, triggering a cascade of neuromuscular mechanisms. Thousands of neurons fire along miles of nerve tracks, which excites numerous muscle fibers deep along the spine to twitch in "anticipatory" contractions. At the very same time, other body systems prepare for action. The heart speeds up to pump more oxygen to the muscles as fuel for the pending motion, the lungs breathe faster to bring in more oxygen for the heart, and the digestive processes are suspended as blood is pumped from the gut out to the muscles.

The self-aware human may or may not notice the shifts that have occurred because what one is aware of depends on where a person points her perceptual organs. The sequences of events that initiate a movement occur at lightning speed, in a millisecond or less. In an able-bodied person these neuromuscular mechanisms operate so quickly and smoothly that they tend to be imperceptible. They do leave traces, however. If the occupant of the body pays close attention, she may notice that the thought of standing triggers a subtle sensation of hackles rising along the backbone as thousands of tiny anticipatory muscles get ready to work.

Suppose this process is occurring inside a man stuck in a desk job he loathes, a man who spends a fair amount of time daydreaming about being somewhere else. If he remains seated while longing to leave, the same sequence may still occur each time he has the impulse to stand up and walk out. The nerves still fire causing the muscles to contract, but the action is aborted. The result is incomplete because the motor responses are inhibited, and the man begins to feel anxious. He is torn between staying and leaving, which creates stress in the system. **Stress** occurs whenever the physiological engine revs up but the body remains motionless. It's like pressing a gas pedal while the car is in park; it wears down the engine. This process happens repeatedly to the modern human who tends to be mentally active yet physically sedentary. During a long day on a sedentary job, most people, unless they love their jobs, have fleeting daydreams about being somewhere else, then wonder why their backs ache and their muscles are sore when all they were doing was sitting.

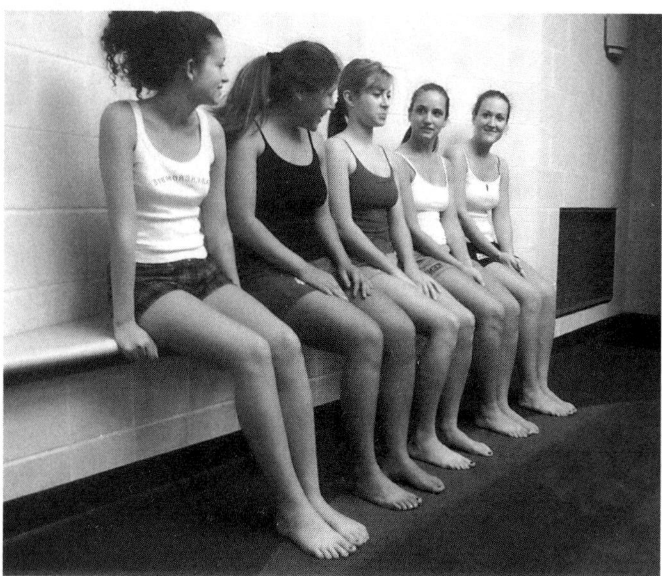

Figure 1.1 Each woman has an individualized pathway to standing (photo courtesy of E. Foster).

But suppose the hypothetical man mentioned above does stand up. The possible ways in which he can rise out of the chair are virtually infinite although he will likely carry his underlying postural tension with him as he stands. Line up 100 people and watch them stand from a sitting position, and it will become obvious that the shape of each movement varies from smooth to awkward, graceful to clumsy, or effortless to strained (Figure 1.1). A person might push with his feet, pull up with his shoulders, use the arms as a crutch, or pitch the head forward. Regardless of the obstacles to an efficient movement, such as pain, injury, weakness, rigidity, poor balance, or lack of coordination, the brain will find a strategy to stand the body up, and, over time, the body will adapt to this strategy. The marvel of the human brain is that it can coordinate convoluted movement patterns that go against our instinctive design. Hence, humans tend to have many awkward body responses that manifest in a number of common faulty body-use habits.

SOMATIC PATTERNING

Most people are unfamiliar with the words **somatic patterning** (SP), yet what this term represents is so fundamental to the life of the body that most will be surprised at how much they already inherently know about the subject.

The late philosopher and Feldenkrais teacher Thomas Hanna coined the term **somatics** in 1970 to describe the emerging field of body-mind therapies that use the body as the primary agent of change. The word "somatic" comes from the Greek root *soma*, which means "the living body in its wholeness."[1] Hannah felt that most people have very little awareness of their body and lack the ability to sense movement in their body. This condition, which he described as **sensorimotor amnesia**, leads to a lack of control over movement and indicates a fracture in the body-mind connection.[2] Poor coordination and awkward body-use habits are outward signs of a lack of awareness, a body-mind split in which the body lacks direction because it functions out of our field of perception.

The medical definition of "soma" is the body distinct from the mind, the torso without the limbs, and all of the body's cells except the germ cells (germ cells are the microscopic organisms that give rise to disease). In this discussion it has a broader, more metaphorical meaning. Soma as used here refers to the conscious, aware, awake body, the living, breathing, moving, and thinking body. **Somatic** encompasses the effects of psychology on the tissues realized in form, attitude, and posture. **Patterning** is such an obvious and natural process that it goes largely unnoticed. People pattern themselves all the time by using careful positioning before heavy lifting to avoid injuries, by using ergonomics to make repetitive work tasks less injurious, or by improving sports performance with efficiency training. And patterning is not just mechanical; people pattern their choices or careers after role models, such as a favorite relative or a teacher they admire.

Why pattern? For many reasons. To begin with, on a biomechanical level the efficiency of any movement depends on the brain's ability to coordinate the order in which thousands of muscle fibers fire. Imagine coordinating ten thousand workers to do a single job. It would be a daunting task for the most highly skilled manager, yet this level of coordination takes place with every single motor act we undertake. Add to this the fact that every movement is a series of motor acts strung together in creative and strategic sequences, and the variety of somatic patterns becomes immeasurable.

If humans were prone to natural movement, it would be okay to leave coordination up to chance. The problem is that by the very nature of our cortical abilities to inhibit instinctual responses, we have designed a whole culture that denies the body's basic needs. Consequently, we suffer from many faulty body-use habits that inevitably lead to pain, poor posture, and the accelerated effects of aging. This has resulted in a proliferation of stressed, weak, wobbly, and tight bodies that can break down at the slightest aggravation. Plus, we live longer than our ancestors; therefore, the ills of faulty posture affect us for many more years. In our modern, automated, and increasingly sedentary culture, repetitive-use injuries and musculoskeletal breakdowns are widespread. In fact, it can be argued that *pain not caused by trauma or illness is nearly always associated with poor posture and faulty body-use habits.* The muscle imbalances inherent in faulty postures and inefficient movements usually go unnoticed until a pulled muscle, strained back, tension headache, or a sudden fall grabs the attention.

The good news is that pain caused by faulty body-use habits can be alleviated with simple patterning exercises, which are so easy they can even be done at work, in the car, or even while standing in line at the grocery store. Webster defines patterning as any physiotherapy designed to improve a malfunctioning nervous system by means of feedback from muscular activity. By this definition, patterning is "neuromuscular" re-education. Patterning is learning how to move differently to correct the faulty muscle-use patterns that underlie awkward movements and poor coordination. In a broader definition, somatic patterning is any system a person uses to change patterns of stress, thought, or movement. Using this definition, relaxation training is a form of physiological patterning, cognitive therapy a form of behavioral patterning, and movement education a form of neuromuscular patterning. Although this book is about patterning and offers many simple and relaxing exercises to correct muscular imbalances and poor posture, it is about more than just neuromuscular re-education. Somatic patterning is broader than just the mechanical repositioning of the posture because poor posture reflects not just a physical problem, but a psychological one. Hence the addition of the word "somatic." In this text, the term somatic will be used synonymously with "body-mind."

Somatic patterning encompasses many diverse body-mind therapies that use movement—either physical or psychophysiological—as a therapeutic tool to change the thoughts, emotions, and defenses that affect posture and movement. The field of SP is broad and inclusive, yet there is one aspect that binds all SP modalities together: *they all use some form of movement education and body awareness to change faulty body-mind habits.* **Movement** includes not only the outwardly observable movement of the body, but also the hidden movement of thought, the largely imperceptible movements of biological processes, and the all-encompassing movement of emotions.

As mentioned before, people pattern themselves instinctively. Somatic patterning is a natural process in which people change the way they use their bodies in order to improve performance and efficiency, ease pain, and avoid injury. SP involves stopping before an action, becoming aware of how one is about to do that action, and finding a new and improved way to do it. Whenever we interrupt our habitual behaviors to find better, easier, and healthier replacements, we are patterning ourselves.

People pattern themselves with each new task. Every new chore we do, every new tool we use, and every new situation we are in requires some kind of patterning process. Since the body is a dynamic, living system that never stays the same, the patterns of movement and posture either improve or digress; there is no status quo. Poor posture and faulty movement will worsen unless attended to. Thus, we either figure out the best way to use our bodies, or we fall back into habitual ways of doing things and rely on faulty habits. In essence, patterning is the adaptation we make to each new situation. These adaptations can be deliberate efforts or subconscious responses.

A Historical Perspective

Before technology became the basis of health care and we came to rely on specialists to solve body problems, people were used to consulting the "healer within" to take care of their ailments. People applied herbs and home remedies to body ills, wrapped wounds and rehabilitated from injuries on their own, and created new techniques or tools to make their labors easier. Tending to body patterns was once a natural part of the process of adaptation to physical challenges and ill health.

Much of this innate wisdom was lost when, more than 300 years ago, Westerners began operating under a mechanistic world view. The seventeenth-century French philosopher René Descartes ushered in this view with his famous statement, "I think, therefore I am." In this paradigm, the body is considered to be like a machine with many parts that can be disassembled and analyzed to determine the causes of malfunctions and disorders. This perspective underlies our current mechanical, cause-effect approach to health care, in which a person takes his or her body to a specialist, much like one would take a car to the shop, and has a "broken" part singled out for "repair." If the part is no longer needed, it is surgically removed; if the part has a systemic malfunction, it is treated with chemicals; if the pain is not understood, patients are often told it's all in their head and sent home to suffer. At least the last scenario points to the possibility of a **psychosomatic** connection—a link between the body and mind.

Today the view that the body and mind are separate is crumbling as evidenced by the public demand for holistic health care, whose popularity has been spreading since the 1960s. Curiously, what is referred to as "New Age healing" is actually a revival of age-old holistic medicine, of ancient healing approaches that developed prior to the body-mind split. The current shift in paradigm is gradually seeping into the medical community, as evidenced by the committed and compassionate physicians who have recognized the importance of the body-mind connection in healing and are embracing alternative therapies. Many innovative doctors are now developing large bodies of research about the efficacy of the alternative healing modalities, such as Chinese medicine and acupuncture; the healing power of prayer and visualization; and the usefulness of movement practices such as qigong, tai chi, and yoga.[3] Also, in 1992 the United States Congress mandated the creation of the Office of Alternative Medicine (OAM) and in 1998 mandated the opening of the National Center for Complementary and Alternative Medicine (NCCAM) at the National Institutes of Health (NIH).[4] Plus, two large medical publishers recently published groundbreaking texts to familiarize physicians with alternative therapies.[5]

All of these changes have been spurred by the revival of ancient and long-used methods of holistic medicine. For example, the Eastern cultures have long recognized the curative powers of circulating "chi"—"the unified vital life energy that permeates and animates all individuals and the universe"—through the body using various mental and movement practices.[6] Also, ancient Greek physicians administered holistic treatments for the ailments of the body, mind, and spirit. During this period, ill people journeyed on foot for days to healing temples where they were given spiritual and physical respite as well as nourishing meals, therapeutic baths, and plenty of time to rest and contemplate the deeper causes of their health problems.[7]

In contrast, the dominant system of Western medicine—allopathy—is built primarily on pharmacological principles. It is the only medical system in human history that operates under the notion of body-mind separation, meaning it tends to treat a health problem in isolation without acknowledging the integral and complex relationships among body, mind, and spirit. Such fragmented treatment modalities often attribute complex health or structural problems to a single cause, curable by drugs or surgery. As a result, more and more Americans are turning to alternative health practitioners for holistic care that allows them to work with healing from within as well as preventive care. In 1997, 42 percent of Americans in a survey said they used some form of preventive or alternative medicine, and collectively spent $27 billion on alternative therapies.[8]

Out of this growing demand, large numbers of therapies and educational methods have developed in Western cultures. They address somatic patterns in what the peer-reviewed journal *Alternative Therapies in Health and Medicine* terms "a rational, individualized, and comprehensive approach to healthcare."[9] The alternative modalities usually discussed in this journal include yoga and martial arts, energy and spiritual healing, chiropractic, hypnosis, music therapy, aromatherapy, cognitive and behavioral therapy, biofeedback, acupuncture, Chinese medicine, psychoneuroimmunology, visualization, therapeutic touch, plus a miscellaneous category of "body-mind" approaches.[10] Many physicians practicing alternative approaches, such as those doctors involved in **complementary alternative medicine (CAM)**, use the term body-mind (or mind-body) as a catch-all phrase for a number of the Western movement therapies such as Feldenkrais and Alexander, as well as for such educational bodywork systems as Rolfing. Unfortunately, research on these modalities is slim at best, and frequently nonexistent. It appears that the body-mind, or somatic, category needs definition, which this text sets out to accomplish.

The numerous body-mind therapies that Western culture has sprouted teach a person how to work with somatic patterns in ways that get results remarkably similar to those achieved by yogis for many centuries. Although often associated with primarily stretching exercises, *yoga* is actually an ancient Eastern spiritual practice based on the mental control of the body, the thoughts, and the emotions. Individuals undertook the ancient art of yoga in the pursuit of spiritual growth. A yogi learns to regulate his or her posture and metabolism with stretching and breathing exercises, and by practicing conscious control over physiological processes such as breathing and heart rate, and over thought processes. An adept yogi achieves a level of self-regulation that heals and purifies the physical body to prepare it for spiritual attunement.

Similar results have been achieved in the alternative modalities that are gaining popularity in the West, such as cognitive therapy, psychoneuroimmunology, and biofeedback. Each of these modalities was developed to teach people how to reduce stress and to heal from stress-induced illnesses. The primary difference between the bodies of somatic practices in the East and the West is that the former came to these practices through religion (more accurately put, through advanced spiritual practices), and the latter through science (with many spiritual underpinnings). It may be that the main contribution of Western somatic patterning modalities is that they provide a renewed link between the mind and body, using the embodied integration of knowledge and experience to promote healing and wellness.

If you were an actor or actress in a play, what part would your posture be playing?

Posture and Attitude

Volumes have been written on the biomechanical features of upright posture and bipedal locomotion. Although both can be measured with great precision, posture and movement are also psychologically motivated. **Posture** is a physical artifact of the mind and the emotions that conveys a temperament or disposition in an observable stance. To posture is to pose, to assume a position, to take a conscious stand, to literally freeze movement. Movement occurs as the outward result of intrinsic motivation driven by biological urges such as hunger or fear, and by mental planning that carries out intention and purpose. To posture is to interrupt organic movement impulses and urges. Posturing is, in essence, a pause that renders control of the body to the mind.

The problem with posturing is that the more we do it and the less we move, the more readily our postures become habitual and fixed. Fixations in rigid postures are a largely human phenomenon made possible by our advanced abilities in self-awareness and the inhibition of movement. They limit movement and underlie a general somatic malaise that plagues the average person. Observe a typical group of people eating in a restaurant and it becomes obvious how common it is for some part of the body to be held captive to a postural fixation. For example, a typical person habitually props the nonmoving parts of his body into a stationary position (usually on the elbows) while the hand feeds the face. In an integrated body, the whole body is active with the trunk subtly rocking and swaying, lending an underlying support to the movements of the arm as well as responding to minute fluctuations in position, thought, and group interaction.

The nature of postural fixations is illuminated by differences between the movement patterns of animals and humans. An animal does not get stuck in a posture; every position it assumes is functional, reflecting the activity it is engaged in. An animal rests while awake in a lying position. It does not get up on all fours unless it is moving into action, usually motivated by an interest in food, in confronting or fleeing a threat, in sharing affection, or in going somewhere. The human being is too industrious to lie down while inactive. Rather, we prop our bodies in a sitting or standing position while busying ourselves with work, whether to sustain a home or earn money. Typical work as a method of earning money used to be defined by exertion of muscles and the creation of sweat; it now refers mainly to mental activities divorced from physical labor.

A human being has a vast repertoire of postures that may or may not have anything to do with the task at hand (Figure 1.2). Posture is usually the outward reflection of the person's thoughts and emotional state. Often it conveys an attitude or belief taken on a long time ago. Every psychological pattern has a corresponding body posture. The postural expression of emotional difficulties, for example, is obvious in a depressed chest, a confident swelling, a

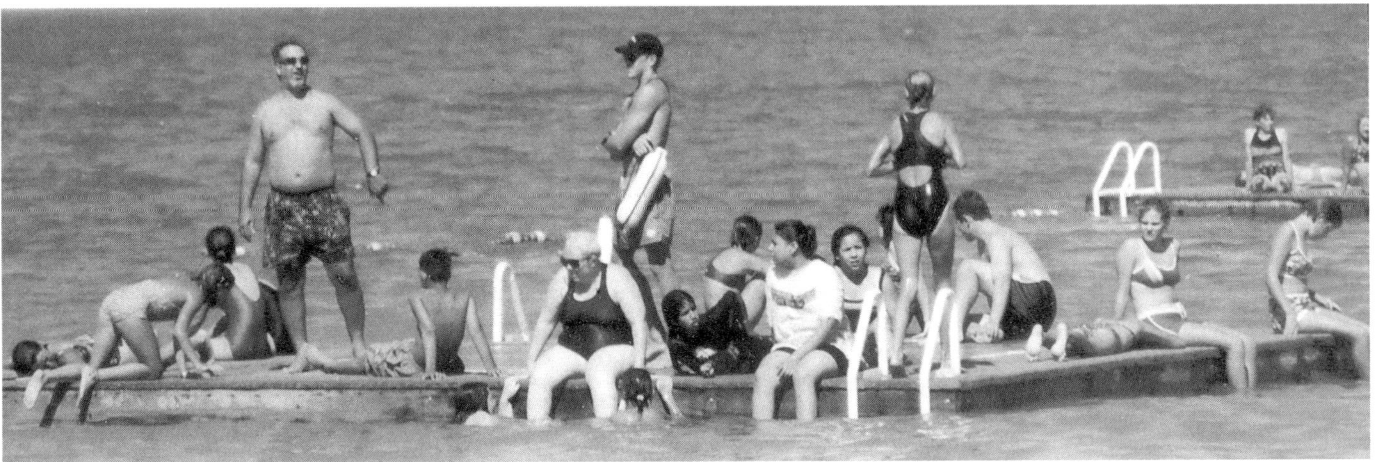

Figure 1.2 The beach is a great place to observe postural patterns.

shamed stoop, an idle slouch, or fearful rigidity. People wear their postures like clothes, and we all know how tight, ill-fitting outfits distort the normal shape of the body. Posture becomes distorted by defense mechanisms known as "muscular armor" (which will be discussed in the section titled "Muscular Armor and Bracing"). In this sense, posture could be defined as the psyche frozen in habitual muscular contractions.

The Human Movement Crisis

The body-mind split, although illusory (for there is no actual space between the mind and body), has had profound implications on the human movement potential. The human body evolved to allow for a broad range of mobility and a high degree of economy, a potential embodied by superathletes, gymnasts, and dancers (Figure 1.3). Sadly, the average person does not even come close to realizing this potential. In essence, *the human body is in the midst of a biomechanical crisis induced by lifestyle and longer life spans*. The tame tendencies of our modern lifestyles, particularly since 1900, have generated numerous "civilized" behaviors that are largely sedentary, causing the body and mind to advance in conflicting realms: the body needs to move while the mind stops to think.

The analytical mind of our technological age has created an unnatural culture, one that sacrifices natural movement, such as walking, running, or doing chores, to positional movement in cars and chairs. In America, where today more than half the people have sedentary desk jobs, movement is relegated to exercise that is accomplished after hours in a gym or sport. Only one out of four adults gets even moderate exercise. (Whether this is the result of weak intrinsic motivation or weak cultural support is a matter of debate.) At the same time, more than half the population is plagued by some combination of back pain, poor posture, mental stress, and stress-induced illness.[11]

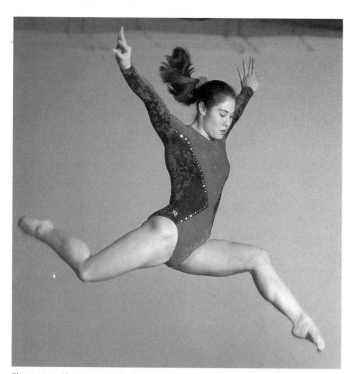
Figure 1.3 The outstanding range of human movement abilities is often realized in gymnastics.

Examining Myths

Myth: Posture can't be changed because it is inherited.

If posture is inherited, does this mean we are stuck with what we have? Although genetic factors determine the shape and physiology of our tissues, posture is largely a learned pattern; therefore, it can be unlearned. Our thoughts, emotions, attitudes, developmental history, and family habits underlie the unique style of each posture—all elements over which we have control.

When a person postures and moves in a smooth and efficient manner, an awareness of the body usually disappears. Errant impulses, chronic habits, and awkward movements remain unnoticed until the deterioration they cause leads to a body problem such as a strain or sprain, a sudden injury, or joint damage. A healthy experience may leave a lingering trace of good feeling, but the unhealthy experience grabs the attention. Body problems jump out in the form of a shooting pain, a sudden tear, or a clumsy stumble. They make us start paying attention to how we use our bodies and remind us that we are aging. They motivate us to stop, to become self-aware, and to use our bodies with more thought and care. They teach us what balance is by showing us imbalance. And they bring us face-to-face with an inevitable truth: *a person gets only one body, and it needs to serve the person as long as he or she lives in it.*

Backtracking is an essential part of the somatic patterning process. In short, a person notices what the body does that causes problems, then forms an image of what would solve the problem, and chooses between the two. Implementing the choice involves inhibiting a faulty pattern and learning or facilitating a better one. Each choice we make is like a rudder that steers the body away from faulty habits toward increased ease. The choice is somatic.

SOMATIC PATTERNING APPROACHES AND PATTERN RECOGNITION

The prevalence of back pain and musculoskeletal imbalances stemming from sedentary and/or overly stressful lifestyles is forcing people to address faulty postural habits and shrinking movement vocabularies. To this end, many therapeutic and educational modalities have developed that provide an assortment of tools with which to change somatic patterns. The complexity of body-mind patterns underlies the variety of modalities that have developed to address somatic patterns, each from a different angle. No one system is bet-

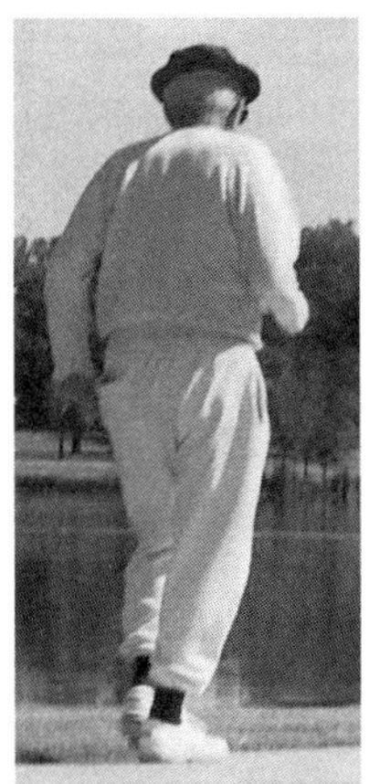

Figure 1.4 We recognize people at a distance by their unique postures and gaits.

ter or worse. Taken as a whole, they constitute a comprehensive body of knowledge designed to alleviate somatic problems and improve body-mind function.

Since 1980 the SP field has burgeoned, and there are numerous variations on each modality in second, third, and fourth generation techniques. Many are slightly different versions or combinations of the same method, which makes it confusing for an SP novice to make an informed choice among SP methods. To help the reader make intelligent choices based on a comprehensive understanding of the primary SP methods and procedures, the SP systems presented in this text provide an overview of a broad range of approaches. The systems surveyed to compile this overview are all first-generation SP modalities, ones that introduced something new to their respective field. The fields are listed in each chapter title in Part 3 ("Integrative Movement Modalities," "Integrative Manual Therapies," "Physiological Patterning," "Behavioral and Cognitive Patterning," and "Body-Based Psychotherapy").

The text offers many SP tools and exercises, but more importantly, it discusses how to choose which approach when, in order to pick the best tool for a given pattern. It is designed to help the reader recognize basic patterns, especially patterns of early motor development, muscular patterns that affect posture and movement, and cognitive and physiological mechanisms that create stress reactions and healing responses.

All forms of life have characteristic qualities and patterns of movement. Other than shape and size, movement is the most readily observable factor in identifying individuals of one species or another. For example, frogs hop, lizards crawl, amoebas flow, snakes slither, and humans walk. Every action, every behavior, every life activity is marked by movement. Humans come in a variety of shapes and sizes, yet each person has a style of movement as unique and exclusive to that individual as a fingerprint or a signature.

An individual's stylized pattern, or "movement signature," is so obvious that we tend to notice it without even thinking about it. A quick glimpse reveals a person's overall pattern. The eye is able to see the complete picture in a flash, capturing the fleeting details of shape, rhythm, and attitude. Because of our innate ability to see whole patterns, we recognize a friend at a distance by how he or she moves (Figure 1.4). A glance, like a snapshot photo, leaves a whole impression and reveals the configuration in its entirety. Yet, the overall picture fades as a focus on the parts increases. In fact, the more the parts are singled out for observation, the more difficult it is to see the overall pattern, in which case we miss the forest for the trees, so to speak.

On the other hand, a person needs to understand the diverse elements making up a pattern to effectively employ pattern recognition in SP. The hardest part of pattern recognition is being able to see a pattern that is not understood, to keep the field of observation open. Therefore, a person needs to be able to see both the forest and the trees, to recognize both the overall pattern and the interacting elements within it. A basic SP axiom and also a fundamental SP skill involves oscillating between the dualities within a pattern to integrate the parts with the whole, and the body with the mind (see Chapters 3 and 4). The most common oscillations are between body and mind, thought and action, awareness and response.

When posture and movement are integrated, the body moves with a natural flow and continuity; the muscles work in an efficient, well-organized synchrony. The shape of the body is dimensionally balanced, the limbs and trunk have proportion, and the core of the torso remains stable and connected. The eye is more readily drawn to distortions in shape and break in flow than to well-integrated patterns. Any break in the continuity of shape stands out. A frozen shoulder or limp seems pronounced, as if it were specially designed by nature as an attention-getting beacon that calls out for help.

A good way to observe the profusion of diverse movement patterns in people is to sit in an airport and watch the crowds go by (Figure 1.5). Each person is focused on traveling with a single destination in mind, so the movements are

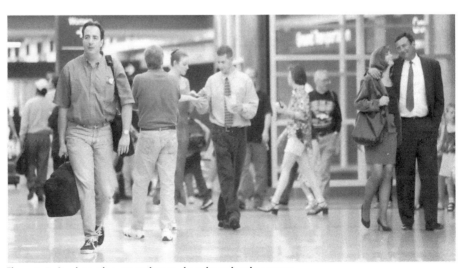

Figure 1.5 An airport is a great place to sit and watch gait patterns.

relatively free of self-consciousness. The group moves in a silent symphony of shapes and rhythms, a sea of bobbing heads and shoulders over a herd of rustling legs. Their bags teeter, clothes shift, and loose hair bounces along with the cadence of each gait pattern. Arms swing, heads rock, and hips sway. Upon close observation, a viewer can see movement flowing *through* certain open and flexible areas of a body, and flowing *around* blocked and stiff areas of a body.

FORCES THAT SHAPE MOVEMENT

Environmental influences shape the world within and around us. Consider the way the wind affects the growth of trees. A remarkable example is found at timberline in the high mountains, where the trees grow bent to one side with twisted trunks. Air currents on the windward side strip the misshapen trunks of all green growth. Environmental influences also shape individual differences among members of the same species. Every tree in a row is basically the same variety, yet each one varies in shape and size.

A newborn baby has minimal patterned movements. As the baby grows, movement tones the body in a cumulative process and forms patterns that progressively become entrenched over time. The infant gradually navigates more and more of his or her inner and outer worlds with creative and often spontaneous movement explorations. Movement shapes muscular and postural patterns, which in turn become the visible, observable aspects of the hidden patterns of the psyche.

The range and quality of movement that people experience sculpt the diverse shapes we each have. Postures and movement preferences are influenced by both external factors, such as relationships and environment, and internal factors, such as thoughts, feelings, and instincts. Changing moods and emotions move through the body like weather patterns, molding our behaviors and manifesting in the personalities of our expressive movements.

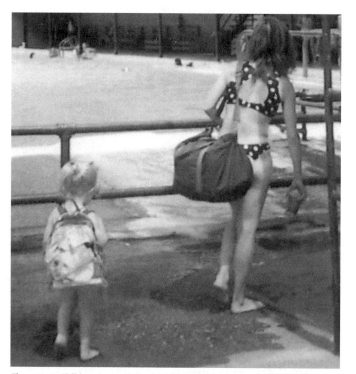

Figure 1.6 Children learn through modeling (photo courtesy of D. Kolway).

Habitual styles of posturing and movement, or lack of movement, pass from generation to generation as children learn from their parents. Similar postural patterns within families are so common that many people assume posture is inherited, yet a child learns a parent's patterns through largely unconscious processes (Figure 1.6). The current trends toward obesity and sedentary lifestyles hasten the degeneration of our collective postural patterns. One need only observe a random crowd to notice that many people suffer the ills of poor body-use habits. This may sound bleak, yet the good news is that even as adults, we can learn new patterns of movement and practice them throughout the course of our lives. It is easier and wiser to change poor body-use habits before they turn into health problems, no matter what our age.

Because human movement is complex, the elements that shape the body early in life must be considered on many levels to effectively change patterns. Every body pattern has an emotional component and a thought pattern that perpetuates it. The deep biological roots and developmental affinities of each person shape the sensorimotor and cognitive dimensions of that person's behavioral patterns. Understanding our roots and primal affinities toward particular movement pathways offers insight into how deeply somatic patterns permeate the very essence of our cellular organization and being, and predetermine all our habitual behaviors. This understanding also points to a place where somatic patterning can begin.

Biological and Behavioral Foundations of Movement

All life is characterized by movement; death, by the absence of movement. Human life begins with predictable patterns of movement. Some 200 to 300 million sperm swim toward the uterus, 300 to 500 reach the site of fertilization, where only one fertilizes the egg. Once this lone sperm penetrates the egg, the fertilized egg implants into the wall of the uterus and begins dividing. The new cell divides into two, then four, then eight cells, and so on, sending a juggernaut of biological forces rolling—beginning a new human life. The process is predetermined, predictable, and automatic; we all go through the same stages of development. Yet there are as many variables to direct the patterns of growth within an individual as there are cells in the human body, and these variables underlie the unique patterns we find in each individual.

In 1859, the British biologist Charles Darwin proposed his theory of human evolution in his book *On the Origin of Species*. In a later book, *The Descent of Man*, he presented his ideas about the laws of variation. These laws hypothesized that organisms develop specific anatomical features in response to functional demands. Conversely, anatomical features no longer needed cease to exist. Other physical structures change as organisms adapt to new conditions.[12]

Adaptations are the structural and functional changes that occur over a period of time to secure survival. Diverse adaptations have taken place within every life form on Earth to ensure the continuation of that species. Human evolution is a unique story. We have undergone a number of specific adaptations that set us apart from animals—the upright posture, neoteny, opposable thumbs, and the evolved cerebral cortex. Along with these adaptations come our unique capacities for self-awareness, reflective thinking, memory, and the ability to inhibit action. The human body has evolved for great mobility and flexibility, yet contemporary culture increasingly eliminates physical activities while demanding more refined mental activities. More and more of us are faced with the struggle of how to adapt to unnatural, sedentary, and overly mental lifestyles. Ironically, the very traits that predispose human beings to an unlimited movement potential simultaneously create the restrictive conditions that result in widespread immobility and pain. This brings up the possibility of losing body functions we no longer use. We know that the more we use a muscle, the stronger it becomes; the less we use it, the more it atrophies. With successive generations of use or lack of use, a structure or function will either adapt or disappear in a species. The quandary is this: How can we adapt to modern lifestyles without losing our diverse yet often unrealized physical abilities?

How we collectively adapt remains to be seen. Perhaps we will build motor vehicles in the future with dummy pedals so that we can exercise while in transport. Or somatic education will become a part of school curricula (another alarming trend since the early 1980s has been the reduction of physical education programs in the public schools).[13] Or perhaps we will build mock pulls or pumps on our machines of convenience so that they require us to perform some kind of muscular effort in order to use them.

How each individual adapts is a matter of choice. Many options exist. One option is regular exercise, which a person needs regardless of whether he or she practices somatic patterning. Another option is to actually do physical labor for a living, although even laborers suffer from pain and injury caused by poor body mechanics and are often in need of neuromuscular re-education. Although this text offers no single solution, many SP choices are introduced throughout the rest of the book.

Upright Posture

Our **upright posture** is a direct outgrowth of the evolution of our large and sophisticated human brain. We have evolved a vertically orientated backbone that orients the head on top of the body in a forward-facing erect stance. Unlike a dog or cat, our eyes look down on the body from above. This upright alignment tends to reinforce the illusion that the mind operates separately from the body, although in actuality, the two function together in a seamless manner. One could not sustain life without the other.

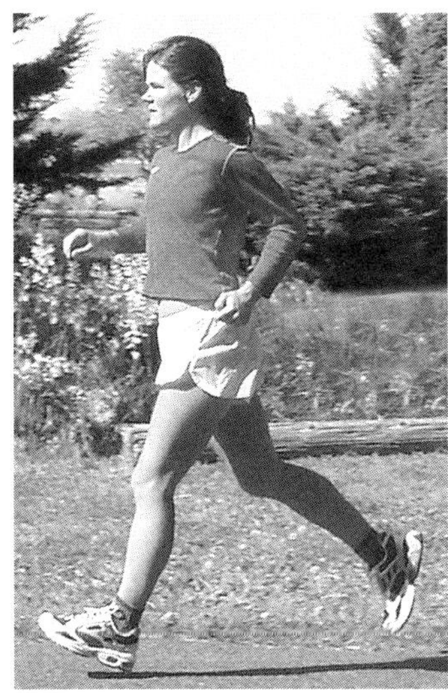

Figure 1.7 Humans walk and run with a bipedal gait.

Upright posture gives humans the advantage of being able to freely turn and look around, to efficiently scan and assess the surrounding environment, and to run in an incredibly efficient bipedal gait from any survival threat (Figure 1.7). This unique range of motion allowed our ancestors to adapt to, survive, and actually thrive in the many life-threatening situations that had already extinguished numerous other species. However, these benefits came with losses. For example, three tiny muscles around the ear are mere remnants of the telescoping muscles around an animal's ear that allow it to point its auditory shell in the direction of danger. The *platysma muscle* in the neck is also a remnant of the subcutaneous muscle that covers an animal's entire body and allows it to twitch to ward off flies. The most profound loss, which is also a great gain, is that we became civilized in the sense of developing organized communities for living. The human race literally stood up, began assessing the environment, and gradually recreated it in our image. Yet with civilization came the loss of numerous instinctual responses and diminishing contact with the natural world.

On a psychological level, many aspects of human cognition—ambition, desire, creativity, curiosity, objectivity, and dominance—motivate our upright posture. On a physiological level, the body is teeming with an ongoing stream of dynamic reflexes and modulating forces that maintain an upright equilibrium and poise in the human spine. A few, which will be covered later in the text, are optical righting and head righting reactions, phasic and tonic balance, and the fluctuating oscillations of postural sway.

Although the base of support of the bipedal human is much narrower than that of a quadruped, our upright posture is remarkably adept and dynamic. It takes far fewer muscles to balance and walk around one spinal axis over two legs than it does over the four-point base of quadrupeds.[14] Consequently, the human body has evolved for highly efficient weight-bearing and locomotion.

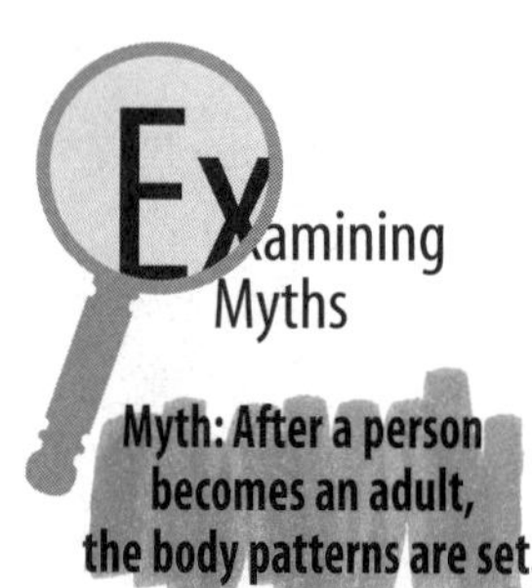

Myth: After a person becomes an adult, the body patterns are set.

Never assume it is too late to change somatic patterns. Humans have the most pliable nervous system of any species. We have the power to change seemingly fixed patterns of the body and the mind. Even if a person is a senior and has never exercised or developed body awareness, that person can still develop his or her body, learn to release tension, and increase strength, endurance, and coordination. As opposed to the old adage, it is never too late to teach an old dog (or even a stubborn human) new tricks.

Humans are well adapted for long-distance walking and running, an innate ability realized by the long-distance walkers and 100-mile ultra-runners.

Opposable Thumbs

Very few mammals have the ability to grasp and take hold of objects. This rare ability is made possible by the evolution of **opposable thumbs**, a development that enables humans and apes to manipulate the environment within a broad three-dimensional range of arm movement. The prehensile abilities of the human hand evolved into an appendage capable of enacting the innovative creations of the human brain, such as surgery, art, or music. The hand and arm emerged subservient to inventions of the brain. The shoulder girdle has a shallow socket that makes it highly mobile and able to reach all around the body, giving the hand even greater range of function. The opposable thumbs make the hands incredibly articulate, not only in a wide range of fine motor tasks, but in expressive gestures. The breadth of range of the thumbs is reflected in the size of the thumb on the motor cortex in the descriptive illustration in Figure 1.14.

Opposable thumbs enable us to dismantle and rebuild our environment as no other species can. We are thus the only species that continually adapts our surroundings in elaborate ways for comfort and convenience. Our inventions may make us more comfortable, yet for every machine we create to do a job for us, we collectively lose the physical coordination and strength to perform that job on our own. Ironically, our highly mobile arms, which gained mobility once freed from the weight-supporting functions of the front legs of quadrupeds, lose mobility as we limit their use. The irony lies in the fact that at the height of our evolved mobility, we are less mobile than perhaps ever before thanks to the modern applications of our sophisticated mental abilities.

Neoteny

Whereas a newborn foal is "hardwired" to stand and run the first day of its life, a human being must go through many stages of motor development, often in trial and error, to learn how to walk. Unlike other animals, humans are born "softwired," with only the capacities to suck, swallow, cry, and eliminate; all other human skills must be learned. Therefore, human children require a longer time to mature than animals, physically as well as intellectually and emotionally. Humans also retain childlike characteristics into adulthood, a human adaptation called **neoteny**. Neoteny means we are born ignorant yet have the capacity to continue learning throughout our lifetimes. What and how we learn shapes our body and mind. Since our period of maturation is long (18 years average), we also have a longer period in which to learn good and bad habits. When the caretakers continue to learn and grow, their offspring mature. Without continual learning by both parents and children, family patterns stagnate and unconscious, faulty habits pass to subsequent generations.

Since human development occurs throughout a lifetime, neoteny is apparent in the recurrence of developmental stages. For instance, an adolescent repeats the developmental stage of individuation during the typical teenage phase of rebellion, referred to in its first incarnation as the "terrible twos." Our neotenous nature makes our nervous system extremely malleable, and anything we have learned we can

Patterning Exercise #1: Family Trends in Somatic Patterns

This exercise illuminates how your family patterns have influenced your somatic tendencies. Write down your answers; then, when you finish this book, come back and look at your answers again. Ask yourself then: Would you still answer these questions the same way?

1. What skills do you have that your parents and grandparents lacked? Are your skills mental, physical, intuitive, artistic, etc.? How do you use your body with these skills?
2. What skills did your parents and grandparents have that you lack? Were their skills physical, mental, artistic, etc.?
3. How is your lifestyle more or less physically challenging than your parents' and grandparents'? More or less mentally challenging? More or less emotionally challenging?
4. What was the level of physical activity for your parents and/or grandparents? Is your level of physical activity greater or lesser? How do your activities differ from theirs?
5. What were the postures of your parents and grandparents like? How is yours similar or different?
6. Are you beginning to see family patterns? If so, which patterns are healthy and which patterns are maladaptive? How do your family patterns affect your posture and your levels of physical activity?

EMSPress.com

Patterning Exercise #2: Contrasting Reflective and Reflexive Movement

1. Tie your shoe without thinking about it.
2. Next, stop and think about the steps that it takes to tie your shoe. Then untie your shoe and retie it slowly, differentiating each step as you go, as if you were going to draw a picture of each step or explain it to another person.

Feedback: Compare tying your shoe the first time with the second. What was the difference? Which was easier?

3. Take a brisk walk for several minutes.
4. Next, walk very slowly, paying close attention to how you walk. Observe how you roll through your feet and shift from the heel to the toe. Feel how your toes bend. Sense the exact point at which your weight transfers from one leg to the other. Is your standing leg and hip straight or bent? At what point does your knee bend? Where are you looking: down, straight out, or up? What are your arms doing? Keep walking, taking at least four steps. Notice each of these elements on each step.

Feedback: Compare walking briskly and walking slowly while paying attention to each minute aspect of a gait pattern. Which do you prefer?

6. Now walk quickly again for several minutes. Does a brisk walk feel different than before?

Note: It may have improved because by slowing it down and paying attention to the minute elements of your gait, you probably identified where along the chain of action there were inefficiencies and instinctively corrected them.

EMSPress.com

unlearn. Therefore, it is never too late to learn something new, which holds true for sensorimotor as well as cognitive learning. Anyone of any age can undertake somatic patterning, including seniors and those who have never engaged in any physical activity. In fact, these population groups could greatly benefit from SP because SP exercises are gentle, easy to do, and require only one thing—a willing person.

The Cerebral Cortex

All of the previously mentioned adaptations were made possible by a single one that sets us apart from all other species. It could be said that most political and social achievements as well as problems stem from the phantasmagoria of inventions conjured up by our most accomplished and recent adaptation, the evolved cerebral cortex. The reflective abilities of the human **cerebral cortex** are a relatively new part of the brain that provide humans with an innate ability to project thought into the future and retain thought as retrievable memory (Figure 1.8). It gives us the capacity to think creatively, making us a species of diverse inventions. And it allows us to project the mind (or field of thought) away from the body into memories or desires—basically, to separate the body and mind with reflective thought.

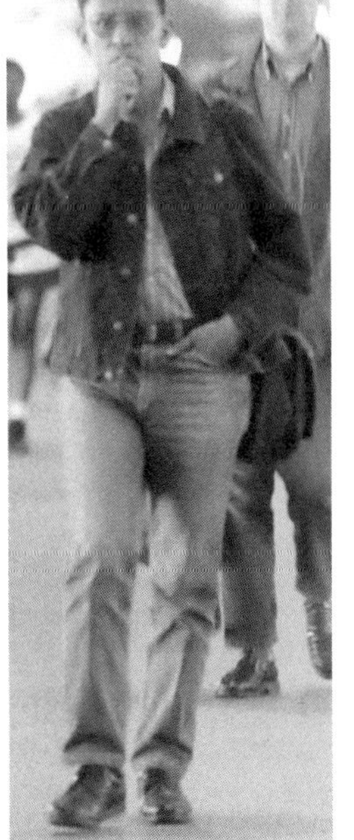

Figure 1.8 A reflective moment

Reflective thinking is an essential feature of human consciousness. It sets human movement apart from animal movement because we can stop action to observe ourselves reflecting. We can be aware of awareness. This state of consciousness comes with a major liability, however, one that can override all other human adaptations. With our unique aptitude to think analytically, to plan and implement ideas, we are prone to stopping action with thought and inhibiting natural body movement. Doing this has the tendency to take a person out of a present moment experience of the body. To realize how integrally related posture and movement are to machinations of the cerebral cortex illuminates the magnitude of this dilemma. In essence, human evolution could be summed up as a story of how the mind became more active while the body became more sedentary. Is our collective repertoire of human movement abilities shrinking at the same rate that our mental abilities expand? If so, the cerebral cortex may prove not to be the best adaptation for human survival.

Although the ability to think reflectively has spawned lifestyles that limit the human movement potential, it also holds the key to enhancing that potential. By being able to reflect on posture and movement, we have the capacity to stop and

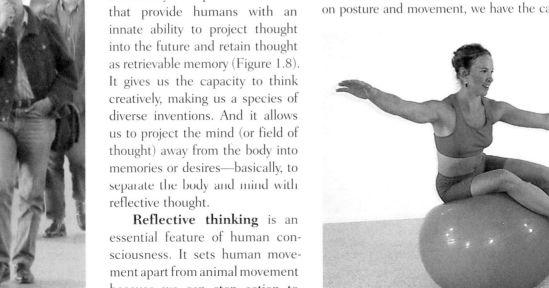

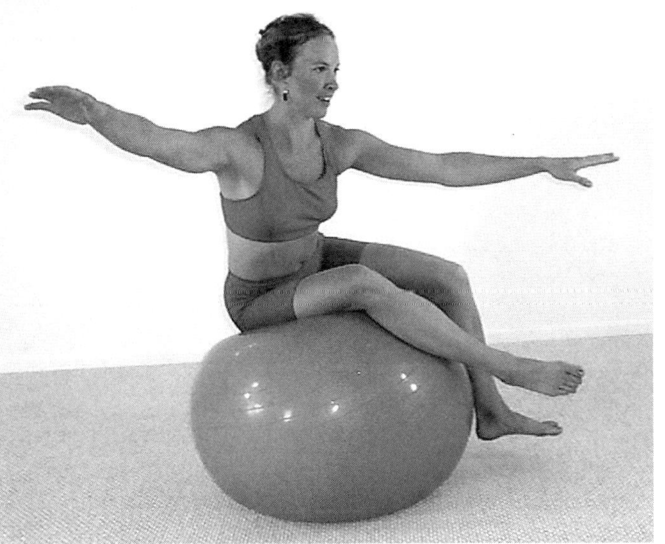

Figure 1.9 A reflexive movement

analyze where a postural pattern can be improved, or where a chain of movement is inefficient, and then use this information to restore balance and mobility. In other words, we have the power to figure out what has gone wrong with the evolution of somatic function and redirect its course.

Most people assume that the mind controls the body, yet 95 percent of all movement patterns are carried out on a subconscious level in automatic, reflexive patterns coordinated by hindbrain and spinal cord reflexes (Figure 1.9). A **reflex** is an automatic and inborn response to a stimulus, usually along a glandular and neuromuscular pathway, that is generally unconscious. A reflex differs from a reflexive movement in that the neural pathway for a reflex is hard-wired, preset in our neuromuscular circuitry, whereas a **reflexive movement** is any automatic movement that becomes habitual. This distinction will be revisited in the discussion about the startle reflex later in the chapter.

The reflective abilities of the cerebral cortex provide direction for human behavior. Yet while thought initiates action and gives movement direction, purpose, aim, and intention, most body movement is coordinated on an unconscious level.

Sensorimotor Learning

The differentiated channels of experience that adults have available to them—tactile, gustatory, auditory, visual, verbal, and cognitive—come bundled together in a newborn as an undifferentiated potential for learning. The infant's primary channel of learning and expression is sensorimotor. In the first couple of years, all learning takes place on this most rudimentary level, through the sensorimotor processes that occur within movement explorations. Since sensorimotor processes are the foundation of all learning processes and build a foundation for all channels of experience, movement is the integrating element of all somatic processes. Therefore, the foundation of somatic patterning is **sensorimotor (SM) learning**.

The famous learning theorist Jean Piaget, in his theory of cognitive development, identified sensorimotor processes as the first in a series of stages.[15] In the SM stage, children's reality is made up of that with which they interact directly (Figure 1.10). Objects only exist if they can be seen, touched, or moved. An infant constructs reality through constant and intricate sensorimotor explorations, either perceiving an object then moving it, or moving an object and then perceiving the motion.

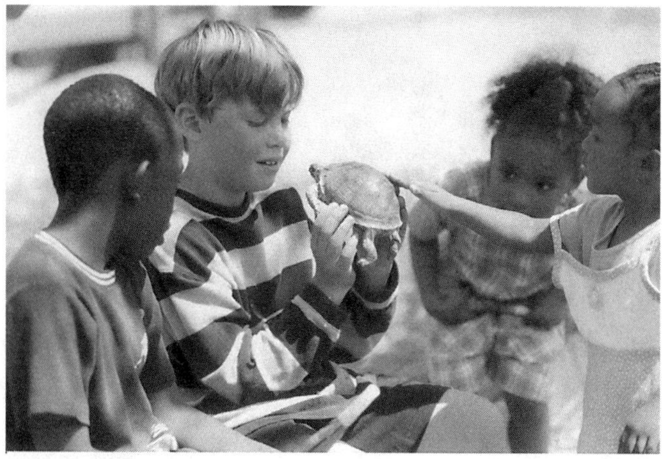

Figure 1.10 Children's reality is made up of that with which they have direct contact.

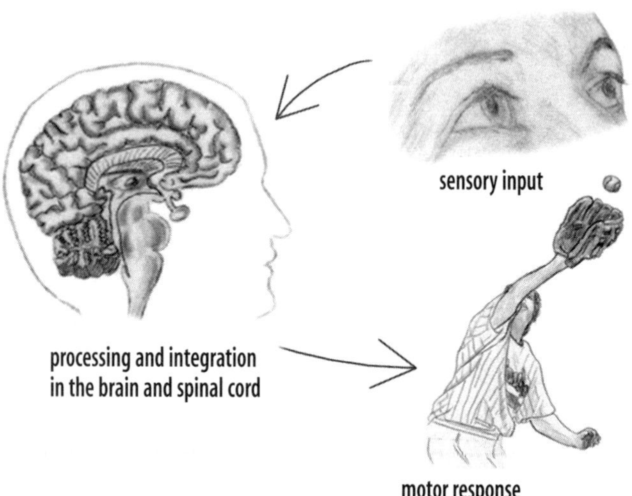

Figure 1.11 A schematic of the sensorimotor loop

Newborns spend an enormous amount of time exploring tactile and sensory delights. When an infant places an object in his mouth, a new sensory experience is created, which leads to a shift in perception. This new perception leads to another motor action, which creates a new perception, which then leads to another motor action, and so on. The constant movement explorations that occur during SM learning gradually build more and more complex neurological pathways. Each learning experience builds upon previous learning, and the whole process is stimulated and perpetuated by motor activities.

Thought, emotion, sensation, and movement are undifferentiated at the beginning of the sensorimotor stage. A newborn cannot yet differentiate the parts of an experience; he gets the same kind of pleasure playing with a toy as he does playing with his genitals. Learning is stimulated by **proprioception**, which is the reception of stimuli within an organism. Proprioception is stimulated by all of the rudimentary senses, from movement and touch to smell and taste, then to sound and vision. Each new proprioceptive stimulus affects neural pathways in an ascending order, with movement and touch being the most primitive.[16]

An infant responds to his mother's whole pattern: her scent, the inflection of her voice, the quality of her touch, and the sensations that occur while he is being handled. Sensory information comes in through the rudimentary proprioceptive channels, and motor responses follow, creating a new sensory experience, perpetuating infinite cycles of the **sensorimotor (SM) loop** (Figure 1.11). Physical contact influences emotional development. An infant feels secure during a soothing song and a warm embrace, or feels fear when hungry or cold.

The sensorimotor stage continues until the next level of cognitive development identified by Piaget, the **preoperational stage**, which still precedes cognition. This period begins at about age two, when the child starts to develop skills for using symbolic language to describe the sensations or feelings she is having. Prior to this period, sensations and emotions had occurred simultaneously. Now the ability to think in symbols enables the child to separate thoughts from feelings and actually describe her feelings. The child begins to differentiate ideas from actions. She is now able to stop her activities to describe them. During this stage, a child begins to assign symbols (names) to objects and people and calls them so. The toddler's grasp of symbolic thinking and language expands with imaginative play throughout this stage.

The child's use of language is limited until age seven, at which time the average child learns to represent states of being and is able to describe how things change. Piaget discovered this stage of **concrete operations** during a famous experiment in which he poured the same amount of water into both a tall, narrow glass and a broad, wide glass, then asked a group of children which glass had more water. The children under seven judged the amount of water by its height in the glass, claiming the narrow glass had more water. The children over seven were able to tell that although the quantities appeared different, the amount of water in each glass was the same.

In the final stage of **formal operations**, a child is able to grasp abstract thought. This stage usually begins at about 11 or 12 years of age, but it can begin later or not at all, in which case a person may fail to develop reflective thinking skills. During this stage, a child learns to think rationally and reason things out. Many adolescents become idealistic during this phase as they exercise this new level of cognitive development and work out solutions to social problems.

Although they occur progressively, all four stages are always present in adult behavior. They crystallize during different activities, and the strength of the latter three is built upon the SM foundation. When the SM patterns are weak or there are gaps in motor development, subsequent cognitive and intellectual development can be affected. To understand how SM development can create somatic problems later in life, let's look at a fictitious example described by occupational therapist Jean Ayres in her groundbreaking book, *Sensory Integration and the Child*. One child at age ten has difficulty figuring out how to climb a ladder. Another ten-year-old, with a healthy SM foundation, takes a quick moment to assess how he will climb, then scrambles up the ladder (Figure 1.12). Since the first child has poor SM integration skills, he most likely will grow into an adult who has poor coordination and guarded movement patterns, and may eventually develop other problems resulting from earlier gaps. These problems may include movement limitations, distorted postural patterns, and emotional difficulties accompanied by feelings of excessive fear.[17] The point of this example is that movement not only shapes the journey through motor development, it underlies emotional and cognitive development as well.

Movement Precedes Sensation and Perception

Early motor responses actually precede the perception of these responses. Movement precedes the awareness of movement, which becomes obvious when looking at the physiology of nerves. As the nerves develop, they become *myelinated*, or become wrapped in a fatty sheath called *myelin*. These fatty sheaths serve as conduction highways along which neural impulses flow. The thicker the myelin sheath, the faster the conduction.

The cranial nerves myelinate in the order of their importance for survival. The development specialist Bonnie Cohen points out that the first cranial nerve to become myelinated, the *vestibular cochlear nerve*, is a motor nerve that registers proprioception, suggesting that movement is the most important function that manifests in order to ensure survival.[18] Since the infant moves before she is able to perceive movement, it could be argued that the body develops before the mind, although the process is circular. Motor activity stimulates the development of the sensory neurons. Each time the brain registers a movement, a neurological pathway is either formed or strengthened, and SM

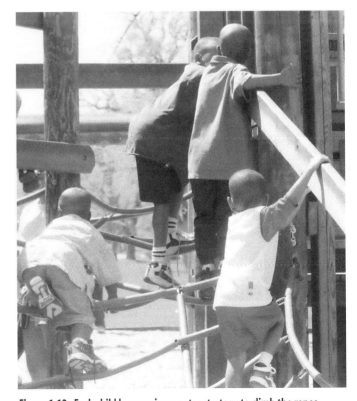

Figure 1.12 Each child has a unique motor strategy to climb the ropes.

learning occurs. In the same way a body requires food to grow, the nervous system requires movement to develop.

Each new movement pattern the child goes through marks another step in the long process of human development. Because our complex nervous systems need ample time to develop, humans take longer to reach maturity than any other animal; hence we are innately neotenous—we continue to learn throughout our lifetimes on all levels, through all channels.

Even in adults, motor responses precede a conscious awareness of stimuli. This was verified by Michael Gazzaniga, a neuroscientist who, after many years of research, found that people react to outside stimuli before they know *why* they react as they do.[19] After the reaction, what Gazzaniga calls the interpreter part of the brain provides a reason for the reaction. Cohen described this phenomenon succinctly in her comment, "the nervous system is the last to know, yet the first to remember."[20]

SM learning is a bottom-up process in which experience precedes thought. In the opposite learning style, the top-down approach taught in most public schools, thought precedes action (or is devoid of action). It is interesting to note that children begin school once the brain has developed the ability to interpret through symbols and learn from the top down. Yet until first grade, most learning has occurred from the bottom up. The transition from SM learning to cognitive learning can be abrupt for the child who is forced to sit still and think, which may help to explain why some young children become hyperactive when they start school. Still, the transition between SM learning and cognitive learning can be eased if the child is still able to follow internal movement impulses while learning to gradually adapt to external structures.

Imprinting and Family Patterns

A child recognizes the gestures or innate characteristics of a parent or caregiver and learns to imitate them. The famous ethnologist Konrad Lorenz identified this method of learning as **imprinting**. In an attempt to understand why mallard ducks would not imprint upon him when they saw him immediately after their birth, Lorenz perfected their quack. When the ducks were born, he stood by patiently quacking to them in their own language and immediately became their surrogate parent. His ducks followed him around and became distressed if they could not hear his quack. Lorenz realized that mallards imprint aurally, through the auditory channels. Human imprinting is much more complex and occurs through multiple channels.[21]

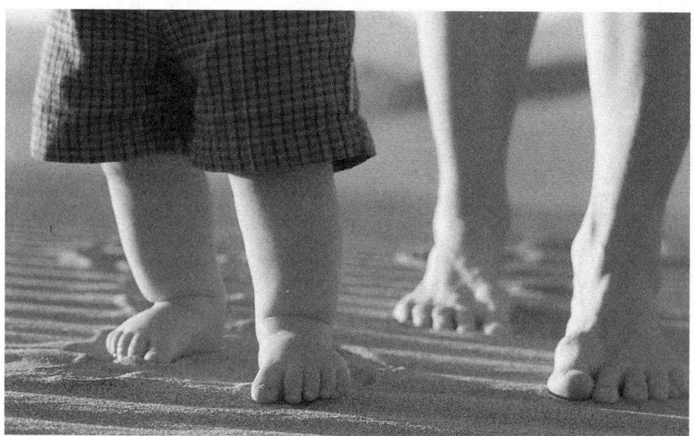

Figure 1.13 Children learn motor patterns through imitation.

During early development, a deep somatic exchange occurs between parent and child in which the child seemingly absorbs the personality characteristics of the parent. This process goes undetected by most people because it is largely an unconscious and invisible process, yet the magnitude of what is going on is huge. The younger the child, the more impressionable she or he is. We see imprinting when we watch a baby imitate her caregiver's mannerisms and gestures. The parent's smell, touch, voice, and movement characteristics shape the infant's somatic rhythms. The infant matches and internalizes the subtleties of her parent's gestures, speech patterns, and behaviors, modeling with an astonishing and sometimes startling accuracy.

The parent is always teaching the child something, whether the parent's behavior is intentional or habitual, conscious or unconscious. Every interaction between parent and child communicates a value or behavior that the child learns and internalizes. The extent of this exchange is profound, particularly when we observe a child's ability to precisely mimic the movement and speech patterns of the parent (Figure 1.13). Whenever the child can successfully imitate the somatic patterns of the parent, a strong connection occurs between the two, and this connection deepens the bonding between the two.

Somatic patterns are passed down in a family largely through imprinting and imitation, and can be observed in the postural and gestural characteristics unique to each family. For example, an active or athletic mother models patterns of movement that her child will be likely to repeat. Conversely, a sedentary parent models patterns of immobility. Although we inherit genetic similarities that predispose us toward the similar body types and movement styles of our birth parents, we are innately predisposed to learning through imitation and can recreate the subtlest shapes and postures. This means that most faulty patterns are learned and can be unlearned.

Body Awareness and Self-Image

> Each one of us speaks, moves, thinks, and feels in a different way, each according to the image of himself that he has built up over the years. In order to change our mode of action, we must change the image of ourselves that we carry within us.[22]
>
> —Moshe Feldenkrais

Awareness can be based on body sensations coming from an actual physical sense of the body or from an image the mind has formed of the body. **Body awareness** arises from direct experience of the body through sensations, feelings, and the proprioception of motor acts. We feel our bodies by sensing changing tensions in our muscles via contraction or elongation, and sensing the changing tone in our physiology, which spans from a relaxed state to an aroused state. Without movement, the body is difficult to sense; hence, prolonged immobility has a numbing effect on body awareness. Immobility also has deep psychological effects: paralysis not only creates dependence on others to meet one's basic movement needs, it often leads to depression. A person needs movement to stimulate psychological health. This is why exercise is a natural antidote for both depression and low self-esteem.

Self-image differs from body awareness because it is largely a mental process. It is an indirect, secondhand awareness of self, one step removed from direct experience of the body. Self-image is, essentially, the mind reflecting upon the body and the personality, and then forming a picture of them. Many people confuse self-image with body awareness, thereby distorting a direct experience of the body.

The foundations of body awareness and self-image are established during early motor development when a baby forms a sense of self in relation to her physical communications with others. Since an infant has not developed the capacity to use symbols or language, communication is based on motor acts. As infants grow into toddlers, communication gradually expands into verbal channels, as body experiences and feelings are translated into ideas and words. This explains why "body language" is so accurate. Since the foundation of personal expression was established in early sensorimotor pathways, all our postures and gestures reflect the content of our communications.[23]

It is estimated that only 5 percent of the cerebral cortex, the site of cognitive abilities, is developed in the average person. On a parallel note, does the average person use only 5 percent of his or her movement potential? And, does the shape of the homunculus change with the development of motor skills?

The size of areas in the motor cortex devoted to the control of movement in a specific part of the body is illustrated in a *somatotopic map* (Figure 1.14). The size of each part is proportional to the motor skills performed by that area; therefore, the thumb and lips are huge, whereas the legs and trunk are small. Moshe Feldenkrais, the physicist who pioneered a popular movement therapy described in Chapter 11, theorized that a somatotopic map or "homunculus" is the closest concept we have to a neurological map of body image.[24] He speculated that self-image has a direct relationship to the level of a person's motor development and the size of the motor cortex in the brain; therefore a person with a broad base of motor skills has a broad self-image. Conversely, a poor self-image grows around awkward, uncoordinated, and limited movement patterns.

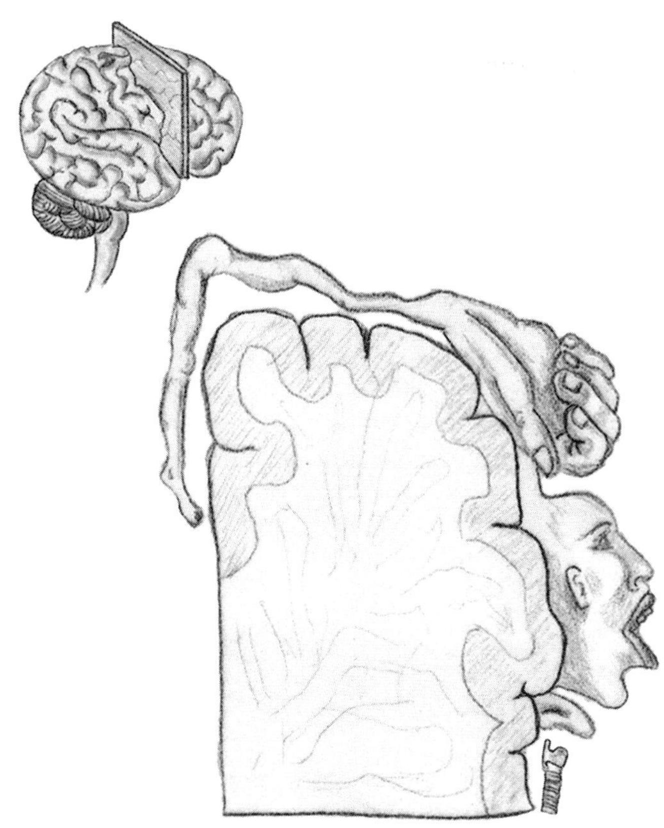

Figure 1.14 A somatotopic map of the motor cortex shows the relative size of the cortex devoted to motor control over each body part.

Ideally, there is congruence between self-image and body awareness, with one reflecting the other. In this case, people are who they see themselves to be, and, when asked to describe themselves, their descriptions match how they look and how they move. Conversely, a lack of congruence between body awareness and self-image points to fixations in psychological development. For instance, a small, clingy person may have a self-image of being strong and independent, or a large, muscular person may see himself as weak and needy.

It is best if children can develop self-image through sensorimotor exploration without too much negative interference from the outside world. Development begins with a normal sequence of sensorimotor processes, which establish a sensorimotor foundation for a sense of self rooted in intrinsic awareness. Yet many children have their sensorimotor explorations interrupted and are forced to cope with the outer world before their inner somatic world is firmly

Conforming the Body to Ideals and Images

Many faulty body patterns develop according to a person's ideas about how he or she should look. For example, a client named Tom had chronic jaw pain. He also had strong beliefs about how inappropriate it was to be seen with his mouth open. Tom had developed a tight jaw in his efforts to maintain his image of how a face "should" look. He would also become extremely angry with his teenage children when they let their jaws hang open. Upon examination, Tom found that both his behavior and his jaw tension masked deep feelings of insecurity and rage. With this insight, he was able to feel more compassion toward his children and stopped nagging them about their slack jaws.

Another client named Beth did everything she could to not be like her mother, whom she disliked immensely. Beth had developed an image of herself congruent with her father's qualities, adopting his masculine style of movement, behavior, and language. During patterning sessions, Beth realized her somatic patterns did not really express who she was. This realization began a lengthy process of first disassociating from her father's patterns by telling herself that, when she felt his patterns, she was feeling a pattern she took on that was not her true self. Beth gradually developed a body awareness that was based on her own intrinsic sense of self. Eventually she developed a more poised posture and had more spontaneous movements that were absent of the self-consciousness she had felt when trying to emulate her father.

A third client named Julie had a pattern of collapsing her body below the right side of her diaphragm, around the area of the liver. When asked about this pattern, Julie spoke of how she had had a cancerous section of her large intestine removed. After the surgery, she formed a body image of literally having a hole in the area where the part of the organ had been taken out, and collapsed her body to accommodate the image. When asked to sense the area, Julie realized that there was not really a hole or hollow space there. As she realized this, her torso began to relax and elongate, filling out the collapsed posture.

established. Many events can interfere with normal development, among the stronger influences being physical and emotional trauma and neglect. A positive self-image grows with each positive experience of body awareness, such as the achievements a child makes in sports, dance, and physical activities. Successful and gratifying physical activities and awareness can be cultivated any time in a person's life to build a positive self-image, which is the essence of what occurs during somatic patterning.

Movement Initiated by Input from Sense Organs

We take it for granted that we are in control of our body movements, yet most movements are initiated by sensory processes that occur naturally and unconsciously. Movement initiates as a response to our immersion in somatosensory experiences. In other words, we continually make subconscious responses to the deluge of sensory input that floods our awareness on a constant basis. Sensory input comes from internal physiological processes such as digestion and hunger, from muscular activity, and from the continual environmental stimuli received through the sense organs, such as tastes, smells, sounds, sights, tactile stimulation, and vibrational shifts.

The earliest movement patterns initiate in response to internal processes. For example, activity in the digestive track creates intrinsic sensations to which we may find ourselves responding on a subconscious level. These natural responses are most obvious in newborns, who silently wiggle and squirm as digestive processes move between the head and tail and crystallize every now and then in a burp, gurgle, or gas.

We also make continual responses to sensory input coming from the environment, which we may or may not be aware of. Again, these responses are most obvious in infants, who spend the bulk of their waking hours making subtle spinal undulations as they explore the environment through their mouths and tactile and visual senses. A reach to grasp an object with the hands or mouth may initiate a transition from flexion to extension and may even spontaneously roll the infant over. Or a baby may turn his or her head toward a pleasant sound or away from an unpleasant one. When auditory responses engage, the ears "perk up," the head turns toward the sound, and the body follows. The trunk extends, which brings more spatial support to the spine. Or a strong scent lifts the head up and forward, bringing length to the trunk and buoyancy to the sinuses.

Most mammals navigate their territory with their noses, sniffing and following scents. In contrast, vision could be said to be the most active sense organ and the most predominant coordinator of spinal movement in humans. Again, the support of vision in spinal movement is most obvious in the formative stages. A baby receives a large degree of neurological support for a proportionally large head from the **optical righting reaction,** which maintains the head in a vertical position when the body is tilted in any direction. Optical support can be seen when the infant lifts his large head to look at something (Figure 1.15). As the head turns or moves to focus the eyes, the spine follows. Watch a person walking

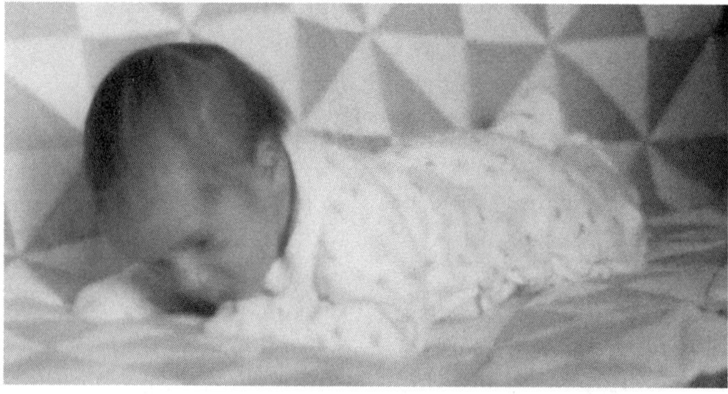

Figure 1.15 Optical support assists this newborn (3 1/2 weeks old) in lifting his head (photo courtesy of L. Bright).

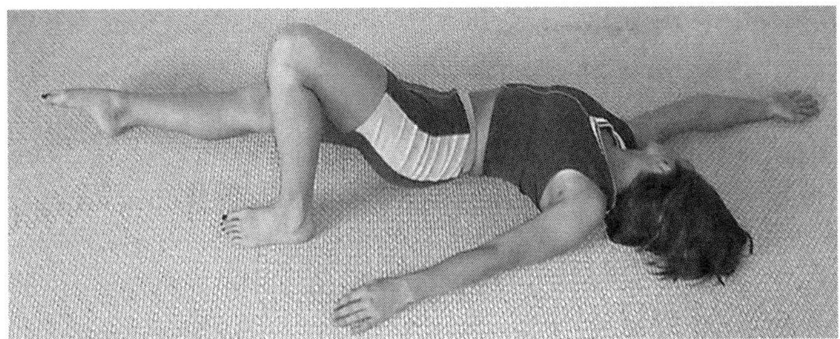

Figure 1.16 As the eyes focus on one hand moving above the shoulder level, that entire side of the body goes into extension.

around a grocery store shopping and it becomes obvious how each change in direction initiates in the head. The head turns and looks, and the body follows. The **horizontal scanning** of the eyes as well as hand-to-eye reflexes, both of which turn the head and rotate the spine, initiate homolateral movement—flexion on one side of the body with extension on the other (Figure 1.16).

The bulk of our daily movement repertoire is initiated by the constant sensory stimulation we encounter, often below the radar of awareness, which leads to a myriad of spontaneous motor responses. The body relies on sensory input, both from the environment and from the body (such as hunger, cold, or pain) to regulate function. The sense organs and the proprioceptors of the muscles and joints create a vital link between the body and the outside world. Without them, we would suffer from sensory deprivation, which has been known to delay and even inhibit development. During extreme sensory deprivation, the brain will fabricate reality in the form of hallucinations. The effects of sensory deprivation underscore the importance of sensory stimulation and movement for normal neural development. Even as little as an hour in a float tank cuts off our connection to reality, which, depending on the person, can be either relaxing or disorienting.

Many patterning practitioners believe it is important to consider the order in which tactile, auditory, visual, and cognitive functions develop when deciding where to begin work on changing inefficient patterns or learning beneficial patterns. Feldenkrais discussed the order with which he addressed the various sensory levels in his rehabilitative work with a stroke patient. He pointed out that the earlier a brain function occurred in evolution, the lower it is when considering the entire nervous system within a vertical hierarchy; therefore, dysfunction in lower centers can put a brake on higher centers.[25] With this in mind, a bottom-up approach to patterning could begin by reawakening tactile receptors in the skin with such exercises as rolling around on the floor and sensing the changing contact that the body makes with the floor.

Two other sensory elements are important to consider in somatic patterning: *weight* and *space*. The body is anchored to the earth by the pull of gravity, which gives its mass weight. The body receives an upward lift from the numerous reflexive mechanisms in the head and the sense organs that orient the spine in space. During somatic patterning, we increase our feeling of support by increasing an awareness of sensations of body weight and of where we are in space. Feeling sensations of body weight can evoke an intrinsic awareness of the body and a relaxation response, whereas sensing where the body is in space develops an extrinsic awareness and tends to make a person more alert. It is usually easier to feel body weight while resting into a supporting surface when the eyes are closed to shut out visual distractions. It is easier to feel spatial support by sensing the environment around the body or extending the limbs into the space around the body, like a person would do to stand taller or stretch. Different cultures have different spatial awareness; for instance, in an overpopulated area, people tend to have an awareness of the space behind them although their visual focus may be in front of them. Where people are used to wide open spaces, spatial awareness is probably more expanded yet may not be refined in crowded situations.

Patterning Exercise #3: Optical Support and Optical Righting

1. *Optical support:* Lie on the floor on your belly with both upper arms out to the side, palms flat, and elbows bent at a right angle. Rest your head on your forehead and relax into the position with your eyes closed.

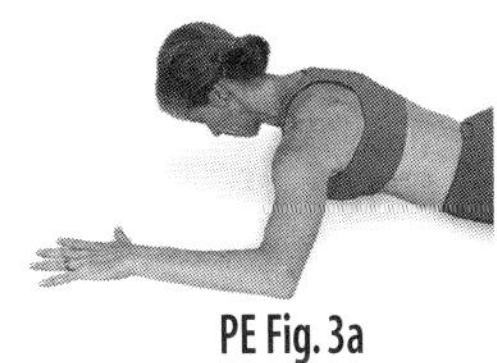

PE Fig. 3a

2. Open your eyes and look at the floor directly below you. If you have elicited optical support, you will be able to lift your head while keeping your neck long and hold it there with minimal effort (PE Fig. 3a).
3. *Optical righting:* Lie over a physioball. Close your eyes and relax your neck and spine (see PE Fig. 3b).
4. Now open your eyes and look at the floor. Again, you should be able to effortlessly lift your head with optical support. You will also feel tone subtly increase along your entire spine (PE Fig. 3c).

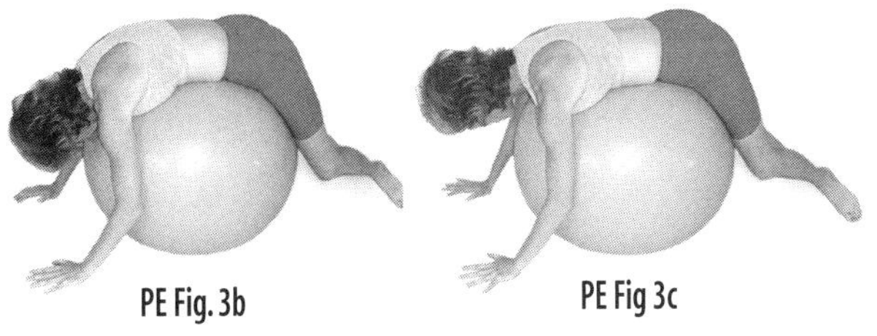

PE Fig. 3b **PE Fig 3c**

Defense Mechanisms

Somatic processes are the same in some respects for all living organisms. The processes common to the smallest organisms, microbes, and the most complex, humans, give us insight into the roots of our most primitive movement patterns—those of survival. The survival of any animal is based on its ability to move. Without movement, we could not gather food and prepare it, we could not procreate, and we could not feel, respond to, or defend ourselves. To expand our understanding of the motor learning processes that shape our multicellular bodies, we can contrast the somatic processes of microorganisms with those of humans.

The *vorticella*, a type of microorganism called a ciliate, attaches to rocks and vegetation under water and quickly contracts into a closed posture when protecting itself from predators (Figure 1.17). The vorticella's defensive response is triggered by such stimuli as mechanical vibrations and rapid water currents, and, when engaged, causes the microbe to lose valuable feeding time. Similarly, humans respond to danger signals with a defensive reaction that has a systemic effect, meaning it affects every system and cell in the body. Our defenses are more commonly known as "fight, flight, or freeze" responses.

Fight, Flight, Freeze Responses

Our primitive ancestors needed quick defenses in order to run from real dangers, such as a bear or tiger. In the modern world, defense responses affect people similarly, although the triggers, rather than being external, are often internal. Rarely does the city or suburban dweller need to flee from wild animals, although human predators and out-of-control cars can and do threaten people on occasion. *A perceived threat*, whether real or imagined, usually causes stress today. (This is not meant to discount the very real stress incurred by the many dangerous situations people encounter in wars, violence, and natural disasters.) This point needs to be underscored because it is the basis of stress, which is believed to initiate or exacerbate many disease processes. Two people can be in the same stressful situation but be affected totally differently by it, depending on their outlooks. A negative attitude, such as worry or fear, increases stress while a positive outlook, such as optimism or a healthy detachment from discomfort, reduces it.

Perceived threats and emotional reactions trigger a fight-or-flight response that puts the body on alert to prepare for defensive action.[26] This primary **stress response** revs the physiological engine, sends adrenaline rushing into the bloodstream, accelerates heart rate and respiration, and triggers muscles to contract into a state of readiness. But since there is usually no bear to run from, the physiological fuel floods out and courses through the body while the person undergoing stress freezes. In essence, stress from a perceived threat that is not carried into some kind of action causes an incongruity between inner and outer processes. The physiological motor races while the muscular readiness locks the body into a contracted grip. This type of reaction wears down the system, yet the body gradually adapts and each threat needs to be a little bit stronger to elicit the same level of response. If a person is unable to adapt, each threat creates a stronger reaction, and the stronger reaction creates more physiological damage in the body. Without adaptation, survival is threatened.

Muscular Armor and Bracing

Defense reactions that are patterned early in life shape both personality development and postural aberrations. The renegade psychiatrist Wilhelm Reich advanced this idea by describing how chronic muscular contractions occur in conjunction with psychological defenses to create the personality structures. In Reich's view, we wear our defenses like a suit of protective clothing that he called *muscular armor* (see Chapter 15), made up of specific configurations of chronic muscular contractions that tend to remain unconscious and, over time, feel habitual and normal. Reich identified a handful of contraction patterns that are associated with personality types, such as *schizoid* or *masochistic*. Each type has a specific postural fixation in which a person becomes stuck. Although muscular armor seems crucial for survival the first time a threat appears, the energy we use to habitually armor ourselves to avoid emotional pain eventually reduces and may deplete the energy we need for other life processes.

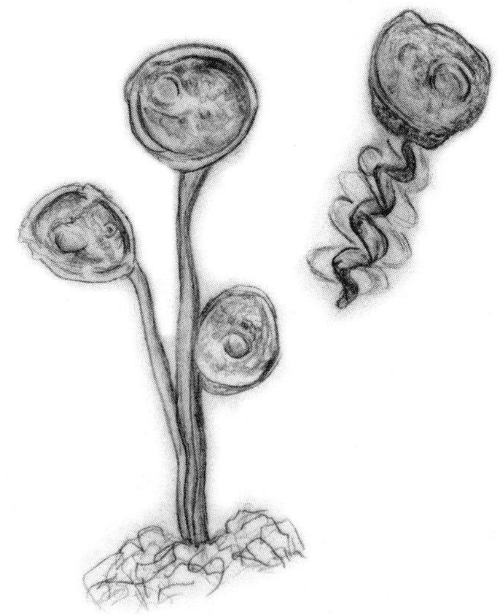

Figure 1.17 One vorticella retracting from a clump

Fear triggers muscular contraction. When there is a perceived danger or threat in the surrounding environment, the body goes into instinctive defensive response, preparing for fight or flight. If neither of these alternatives is possible, the body freezes. Even the mere thought of danger can trigger muscular contractions. A person who thinks obsessively about perceived dangers subconsciously assumes a defensive posture. Edmund Jacobson, the psychiatrist who developed the term *muscle bracing* (see Chapter 13), calls this dynamic the "inciting role of imagery" in emotional reactions.[27]

Fear is one of the most powerful and prevalent biological responses to many life situations. It plays a large role in the formation of chronic muscular contraction. Children raised in an environment of physical, sexual, or emotional abuse often develop contracted postures in reaction to the threats they face; they cringe or cower, or toughen into defensive patterns. Even mild criticism can induce a cascade of physiological and muscular responses in a child, which then underlie many of the mysterious aches and pains the adult suffers later in life.

Habituation and Holding Patterns

Our complex human bodies have retained the biological functions found in microorganisms; therefore, habituation remains our most primitive and subconscious level of learning. Microorganisms learn through **habituation**. This process was observed in experiments in which mechanical and electrical shocks were applied to ciliates. They all contracted at the first shock, but after 10 to 50 shocks, 50 percent stopped responding.[28]

Each cell in the human body retains the primitive nervous system found in a single-celled organism. Microbe learning occurs within a rudimentary nervous system of several hundred neurons, whereas human learning is much more complex because it occurs in a multicellular environment of billions of cells per person. Thus, human learning requires elaborate circulatory and nervous systems that extend over a comparably large surface and allow complex, multilevel neurological communications to take place. Microbes lack the sophisticated sensory and circulatory systems that connect billions of human cells within an elaborate circuitry.

While habitual learning is the most primitive type of learning, it is also the fastest. We need habituation to filter the enormous amount of sensory stimuli with which we are constantly bombarded, such as annoying noises in a crowded room, yet habits can also dull the senses. For instance, addictions are built upon habituation: each repetition requires a stronger stimulus or "drug" to achieve the same results. Likewise, habitually ignoring pain signals or structural imbalances in the body can lead to a greater tolerance for pain with a simultaneous reduced perception of the imbalance. This is why severe body problems may seem to appear all at once: the milder warning signs leading up to the problem went unnoticed.

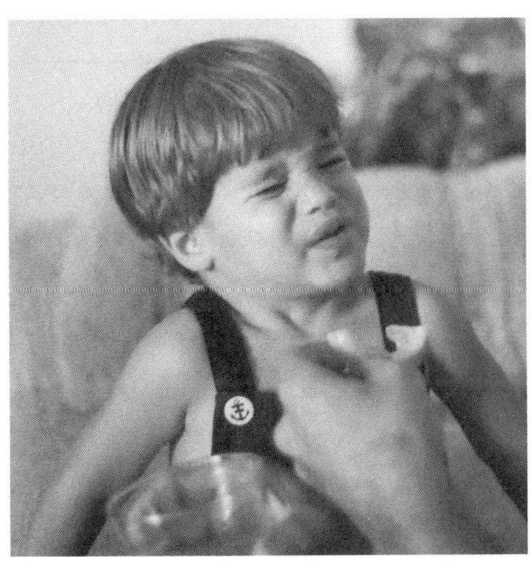

Figure 1.18 A sour lemon triggers a startle reflex (photo courtesy of L. Bright).

Defenses are systemic. They occur in a millisecond as a rush of adrenaline floods all the body systems, affecting every part of the body, inside and out. During this millisecond, a person responds to a threat by calling up the strongest defense available—the one that has become habituated along a well-worn, highly myelinated neuromuscular pathway. The entire process occurs below a level of conscious awareness in the centers of the brain that regulate emotions and instinctual responses. Because defenses form so fast, we often think of them as habitual muscular contractions over which we have no control and therefore cannot change. Yet by becoming aware of the inception of a defense, we can change the series of events that follows. Awareness is the key to interrupting a habitual and chronic stress response. Using somatic awareness, we can sense the *moment* a defense reaction is triggered, *what* sets it off, and *where* in the body it begins, then take the steps we need to inhibit and counteract the response, or to act on it appropriately.

Once a person's posture is tangled up in a habitual defensive pattern, the pattern tends to get stronger until there is significant reason to change. Habitual defense patterns gel, over time, into **holding patterns,** a literally "stuck" body state maintained by chronic muscular contractions and marked by postural imbalances and movement restrictions. Although we rely on reflexive, largely automatic movements to carry out our neuromuscular programs and coordinate most actions, habits differ from reflexive movement in that they are often dysfunctional patterns. Habitual holding patterns wear a groove in the neuromuscular pathways. Their well-worn pathways function like superhighways, speeding impulses along a singular route to the exclusion of many other possibilities.

The process is circular. Habituation perpetuates holding patterns, and holding patterns perpetuate bad habits. Once the muscular habit and its neuromuscular pathway is established, the nervous system tends to favor this pathway and continues the same faulty pattern over and over again. Unless we consciously inhibit dysfunctional habits and learn new ways to posture and move, these over-trodden pathways dominate. Eventually they take their toll, creating undue wear and tear on the body, particularly on the musculoskeletal system, and may flare up in problems like repetitive-use injuries. Old habits do die hard, particularly the primitive, survival-based pathways established during early motor development.

The Startle "Reflex"

A newborn arrives in the world naked, literally and figuratively. The first time the child's defense alarm rings, it has a deep physiological effect because the infant is without defenses. She cannot just stand up and run away like an animal because she is softwired—she learns her defenses over time. When threatened, an infant must mobilize a defense pattern and do so quickly. A frightful or startling experience triggers the infant's first call to arms. In this case, defenses are prematurely rallied and hastily patterned before the infant has developed enough muscle tone to adequately defend herself. Eventually another threatening experience jars the infant, and she is startled again. Once startled a third or fourth time, her defense reaction becomes so automatic that it looks like a reflex; hence it has been called the **startle reflex** (Figure 1.18).

Tabor's Medical Dictionary defines this reflex as "the uncontrollable startle reaction that follows any stimulus for which there is no adaptation, such as a sudden noise, flash of light, or touching a person. This causes a stiffening of the body, a flexion of the arms, and sometimes a shout or fall to the ground."[29] Although being startled triggers a reflexive, automatic movement, the startle reflex is not an actual reflex, but a reflexive movement. Because it is a learned, adaptive response, the startle reflex varies in each person. The number of movement responses in a baby's repertoire at the time of the first startling experience determines the shape of the response. It is weak in some and strong in others, ranging from an isolated reaction of pulling the shoulders in to a full-body retraction. The earlier the startle reflex develops, the more likely it is to be a full-body, systemic response, and the more likely it is to be coupled with anxiety, shaping the psychic structure and emotional predisposition of that person.

Each time an overly stressed person feels fear, a charge builds. If a defensive charge—an intensification of tense energy in the body—has built up into an overly strong startle reflex, the level of charge influences the degree of reactivity a person has. A stimulus that goes unnoticed by a calm person may send a highly stressed person into a panic. This creates a powder keg situation in which a relatively small trigger can set off a full-blown defense reaction.

Peter Levine, a trauma specialist, explains why a person can explode in a traumatic reaction with little provocation. Levine studied what triggers flashbacks in Vietnam war veterans and found that each memory of a traumatic event, or series of events, builds a cumulative charge, gradually increasing physiological stress. He describes this phenomenon as the "kindling effect." After the original trauma, an experience that triggers a traumatic memory also triggers the same physiological response. With each memory the person relives the original terror; the body has the same physiological responses—a sweat breaks out, the heart races, and panic sets in. Each repetition builds more heat, like hot kindling smoldering when stacked in a pile. Eventually, the pile reaches a critical charge, and the next piece of kindling, the next traumatic memory, ignites the entire pile.[30]

Every person has some kind of startle pattern. Because it is a learned pattern, every startle is somewhat different. Some people hike their shoulders, others shrink their head into the shoulders, and others cock the fists back. When a person's holding pattern takes the body into flexion, the startle will cause the body to thrust out in a strong, explosive extension. When a person's holding pattern takes the body into hyperextension, a strong startle will cause the body to retract and pull back into flexion. The later the startle reflex becomes habitual, the less apt it is to be a full-body reaction, and the more likely to be an upper-body reaction.

Thus the startle reflex moves the body in two primary directions: a person either goes into flexion or hyperextension. Flexion underlies a collapsed or compressed posture in which a person curls to retreat or withdraw. Hyperextension underlies an arched, rigid posture in which a person chronically contracts muscles along the spine, pulling the body up and back in preparation to move. The nicknames somatic philosopher and teacher Thomas Hanna gave these two common patterns clearly describe their purpose. In the *"protective red-light reflex,"* the body retracts away from the stimulus, creating contraction and flexion along the front of the body. In the *"assertive green-light reflex,"* the body moves into action toward the stimulus, creating contraction and extension along the back of the body (Figure 1.19 a-b).[31]

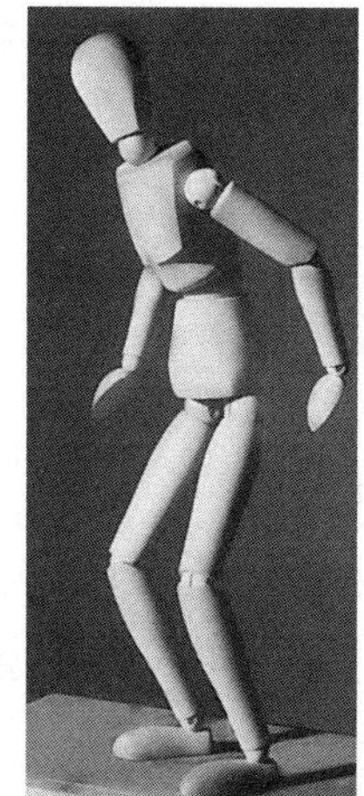

Figure 1.19a Flexion

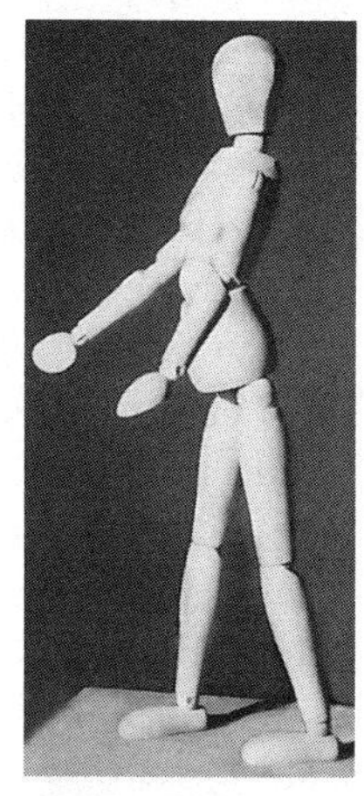

Figure 1.19b Hyperextension

The startle reflex is normal and occurs many times over the life span. It becomes problematic when it dominates other responses, limits movement, and distorts posture, pulling the body in front of its center or dragging the body behind its center. Ideally, the startle reflex is tempered by a diverse array of motor development. If not tempered, it can affect a person so deeply that it perpetuates low-grade anxiety and reduces the efficiency of a person's function throughout a lifetime. The earlier it is wired into the nervous system, the more deeply embedded it becomes.

Fortunately for many of us, we have miraculous bodies that can tolerate movement inefficiencies with creative compensations. And as adults, we can always go back and relearn developmental movement patterns that are weak or undeveloped because of an overly strong startle pattern. The startle reflex holds the crucial link between the physical and emotional body—a link that, if clearly understood, can initiate deep change in chronic holding patterns.

Emotional Tone

Emotions color the tone of posture and movement. When people allow their bodies to display qualities of **emotional tone**, such as the soft fullness of vulnerability, movement takes on another dimension. Without the enlivening influence of emotions, movement appears flat, like the mechanical motions of a robot. Theater critics often praise actors for performances that are full of feeling, vitality, and energy. It is possible to dance, move, and act without feeling, divorcing the body from the enlivening influence of emotions, although it is doubtful a professional dancer or actor would be successful without the filling dimension of the emotional body.

Feeling emotions, expressing emotions, and blocking the sensations of overwhelming or unwanted emotions are three different experiences. Which one dominates underlies the emotional tone in the body. Initially, it takes a considerable amount of energy to block feelings. Many of us have seen small children try to hold back tears and have felt sympathy for them. If strong emotions are consistently blocked over a long period of time, eventually they create deep holding patterns that reflect the core of a psychological issue.

A person feels emotional tone in many ways, in the gripping sorrow of grief, in the expansive lightness of joy, or in the harsh heat of anger. Emotions move through the body the same way any other movement impulse does, although emotions move and may be processed through expressive movement. To move emotions through the body, first a person must feel the sensations or tone of emotion in the body, then embody it and move it with expressive movements. **Embody** means giving body to something, personifying, incarnating, and incorporating some aspect of ourselves into our body experience. The term is widely used in the field of somatics to denote the act of allowing a thought or feeling or expression to manifest and sequence through body experience.

When your defenses are triggered, what shape does your posture take? Does your spine go into flexion, extension, or a combination of the two? What happens in your limbs?

The important thing to understand about emotional tone in the body is that emotions, particularly if they are unresolved, tend to trigger stress responses. When unresolved, emotions can literally "eat away at a person," affecting the body in the same way that any stress-inducing situation would. In fact, a person can become stuck in an emotional holding pattern, which develops in one of two primary ways: emotions either cannot fully develop in the core or they do not sequence between the inner and outer layers, out to the limbs. Feelings may not be given the time or attention needed to develop, or a person may not be able to allow the emotions to sequence in an expression of feeling. A person who cannot speak about her feelings may block the energetic flow in a clenched jaw or pursed lips. An angry person may block the full expression of anger midstream in a kicking or stamping gesture that does not travel from the core to the foot.

Healthy emotional processing and expression occur in a sequence, with a beginning, middle, and end. At the end of a successful resolve, a person has a feeling of completion or satisfaction. As discussed earlier, psychological issues develop early and run deep. Therefore, getting to the root of psychological problems uncovers core issues, which tend to color all behaviors. For example, a person may have a deep underlying belief that he was never good enough. For whatever reason, he learned that nothing he did ever met up to anyone's expectations. Perhaps his parents harped at him about being lazy, or told him he would "never amount to anything." Gradually, a beat-down posture grows around this core issue and behaviors develop to reinforce and defend it. The man goes through life seemingly failing at one thing or another. And until he resolves this core issue, the situation will probably remain the same.

Conversely, we would like to think that a person's core strengths and psychological health usually boost the energy level, bring integrity to the posture, and show up in confident, strong, and balanced patterns of movement. Many somatic psychotherapists link psychological health with posture. From a psychosomatic perspective, core psychological issues tend to be associated with "backbone," which, in a healthy person, reflects not only *behavioral* but also *physical* integrity and strength. In short, integrity and strength of character are thought to manifest in the postural integrity of the actual spine. If this belief fails to be true, then a person's psychological state and posture can be incongruent, although most somatic psychologists hold to the axiom that the "body never lies." Even a lay person can easily recognize an inflated ego in a rigid pumped-up spine, or patterns of grief in a sunken chest that folds around the heart. All core strengths and issues color posture and movement with an emotional tone.

Links to Practical Applications

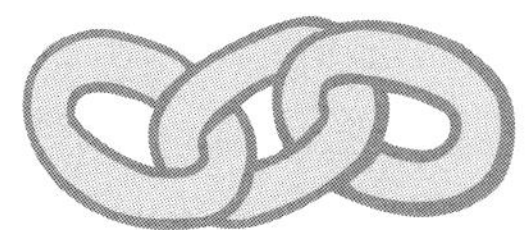

Working with Chronic Muscular Contractions

Novices to somatic patterning tend to work very hard to get rid of pain or the chronic muscular contractions that are causing pain. But it is important to realize that your contractions developed for a reason, often as part of an innate psychophysiological defense. If this is so, they will keep coming back until you no longer need the defense. Therefore, when you experience chronic contractions, begin by just feeling them without expending any energy to get rid of them. Awareness alone can help you to relax your muscles and begin to understand the dynamics underlying your defenses.

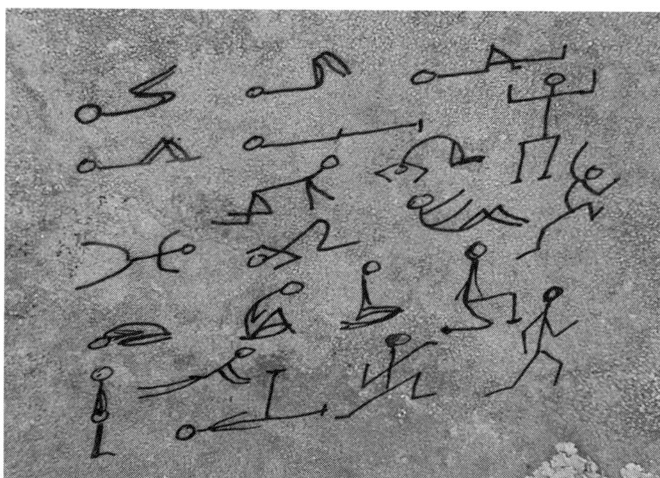

Figure 1.20 If our ancestors had etched the fundamental movement patterns on cave walls, they might have looked like this.

Parallels between Human and Other Animal Movements

The motor development of an infant from conception to walking reflects the development of simpler forms of life. The developmental stages that each person goes through recapitulate the patterns of all the life forms that preceded us in evolution. For example, newborns go through a stage of radial, jelly-like movement similar to that of the single-celled protozoa. Infants also cycle through stages of homologous movement (in which either both arms or both legs move simultaneously) similar to that of amphibians such as frogs. The series of early motor patterns create a continuum of shapes that reflect our animal heritage. Each shape resembles the primary movement of a specific species along an ontological continuum of development. Our ancestors etched many of these shapes on cave walls, perhaps to remind us of our biological heritage (Figure 1.20).

To understand these principles more fully, let's first examine cell physiology and its relationship to evolution. The research of the distinguished physiologist Sir Charles Sherrington established a broad foundation for understanding the physiological mechanisms of reflexive movement. He identified "cell-theory and the doctrine of evolution" as the basis for understanding problems of function or disturbances in body patterns.[32] The neuromotor pathways of a living organism, from the single-celled creature to the human, become increasingly more complex with each subsequent species, yet every species retains the neurological pathways of those that evolved before it.

Prevertebral Patterns

"Pre" means "before" and "vertebrate" means bony spine; thus prevertebrate animals developed before bony skeletons, the smallest of these being the single-celled creature. The **prevertebral patterns** are the movement patterns of prevertebrate species that mark each evolutionary phase. In the smallest prevertebrates, the unicellular organisms, physiological events occur either inside or outside the cell. The cell wall (*plasma membrane*) is a defining structural element, a membrane across which substances flow. The surface of separation divides the inner fluids of the organism from the surrounding environment. In multicellular organisms such as humans, each cell is surrounded by an extensive network of extracellular spaces. These spaces are filled with *interstitial fluid*, which creates an inner "ocean" within the multicellular organism. Our billions of cells communicate with each other through this ocean, via a multitude of floating chemical messengers such as hormones. Because the cell membrane is semi-permeable and selective, allowing some substances to pass through it while keeping other substances out, it functions as a primitive nervous system. The cellular permeability of the protozoa is reflected in human patterns of **cellular breathing**, or cellular respiration, in which oxygen and waste products, as well as hormones and other substances, pass between the interstitial ocean and the cell membrane.

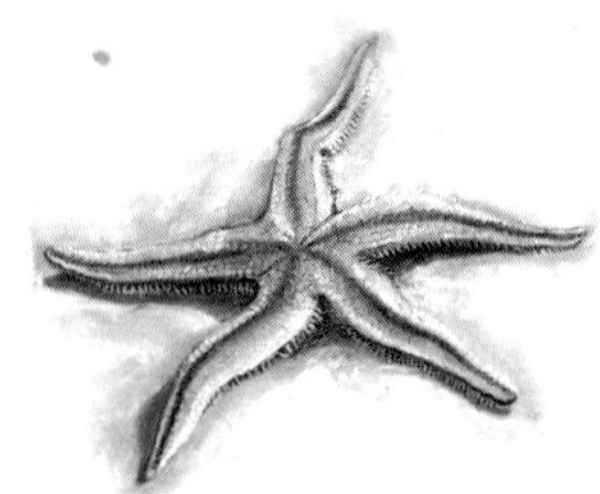

Figure 1.21 The starfish

A species more complex than protozoa, the starfish, is an *echinoderm* with five distinct limbs that move in patterns of radial symmetry, where all limbs function in equal relationship to the center (Figure 1.21). In humans we find parallels to the starfish in patterns of **navel radiation**, where all limbs—spine, arms, and legs—simultaneously flex and extend from the navel. This pattern is strong in infants, who may extend the arms, legs, or spine in an action that initiates in the navel (Figure 1.22a-b). The abundance of sensory nerve endings in the *endpoints* of each limb—the fingers, toes, face, and pelvic floor—reflects the photoreceptors on the ends of starfish limbs. This configuration enables the limbs to extend into the environment to gather sensory input.

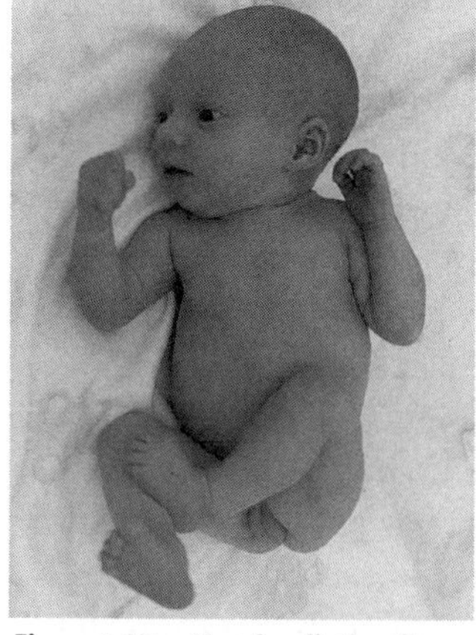

Figure 1.22a Navel radiation flexion phase (both photos courtesy of D. Radandt).

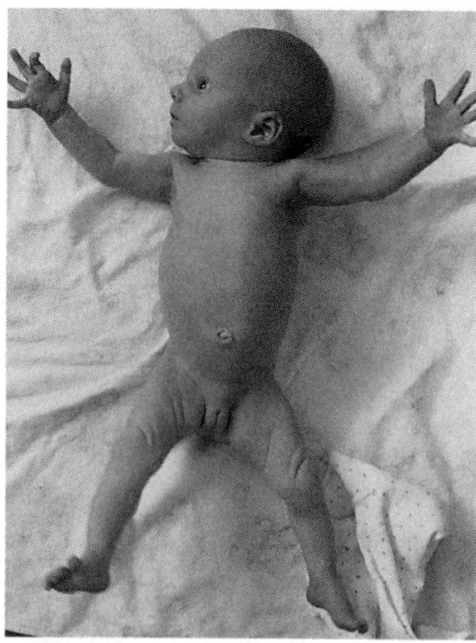

Figure 1.22b Navel radiation extension phase

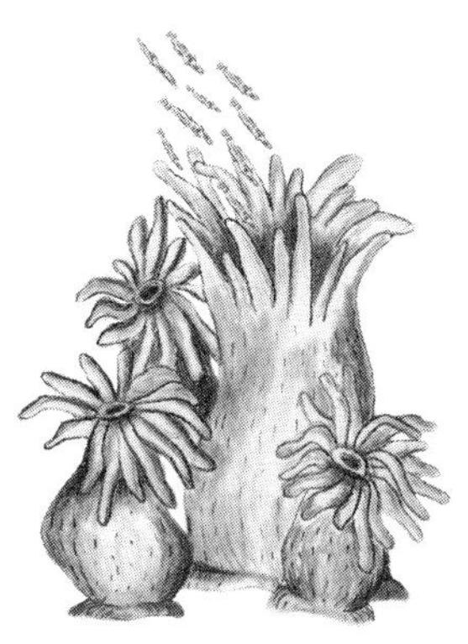

Figure 1.23 Sea squirt (anemone)

The *sea squirt*, another prevertebrate, filters food and waste through a tube-like body that is anchored on the floor of the ocean. Its simple feeding patterns involve gathering food and eliminating waste products through its alimentary opening. Even its offspring are birthed out this opening (Figure 1.23). The sea squirt's level of neurological development is reflected in the human **mouthing** patterns. Its intestine is a primitive organ tube. Our digestive tract is a more sophisticated alimentary tube that begins at the mouth and ends at the anus. During the first few months of life a human infant is totally dependent upon its caretakers for nourishment. To ensure survival, sucking and swallowing reflexes are hard-wired, and a newborn is able to root (search for the nipple) immediately after birth.

As life forms become complex, communication networks become specialized within their rudimentary nervous systems. The *notochord*, a flexible rod that is the precursor of the spinal cord, is found in multicellular organisms such as the *lancelet*. This eel-like invertebrate moves with snakelike undulations along its notochord (Figure 1.24). Its **prespinal movement** is reflected in the soft spinal undulations that can be observed in newborns, or in the rippling spinal waves of a belly dancer. The prespinal quality of movement underlies fluidity and ease in subsequent patterns of the bony spine. (Patterning exercises for the prevertebral patterns are found in Chapter 7.)

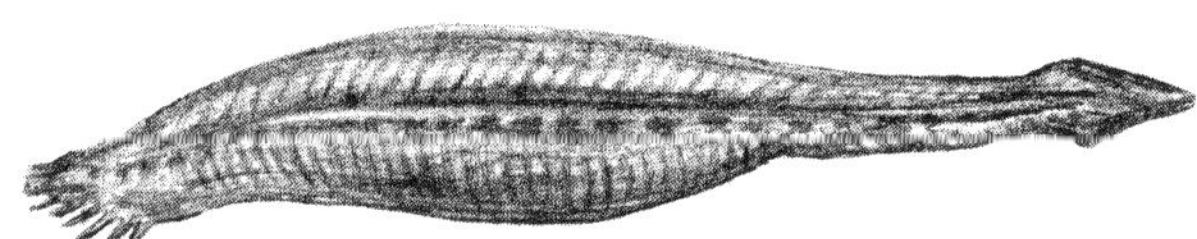

Figure 1.24 Lancelet

Vertebral Patterns

Animals with bones move in what are called **vertebral patterns.** The human body echoes the shape of the starfish but with six limbs—two arms, two legs, a head, and a tail. With maturation, movement differentiates along the various bony pathways between the six endpoints, making up four major vertebral pathways that reflect the neurological development of the brain:

- Movement between the head and tail is **spinal movement**, establishing a core axis and differentiating the front of the body from the back.
- Simultaneous movement in either both arms or both legs is **homologous**, establishing a top-bottom differentiation in the torso.
- Simultaneous movement in the arm and leg on the same side is **homolateral**, establishing the right-left differentiation.
- Movement that sequences from one arm to the opposite leg is **contralateral**, establishing the diagonal differentiation seen in cross-crawl patterns.

With each evolutionary step, the nervous system evolves one more function, and movement patterns become more complex. Each pattern reflects a level of neurological development. The spinal movements of the fish are associated with spinal cord development (Figure 1.25a). These spinal movements literally create pathways for energy and motion to flow along the vertical tracts of the spinal cord (Figure 1.25b). An infant develops a broad range of undulating spinal movements through the soft tissues before pushing and reaching with the head and tail. A mother pushes down through the tail during childbirth; a baby pushes with the tail to defecate and with the head to nuzzle. Each spinal push compresses the spine, gradually building strength and integrity in the bony vertebral column. Conversely, each spinal reach with the head lifts and lengthens the entire spine.

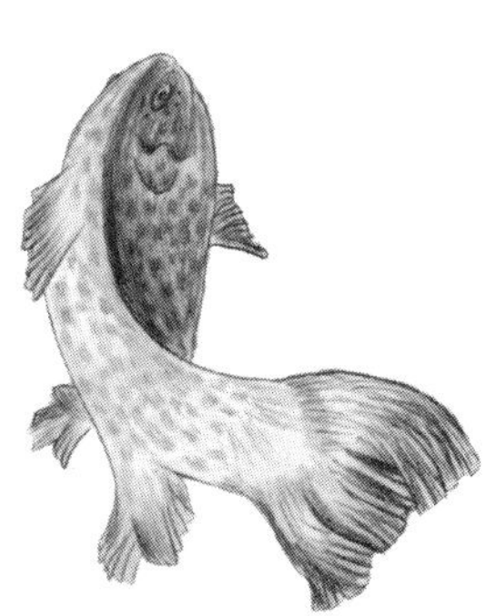

Figure 1.25a The fish

The homologous movements of the amphibian—in which both arms or both legs are doing the same action—allow the frog to jump back and forth between water and land (Figure 1.25c). Homologous movement is associated with hindbrain development, a part of the brain that first appeared in amphibians. A homologous push with both arms compresses the arms into the spine, whereas a homologous reach with both arms extends out from the heart area (Figure 1.25d). We use a homologous push with the legs to spring off a diving board, or to figuratively "stand our ground." A baby might use a homologous

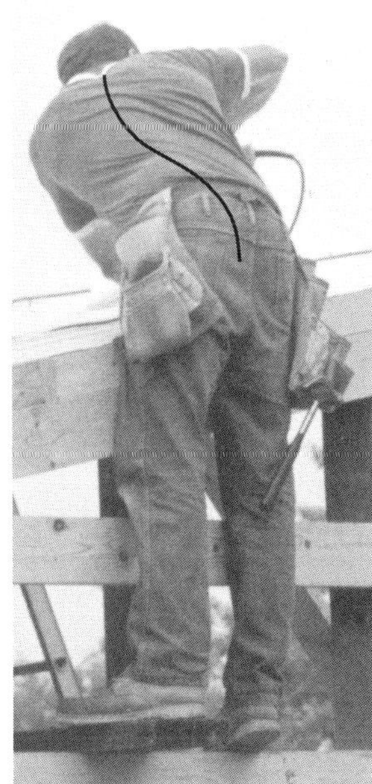

Figure 1.25b Spinal movement

reach with both legs to slide backward off a lap or down from a step; the action is less common in adults.

In the homolateral movements of the reptile, the lizard crawls by alternately pushing through one leg, then the other (Figure 1.25e). The pushing leg extends that side while flexing the other side, creating a right-left slithering motion that shifts the body's weight between the two sides. The homolateral pattern is associated with the integration of the brain's right and left hemispheres. In a homolateral pattern, one side of the body flexes while the other side extends (Figure 1.25f). For example, a shot-putter throws the ball with a homolateral push. There is no homolateral reach pattern because when one arm or leg reaches, it sequences diagonally across the body into the opposite corner and becomes a contralateral reach.

The contralateral pattern shows up in the gait of four-legged mammals such as felines and monkeys. Contralateral movement sequences diagonally across the body, pulling the opposite arm and leg through coordination best seen in the slinky stride of a stalking cat (Figure 1.25g). This diagonal pattern is associated with the diagonal connection between the two hemispheres of the brain, a crossing found at the *corpus callosum*. Humans walk and run in a contralateral gait pattern in which the legs and arms swing in opposition (Figure 1.25h). An unnatural homolateral gait such as the one seen in the Frankenstein monster is atypical and indicative of some sort of developmental delay or disability.

The efficiency of each vertebral pattern depends on the strength of the underlying patterns. For example, weak spinal pushes might show up in a collapsed spine, and weak spinal reaches in a rigid, overly compressed spine. A collapsed spine tends to buckle into a zig-zag shape due to lack of deep muscular support, whereas a compressed spine becomes more compact due to chronic contractions that prevent it from extending. Both patterns affect the sequence of motion through the many vertebrae of the spine, a translation required for the more complex patterns, such as crawling or walking, to be efficient. A weak spinal connection can create an instability that underlies the back pain someone feels while doing twisting contralateral movement, such as exercising on a Nordic Track. This person might exercise more efficiently on a machine requiring homologous patterns that stabilizes the spine, such as a rowing machine.

INTEGRATED MOVEMENT AND POSTURE

Somatic patterning modalities are the common and general methods taught in somatic schools. Some SP modalities are purely experiential, meaning a person learns about somatic patterns by exploring diverse ranges and qualities of movement. Experiential modalities often use improvisational movement explorations that will expose a person to many diverse sensory experiences derived from the body. Other

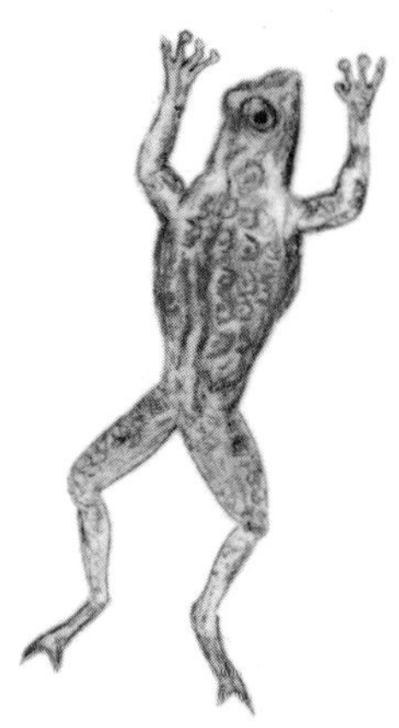

Figure 1.25c The frog

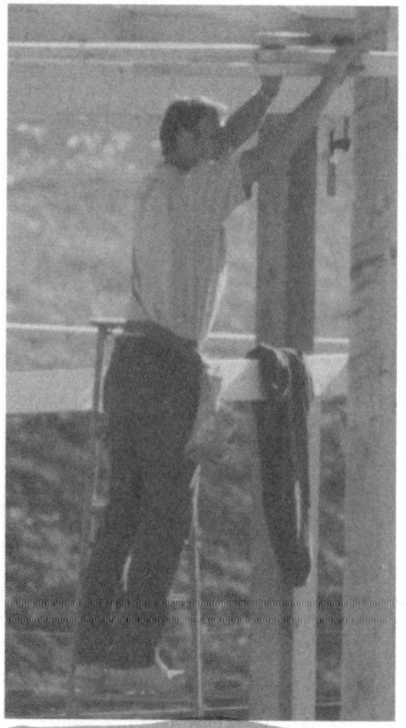

Figure 1.25d Homologous pattern

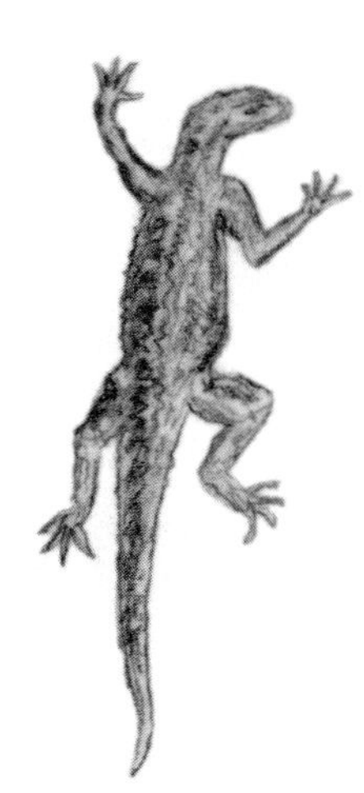

Figure 1.25e The lizard

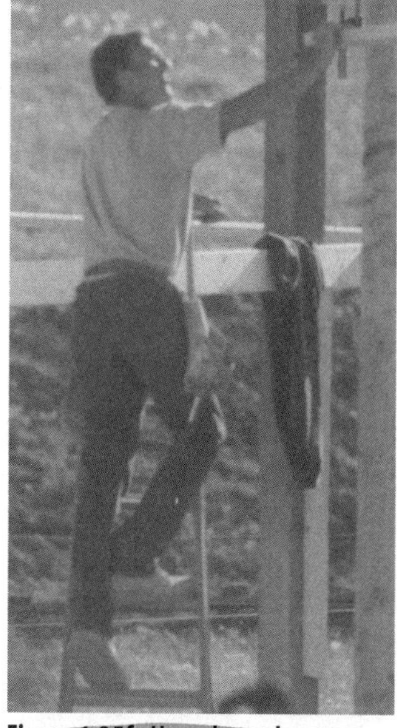

Figure 1.25f Homolateral pattern

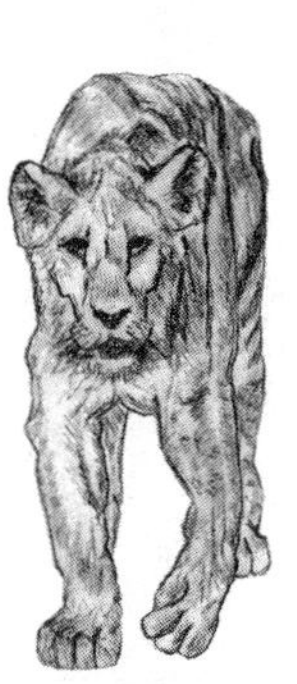

Figure 1.25g The lion

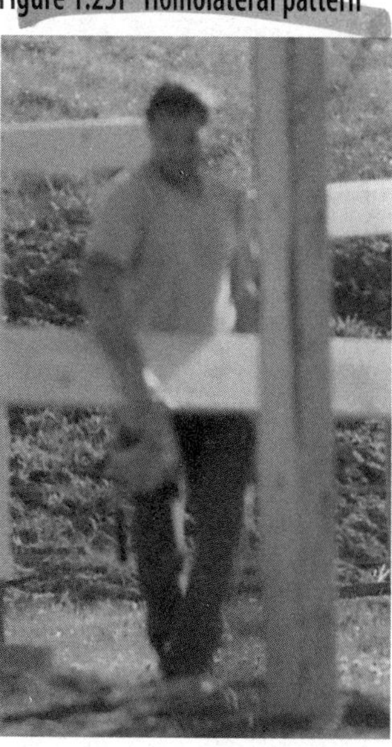

Figure 1.25h Contralateral pattern

Patterning Exercise #4: Differentiating Spinal Pushes and Reaches

1. Sit or stand in a comfortable position. Put your hands on top of your head. Making sure your head is aligned over your neck, gently push down with your hands, and push back up with your head (PE Fig. 4). (Be careful if you have neck problems or get headaches.) Sense the compression traveling down your spine through each vertebra.

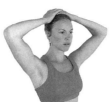

PE Fig. 4

2. Release the push, and reach up with the top of your head. Sense the reach pulling your head and neck up, elongating your entire spine. Can you feel difference between the push and the reach of the head?
3. Change your focus. Push down through your tail (coccyx) and pelvic floor (an action that you probably use to defecate). If you are sitting, push your tail into the surface under you. If you are really pushing, your tail will curl under toward your pubic bone.
4. Relax the push with the tail. Begin to reach with the tail. This action is often difficult to feel. We do it when we are walking in the dark or searching for a seat in a dark theater. In fact, stand up in front of a chair. Reach with your tail to initiate sitting down. You might imagine having a flashlight on your tail and shining it down below you. If you are truly reaching, your tail will feel light and your entire spine will lengthen down.

Feedback: Which action is the easiest for you, push or reach? Can you feel the difference between the opposite actions? (The push compresses the joints and the reach elongates the joints.) Humans have a natural affinity toward reach with the head and push with the tail.

EMSPress.com

Patterning Exercise #5: Exploring Core Connections to Vertebral Patterns

There is not a right or wrong way to do any of these movements. The exploration is simply to help you begin to feel different pathways of movement. The same sequence could be done lying on the belly, which makes some of the patterns easier and others harder.

1. Lie comfortably on your back. Extend your arms and legs out into the shape of a large X (PE Fig. 5a). Imagine your navel connecting through your torso into the floor; feel or sense your navel as the core of all your limbs.

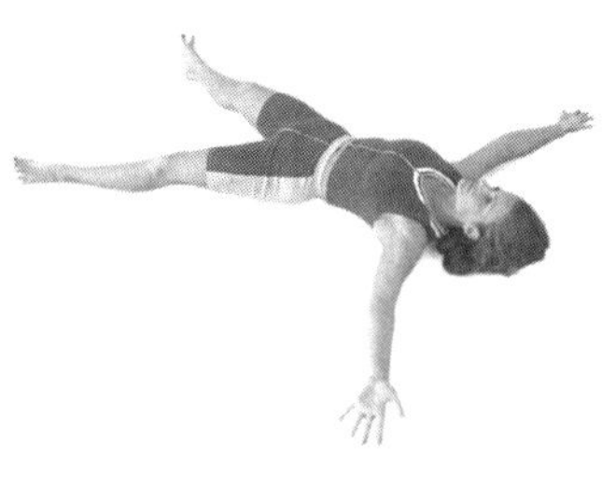

PE Fig. 5a

2. Sense your whole body like a six-pointed starfish, with the navel as the center. Imagine or sense energy traveling from your navel out your fingers, toes, head, and tail. Note which pathways you tend to be aware of and which pathways feel dull.

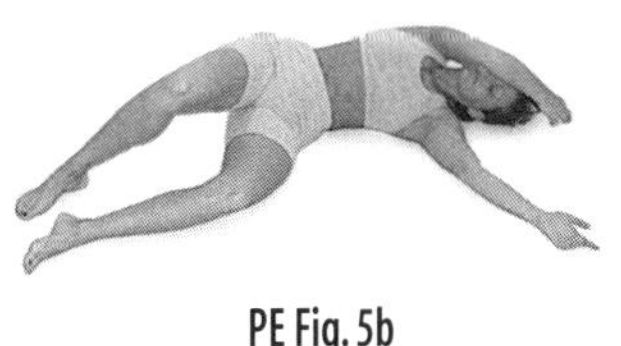

PE Fig. 5b

3. One at a time, gently reach through each limb. Extend that limb from your navel. Imagine your muscles like fabric. Allow the reach to take the slack or wrinkles out of the fabric and extend your joints. Begin with your right hand, then left hand, right foot, left foot, head, and tail. In which limb do you feel the strongest connection to the core? Which is the weakest?

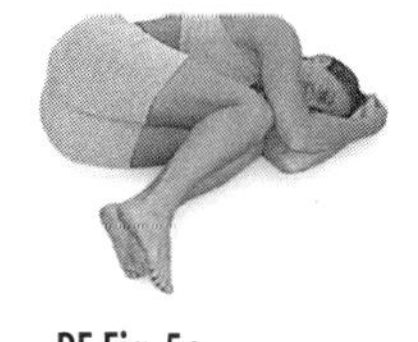

PE Fig. 5c

4. *Navel Patterns*: Simultaneously reach out through all six limbs. Then pull them in and roll to your side into a little ball (PE Fig. 5b-c). Reach out again and roll onto your back. Pull the six limbs in again and roll to the other side. Repeat until the movement is smooth.
5. *Homologous Patterns:* Reach through both arms. Are they symmetrical? Reach through both legs. Are they symmetrical? Push both palms into each other or into the floor. Sense the push travel from your hands into your arms, spine, and navel. Release. Then bend the knees and push both feet into the floor. Again, sense the push travel through both legs into the hips and spine (PE Fig. 5d). Then release.

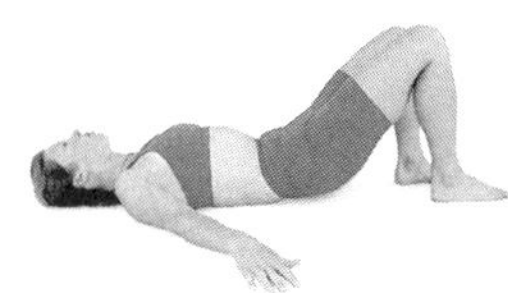

PE Fig. 5d

6. *Homolateral Patterns*: With one leg bent and the other straight, push with the foot of the bent leg. Does it extend that side of your body? It may even roll you over. Now bend the other leg and push with that foot. Keep your palms and forearms flat on the floor as you push with your leg.
7. *Contralateral Patterns:* Start in the big-X position. Reach through one hand and let the reach pull through your navel across to your opposite leg (PE Fig. 5e). Do the same with each limb: reach through the other hand and arm, then one foot and leg, then the other.

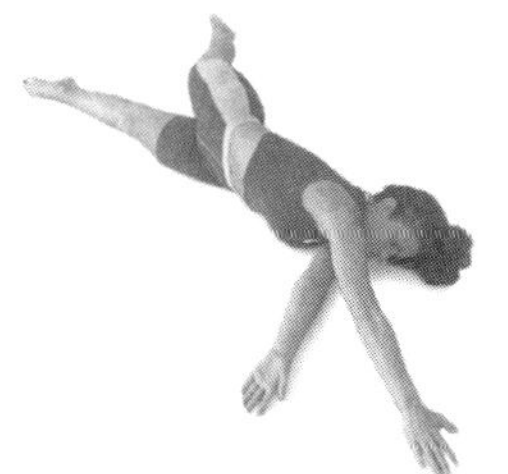

PE Fig. 5e

EMSPress.com

Links to Practical Applications

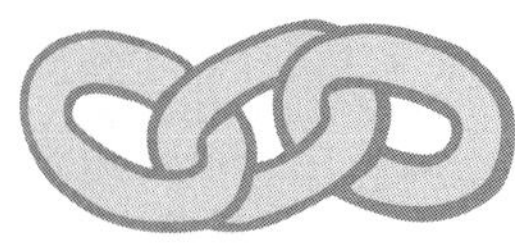

Surviving a Sit-Down Job

If you have a sit-down job, figure out ways to keep your body active and your tone up as you work. For instance, whenever you reach across the desk for something, stretch the arm and opposite leg. Or rock back and forth on your pelvis as you type. Be creative!

Stand up every 20 minutes for at least a full minute. Bend over and touch your toes. Stretch your arms to the ceiling, then to each side. Swing your arms, then legs, for a few seconds to get your blood circulating. Rise on the balls of your feet and lower at least six times to get the blood pumping in your legs.

modalities offer models of the elements underlying integrated posture and movement, and teach patterning exercises based on these ideals. Practitioners of each modality tend to use the models put forth by the founders of each method, yet in the absence of a model, it is common for the human mind to conjure one up. Integration sounds simple enough, but let's look at what it really means.

Integration has become a popular word in many somatic therapies, particularly since many somatic practitioners address body patterns on multiple levels. Defining this broad term is as elusive as narrowing down the definition of health or happiness. Somatic integration is a condition in which an organism functions so that all the parts and body systems work together in a synergistic manner, one that contributes to the overall health of an organism.

The combined effect is that the function of all the parts together is greater than the function of any one of these same parts individually. All parts and systems share equally in keeping a person in a state of health. No single part does the job of another, yet all parts rely on each other for integrated function. For example, muscles do not function in isolation. Integrated movement occurs when each muscle contributes proportionally to the movement of the whole body. On a mechanical level, integrated movement sequences along a series of joints forming a chain of action, all the way from the foot to the spine, or the spine to the end of a limb. Integrated movement initiates from a relaxed resting place; its foundation is balanced autonomic tone, which requires an ability not only to recover from stress, but to be strengthened by it. On a psychological level, integration manifests in a congruency between a person's posture and movement, and between his words, thoughts, and feelings.

Most somatic practitioners can see and sense integrated movement and posture on an intuitive level. Most people recognize integrated movement and posture when they feel it. A person might describe it as a feeling of ease, grace, balance, stamina, and vitality, as hitting one's stride or achieving a top-notch performance. And by recalling the feeling or sensation of an integrated movement and posture, a person can recreate it.

Body-Mind Integration

Consider this: the body and mind are so seamlessly integrated that every thought we have and every activity we do patterns the body, whether it is meant to or not. The triathlete trains the body for endurance, speed, and agility; the "couch potato" trains the body for detachment, immobility, and decline. We tend not to think of prolonged sitting as training, but a sedentary person usually becomes adept at ignoring the signals coming from the body. Regardless of how much mental endurance a person has, ignoring the body's need to move eventually leads to some type of physical and mental limitation and may escalate into a serious problem.

Movement is the integrating factor in making the body-mind connection. Within the context of integration, movement is broadly defined. It is movement of the body, of thoughts, of energy, of consciousness, and of physiological processes. If a person tends to ignore her body, by simply moving her awareness to the ongoing physiological processes within the body, such as breathing, she will begin to make a body-mind connection. Most people understand this connection in pathological terms, as psychosomatic. Many people with seemingly unsolvable health problems have been told by their physicians, "It's all in your head." Consequently, the word has taken on a negative connotation. Yet psychosomatic conditions indicate a degree of integration between the body and the mind—thoughts do affect the health of the body.

One might wonder why, in a book about somatic patterns, there are so many references to psychological patterns. This is because a person's psychology is probably the strongest influence that shapes body patterns; therefore, this background is necessary in order to take a holistic approach to somatic patterning. Body patterns will not change unless all aspects of them are addressed: short of injury, illness, or genetic weaknesses, most body problems have psychological roots.

Many psychotherapy clients come to somatic patterning to catch up their body patterns with the cognitive and emotional growth they have gained from psychological work. Conversely, many bodyworkers access deep emotions underlying psychological issues in their clients as those clients release physical tensions. Postural patterns rooted in the psyche will only change if the psychological patterns are also addressed. Hence, bodyworkers often recommend psychotherapy to help their clients address psychological issues that underlie the body problems that come up in bodywork sessions.

Postural Integration

Although postural integration involves physical, mental, and emotional well-being, we can both observe and measure it in the alignment of the bones and the activity of postural muscles. In **kinesiology** (the study of movement) there is a fundamental axiom stating that *as mobility* *increases, stability decreases proportionally, and vice-versa.* As mentioned earlier, the upright human posture requires less muscular effort than the posture of any other mammal. The drawback of this efficiency is that any slight variance from plumb throws the body off balance disproportionately. In light of this, the unique postural challenge given humans lies in staying fluid without becoming wobbly or unstable. We need to be fluid because our bodies are in constant motion, even when we try to hold ourselves as still as possible. Remember playing statue as a kid? This game exaggerates the impossibility of standing completely still, which will cause a person to faint eventually.[33]

Variances from vertical postures occur for many reasons, but all are associated with faulty body-use habits. In sum, what we gained in mobility and control with our upright stance, we lost in postural stability and instinctual movement. The most common solution to a perceived postural misalignment is to position the body by chronically holding certain areas, perhaps pinching the shoulders back and sucking the gut in. This may or may not work. The prevalence of chronic pain despite such attempts suggests that it does not. Plus, most people struggle not with maintaining a good posture, but with finding a pain-free posture.

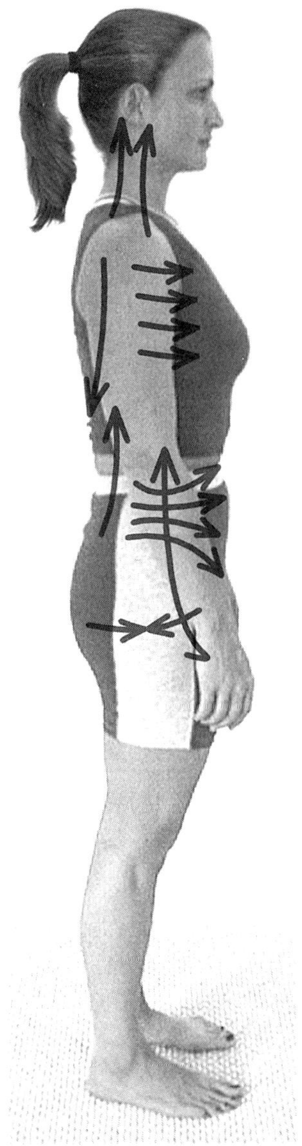

Figure 1.26 Each arrow is placed over a primary postural muscle (see Chapter 9).

Another common solution to alleviate poor posture and chronic back pain is to exercise. The human body evolved for movement and needs exercise every day to be healthy and strong. The muscles need to push against resistance, and the heart needs to power the body at high speed on a regular basis. Yet less than 25 percent of adults get enough exercise.[34]

And exercise does not guarantee good posture. The muscles that maintain postural balance do not necessarily work during ballistic or aerobic exercise. This is why a great athlete can have poor posture when off the track or playing field. Postural muscles work differently than muscles that generate movement. They contract to stabilize, but not move, joints. They pull the two bones in a joint together rather than bending or twisting the joint. Postural muscles can be developed with a focused awareness and **isometric contractions** (contractions done in place), a topic that will be revisited throughout the book, especially in Chapters 8 and 9. Poor posture puts a person at higher risk for pain and injury, including people who exercise regularly. Exercise may reduce the risk of injury and help relieve joint and muscle pain, but it is not guaranteed to improve posture. On the other hand, good posture will most likely improve performance in any sport, dance, or physical activity.

Examining Myths

Myth: Strong muscles ensure good posture.

Although strong muscles certainly help, the muscular development that underlies strength is different from the muscular development required for postural stability and coordination. Therefore, a bodybuilder can have terrible posture and lack coordination. Timing (recruitment order) and balance are more important than strength for coordination. Plus, postural muscles need to be trained to function in light, sustained contractions. The powerful bursts (contractions) of a weight lifter's or athlete's movements do not necessarily develop postural muscles.

What is good posture? Postural integration is a result of overall **postural tone**—the tone of the postural muscles that support and align the body in an upright posture (Figure 1.26). Ideally, all the postural muscles work together in harmony to maintain the vertical integrity of the body, particularly of the spine.

In an overly simplistic analogy of the job of postural muscles along the spine, think of the spine as an upended beam. Specific muscles along the spine work in continual contractions to stiffen the joints in order to keep the beam aligned in an upright balance. This is akin to securing the luggage on a plane before take off so that nothing slips or slides. Likewise, if our joints are stabilized in an aligned posture when we are stationary, we can carry this underlying postural stability into motion.

Also, if the spine is truly stable while sitting or standing, it will feel effortless; any slight variation from plumb will not cause the spine to buckle or the back muscles to ache. This description of postural integration may sound stiff, but good posture is not. The body is a dynamic, organic, breathing system of living tissues composed of mostly fluid, or plasma. It is, basically, a shape-shifter, teeming with a continual sea of intrinsic metabolic and homeostatic processes. Although good posture appears steady and positional, a closer look at a relatively stable posture reveals a subtle underlying sway.

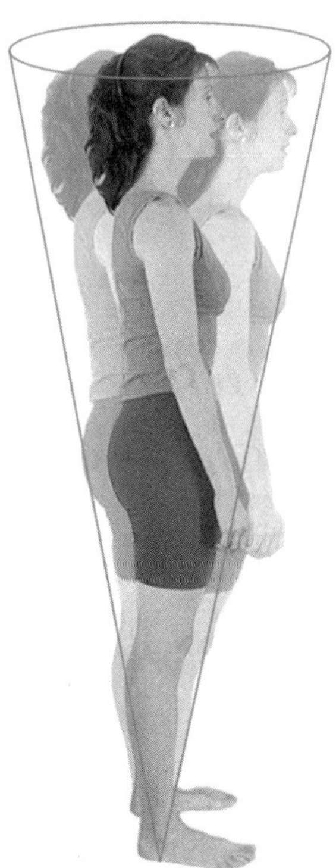

Figure 1.27 The range of postural sway

It is literally impossible to stand completely still. Even when we are standing in a stationary posture, the body teeters back and forth around its vertical axis. This subtle oscillation is called **postural sway**. When a person stands relatively still, muscular reflexes continually balance and rebalance the body around its central axis. As the body leans to one side, the muscles on the other side lightly contract to pull it back. Then the body leans in the opposite direction and the opposite muscles work to reposition it (Figure 1.27).

The sway is maintained by a **stretch reflex** in the muscles that protects them from overstretching by causing muscle fibers to contract after being put on a stretch. As the body sways, muscles on one side and the other work as coupled pairs, subtly contracting then relaxing to continually rebalance the body around its vertical axis. To get a picture of this dynamic postural function, imagine the muscles like a diverse group of workers whose job it is to keep the body upright. Each worker holds the end of a pliable guyline, letting it out or pulling it in to adjust for any sway that tips the plumb. Any minor imbalance in the length or strength of any one guyline reduces the effectiveness of the entire posture and alters the overall balance of the plumb.

Postural sway occurs naturally and involuntarily. It creates a subtle muscular pump that assists the return of blood to the heart and the circulation of blood into the brain. Postural sway creates a continuous spiral-shaped motion, maintaining a mobile and dynamic posture rather than a static posture. Postural sway also creates a neutral, fluid stance from which the body can move freely in any direction.

During postural sway, the weight of each body segment needs to shift as close to its center of gravity as possible if the spine is to remain aligned. This occurs when one body mass is balanced over another in a neutral standing posture. The head balances over the thorax, which balances over the hips, which balance over the feet. Gravity creates an imaginary line that falls as close to the center of each body mass as possible. When viewed from the side, the line of gravity drops from the earlobe to the center of the shoulder, hip, knee, and ankle. In a sitting posture, the same relationship remains in the torso, although the "sit bones" (the bones upon which we sit) take the place of the feet. Ideally, in a seated posture, there is a plumb between the sit bones and the top of the hip bones, although many people tend to slump off of their base of support (Figure 1.28).

The more aligned the body is during postural sway, the more efficient any subsequent movement will be. A person can push off from a dynamic posture in such a way that the center of body weight is thrust ahead of the base of support. The body neither drags behind nor falls ahead. If, in a neutral posture, a person either leans back or spills forward, she usually carries this postural instability into motion, making the motion uncoordinated and awkward. The person either has to drag the backward-leaning body to pull it forward, or she falls ahead of the forward-leaning body and trips or lurches to regain balance.

Models of Somatic Integration

Integration is easier to see in others than to feel in oneself. When watching a team sport or the Olympics, most spectators can naturally single out the well-integrated athlete as a favorite, being naturally drawn to the balance, agility, strength, fluidity, and coordination on an intuitive level. When asked why this athlete draws attention, the average person will have some vague idea and may even mention one or two of the qualities described, but will not really understand why.

Most people have an experience of what their bodies feel like when they have a faulty or painful pattern, yet the sensation of integration is elusive. The descriptions of pain far outweigh descriptions of health, which clients generally sum up in one short phrase: "I'm feeling good." Describing what feels good can be a difficult process because when the body is functioning in an optimum manner, our awareness of it disappears. Integration is marked by an absence of overt sensation. But with practice and an expanded vocabulary, integration can be felt and described; at the very least, a person can learn to spot it in others.

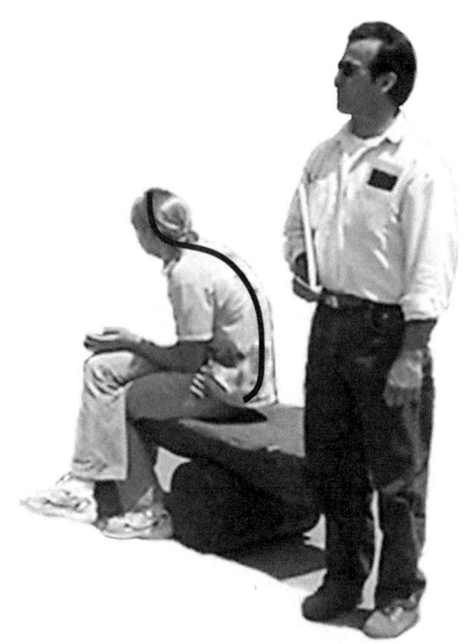

Figure 1.28 Contrast the verticality of his spine with the slouched curve of her spine.

Seeing integration in movement and posture in others and feeling it within oneself are two fundamental patterning skills. By feeling integra-

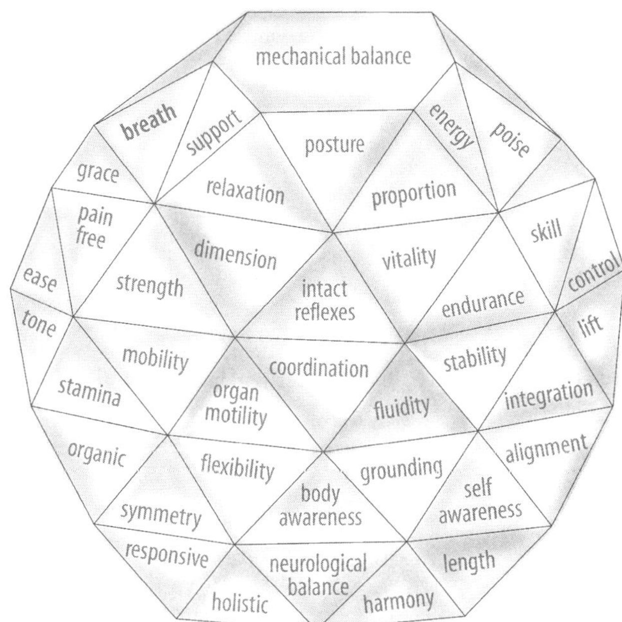

Figure 1.29 The elements of integration are like the facets of a diamond.

tion, we experience it and embody it. By seeing integration, we tune up our visual skills. Understanding what we see and feel is an even more advanced cognitive patterning skill. By simultaneously understanding it and feeling it, we connect cognition to experience, connect thought to feeling, making the ultimate body-mind connection.

A well-integrated body, like a well-cut diamond, is multifaceted (Figure 1.29). Many different facets reflect the diverse components of integration. Idealistic models for posture and movement naturally arise out of the human structure we all have in common, yet the problem with an ideal is that we run the risk of getting stuck trying to create an image of how we "should" be rather than feeling how we are. On the other hand, models provide images that can be used to guide patterning toward our optimum human movement potential.

Integration is not only a state of being, it is a process. At any given moment, the body is moving toward or away from integration. For most people, it swings back and forth between organization and chaos in a narrower or wider range. The posture and tone of the body reflect the *state* of integration; the pathways of movement reflect the *process* of integration.

In Part 3 of this text, on the history of somatic patterning, the models of integration specific to each somatic patterning modality are presented. Each modality approaches body integration from the perspective of the model with which the practitioner is working. If we look at the various models all together what emerges is a larger, more holistic picture of somatic integration. This integration is inclusive of a healthy connection and congruent expression of the body and mind together, as well as postural integrity in both stationary and moving activities.

SUMMARY

This chapter introduced what somatic patterns are, the biological roots of somatic patterns, and how human patterns of movement are unique in several adaptations. We have not only evolved into an upright posture, but we differ from other life forms because of our unique adaptation—the advanced cerebral cortex. We have the ability to be aware of awareness, which has its benefits and liabilities. In regard to posture and movement, we are able to change our faulty habits by directing our movements with mental control. The downside to this ability is that most people stop moving to think, interrupting and hindering natural movements. Consequently, our advanced cerebral capacities often lead to faulty body-use habits in the first place.

Somatic patterning is a natural learning process based on body awareness and sensorimotor education. SP usually begins when discomfort or pain reminds us that we need to start paying attention to how we use our bodies. The desire to avoid injury and pain is often the first motivator for stopping and thinking about changing faulty posture and movement habits, then starting to use common sense to notice how we sit and bend and lift.

The next chapter focuses on the diverse reasons that people use somatic patterning. It examines the causes of

Patterning Exercise #6: Dynamic Postural Sway

1. Stand comfortably, with your eyes closed. Maintain this position for one minute or more. Notice the swaying motion caused by various physiological rhythms balancing and counterbalancing your body around a vertical axis, the same way a level indicator on a ship sways back and forth indicating the boat's relationship to the horizon. There is a continuous interplay between the supporting and moving functions of the tensional structures.
2. Continue to stand, and sway back and forth. Sense your weight shifting between your heels and your toes. Sense when your thorax comes over your pelvis, and when it goes behind your pelvis. If you are used to leaning back, when you find a plumb posture, it will feel like you're leaning forward.
3. Stand sideways to a mirror. Check your normal posture. Now close your eyes and find your dynamic postural balance. Feel when your head, thorax, and pelvis sway close to the vertical line. Then open your eyes and again check your dynamic posture in a mirror. Are there changes? If so, what are they?

EMSPress.com

holding patterns, their neuromuscular components and associated behaviors, and what we can do to change them. It also presents some of the primary issues that arise when using somatic patterning to alleviate pain patterns. Last, and most important, it offers methods to release holding patterns, particularly when they limit function and cause chronic pain.

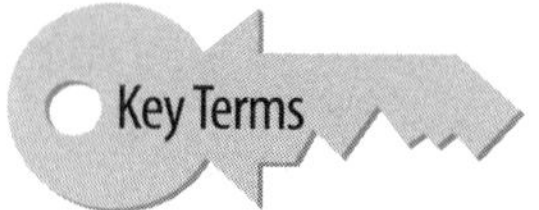

adaptation
body awareness
cellular breathing
cerebral cortex
complimentary alternative medicine (CAM)
concrete operations
contralateral
embody
emotional tone
formal operations
habituation
holding patterns
homolateral
homologous
horizontal scanning
imprinting
integration
isometric contraction
kinesiology
mouthing
movement
navel radiation
neotony
opposable thumbs
optical righting reaction
patterning
postural sway
postural tone
posture
preoperational stage
prespinal movement
prevertebral patterns
proprioception
psychosomatic
reflective thinking
reflex
reflexive movement
self-image
sensorimotor amnesia
sensorimotor (SM) learning
sensorimotor loop
somatic patterning (SP)
somatic
somatics
spinal movement
startle reflex
stress
stress response
stretch reflex
upright posture
vertebral patterns

OVERVIEW OF CHAPTER 2

Movement Problems, Holding Patterns, and Pain

2

> **The harder we look at our aches and ailments, the more we will be startled by the painful truths they are trying to convey about our dangerously disembodied way of life.**
>
> ***—Marion Woodman***

The automatic processes of the human body are extraordinary. The soma is a markedly well-functioning organism, able to live and breathe and move with only a minimum of self-awareness or conscious direction. It is a self-contained ecosystem with an array of built-in homeostatic mechanisms all geared toward self-correction, rejuvenation, regeneration, and healing. Of course, we all have bad habits that could be changed to improve how we feel, and many times these habits lead to painful problems. Yet bodies function remarkably well given the abuse that people often subject them to.

Since our bodies operate on automatic pilot most of the time, our minds would not even know where to begin if we had to think ourselves through the processes of digestion or circulation or tissue repair. Yet when something goes wrong, we think we can step in and remove the problem, much in the same way as we would cut bruises off an apple. But this orientation is a fallacy because if we relied on it, soon there would be no apple, or body, left.

The issue lies not in the fact that upon an accurate analysis of a somatic problem, logical and effective solutions can be found. Instead, the problem lies in the focus that a person takes. If the focus on figuring out and fixing a somatic problem is greater than the focus on *feeling the embodied solution*, a person can fall into a fix-it trap. This trap is akin to running on a hamster wheel: the process turns in circles but does not go anywhere. In this case, a person works so hard at getting better that the problem can actually become worse.

The point is that for somatic patterning to be successful in helping a person overcome a body problem, the person needs to respect the body's many highly effective and natural processes and use them to build a healthy state of being. The focus needs to be on building an awareness of healthy function. Granted, people are usually driven to somatic patterning because of pain and suffering. But it is imperative that the focus on what *works* be greater than the focus on what is wrong in order to step into the healing current that already exists within us and tap its potential. If we focus only on the problem, we can actually grow the problem because a fixation on pain will actually increase the pain, and a fixation on neurotic habits will eventually turn them into obsessions.

The reason that this point is being underscored—to approach somatic patterning by cultivating an awareness of the self-corrective homeostatic mechanisms within us and building upon them—is that this chapter is about what goes wrong with the body. Specifically, it is about holding patterns (first introduced in Chapter 1): the complex physical, physiological, psychological, and emotional conflicts that manifest as habitual behaviors, chronic muscular contractions, and chronic pain. Holding patterns cycle in repetitive loops, manifesting as annoying twitches, compulsive thoughts, recurring emotional problems, and chronic muscle spasms. They distort posture and interrupt the flow of movement. They also mark us with a distinct posture and gait that become so familiar we no longer notice them (Figure 2.1).

One of the primary applications of somatic patterning is to alleviate the movement problems and persistent pain caused by holding patterns. Understanding how holding patterns develop is a first step in breaking out of their degenerative grip. In this chapter, we will discuss the causes and effects of holding patterns. We will focus on the body problems that lead a person to somatic patterning, defining, for now, the problem but not the solution. Patterning solutions are presented throughout the book, with specific emphasis in Part 2 on practice.

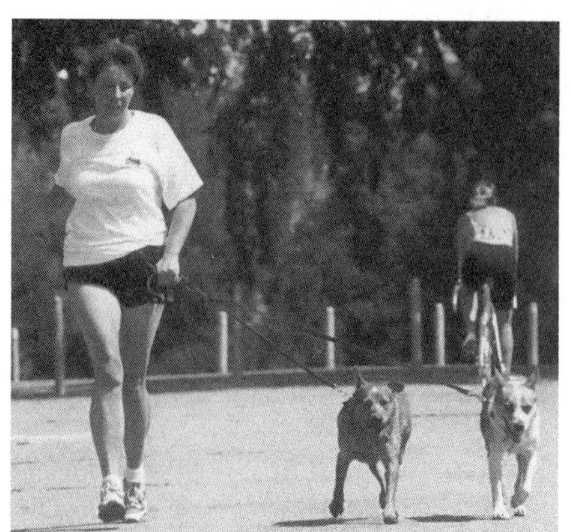

Figure 2.1 Each individual has a distinctive gait.

HOLDING PATTERNS

The words "holding pattern" evoke diverse images or muscular responses in different people. Some visualize an airplane circling the airport, waiting for its turn to land. Others pull their shoulders to their ears to flinch as they remember an argument or conflict with another person. Still others become self-conscious of the remnants of a limp or painful posture from an old cast, injury, or surgery. Probably the most familiar use of the term is by newscasters and political pundits who describe political conflicts as "holding patterns." Although most people have a sense of what holding patterns are, how do they relate to somatic patterns?

Any habitual activity or repetitive movement creates an environment ripe for chronic muscular holding. On a physical level, a holding pattern develops when the body wars with itself, with some muscles overworking while others become rigid from being held in chronic contraction. Holding patterns are most obvious when one part of the body moves in the opposite direction of another part. One group of muscles remains frozen while another group strains and pulls against the first. For example, a person might lean back to move forward, or depress the chest while reaching up. The place between the moving part and the held part becomes a point of conflict, a place where tissues literally pull or drag against each other, culminating in excessive wear.

When the body performs an inefficient movement over and over again, chronic muscular contractions form and eventually immobilize certain parts of the body. Motion travels around, rather than through, the contracted areas, and movement efficiency begins a downward spiral. At the same time, the moving areas become hypermobile and unstable from additional wear and increased friction. Instability leads to shearing forces, and eventually the weak link in the chain breaks, resulting in injury and pain. Over time, the faulty body-use habits that create holding patterns often lead to chronic pain and injury.

Body problems caused by holding patterns are widespread. Pain is the number one reason people seek either conventional or alternative methods of healthcare. Chronic pain—defined as pain that lasts three months or longer—accounts for 75 percent of overall healthcare costs. Eighty percent of the population suffers from back pain at some point in their lives, and pain is the third leading cause of disability.[35] Low back pain alone accounted for 93 million lost workdays in the United States in 1998, at a price of about $5 billion in healthcare costs and lost productivity.[36] Although not all conditions of chronic back pain are caused by holding patterns, holding patterns develop whenever there is pain and often precede conditions of chronic pain.

Holding patterns also have emotional and physiological components. Unmanageable emotional responses can trigger muscular contractions that underlie psychological muscular armor (see Chapter 15). Chronic contractions wear not only on the muscles and joints, but also on the adrenal glands. Most people know this condition as stress.

FUNCTIONAL ANATOMY

Movement is a vital force for normal human function. It stimulates bone growth, increases lymph and blood circulation, reduces fibrous build-up, and strengthens both the muscles and the immune system. Movement also has a psychological effect, demonstrated by the fact that most people become depressed when they are immobilized because of injury or illness. All of the body-mind functions suffer without movement. Any type of chronic muscular holding leads to a mechanical imbalance in posture or movement. Chronic holding in the muscles manifests in both poor posture and faulty mechanics, and it restricts movement. On a physiological level, chronic holding patterns show up as fatigue, poor digestion, sluggish circulation, chronic colds, or other minor illnesses, all of which have been associated with depressed immune function that can make a person more susceptible to stress-induced disease.

Human anatomy is usually studied by observing a stationary body. Anatomists rarely observe the movement of the body in action; rather, they dissect the artifacts of once-living tissues in cadavers, absent the dynamic interchange of life processes. Functional anatomy is the study of the moving body. Studying functional anatomy requires a different orientation to learning: it involves learning to observe and feel movement patterns as they happen, not only in others, but within oneself. A study of functional anatomy is akin to watching wheels turn as part of the overall workings of an engine or tracking signs of electricity flowing in a circuit. It is further complicated by the interaction of the diverse dynamic biological processes that take place within each system in the human body.

Form and Function

The forces of movement shape our changing bodies moment to moment. (In this context, movement involves not only the muscles and the joints, but the myriad of organic processes such as digestion and breathing, and even the movement of thought.) More simply put: *form follows function*. How a person postures and moves leaves artifacts in the structure that can be seen in the resting tone of the musculoskeletal system. Certain muscles might have high tone, while others have low tone, creating an overall muscular imbalance that is reflected in the asymmetry of the body and its movement patterns. As anyone who has had extensive bodywork knows, when the alignment of the body improves, so does the efficiency and effectiveness of movement. (At least until the person's faulty muscular habits return, which is why neuromuscular patterning along with bodywork creates more lasting change. Bodywork changes the structure, or form; patterning changes the function.)

Form not only follows function: *function follows form*. They are opposite sides of the same coin: one generates and perpetuates the other. Therefore, if movement efficiency improves, so will the structural integrity of the body.

The fields of orthopedics and physical therapy have thoroughly delineated the many biomechanical problems that occur in the body. In fact, there are so many classifications for the specific structural and functional problems involved in injuries that most people believe that musculoskeletal breakdowns are caused by some inherited or structural flaws in their joints or soft tissues. We do inherit genes that can predispose us to structural weaknesses, although believing that this alone determines biomechanical health is a misleading notion. Structural problems do not just happen; we create them by how we use our bodies, which in many cases means with our movement, or nonmovement, habits.

We must move a lot to remain healthy. Movement improves circulation, keeping the heart and lungs healthy and moving out metabolic by-products. Movement stimulates digestive processes. Movement keeps muscles supple, strong, and healthy, particularly if the muscles work with exertion, either moving heavy loads or lifting weight. And movement puts mechanical stresses on the bones, causing the build-up of new tissue along the lines of stress, which, in turn, strengthens and hardens bones.

Conversely, with minimal use, muscles and bones atrophy at a rapid rate. When a person is completely immobilized—in conditions such as total bed rest or paralysis—muscular strength decreases at the rate of 5 percent per day.[37] After even brief periods of immobility (as little as one hour), fiber builds up in muscles causing them to stiffen. Immobility also weakens bones, making them more brittle. Bone loss occurs at the dramatic rate of about 1 percent per week in a bedridden person.[38]

On the other hand, inefficient movement causes premature wear and tear on the soft tissues and the joints. Faulty movements predispose a person to injuries from forceful exertions, awkward postures, and repetitive motions.[39] Short of injury or neurological dysfunction, muscular imbalance is the source of bilateral movement problems. The asymmetrical use of the muscles causes strain on the body and prematurely ages it. Add to this the stress caused by immobility, and the problem is compounded. Sedentary people will inevitably suffer from muscular imbalances and the joint and movement dysfunctions that follow.

Normal Spinal Alignment

The human spine is made up of five curves—head, neck, ribcage, lower back, and pelvis, respectively the cranial, cervical, thoracic, lumbar, and sacral curves (Figure 2.2). Since a curved column is stronger than a straight column, the combined curves of the spine make it a much more resilient column, capable of withstanding far more stress than a linear spine could handle.

When the spine is truly upright, it moves from a balanced **position of mechanical advantage**. In this position, the three body masses, or blocks—head, thorax, and pelvis—are aligned one over the next and maintain this alignment during movement. The **neutral position of the spine** is extended and upright, in what is commonly referred to as the *anatomical position*. The terms flexion, extension, and hyperextension need to be clarified because they can be confusing when used in different contexts. Flexion and extension are terms used relative to a joint or relative to a part of the body. For example, **flexion** closes the angle of a joint; **extension** opens the angle of a joint. **Hyperextension** is extension past joint neutral, which can damage joints that lack this range, such as the elbows or knees. The hips and shoulders hyperextend when the limbs move behind the body, and the spine hyperextends when we arch over backward.

When a neutral position of the spine is viewed from the side, a plumb line passes from the ear to the tip of the shoulder to the center of the hip. The curves between each

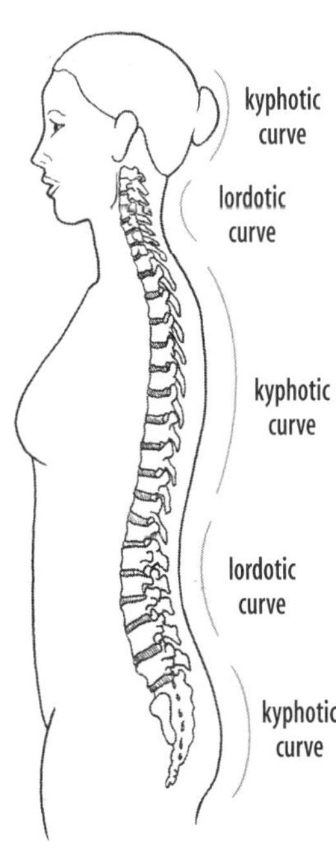

Figure 2.2 Spinal curves

body mass—the cervical and lumbar curves of the neck and lower back—function as up-ended yet bowed bridges between the large skeletal masses of the pelvis, thorax, and head. Ideally, the cervical and lumbar curves are as elongated as possible. Yet, if one bony mass rests in front of or behind another, chances are that the curves in the neck and lower back will compress, bow, and shorten, which puts undue stress on the spine.

Myofascial Restrictions

Chronic misalignment in the spine creates distorted pulls on the soft tissues attached to it. In fact, most physical pain comes from chronic stress in or injury to the *myofascial system*, which includes all the skeletal muscles and the fascias that cover, connect, and separate them. Most people are familiar with the thin, milky coverings found in chicken, fish, and beef, a connective tissue called *fascia*. The word **fascia** is from the Latin word for "band" or "bandage." Ida Rolf, the founder of a bodywork system that reorganizes myofascial balance, calls fascia the "organ of support" because the fascial network binds, supports, and protects every structure within the body. Fascial wrappings are both general (broad sheaths that encase organs and muscles, and bind groups together in bundles and compartments), and specific (sheaths and tubes wrapping and connecting microscopic parts, such as every muscle or nerve fiber, every circulatory tube, and every cell).

The fascial network creates a complex, three-dimensional matrix of non-living *collagen fibers* that permeates every tissue and cell. For example, fascia wraps every individual fiber within a muscle, every muscle, and even groups of muscles. It also separates muscles and their tendons into compartments, as well as organs. (The abdominal organs are situated in one compartment, the lungs and heart in another, and the brain in another.) Like layers of fabric, fascial planes are continuous from one part of the body to the next. For instance, the fascias of the jaw are continuous with fascias along the front of the neck and chest, and the fascias of the deep lumbar muscles are continuous with the fascias of the muscles along the inner thigh and muscles of the pelvic floor (Figure 2.3).

Fascia is made up of sheet-like layers of collagen fibers that are embedded in a viscous ground fluid (scar tissue is a conglomeration of collagen fibers). When muscles con-

Links to Practical Applications

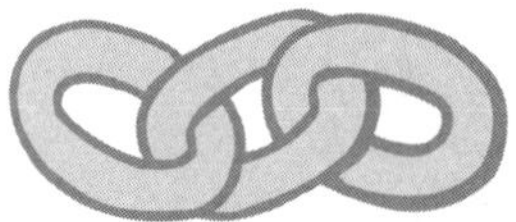

Improving Posture

Whenever you find yourself sitting for long periods, practice subtle spinal alignment exercises, such as rocking over your sit bones, lifting and lowering your chest, rocking your head, or turning an imaginary wheel on the sides of your hips to flex and extend your spine. As you do these exercises, sense where you feel your body masses—hips, ribcage, and head—aligned one over the other.

Patterning Exercise #7: Finding a Neutral Position of Mechanical Advantage

1. Sit comfortably in a chair, in a neutral position, with your head over your thorax over your pelvis (see PE Fig. 7a). If possible, sit sideways to a mirror so you can check your alignment in the mirror.
2. *Finding neutral in the pelvis:* Put your hands on your pelvic bones. Rock back and forth on your sit bones as though you were turning a wheel with its pivot on the sides of your hips (PE Fig. 7b). At what point are the tops of your pelvic bones directly over your sit bones? Rest at this point. If possible, check the mirror to get feedback on your position.
3. *Finding neutral in the head:* Nod your head back and forth (PE Fig.7c). Stop at a neutral place, where your head is on top of your thorax. Now move your head forward, back, then to the center. Check the mirror to see if what you feel is aligned.

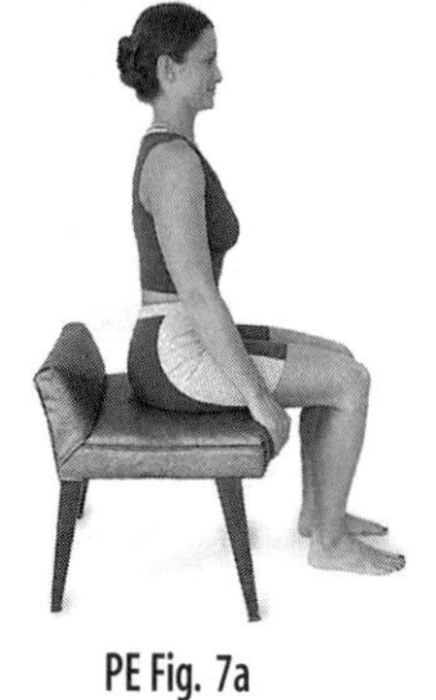

PE Fig. 7a

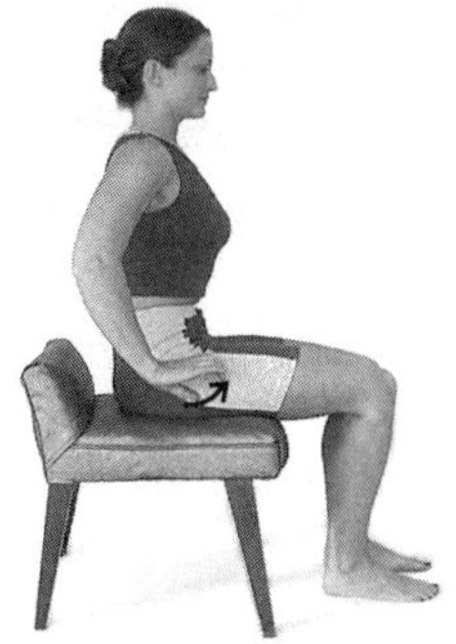

PE Fig. 7b

4. *Finding neutral in the thorax:* Keeping your head and pelvis still, lift then depress your sternum (PE Fig. 7d). Stop where your ribcage feels balanced over your pelvis and below your head. Once again check the mirror to see how you are aligned.
5. *Finding neutral in the entire spine:* Rock your entire spine forward and back over your hips. Sense when you are behind your hips and when you are over your hips, then come to a neutral resting place in between. Again, check the mirror to see if your senses are accurate in letting you know what a position of mechanical advantage feels like.

Application: Familiarize yourself with this neutral, upright posture while you are sitting and standing so that you can recognize when you are or are not in a position of mechanical advantage during your daily activities.

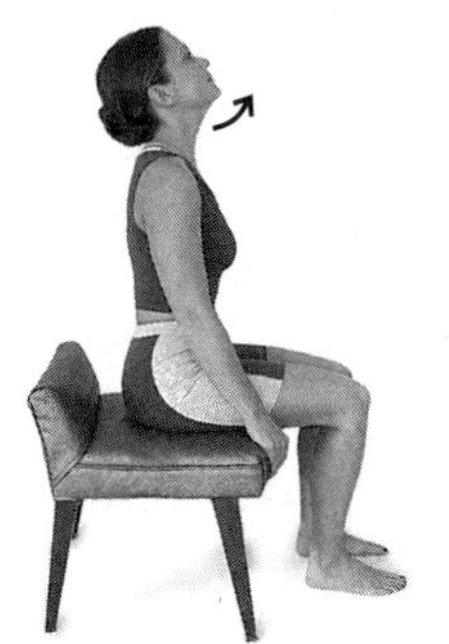

PE Fig. 7c

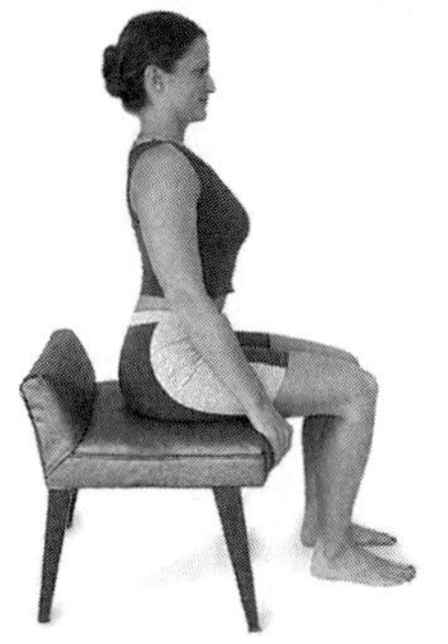

PE Fig. 7d

tract and relax, their surrounding fascial pockets also change shape to conform to the action of the muscles. Myofascial sheaths and cords are so pervasive and interconnected that a pull or shrinkage in one area can translate to another area, similar to how a snag pulls a sweater out of shape. When the muscles are tense or chronically contracted, fibers tend to build up in the surrounding fascia, dehydrating it and making it stiff and unyielding. Fibrous build-ups can develop in an immobile area under stress in as little as 20 minutes, clumping like a pseudo-stiffening material to shore up unstable or stressed areas.

The common stiffness that people think is due to tight muscles usually comes from a combination of chronically contracted muscles plus tight fascia. Thickened fascia tends to "glue" together adjacent muscle groups, creating myofascial adhesions, thereby restricting movement between them. Myofascial adhesions can also compress and irritate peripheral nerves, causing pain.

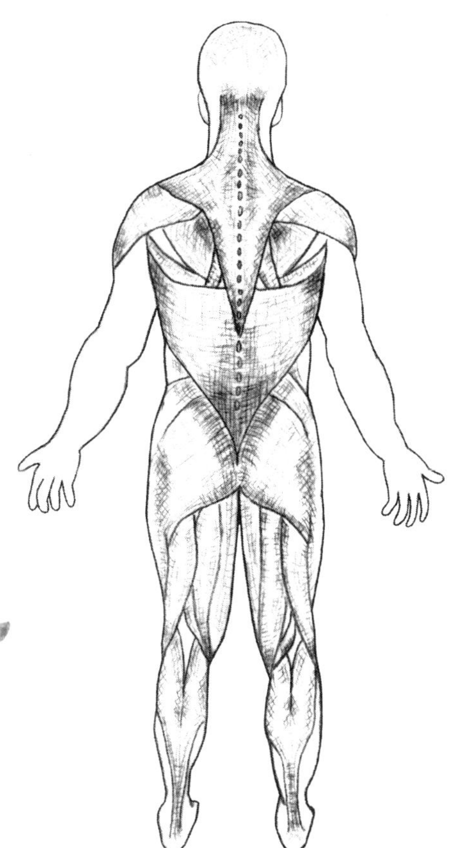

Figure 2.3 Fascia over the superficial muscles

Weak, overstretched muscles often become taut and ropy because the body lays down collagen fibers in them to stiffen and protect them. In an area where a flat muscle is under extreme tension, usually from the pull of an overactive antagonist, the fibers may become so thick that they feel like a cord, a sort of makeshift protective tendon, in one fascicle of an oblique or rhomboid-shaped muscle.

A commonly used bodywork technique called "myofascial release" is an effective method to manually stretch tight myofascia, which usually relieves pain caused by it. Rolfing is a popular form of bodywork that balances the body by systematically releasing myofascial restrictions in an orderly, ten-session series (see Chapter 12).

Stretching can also release tight myofascia, although it is important to differentiate between stretching muscle and stretching fascia because each responds to a different type of manipulation. Stretching fascia is a mechanical process by which a tight area is put in a position of elongation and held there. Stretching muscles is a neurological process. It requires first turning off nerve signals that trigger contractions in order to relax a muscle before stretching it (see Chapter 8). This explains why pain caused by muscle spasm can become worse after stretching or after a deep massage: the fascia may have stretched, but since the nerve impulses causing the muscles to contract have not been addressed, the muscles tighten up even more.

Patterning Exercise #8: Partner Touch Exploration with Myofascia

There are many different ways to explore myofascia with touch, a few of which are listed here. Use this exploration to begin tracking the tone of the muscles and to match your quality of touch with the quality of tone in the myofascial tissues.

1. *Trace the muscles*: Use a muscle chart to get a clear image of the shape and direction of the striations in the muscles. Touch your partner and follow the muscle striations of the muscles, feeling the three-dimensional spiral forms in them. Sense the resting tone of the tissues you are tracing. Sense the density and associated fascias. Keep tracing along kinetic chains, passing from one muscle group to the next across joints.

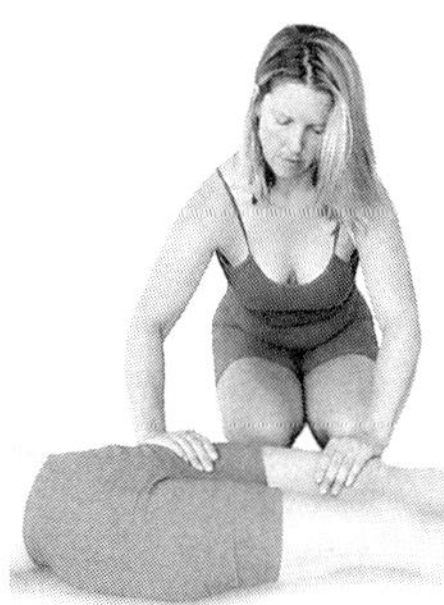

PE Fig. 8a

2. *Approximate a muscle.* Isolate one muscle and place each hand on either end of it (PE Fig. 8a). Slowly compress the muscle by bringing your hands closer together (PE Fig. 8b). This will simulate a contraction. When you have reached maximum compression, slowly pull your hands out and stretch the muscle to approximate relaxation and stretch.
3. *"Putty" the myofascia:* This exercise is to help you match the quality of your touch to the quality of the myofascia. To do so, imagine your partner's superficial layer of myofascia as a layer of putty over the body. Slowly knead the putty, gradually working over his or her entire body. Feel the continuous nature of the myofascial system as you move from one area to the next.

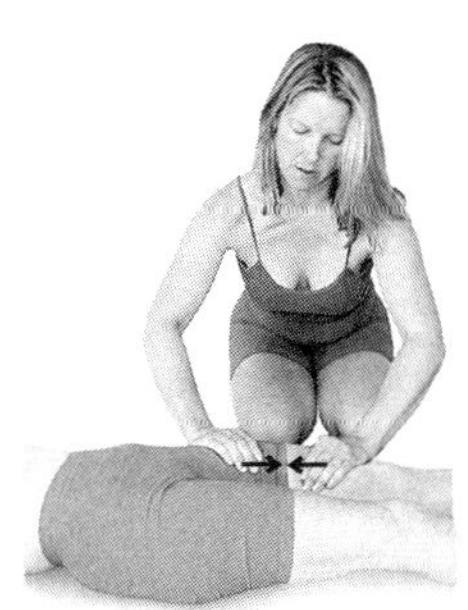

PE Fig. 8b

Musculoskeletal Imbalances

Muscular imbalances develop for many reasons: as the result of injury, stress, developmental movement gaps, muscular armor from psychological issues, or faulty body-use habits. Muscular imbalances caused by purely structural problems, such as injuries, can usually be treated with some form of manual therapy such as bodywork, chiropractic, or physical therapy. Imbalances either caused or sustained by functional problems such as faulty movement patterns require some form of patterning to reorganize the neuromuscular pathways. It's important to note that even though structural treatments can release chronic restriction in the myofascial system, once the person starts moving with faulty patterns, myofascial restrictions are likely to build up again.

Figure 2.5 The skeletal muscles wrap the body in a continuous layer below the skin.

Dysfunctional muscles affect joint stability, mobility, and health. The forces created by muscular pulls pass through a series of adjacent joints that function as links along a **kinematic chain**. Because the joints are linked together, movement in one joint produces predictable motion along the entire chain. In an **open kinematic chain,** the end of a limb is free to move without necessarily causing motion at another joint, such as with gestures of the hands and arms. But in a **closed kinematic chain**, the end of the moving limb is fixed against something and/or weight-bearing. For example, during walking the legs alternate between closed chain in the stance leg and open chain in the swinging leg (Figure 2.4). If any one joint along a kinematic chain is misaligned, especially in a closed chain, the misalignment can translate to other joints along the chain and disrupt the continuity by which movement forces pass through that area.

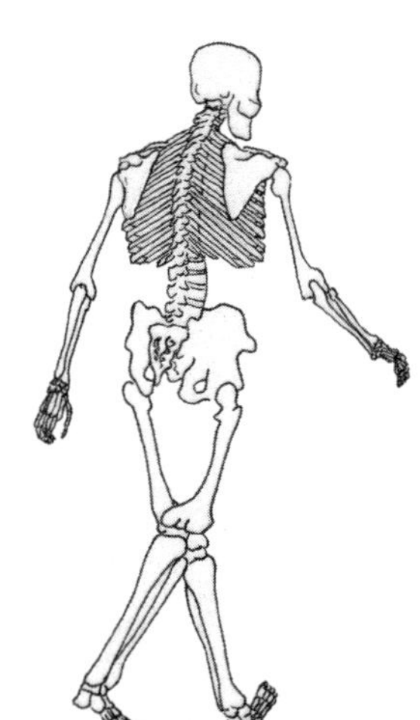

Figure 2.4 The arms swing in an open kinematic chain while the legs work in a closed kinematic chain against the ground.

Skeletal Muscles

The more than 600 skeletal muscles of the musculoskeletal system account for about 40 percent of the body's weight. The extrinsic skeletal muscles wrap the entire body in a continuous layer under the skin, containing the body with a web of elastic tissue much like a form-fitting wet suit (Figure 2.5). Skeletal muscles have an extraordinary level of adaptability. They can vary greatly in strength, speed, and type of contraction. For instance, the muscles of the hand can reduce their force to a fraction of an ounce to pick up a stamp, or increase their force to over 100 pounds to pick up heavy bricks.

Movement occurs as a result of the changing lengths and tensions that are generated by skeletal muscle contraction and relaxation. Muscular contractions generate pulls on the bones to which they are attached. While all three types of muscle—*smooth, cardiac,* and *skeletal*—have the ability to contract and relax, skeletal muscles are the only type under our voluntary control, which makes them a highly accessible system for changing patterns. For the remaining discussion of muscular movement, "muscle" will be used to refer to skeletal muscles unless otherwise stated.

Regardless of the cause, the dynamics of muscular imbalances are the same. Some muscles are weak, some overwork, some fail to contract in sequence, and some just fail to contract. To understand the effects of weak or nonworking muscles, consider that opposing muscles work in **coupled pairs** similar to two ropes on a pulley. The **agonist** muscle functions as **prime mover**, the muscle that does the majority of work in a movement. The **antagonist**, the muscle that opposes the prime mover, counters its motion to control the range and speed of the action.

In a typical action, the agonist muscle shortens with a **concentric contraction,** which pulls the two ends of a muscle closer together. The antagonist muscle usually functions in an **eccentric contraction,** which gradually lengthens the muscle. Eccentric control prevents a movement from going too far. For example, when a person lifts a glass of water to drink, the biceps is the agonist or prime mover. The triceps is the antagonist, controlling the rate at which the glass is lifted (Figure 2.6). Without the modulating force of the antagonist, the strong pull of the biceps would slam the glass into the unfortunate model's forehead!

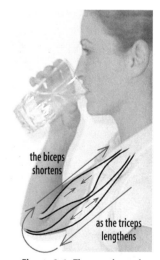

Figure 2.6 The agonist and antagonist muscles work in opposition to move a joint.

Patterning Exercise #9: Agonist/Antagonist Balance

You can use this exercise with any muscle pair, in any position. As you move, imagine your muscles like pulleys, shortening on one side of the body while they lengthen on the other.

1. Stand in a neutral posture. Lift one knee. As you move, guide your muscles with your hands. Sweep up the agonist muscles along the front of the thigh as they shorten, and down the antagonist muscles along the back of the thigh as they lengthen (PE Fig. 9a).

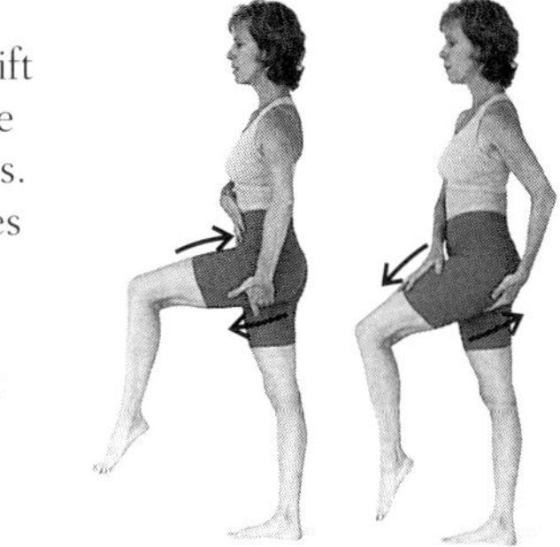

PE Fig. 9a PE Fig. 9b

2. Now reverse the action, sliding your hands in the opposite direction as you lower your knee (PE Fig. 9b). Sense the muscles along the front of the thigh lengthen as the hamstrings shorten to extend the hip.

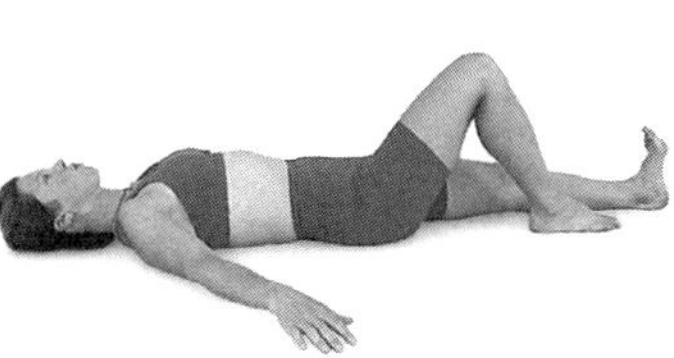

PE Fig. 9c

3. Lie on the floor on your back, with both knees bent and feet on the floor. Slide your heel along the floor and extend your hip and knee (PE Fig. 9c). As you move, feel the flexor muscles over the front of the thigh lengthen while simultaneously feeling the extensors muscles on the back of the hip shorten.
4. Reverse the action, sliding your heel along the floor and flexing your hip and knee (PE Fig. 9d). As you move, feel the hip flexors over the front of the hip shorten while the hip extensors along the back of the hip lengthen.

PE Fig. 9d

5. *Partner Variation:* Use this exercise to help your partner feel counterforces in coupled pairs of muscles during a movement. To give your partner a sense of a concentric contraction on one side of a joint and an eccentric contraction on the other side, place your hand on both sides of an area that your partner is about to move. Move one hand up to shorten the agonist, and the other hand down to lengthen the antagonist. For example, have your partner lie on his or her back. Place one hand under the back of the hip, the other along the front of the hip. While your partner flexes the hip and knee, lengthen the muscles along your back while sinking along your front (PE Fig. 9e).

PE Fig. 9e

EMSPress.com

Like two hands turning a wheel, the stronger muscle in a coupled pair turns the joint in its direction. Ideally both pulls are even, centering the joint. If a weak muscle becomes overpowered by a stronger opposing muscle, these uneven muscular tensions will pull a joint off center similar to how a dominant hand turns a wheel. This type of muscular imbalance is involved in most, if not all, holding patterns.

Smooth and Cardiac Muscles

The skeletal muscles that move our joints are under our conscious control, whereas the smooth muscles making up the sacs, pouches, and tubes of the organs are not. The effects of holding patterns in skeletal muscles are familiar to most people—muscle spasms and chronic contractions. Holding patterns can also settle into the smooth muscles. The most common examples of this show up in the digestive tract, resulting in such conditions as digestive problems, constipation, spastic colon, or a stomach that feels literally tied in knots. Although the contractions of our organs are regulated automatically, we can still learn to relax them through autonomic patterning such as biofeedback or relaxation exercises.

Cardiac muscle is found only in the heart. It differs from smooth and skeletal muscle in that it is powered by local neural stimulation of a pacemaker, made up of the *sinoatrial* and *atrioventricular nodes* that keep the heart beating. Although we usually do not think of the heart as being under our conscious control, a person can strengthen the heart with cardiovascular conditioning and relax the heart by consciously slowing it down, both very important skills to maintain healthy cardiac tissue.

On a metaphorical level, the heart is felt to be the source of loving and compassionate feelings, while the digestive organs are felt to be the place where we process "deep, gut" emotions. Since both the heart and most abdominal organs have muscle tissue within them, perhaps it is possible to improve the health of these vital organs and influence their metaphorical functions by actually focusing on the muscle tissue within them with the intention of relaxing or energizing it (see Patterning Exercise #10).

Stabilizer and Mobilizer Muscles

Many people work hard to develop muscular strength, but strength does not necessarily ensure good posture. This is because the muscular groups developed with bodybuilding or sports are not necessarily the muscles that work to maintain good posture or postural stability. For this reason

Patterning Exercise #10: Releasing Chronic Holding in the Organs

If you feel tightness and tension in your gut, it may be coming from chronic contractions in your organs.

1. To release tension in the smooth muscles of the viscera, lie in a comfortable position on your back and put your hands on the middle of your abdomen.
2. Probe around and locate the areas that feel tight. Spastic intestines may feel like hard lumps under your hands.
3. Rest your hands on the tight areas for feedback, and relax your intestines (PE Fig. 10a). Imagine or feel warmth radiating from your hands into your gut, melting the tension there.
4. Place your hand right above your pubic bone, over your bladder (empty it first if you need to). Again, using feedback from your hands, relax your bladder.
5. To relax your kidneys, lie on your back and bend both knees so that the kidneys sink back.
6. Sit up and place both hands, one on each side, below your lower ribs on the back of your body (PE Fig. 10b). (This approximates your kidneys, which are located behind your lower ribs in the back of your body.) Sense or feel your kidneys sinking into your back and into the floor.
7. To relax your heart, place your hands directly over it. Listen for and feel your heart beat. Use the rate of your heartbeat for feedback. Lean forward slightly and imagine your heart sinking into your hands (PE Fig. 10c). Put forth the intention of slowing your heart down.
8. To relax your lungs, put your hands on each side of your ribcage. Again, feel or imagine your lungs sinking down. Allow warmth from your hands to radiate into your lungs and melt any tension in them. Move your hands around to any areas of the lungs that you want to relax.
9. Use this process—consciously relaxing the organ while resting your hands on top of it—with any organs in which you sense or imagine tension.

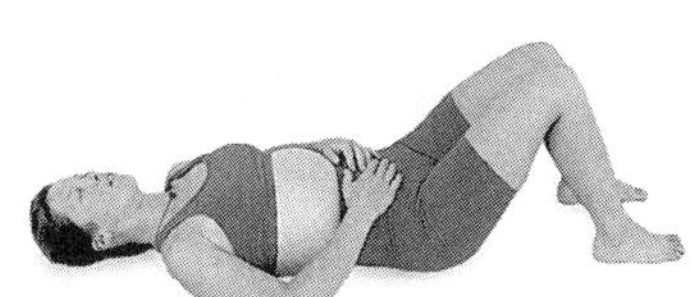

PE Fig. 10a

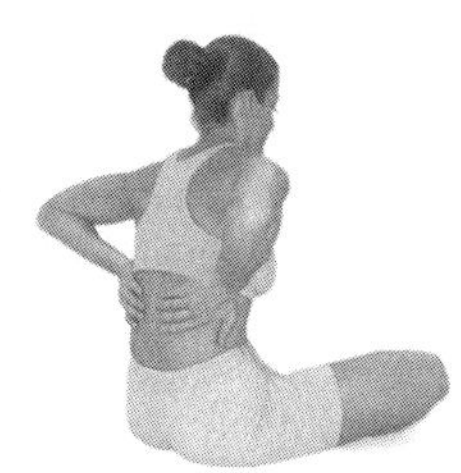

PE Fig. 10b

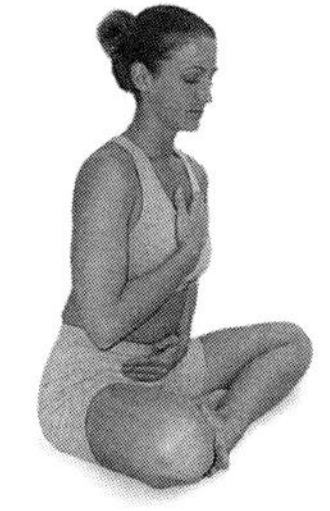

PE Fig. 10c

an athlete can have poor posture and a person with well-aligned posture can be weak in sports.

Probably the most prevalent type of musculoskeletal imbalance occurs when a postural muscle is **inhibited**—meaning either turned off or not firing when it should. The postural muscles, also called **stabilizers,** work to stabilize a joint in a neutral position.[40] They do not produce movement; they stiffen a joint without bending or twisting it. Their inhibition can result in joint instability, which inevitably leads to joint damage, chronic pain, and weak structural integrity (poor posture). The stabilizers are developed by learning to control them with slow, sustained contractions. Because their contractions are **tonic,** sustained and constant, the muscles that work as postural stabilizers have **tonic function** and are commonly called "tonic" muscles.[41]

Figure 2.7 Stabilizer muscles along the spine increase axial compression.

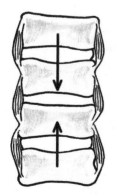

The small, intrinsic stabilizers that lie close to the spine contract in a sustained manner to stiffen a joint by pulling two vertebrae in that joint closer together. Their contractions increase **axial compression** (vertical loading) of a joint within a neutral position, pulling its articular surfaces together (Figure 2.7). Ideally, a joint functions within its normal range of vertical displacement, called a **neutral zone**—the range in which a joint can move without restraint from surrounding muscles, ligaments, or the joint capsule.[42] If the stabilizers are not working to stiffen a joint, the joint will have too large a neutral zone and will lack stability, which makes it susceptible to injury because it can be easily displaced beyond its physiological end range of motion.

In contrast to the stabilizers, the larger, mostly extrinsic muscles cover longer distances and have stronger pulls. Since they work to move bones through space, they are called **mobilizers**. Because the mobilizer muscles span two or more joints, they work as strong lever arms; their contractions generate joint motion. They work in coupled agonist and antagonist pairs to pivot a joint around its central axis, an action similar to two hands turning a wheel. The mobilizers are often referred to as "spurt" muscles because they produce fast contractions, obvious in the pumping action of a weight lifter. **Phasic** means fast; hence, the mobilizers are often called "phasic" muscles. When dysfunctional, a mobilizer can be **over-facilitated**, meaning that it fires too often and overworks, a condition that lead to muscular imbalances.

The progression in which muscles contract is called the **recruitment order**. Coordination depends on the order in which a series of muscles fires. In a coordinated movement, the stabilizers contract before the mobilizers to ensure joint stability during motion. The contraction of the stabilizing muscles has the effect of "battening down the hatches" prior to a movement, literally buckling together the joints to avoid jars and spills once the "ship" starts moving. Thus, when the body does move, the stronger contractions of the mobilizers pull the body through space.

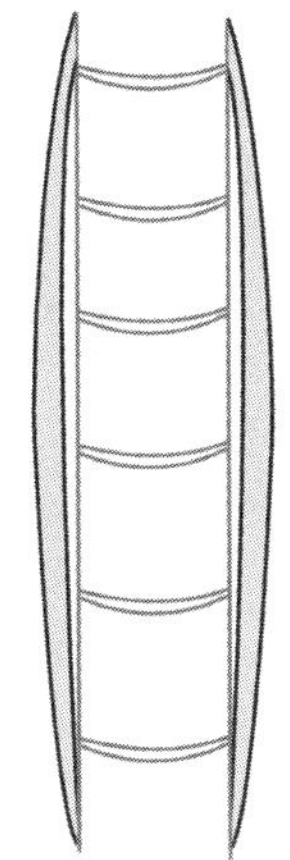

Figure 2.8a In neutral, opposing muscles along the spine rest at the same length.

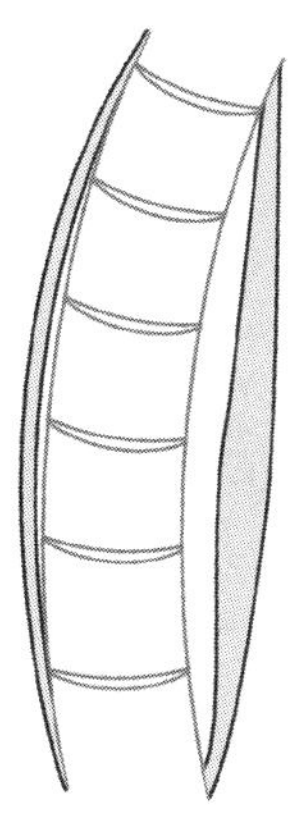

Figure 2.8b Contraction on one side results in elongation on the opposite side.

Muscular imbalances occur when the recruitment order is not in an optimal sequence. Certain muscles may fail to fire at the right time, other muscles overwork, and still other muscles may be locked in either a chronic contraction or chronic inhibition. If the stabilizers fail to contract first, when the body moves, the powerful pulls of the mobilizers will bend unstable joints beyond their normal range of motion. The overall result is a wobbly, poorly coordinated movement, a dynamic that can lead to joint and soft tissue damage.

Ideally, the stabilizing muscles give the body support, and the mobilizing muscles are free to move the body. If the stabilizers are not working, the mobilizers take over their job, chronically contracting to provide postural support, a job they are poorly suited for. Since the mobilizers are usually *biarticular* (spanning two joints) or *multiarticular* (spanning three or more joints), they pull on a group of joints rather than just one segment. Normally, when muscles on one side of the spine contract, the muscles on the other side lengthen and the spinal joints flex or extend with even and stable joint motion. If the mobilizers contract without the underlying stiffening effect of the stabilizers, the vertebral joints at the apex of the motion can bend beyond their neutral range (Figure 2.9a-b).

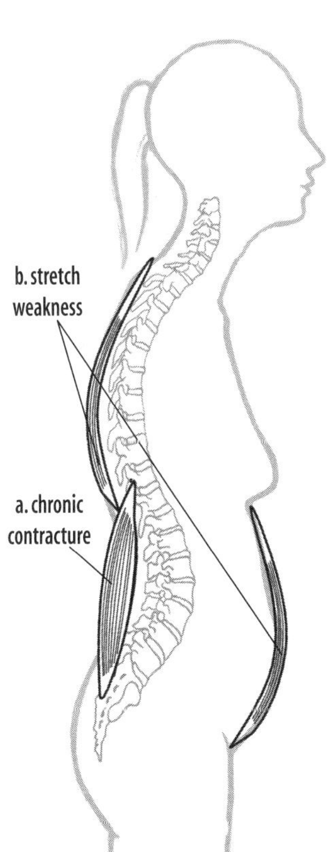

Figure 2.9 In the lordotic-kyphotic posture, (a) some spinal muscles are in chronic contractures, while (b) others are overstretched.

For example, consider the large extrinsic muscles along the lower back. They span four to six vertebrae. When they contract an unstable spine, they hyperextend the lumbar spine, bending the lumbar curve into an exaggerated **lordosis**, the abnormal forward curvature of the spine that most people call a "swayback" (see Figure 2.9). This posture compresses the back of the spine while overstretching the front of the spine, which may lead to soft tissue damage and chronic pain, as well as a stability dysfunction.

Chronic contractures in the mobilizer muscles are often accompanied by a **stretch weakness** in the opposing muscle group, weakened by being held in the overextended position (Figure 2.9a-b). A stretch weakness is particularly damaging to the spinal muscles because they are chronically contracted in an elongated position, becoming taut and weak. Also, the *intervertebral joints* bend like a hinge, which pulls them beyond their physiological range. This can damage their joint capsules, impinge spinal nerve roots, and overstretch already strained ligaments. This is common in an exaggerated **kyphosis**, or "hunchback" posture.

Keep in mind that the process of muscular imbalance tends to progress and layer below a level of conscious awareness. Eventually, the weak link in the spine breaks, and, all of a sudden, a person has a back problem that seems to appear out of nowhere. In truth, the symptoms were probably there all along, but since most people are not oriented toward feeling or understanding postural mechanisms, this sort of problem seems to sneak up on people all too frequently.

Muscular Responses to Chronic Pain

Chronic pain creates double trouble: it triggers muscle spasms in the mobilizers and has also been found to inhibit the stabilizers.[43] This potentially injurious combination can escalate pain by perpetuating the spasm-pain-spasm cycle, and by increasing injuries from light movements performed while in an unstable posture. The inhibition of the stabilizers alone creates several problems. Without the underlying stability in the spine, a person can literally give herself whiplash with a strong or quick movement. Plus, the whipping action stimulates the sensory nerve receptors around the joint, causing pain. As a result of pain, new muscle groups spasm to guard against more pain, which creates another layer of imbalance, and a chronic pain cycle builds in intensity.

Also, when the stabilizers are inhibited, the mobilizers attempt to shore up the unstable structure by becoming locked in chronic contractures and therefore unavailable for movement. Chronic contractures result in cumbersome, rigid movement patterns that lack agility and efficiency. Chronic contractures also fatigue the mobilizers because their fast-twitch fibers are suited for quick, strong contractions rather than sustained, postural contractions. They tire easily when held in sustained contractions, which is why people with poor posture often feel fatigued at the end of the day.

Structural and Functional Patterns

The muscular and joint imbalances that were just discussed affect the body's structure by distorting postural alignment. They also affect the body's function by reducing the efficiency of movement and coordination. From this view, structural patterns are observed in a stationary posture while functional patterns are observed in the quality of movement. In an expanded view, structural patterns are associated with the mechanics of the movement generated by the musculoskeletal system, including patterns of both posture and movement, while functional patterns are associated with metabolism (how our bodies run), encompassing both physiological and emotional patterns.

It is important to understand this difference between structural and functional patterns when working with holding patterns because holding patterns may involve more than just muscular imbalances. Emotional and psychological components that affect psychophysiological functions can also contribute to holding patterns. Both structural and functional patterns need to be addressed, but the one that is overriding should be addressed first. For instance, a person suffering from back pain may have a structural problem that has a local cause, such as muscular imbalance in the lower back. In this case, neuromuscular patterning to address the mechanics of muscle and joint function is called for. Conversely, the pain may be rooted in high levels of stress, nervous tension, and emotional distress. In this case, autonomic patterning that calms the body is called for.

Most holding patterns involve both structural and functional elements, which can be understood by assessing which part of the nervous system that the pattern affects the most. There are two main parts of the nervous system. The **central nervous system** (CNS) is made up of the brain and spinal cord; the **peripheral nervous system** (PNS) is made up of the *autonomic nerves* and *ganglia* (nerve cell bodies located outside the brain), plus all the spinal and cranial nerves (Figure 2.10).

One part of the PNS is the **autonomic nervous system** (ANS). The ANS regulates the involuntary functions of the organs and the instinctive responses associated with emotional tone and psychophysiological activity. It has two divisions: **parasympathetic** (which controls relaxation responses), and **sympathetic** (which controls fight-or-flight responses). The other part of the PNS, the **skeletal nervous system** (SNS), innervates all the muscles, bones, and joints. The SNS is sometimes called the *somatic nervous system* because it controls skeletal muscle movement and the neuromuscular mechanisms involved in all movement responses.

Autonomic and Skeletal Nervous System Balance

The SNS organizes the mechanical aspects of movement observed in muscle and joint function. The ANS gives movement an emotional quality, a mood or feeling tone. Emotional tone can be trained out of a sport or dance, or it can be integrated into the mover's performance. For example, a technically proficient dancer can be quite boring when devoid of passion or feeling, or she can dance with emotional depth that "moves" the audience, eliciting tears or joy. In the former case, the ANS and SNS are not integrated in movement; in the latter case, they are.

Although neuromuscular pathways are coordinated by the SNS and psychophysiological processes are regulated by the ANS, the two systems are inextricably interconnected. Patterns in one affect the other. ANS impulses initiated by emotions and instincts are relayed to the SNS, where they are either carried into action by the muscles or are inhibited. For example, a person feels fear or anger, then either acts on the emotion with a movement or suppresses taking action. The SNS and ANS are so integrally connected that imbalances in one often underlie imbalances in the other, which blurs the edge between what feels like emotional pain and what feels like physical pain. In short, neuromuscular imbalances can greatly compound nervous tension and emotionality, and exacerbate functional movement problems. On the flip side, nervous tension and psychophysiological stress can reduce neuromuscular efficiency and exacerbate structural postural problems.

Typically, functional dysfunctions are considered body problems caused by poor biomechanics, and structural dysfunctions are considered body problems caused by structural abnormalities. In this discussion, structural and functional patterns are being used to refer respectively to biomechanical and psychophysiological problems. Traditionally, structural problems have been treated with the biomechanical therapies used in orthopedics and

Can you think of examples when structural patterns complicate functional patterns? When instinctive impulses override rational choices? When reason inhibits acting on impulse or even acting on signs of physical distress?

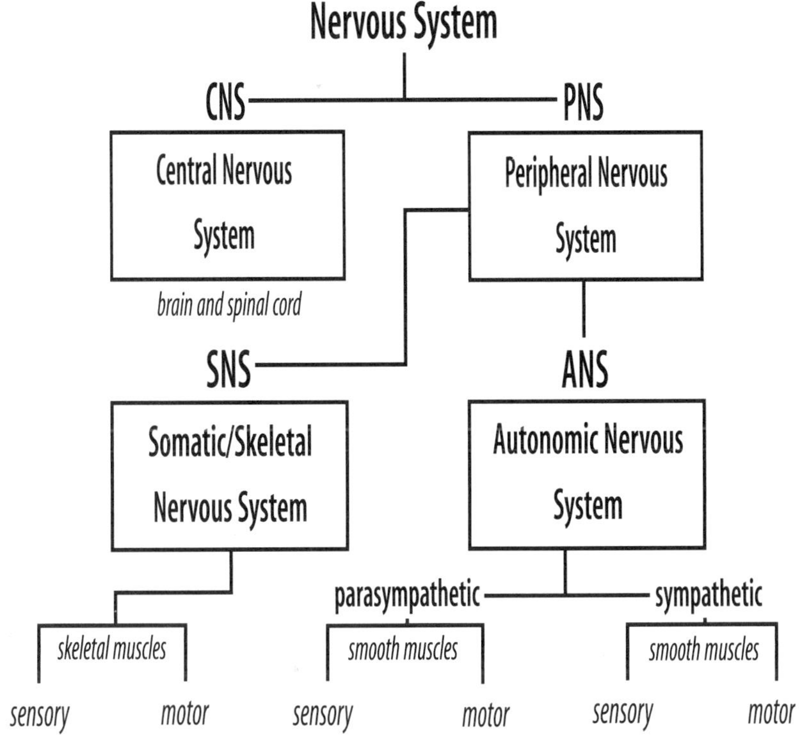

Figure 2.10 A general schematic of the nervous system and its divisions

physical therapy, while functional or psychophysiological problems have been treated using the biological therapies found in psychiatry, with both cognitive therapy (talk therapy) and physiological interventions (drug therapy). But the polarities of the biomechanical and biological approaches are becoming more integrated as people realize that all body patterns have mental, emotional, and even physiological components to them, and begin to use somatic patterning to address the connections among them.

The Sensorimotor Loop

The human body is a **dynamic system**: it has no static properties. It is made dynamic by a kaleidoscope of interactive feedback loops that regulate function and physiological equilibrium. A dynamic system is constantly seeking to improve itself. It evolves by means of a two-way flow of information or energy.[44] Holding patterns develop when the dynamic systems of the body are interfered with or blocked, causing a person to receive inaccurate sensorimotor feedback necessary for normal body functions. The sensorimotor (SM) loop, a continuum of incoming sensory information and outgoing motor responses, can become stuck in several places (Figure 2.11).

For example, a person might receive sensory signals that she cannot act on or process with a movement response, in which case, sensory input piles up. This person is unable to process signals in order to complete an action and may suffer from a feeling of being overloaded, of not having enough time to work things through. People stuck in a holding pattern on the sensory side of the loop, as described here, tend to have nervous tension coupled with a held posture. It is as though their nerves are frazzled on the inside and their muscles frozen on the outside. Releasing this type of tension can feel like an explosion, so it needs to be done slowly.

On the other side of the loop, a person busies the nervous system with motor activities in the physical movement of the body and the mental movement of thought. It may be confusing to think of thoughts as motor activities, which they in fact are not, but a person can be busy mentally as well as physically. Plus, thought causes nerves to fire that can then cause muscles to fire, whether or not a person is actually moving. A receptive mind, as opposed to a busy mind, is quiet in the absence of thought, a state sought by many in meditation. Similarly, the receptive body is also somewhat quiet; it is open to input and can sense itself.

The more activity or noise the system generates, the less receptivity or sensory awareness it has. A person stuck on the motor side of the loop can become too busy to feel body sensations or emotions. In an analogy, a moving vehicle cannot pick up passengers. Any physical sensation that arises from psychophysiological or musculoskeletal

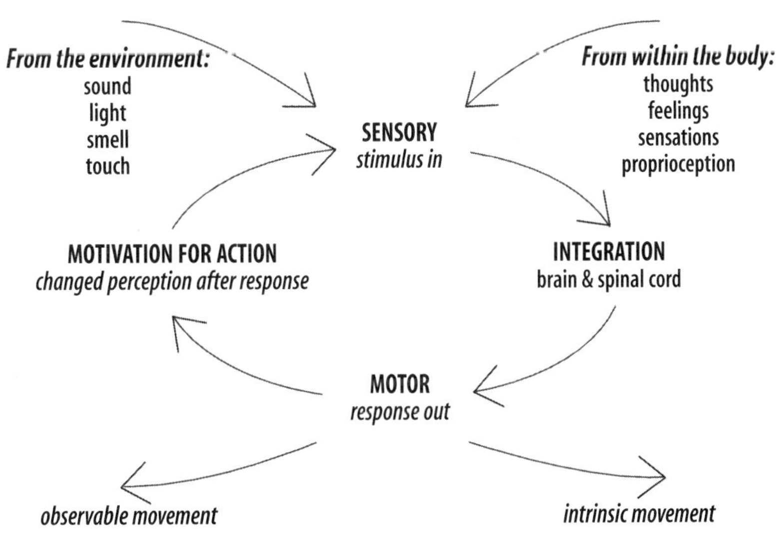

Figure 2.11 A schematic of the sensorimotor loop

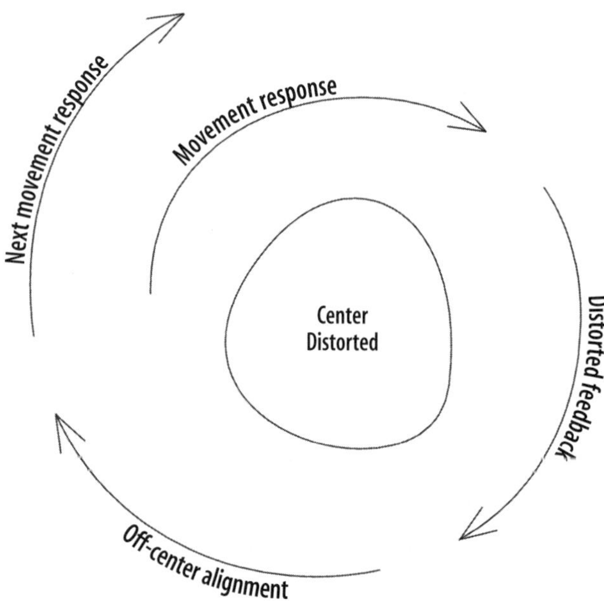

Figure 2.12 A schematic of how distorted perceptions affect movement responses

input is drowned out by a flurry of activity. A person stuck in this type of pattern usually runs out of gas sooner or later, especially if the output is driven more by thought than by physical activity. When a person with an overactive mind does let down and rest, the body can crash into a state of deep exhaustion from which it may take a good deal of time to recuperate.

On a more positive note, a person who ignores body sensation but participates in rigorous daily sports is likely to be healthy and well balanced for two reasons. First, the channels for motor response are open. And second, when a person uses the body for what it was designed for—lots of rigorous physical activity—the body grows healthier. Still, ignoring the signals coming from the body is dangerous because a person could have a serious injury or illness that becomes more serious when undetected, or the pressure of unresolved negative emotions could build up and cause harm in many ways.

It would be impossible to do justice to the complexity of sensorimotor processes in a discussion as simplified as this one. The neural circuitry in the body is a complex net of neuromotor pathways moving signals move so fast that the myriad of sensorimotor processes appears simultaneous while in actuality millions of millions neurons coordinate information along separate pathways at one time. Although we can say, "Now I'm feeling sensation, now I am moving," and separate our awareness of each, in reality we are only feeling a glimmer of the SM process. Also, what we choose to feel and where we choose to point our attention changes the very process we are looking at. Still, each moment of awareness we have of sensory and motor processes makes a body-mind connection, and these connections accumulate and gradually reconnect the body-mind split.

Whenever the sensorimotor loop habituates on one side or the other of the sensorimotor loop, **proprioceptive feedback** coming from inside the body or from positional shifts in the body becomes skewed. A person is then unable to accurately feel which muscles are contracting or stretching, or where the body is positioned in space. When the feedback is inaccurate, a person will invariably pull a muscle or fall down because he is confused about where he is located, how he is positioned. Distorted feedback alters proprioception so that crooked posture feels straight, inefficient movement and off-center alignment feel normal, and holding patterns become more ingrained (Figure 2.12).

Separation

The essence of holding patterns lies in separation. In fact, the idea that the body and the mind are separate could be viewed as a cultural holding pattern. Most of our cultural medicines are based on the notion that body and mind operate as separate entities. Hence, the body and mind develop codependent tendencies; they work against each other. The word "codependency" was developed in treatment modalities for alcoholism, where it was discovered that "enablers" (often the spouses of alcoholics) would sacrifice their personal and emotional needs to meet the needs of the alcoholic. The same codependent dynamics occur within an individual in holding patterns. One part of the body becomes overworked while another part is ignored, abandoned from awareness, or frozen in chronic muscular contraction. For example, a person who exercises regardless of pain sacrifices the body's safety to the mind's authoritative control. A person who overworks regardless of the warning signs of deep stress sacrifices physical and mental health to a work ethic. Eventually, the body reaches a breaking point, and an injury, illness, or mental breakdown calls the faulty pattern to the person's attention.

Purely structural problems rarely develop absent of psychological patterns. Rather, they develop slowly, usually below the radar of body awareness, and are entwined with and complicated by psychosomatic factors. After a long period, the functional imbalances such as chronic stress or emotional angst manifest in faulty mechanics, pulling and weakening the myofascial fibers which in

Links to Practical Applications

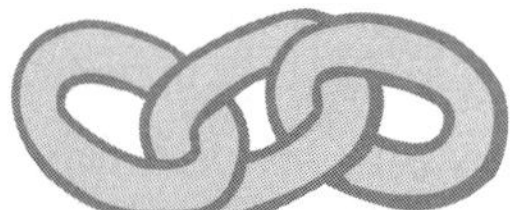

Observing Holding Patterns

To observe how people abandon parts of their bodies, sit and watch people walk by and notice which parts of their bodies do not move, or which parts look like they are being carried like a spare, nonattached part. For example, many seniors hold their elbows behind the body rather than letting their arms swing naturally. Why they do this is a matter of speculation, perhaps because they subconsciously fear falling.

turn stresses muscles and joints, causing scar tissue to build to shore up the faulty structure, which inevitably entraps peripheral nerves. Eventually, functional imbalances culminate in structural problems. These problems may go unnoticed for years, until they reach critical mass. The sad truth is, most people do not pay attention to patterns of posture and movement until they hurt. Imagine using a car for 25 years without looking under the hood!

To effectively look under the hood and heal the split, a person can become more aware of personal tendencies in sensorimotor process. A more fully realized sensorimotor loop leads to more complete movement sequences, in which a person is able to feel or sense something, then respond accordingly with a motor action. A helpful antidote for someone stuck on the sensory side of the loop can be found in the practice of organic movement. In this improvisational movement practice (see Chapter 6) a person explores spontaneous body movements that release tension from a build p of inhibited responses while waking up dormant motor pathways. Someone stuck on the motor side of the loop has troubling feeling sensation. This person would benefit from sensory awareness exercises and relaxation training, as well as organic movement done slowly enough that he or she could begin to feel the body while it is moving in order to restore sensory awareness during a motor activity.

When you sit in a chair, does your body form to the shape of the chair? Or does the chair shape around you? What kind of chairs do you tend to slump in? What kind gives your body optimal support?

THE ROOTS OF HOLDING PATTERNS

Although researchers have thoroughly delineated what constitutes good posture and low-stress lifestyles, and have established many guidelines for achieving both, this information is either not reaching the general public or people are not applying it. Many people still suffer the chronic pain caused by postural holding without realizing how they are actually creating their own problems via the inefficient and unconscious use of their bodies.

Why is this tendency so pervasive? Perhaps because muscular habits develop rapidly—often below the level of conscious awareness. A normal nervous system establishes movement pathways so quickly that one simply needs to imagine a movement or postural characteristic and it will soon be habitual. This is not to say that all habits are bad. We rely on habit to organize the many complex movement patterns we use each day. Imagine the work involved if we had to stop and think about coordinating each step we take. Anyone who has had to relearn how to walk after an injury can appreciate how much of our movement is coordinated below conscious awareness. Our muscles adapt to new furniture, new tools at work, new shoes, and new clothes by establishing new habits. Habits form so quickly that we are often unaware of them until we feel the pain that bad habits create.

Structural holding patterns develop from many mechanical situations, such as injuries, nonsupportive furniture, ill-fitting clothes or tight shoes, sedentary lifestyles, positional postural models, and the most prevalent source of all, faulty body-use habits. Structural holding patterns are easier to change than functional holding patterns because they are usually not enmeshed in the psyche. Purely structural imbalances can be alleviated with mechanical remedies such as postural education, changes in workstation ergonomics, or simply getting shoes that fit properly or furniture that is supportive.

In contrast, functional holding patterns require a deeper inquiry into psychological patterns and how they were shaped by early development. For most people, this involves stirring up emotional and relational issues, plus resolving conflicts based on family history. Doing so may shake up the status quo, which can be both overwhelming and painful. Plus, working honestly with functional patterns involves taking an objective look at the psychology of our own posture and movement abilities. Most people, particularly those who habitually avoid looking objectively at themselves, are usually adept at criticizing how they are shaped, which in itself causes self-inflicted emotional pain. This type of self-flagellating behavior tends to make somatic patterning more difficult. On the bright side, by understanding how the psyche acts out in somatic patterns, a person can use somatic patterning to get a handle on the physical manifestation of psychological issues, and to monitor psychological growth through positive physical changes.

Muscular Splinting

The body responds to pain and trauma by **splinting** an injured area with adaptive muscular spasms. These spasms provide a built-in cast or sling to immobilize an injured area to prevent further injury or irritation while it heals (Figure 2.13).

Ideally, once the injury heals the protective spasms release. In actuality, the splinting pattern usually remains long after the tissues have healed. Chronic muscular splinting restricts movement and blocks circu-

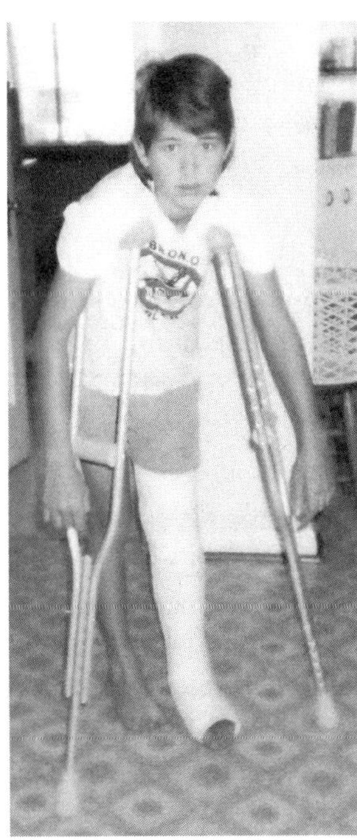

Figure 2.13 Adaptive muscle patterns and postures develop around injuries.

Patterning Problems with Deep Tissue Work

Areas of instability tend to have more pain than areas of rigidity. The problem is further complicated when we mistake the pain of instability for tightness and massage painful areas, which loosens them even more. This is a blind spot in the bodywork field, especially since myofascial release and joint mobilization techniques have become popular. As bodyworkers, we often learn a myriad of techniques for releasing and mobilizing tissues, yet we receive little or no training in assessing which joints are restricted and which are unstable.

Another common problem is that deep tissue work loosens the extrinsic muscles, which can lead to trouble if the intrinsic muscles are not firing. If a client depends on the extrinsic muscles for postural support and they are released, when that client stands up, the body lacks its previous support, which can send the extrinsic muscles into a panic and trigger muscle spasms.

As a rule of thumb, after doing deep tissue work, have your client do sustained contractions in the stabilizers while still lying on the table. If this is not possible, the client can do subtle, intrinsic movements, such as small pelvic tilts, or nodding and turning the head, which will help organize postural muscle control prior to sitting and standing. To engage intrinsic support, make sure the client sits up slowly and with awareness.

lation, eventually leading to new types of pain. In compensation for splinting patterns, a different group of muscles spasm to immobilize the newly pained area, creating a new movement aberration. Because of the layering tendency of splinting patterns, injury rehabilitation involves not only healing tissue trauma, but also releasing the splinting patterns and restoring movement around and through the injured area.

Once certain numbers of muscles (the number will vary from one person to the next) are busy splinting an injured area, fewer muscles are available for the overall coordination of movement. Inevitably, another group of muscles takes over the job abandoned by those in spasm. As a result, movement patterns reroute *around* rather than *through* the injured or painful area in what is called an **adaptive pattern**. Wilson and Schneider, who researched the muscular activity of clients recovering from injuries, found that the new pattern is usually asymmetrical.[45] Muscles are bilateral, meaning that a specific muscle on the right has a counterpart on the left that mirrors it, giving the body right-left symmetry. Asymmetries occur when one muscle of a bilateral pair becomes chronically contracted. By placing electrodes in the muscles two weeks after painful but ignored injuries, Wilson and Schneider found that high levels of asymmetry had developed both at the site of the injury and above and below the site.

Pain from adaptive patterns tends to override an awareness of asymmetrical movement, so that a person feels pain rather than the distortion of movement. As long as the head remains relatively vertical, a person will usually not sense asymmetry in movement. Within a short period of time, the adaptive pattern begins to feel normal and becomes habitual. This occurs more commonly with minor injuries because people tend to brush them off as inconsequential and keep moving around the injured area.

Adaptive or compensatory patterns of splinting are obvious in the limping or hobbling gait patterns of an injured person. The movement aberrations created by the original splinting pattern usually last long after healing has taken place, and the person continues to move with distorted posture in a habitual pattern. In essence, "old habits die hard" because the nervous system likes to route movement down the most well-traveled pathways. Like a rut in the road, splinting patterns quickly habituate along neuromuscular "highways" within our neural circuitry. During the process of habituation, nerves actually change. When nerve cells are repeatedly stimulated, fewer neurotransmitters are released. This has a dampening effect on impulse transmission, and it then takes a stronger stimulus to break the habit. Thus, there is a danger that a person can become susceptible to more severe injuries before noticing the imbalance in movement.

Adaptive patterns develop not only with injuries, but whenever there is pain and chronic muscular holding induced by psychological guarding. Adaptive patterns, in turn, reduce the efficiency of movement and create new stress on the body. They pull joints out of their neutral range, stress tendons and ligaments, and clamp down around nerve bundles, creating new pain centers. With new pain comes more splinting, and the adaptive patterns begin to layer, taking a person deeper into a pain cycle.

Instability and Rigidity

As discussed earlier, a combination of inhibited stabilizer muscles and over-facilitated mobilizer muscles can lead to a condition called a **stability dysfunction**—the inability to control joint play during movement. Stability dysfunctions are marked by excessive joint play in specific joints and the failure of the body to move effectively under low load, such as the load of the body's own weight. Inhibited stabilizers are like absentee or immobilized workers: they bog down the efficient production of movement and neglect their share of the workload, showing up at the wrong time and getting their job done late. People with stability dysfunctions can injure themselves with seemingly benign movements that jar unstable joints.

The natural response to instability is chronic muscular contraction in the mobilizing muscles, which can lead to rigidity. Rigid areas usually develop as an adaptive pattern to unstable areas, particularly when those areas generate pain. Most holding patterns are some combination of instability and rigidity, often with a rigid area adjacent to an unstable area.

The problem with rigidity is that collagen fibers build up in and around chronically contracted muscles, thickening and tightening the areas, blocking circulation, limiting movement, and contributing to a feeling of overall stiffness. People often build rigidity when strengthening extrinsic muscles without first learning to control the intrinsic stabilizing muscles. For example, people with lower back pain are commonly told to do sit-ups to strengthen the lower back, yet sit-ups strengthen the mobilizers without engaging the stabilizers. Muscle strength is important to overall physical health, yet using strength training to alleviate instability can lead to rigidity from overdevelopment of the extrinsic muscles without developing the underlying support of the stabilizers. Also, strengthening large muscles around an unstable joint can compress that joint in a misaligned position and damage it. Still, rigidity is preferable to instability because people with too much joint play run a greater risk of injury.

Abusive and Positional Postures

People often injure their backs doing a movement with the body in a weak or unsupported position. A person can injure a disc or joint capsule by pulling it while it is slightly off center, or strain a tendon or ligament while doing the simplest movement in an awkward position. **Repetitive stress injury** (RSI), in which a person performs the same movement over and over again, is also a common source of wear and tear that leads to injury and is exacerbated by poor postures. This type of injury is common in industrial jobs that require repetitive motion. In fact, faulty postures alone, such as a collapsed spine and a forward head, can lead to repetitive injury; therefore, they are now being called "abusive postures." For instance, a person who sits in a slumped position (a posture common in gangly teens) puts undue strain on the lower back (Figure 2.14). In time, the vertebral discs of the lumbar spine slide in the posterior direction and undergo gradual strain which eventually damages them. (The posterior displacement of lumbar discs is a common cause of low back pain.)

The point to underscore here is that *abusive postures lead to tissue damage from RSI as readily as do faulty movements.* Furthermore, the simplest movement done from a faulty posture, such as bending over to tie a shoe, can lead to injury. This highlights the importance of sound postural education, which requires, at the very least, an introductory understanding of functional anatomy, and more importantly, an ability to feel when the postural muscles are contracted and when the body is in an aligned position.

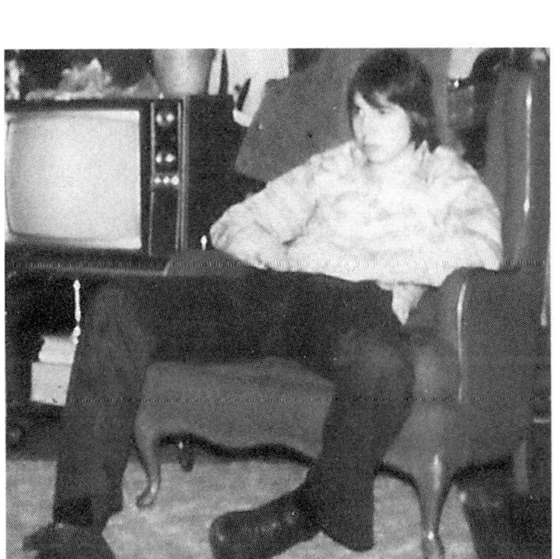

Figure 2.14 A typical teen slouch

Most of us learned as children that posture is a position to assume and hold like a statue. The difficulty we encounter when we try to place ourselves into a "correct" posture is that the body rigidifies into some vague mental image of the proper position. Ask a group of 100 people to stand up straight, and they will assume 100 different versions of "straight." Why? Because most of us understand *what* straight is, but *how* to achieve straight is left to chance.

Since specific postural muscles need to contract in specific ways to achieve a stable yet dynamic posture, postural education is a precise process that cannot be achieved simply by assuming a position. The body responds to commands such as "sit up straight" with quick, strong contractions of the mobilizers, which can override the slower, weaker contractions of the postural stabilizers. All too often, the positional postural response that a person takes on when issued a command to "sit up straight" lasts long after the directive was first issued.

Placing the body in a position does not ensure that the postural muscles will engage. As a result, the body can adapt to a superimposed image of what "good" posture should be, yet the muscles that work to maintain it often pull the body off-center, with one body mass chronically held either behind or in front of its center of gravity. A person either leans too far back or thrusts a part of the body forward. In these stances, the body loses its upward integrity in a series of locked or propped joints. From the side the body may take on a bowed shape, causing the ankles to become stiff from holding in an effort to shore up the leaning, arched structure.

Positional and off-center postures are incredibly common. They are evident in locked knees, forward head or "chin-poke," rounded shoulders, and a tucked or anteriorly tipped pelvis. Off-center postures lack dynamic balance because they always involve chronic muscular contractions that stiffen and bend the vertical axis. Like a bent tree unable to bow to the wind, stiffness blocks the fluidity of postural sway.

A person's posture frequently reflects the type of physical education (or lack of it) that the person received in school and at home. For example, many people have learned to pull their shoulders up and back, pinching the shoulder blades together in a posture that often fails to engage the postural muscles that anchor the shoulders on the back—such as the *lower trapezius muscle* (see Chapter 9). Notice how common it is for a person to pull the body into a compulsive stance to

A Creative Postural Exercise for Schoolchildren

An enterprising first-grade teacher asked her students to imagine they were plants wilting from lack of water, and all the children slumped. Then she went around with an imaginary watering can and slowly watered the group, and the children gradually moved into upright postures. The beauty of this teacher's exercise was that she gave the children an internal somatic experience of gradually increasing their postural tone. The children also learned about concepts of turgidity and fluid pressure by actually feeling these concepts within their bodies. Most importantly, she gave the youngsters a creative way to increase postural tone along a gradual continuum. Rather than snapping into a rigid, straight posture, the schoolchildren learned how to change postural tone gradually, moving through all the places between a slumped and an upright position.

correct what he thinks is wrong with his current posture. The correction usually replaces one positional posture with another. For instance, a person may have the habit of collapsing the chest, then amend it by habitually squeezing the shoulder blades to lift the thorax. The correction merely repositions the collapsed chest. Its sunken shape remains unchanged, and additional problems develop as a result of the muscles pinching the shoulders together. (In a more appropriate correction, this person would learn to straighten the upper and mid back with deep muscles along the spine, and to open the spaces between the ribs with deep breathing.)

Faulty postural habits develop early, often in schools. Children tend to slouch in uncomfortable school desks with curved seats that tuck the pelvis under and provide minimal back support. In this slumped posture, postural tone is low, but it jumps to high when the children are admonished to "straighten up." Since the increase in tone is quick and reactionary, it engages the large, extrinsic muscles that contract to yank the body up, leaving the subtler, sustained contractions that build postural support unrealized. Eventually, the child tires of sitting up straight and gradually slips back into a slump. In the end, all the child actually learned was a compensatory habit to make the posture look straight in an effort to please the teacher or parent, bypassing the intrinsic learning and awareness necessary for effective postural education.

Postural muscle training is almost nonexistent in our schools. In addition, we know that the less general education people have, the less they tend to exercise.[46] Unfortunately, today more people are experiencing repetitive stress injuries from abusive postures and holding patterns in the workplace. Perhaps our growing understanding of the problems that arise from unbalanced postures, lack of exercise, and ergonomic imbalances will seed the broader application of somatic patterning in our society as a system of preventive postural education.

An effective postural education that would be a valuable addition to all school curricula involves cognitive learning about postural muscles and experiential learning to actually learn to engage these muscles. Unfortunately, this type of training is currently limited to injury rehabilitation, although it can easily be undertaken by anyone interested in a healthy dose of preventive medicine. Since the exercises that develop postural muscles are mostly isometric, a person can also practice them during a daily routine—at school or work, in the car, while shopping, and even while watching television. More information about postural stabilization is found in Chapter 9.

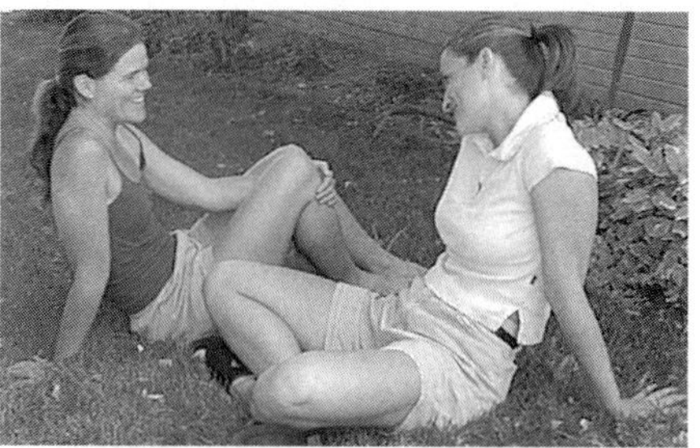

Figure 2.15a Propped up on locked elbows

Developmental Movement Gaps

Although early motor development is complex, and neurological damage can result in severe developmental disabilities and retarded growth, minor gaps in the process are quite common. Every person goes through some developmental stages that are strong and others that are weak. We all pass through roughly the same movement stages, yet each person's journey is unique. Gaps in the process are common and appear to the untrained eye as normal movement.

Fortunately, human beings are softwired and extremely adaptable, able to overcome developmental movement gaps with a multitude of clever compensations. Weaknesses in some stages are balanced by strengths in others. A healthy baby will find its own unique pathway to standing and walking despite many obstacles. Compensations for developmental movement weaknesses underlie the average person's movement signature, forming a personal and distinct style of posture and gait.

Gaps in the developmental movement sequence occur for many reasons. For example, some babies learn shortcuts to sitting and standing and keep repeating them. Or youngsters might favor using one limb or one side more than the other and develop asymmetrical patterns that twist the body and lead to mild lateral curvatures of the spine, such as the s-shaped curve of **scoliosis**.[47]

Premature Demands

Developmental movement specialist Bonnie Cohen speculates that many low back problems in adults are due to the bracing in musculature that occurs when babies are made to sit up before their muscles have developed enough tone to support them.[48] Another source of holding patterns

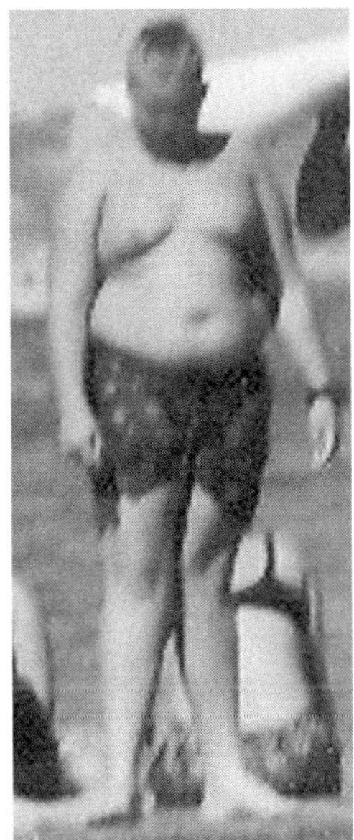
Figure 2.15b Locked knees

is when a young child's body is put under movement demands that he or she has neither the strength nor the coordination to do. For example, many parents stand their babies up before the baby's legs are ready to support weight. Likewise, walkers put babies on top of their little legs before the muscles can adequately support them. As a result, the babies reflexively lock their knees to brace for support. A baby may also be sat up too early, to which she adapts by **bracing** the lower back or **propping** on locked elbows (Figure 2.15a-c). **Hinging,** bending in the middle of the neck, indicates lack of support for the head (see Figure 9.20). Whenever a baby makes level changes on her own, she is developing the strength, coordination, and postural stability that underlie healthy movement patterns. Babies who are sat or stood up prematurely not only learn bracing and propping patterns, they might also miss important stages in motor development. They skip transitions from lying to sitting and standing, which take a baby through the normal developmental series that builds a neuromotor foundation for subsequent learning processes.

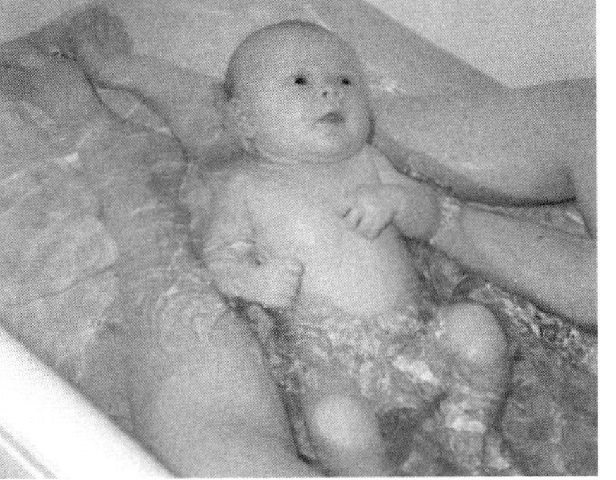
Figure 2.16 A baby negotiating trust (photo courtesy of D. Kolway).

As mentioned in Chapter 1, the nervous system actually requires movement for development. Movement is, literally, food for the brain. Human brain development follows a pyramid-shaped building process with a diverse array of early motor activities establishing a broad foundation. Nature supplies this opportunity by giving infants and children years of playtime to ensure normal development. This long period of sensorimotor development creates a sound neurological base for the narrower, more refined development of the cerebral cortex at the top of the pyramid.

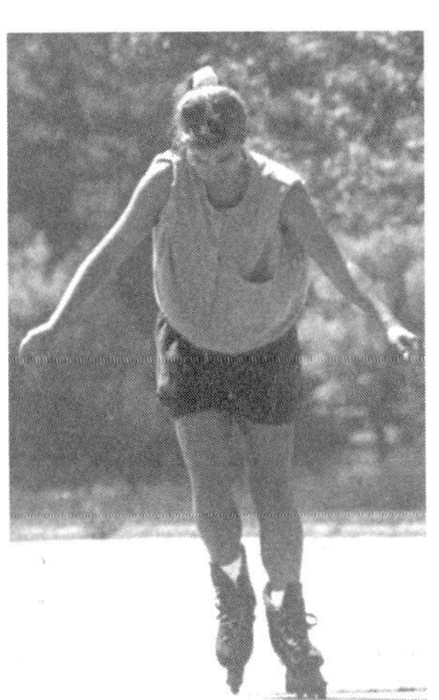
Figure 2.15c Braced shoulders

Unfortunately, extensive television and video viewing disturbs the sensorimotor foundation in babies and youngsters because it places premature demands on the cerebral cortex. Television calls visual centers of the cortex into action before the lower centers involving sensorimotor circuitry have been firmly established. Also, the barrage of external images limits the child's creativity, which grows out of imaginary play based on internally initiated imagery. Thus, television can interrupt crucial playtime during formative years and ingrain sedentary habits in a child at an early age.[49]

The worst types of holding patterns begin when highly inappropriate demands are placed upon a child. For instance, a child laborer is forced to brace both body and mind to compensate for the demands placed on undeveloped muscles, bones, and psyche. Also, physical and/or sexual abuse instills trauma in young bodies that resembles the physical injuries sustained in accidents, yet these injuries are far worse because they are intensified by emotional traumas.

Touch and Early Handling

Dr. Ashley Montagu, the author of a groundbreaking book on the importance of tactile interaction in human development, presents evidence that touch and physical contact are the most basic mammalian needs.[50] The manner in which an infant is touched influences that child's sensorimotor patterning. Movement disturbances resulting from touch deprivation are well documented—they include lethargy, poor coordination, and autistic rocking. Tactile deprivation has also been associated with low weight gain in infants, a reduction in growth hormones, and bone loss; also with schizoid disturbances in youth and adult behavior such as emotional shallowness, detachment, lack of identity, and indifferent social contact.

Infants are motivated to move by a desire to reach out and touch something or someone. Tactile senses develop long before birth and are extremely sophisticated at birth. The primary sensory channel of an infant is touch. All sense organs involve skin receptors of some sort. Skin is the largest organ of the nervous system, and touch feeds neurological development. An infant deprived of touch can lose the motivation to move and may suffer from separation anxiety. Initially, the newborn's body is merged with the mother's. If contact with the mother is terminated too early, or is insufficient to the infant's need for contact, the infant reacts with a stress response, which can result in deep physiological and psychological holding patterns.

The touch that babies receive shapes their budding musculoskeletal system. The quality of touch from early tactile experiences greatly influences overall tone. A baby learns to trust by the care with which he or she is handled (Figure 2.16). Compression from cuddling can increase the tone of a lethargic baby, a soothing touch can calm a stressed and spastic baby, and rocking helps a fussy baby relax. Conversely, an irritating or abrupt touch stresses infants because they have not yet developed the capacity to filter out noxious stimuli or defend against them.

Weak Push and Reach Patterns

As stated in Chapter 1, all babies go through a series of movement patterns during early motor development that include push and reach patterns. Push builds strength in the intrinsic muscles and creates an integrated connection among body parts. Push patterns also send compression through the joints, organizing a **line of force** along a kinematic chain.

People with weak push patterns tend to have collapsed, zig-zag postures, which cause the spine to hinge at the apex of the collapse, stressing the vertebral joints in that area. Weak push patterns also show up in low postural tone, patterns of locking the knees and elbows, a tendency to prop the torso up on the limbs for support, and a line of force that zig-zags through a collapsed or bent structure. When the spinal curves collapse, the force of a push dissipates in the hinged segments (Figure 2.17). People with collapsed postures tend to hike the shoulders while pushing, putting undue stress on the neck. They may even lock the knee or hyperextend the lower back or neck, subconsciously creating a fixed base to push against. The forces of a push put undue stress on the ligamentous cuff around a hyperextended or hiked joint, which can weaken that joint. Ideally, the force of a push travels through the center of joints, which are aligned and stabilized by the intrinsic support of postural muscle contractions.

Reach balances push. Reach extends the body, bringing length to the spine, whereas push compresses it. Reach develops tensional support in the tissues. The perceptual reach of a curious person literally lifts the head and lengthens the neck. Reach patterns also extend the limbs, organizing lines of tension and elongation throughout the body. Weak reach patterns show up in compressed, bulky, or tucked postures, or, when combined with weak push patterns, in collapsed postures. A child may have weak reach patterns because of overprotective parents who pampered him. Or a baby may have lacked stimulation and not been motivated to reach out and explore the environment. Or the child may simply be predisposed to push rather than reach patterns.

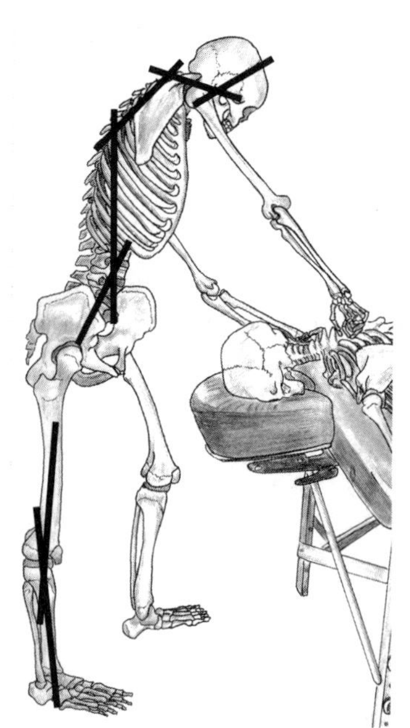

Figure 2.17 Notice how the line of force is bent by the locked knee, braced shoulder, and collapsed spine.

Although it is hard to know exactly why some developmental patterns are strong in some people and weak in others, it is never too late to change patterns established during early motor development. Since early motor processes shape everyone's somatic patterns, and we all have some patterns that are weak, people of all ages can benefit from developmental patterning. (See Chapter 7 for developmental movement exercises.)

HOLDING PATTERNS AND PAIN

Most people want to get rid of pain, yet pain gives us vital sensory feedback that is crucial to survival. Pain is nature's early warning sign that something in the body is injured, diseased, or in need of attention. It signals us to stop and take care of our bodies. Without it, we would risk injury or tissue damage much more frequently. This happens in rare disorders in which people are born without **nociceptors**—the sensory nerves that register pain. Because these unfortunate people do not experience physical pain, they cannot feel when they are injured, and as a result, often die at an early age from the premature accumulation of wear and tear on their bodies.

Holding patterns and pain patterns are intricately related because holding patterns often develop as a response to either physical or emotional pain. Ironically, holding patterns also *create* untold levels of pain. Holding patterns start as chronic contractions that initially develop to help us cope with pain, whether from an injury or psychic trauma. Eventually, chronic contractions create more pain than they originally developed to alleviate.

Physical and Emotional Pain

Pain is psychosomatic. It is both physical and emotional; one exacerbates the other. Physical pain can trigger emotional responses, leading to emotional pain, and vice versa. When distress is both physical and emotional, it is more difficult to localize the source of pain and process it. Pain can arise from the somatic nervous system (SNS) and muscle irritation or damage, from the autonomic nervous system (ANS) and organ dysfunction, or from the central nervous system (CNS) and imbalances in brain chemistry.

Pain from imbalances in the CNS—**centrally mediated pain**—occurs when the tissues are under stress for such a long time that physiological changes occur in the brain that alter brain chemistry and interfere with its ability to process pain. A person might feel exasperated after many tests to determine the source of pain only to be told its source is all in the head, which is partially true. But the problem is not psychological, it is neurological, caused by a processing dysfunction in the central nervous system. Also, the nerves have a certain level of plasticity: prolonged stress can lower the threshold at which nerve impulses occur, making nerve endings more excitable. Centrally mediated pain explains why a person might experience pain from an injury long after that injury has healed.

Another complicating factor is that chronic pain disturbs sleep patterns. A person needs to be asleep at least three hours for the brain to release certain chemicals that heal the body, yet a person suffering from chronic pain might never reach this level of sleep. Therefore, during waking hours this person can become hypersensitive to painful stimuli. Centrally mediated pain tends to have a systemic effect that ranges from a floating discomfort to generalized discomfort throughout the body. This type of elusive pain is difficult to source and often hard to cope with because physical and emotional distress compound each other. This condition is common in people with chronic pain syndromes, a topic that will be discussed shortly.

Nociceptors carry pain signals to the brain's cerebral cortex for rational processing and to the brain's limbic system for emotional processing. The degree of pain a person feels is determined by both cognitive and emotional abilities to process it, which depend on that person's history of sensory processing. A person in a chronic pain cycle often swings between having muscle spasms and having stress reactions. Unable to locate the source of pain, a person may start to ruminate about the possible causes and worry that something serious is wrong, such as having a fatal disease. Rumination can trigger a fight-or-flight response in the autonomic nervous system and create fear that compounds the physical pain.

How can you differentiate centrally mediated pain from localized skeletal muscle pain?

The Pain Cycle

Once the physical sensation of pain becomes entwined with an emotional response, apprehensive thoughts, fear, or panic can trigger defensive spasms and escalate the condition. In this case, one of two things can happen: the brain can respond to the strength, repetitiveness, and duration of the pain signal by sending messages to inhibit the pain and by releasing *endorphins*, substances that calm the emotional responses and thereby inhibit the perception of pain. (Many stories have been told of people who sustain severe injuries in war, torture, or accidents without experiencing pain because of the numbing effect of endorphins.) Or a person can spin into even more pain and become trapped in a chronic pain cycle.

Pain is particularly complex in situations of physical or sexual abuse. Emotional responses become coupled with the physical responses triggered from painful physical injuries sustained in the abuse. One magnifies the other. The body tightens into a defensive pattern because of the physical injury and the emotional injury as well. People with this type of history usually need to process their emotions before they are able to relax and process the physical pain, although emotional processing in itself can escalate the physical sensation of pain. This is particularly true for a person who has a tendency to deal with physical pain before emotional pain and leave "mental health" therapy to the "if all else fails" category.

Pain is easier to process when a person can relax. For this reason, a relaxation massage can have an analgesic effect, producing emotional responses that trigger the release of endorphins and reduce pain. On the other hand, a practitioner needs to be sensitive to variations from the norm. For example, relaxation may be difficult for people with a history of abuse or torture, or for others who have had extremely traumatic experiences, such as war veterans or victims of crime or severe accidents. The reason is that these people often have memories of trauma surface as they relax; therefore, they maintain a certain level of vigilance to manage their memories. An individual working with this type of pattern can learn to relax in increments and work with a psychotherapist to process and learn to manage the painful memories as they come up.

Pain-Avoidance Behaviors

Different people respond to pain in different ways. Some people are able to transcend it whereas others design their whole lifestyle around avoiding pain. Two primary pain-avoidance behaviors are *obsession* with the problem and *denial* of the problem. Each type of behavior requires a different approach in patterning. Generally speaking, people who become obsessed with pain need to learn desensitization skills, and people in denial need to learn to pay attention to pain signals. (*Anyone suffering from chronic pain should seek a thorough medical evaluation to determine the cause of the pain before using patterning to deal with it.*)

Examining Myths

Myth: A person should always rub the spot that hurts.

Rubbing painful area often feels soothing, particularly when we bump an elbow or skin a knee. Yet, when the pain is caused by inflammation, rubbing this area can make the problem worse. A person should avoid massaging inflamed tissues, which are usually hot to the touch, swollen, and may even be red. Also, to keep from irritating damaged tissues, massage should not be applied while the area is in an acute phase of healing during the first three days after the injury.

Wilson and Schneider, who have done extensive research on pain treatment modalities, describe four types of pain-avoidance behavior: hypervigilant, scattered, obsessive, and burned-out. The *hypervigilant type* focuses all her attention externally. All work and no play, she keeps busy, usually as a provider for others, to avoid feeling her body. This type of person often has a history of childhood abuse and alcoholic parents, and learned early patterns of bracing against the world. She is the easiest to treat if she can turn her attention toward herself rather than to others. Her vigilance can be transformed to diligence through self-care, and eventually she can learn to relax her diligence.

The *scattered type* has many ploys to get away from the pain, often going from one healthcare practitioner to another for treatment. This type of person is often emotionally unstable and has a poor sense of self. He is overwhelmed by chaos, having a life pattern that consists of moving from one crisis to the next. Wilson and Schneider speculate that this behavior could be a result of impaired function in the neurotransmitters involved in the processes of sensory perception and sleep, particularly the depletion of *serotonin*. When relaxing, the scattered person often feels a loss of boundaries, which elicits fear and triggers another cycle of chaos. Treatment strategies involve helping this person gain some control over his pain by learning to focus on one thing at a time.

The *obsessive type* is overfocused on getting rid of the pain. The world is viewed in polarities: what is good and what is bad, what gives relief and what hurts. With this overly simplistic viewpoint, the obsessive person becomes rigid and often rages at the therapist. She may also rub the painful area, further irritating it and increasing the pain. The tendency to worry excessively about the significance of any body sensation distorts perception. Increasing body awareness can actually increase the pain. This type of pain-avoidance personality is one of the most difficult to treat and often requires psychological intervention with a highly skilled therapist.

The fourth type of pain-avoidance behavior is the *burned-out type*. This is someone who is exhausted both from the pain and from treatments that have not worked. This type of person usually has had a bad accident and has not recovered. The burned-out individual tends to become passive and dependent, and has usually given up any hope of recovery. Treatment is difficult, often requiring psychiatric intervention and therapy for depression.[51]

Pain is a touchy subject for many people, particularly those who have developed pain-avoidance behaviors that perpetuate their pain and create the appearance that the pain is solely psychosomatic in its origins. With this in mind, it is helpful to understand typical pain-related behaviors and how coping mechanisms can actually escalate symptoms. People who can link behavior and pain levels can begin to modulate their behavior in ways that may reduce their pain. For instance, an overly sensitive person can learn to detach from body sensations, whereas the person in denial can learn how to become aware of painful sensations.

An important part of using somatic patterning in addressing chronic pain patterns is to assess the behaviors that develop around the pain. Some behaviors to consider are:

- the person's perception of pain;
- any pain-coping behaviors the person uses (drugs, alcohol, sleep, obsessive behavior, etc.);
- the person's resources to either reduce the pain or learn to live with it (relaxation techniques, hot baths, massage, positive attitudes, breaks in a busy schedule, etc.);
- the person's level of body awareness of the holding patterns caused by or creating the pain;
- the person's commitment to self-care and treatment;
- and the impact of mood or emotions on pain levels.

Mechanics of the Pain Cycle

Healthy muscles function in alternate cycles of contraction and relaxation, whereas muscles held in holding patterns are caught in chronic contraction. Chronically contracted muscles squeeze off the blood supply to the held tissues, like a pinched straw. Blocked circulation results in **ischemia**, a condition of localized tissue anemia, or lack of vitality, caused by restriction of the blood supply to the tissue. Waste products cannot move out, so toxins accumulate within the muscle and acidity builds up in the tissue. Deprived of oxygenated blood, tissues cannot metabolize normally. The waste products, in turn, stimulate sensory nerves within the muscle, sending pain signals back to the spinal cord. The pain signals trigger reflexes that send nerve impulses back to the muscle, producing a reflex spasm. Thus, a vicious cycle is established whereby the muscle perpetuates its own spasm.

As mentioned earlier, a person tends to move around muscle spasms, increasing asymmetrical movement patterns, which in turn leads to the development of more adaptive contractions, which builds

Links to Practical Applications

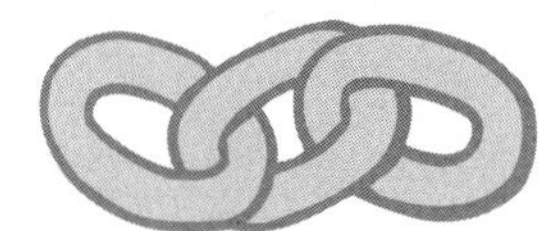

Using Ice or Heat for Chronic Musculoskeletal Pain

Ice promotes healing because it numbs the pain around an injured area. In the absence of pain, protective spasms relax and circulation increases, which, in the long run, allows the tissues to heal. The standard application for ice is 20 minutes on, 20 minutes off, and 20 minutes on again, a regimen that should be repeated on the injured area three times a day. Heat, in the same dose (20 on, 20 off, 20 on), can also promote healing by loosening tissues and helping to relax muscle spasms, particularly chronic spasms. Heat can also be applied before stretching to soften tissue. But heat should never be used on inflamed or swollen tissues because it will make them worse. In such cases, use ice to reduce swelling and inflammation.

deeper myofascial adhesions. The more asymmetry, the more uneven the pulls of the tendons on the bones, and the more misalignment and myofascial restrictions, leading to compression on nerve roots. This compression creates a new area of secondary pain, which is followed by new muscle spasms and a new holding pattern, and the cycle continues.

Each new area of pain stimulates more holding, and a compensatory or adaptive holding pattern develops. Because they tend to build on one another, they create layers of tension in the body's musculoskeletal system.

Tight and shortened myofascial tissues often compress and irritate nerves. A common example is "piriformis syndrome" caused by chronic spasms in the *piriformis muscle*. When in spasm, the piriformis muscle presses on and irritates the *sciatic nerve* (which runs directly under it), causing shooting pain in the buttocks and down the back of the leg (Figure 2.18). The piriformis muscle goes into spasm for a number of reasons, including a chronically turned out leg and toed-out gait, tucking the pelvis under, and reflexively shoring up instability in the sacroiliac joint on that side of the sacrum. The antidote for this syndrome is regular stretching of the area. More importantly, a person with this problem needs to inhibit contraction in the piriformis muscle to get it to stop firing, a process that can be done with inhibitory stretching (see "Stretching Techniques" in Chapter 8).

Chronic Pain Syndromes

Pain is considered chronic when it persists beyond three months or after an injury or illness has healed. As mentioned earlier, chronic pain is a huge medical problem. Although the precise origins of most chronic pain syndromes are generally unknown, most arise from disturbances in the musculoskeletal system, from nerve entrapment, and from chemical imbalances in the brain. Chronic pain sources are difficult to assess because pain often arises from distortions in how we perceive sensation.

There are several types of commonly found chronic pain syndromes, including myofascial pain syndrome, fibromyalgia, headache, and arthritic pain. The symptoms of many of these syndromes have dynamics similar to those of holding patterns. We will examine the ones that can be effectively treated with somatic patterning.

Myofascial Pain Syndrome and Fibromyalgia

Most chronic pain falls under the category of **myofascial pain syndrome (MFS).** Myofascial sources of pain are usually suspected when no skeletal or neurological causes can be found. This type of pain is characterized by generalized aching, localized trigger points, stiffness, and altered sleep patterns. Although the cause of MFS is debatable, it is associated with localized muscle pain and tenderness. MFS often develops after injuries and accidents, when muscles have been subjected to a momentary overload and are pulled or strained, then begin to show signs of trauma.

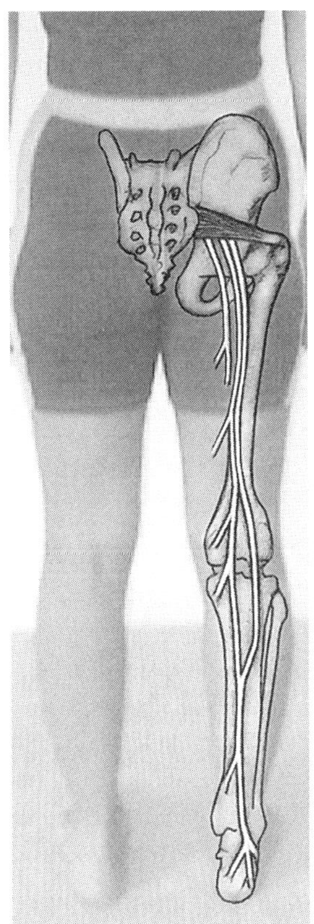

Figure 2.18 The piriformis muscle and the sciatic nerve

Fibromyalgia, which was initially called *fibrositis*, differs from myofascial pain in several ways. Its onset is insidious; it comes on slowly with no apparent reason. It also involves generalized but deep muscle aching spread throughout the body with multiple tender spots in the muscles. This widespread condition is defined by at least three months of chronic pain with local tender points in 11 of 18 prescribed spots in the muscles, tendons, and ligaments.[52] The tender points might also be trigger points, the difference being that trigger points refer pain. Because no evidence of tissue abnormalities or changes in the CNS have been found to identify its source, the etiology of fibromyalgia is unknown and the diagnosis controversial.

People who suffer with fibromyalgia tend to wake up tired and unrefreshed. The exhaustion may also affect the levels of *neurotransmitters* (see Chapter 13 for a discussion of neurotransmitters), biochemicals that act as neural messengers and increase the firing of the nociceptors that relay pain signals to the CNS. The overall effect lowers a person's pain threshold. *Neuropeptides*, a type of neurotransmitter produced by nociceptors, have been found in high levels in the *cerebrospinal fluid* of people with fibromyalgia, so neurotransmitter disturbances may also be the source of pain.[53] Because the production of neuropeptides is so closely related to emotions, an emotional upset in an individual suffering with chronic pain is thought to exacerbate fibromyalgia and other chronic pain syndromes.

Since muscle pain is the primary symptom of both myofascial pain syndrome and fibromyalgia, treatments that release chronic muscular contractions—trigger point therapy, myofascial release work, somatic patterning, exercise, and stretching—may effectively reduce the chronic pain of both, particularly when applied early in a treatment program. Treatments that restore movement to areas immobilized by chronic pain, such as stretching or strengthening, are helpful if they do not contribute to holding patterns and postural distortions that can increase pain. Cardiovascular conditioning helps increase circulation and flush out metabolic wastes that may contribute to nociceptive disturbances, and is particularly helpful in the treatment of chronic muscle pain, although exercise needs to be mild because rigorous exercise can increase pain. People with fibromyalgia need to combine rest with exercise to reduce the exhaustion already stored in the body and to prevent increasing fatigue levels. Postural imbalances and movement asymmetries common in chronic pain syndromes can be addressed with somatic patterning exercises.

Nerve Impingement, Irritation, or Damage

Peripheral nerve roots pass through compartments in surrounding tissues, passing under bones, between muscles, and across joints. Nerves are somewhat elastic so that they can stretch, bend, and slide through surrounding tissues to adjust to changes in position and shape of the body during movement (Figure 2.19). Myofascial and joint restrictions can impinge on the compartment through which peripheral nerves pass, causing a range of symptoms that come with nerve entrapment: tingling; a sensation of pins and needles; diffuse radiating pain; or sharp, electric, shooting pains. Nerve pain usually radiates far from the site of impingement so that an impingement in the neck can create symptoms in the shoulders, arms, and all the way down to the fingers. A restriction in *lumbar, sacral*, or *coccygeal nerves* can create symptoms in the legs and feet.

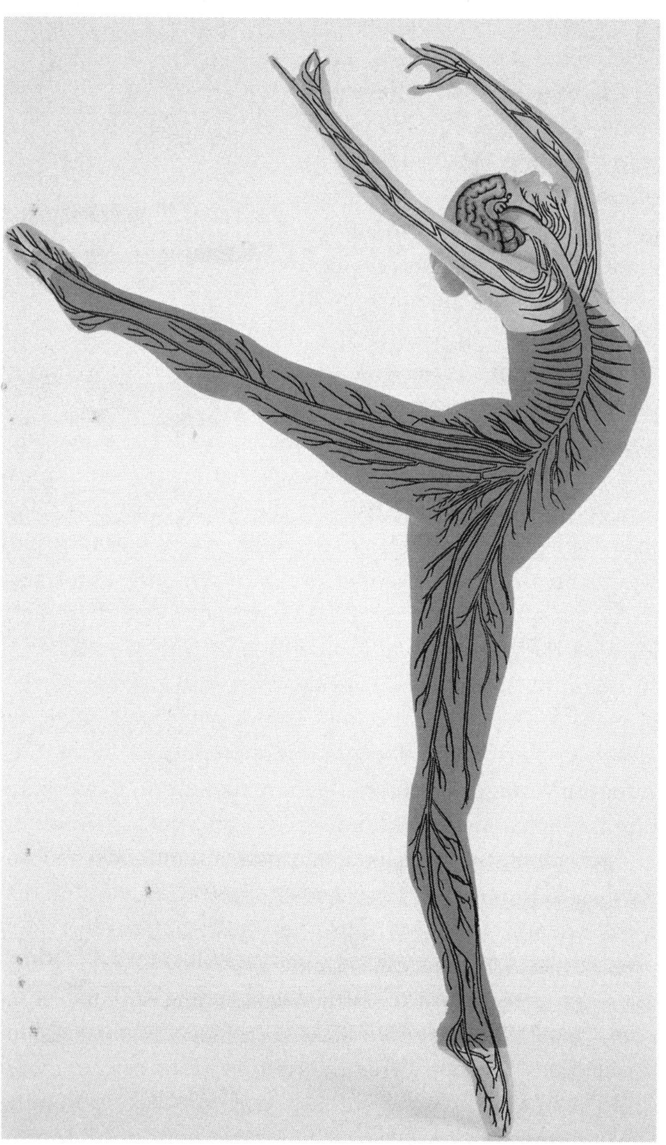

Figure 2.19 The nervous system bends and stretches with every movement. Therefore, the peripheral nerve roots are pliable and extensible; they can elongate to accommodate the pulls and tensile stresses of the moving body.

If injury rehabilitation involves nerve regeneration, spontaneous neural firings may continually bombard the spinal cord with pain signals. The spontaneous firing acts like a broken thermostat, keeping the furnace on even though the temperature is hot. Recovery may take months and even years because nerve tissue, being part of the most sophisticated tissue in the body, heals the slowest. It is important for an injured person to understand this process to avoid becoming discouraged with the amount of time nerves take to heal.

Trigger Points

Most people suffering from chronic pain have **trigger points** (TPs)—localized tender areas in muscles that develop as a result of chronic muscular contraction and adaptive shortening (Figure 2.20). Chronic contractions inevitably block circulation and accumulate metabolic waste products in muscles. This buildup underlies the formation of TPs in the areas of irritation. The TPs build nodules in muscles and are usually tender to the touch. Some TPs are latent, meaning that a person does not feel them until they are pressed. Other TPs hurt all the time and can cause referred pain to other areas of the body.

Whether TPs cause or are created by holding patterns is a cart-and-horse affair; which comes first is questionable. It has been hypothesized that TPs form where myofascial planes intersect and adhere. More important is the issue of how to effectively address these painful nodules, which involves recognition of the role that TPs play in the pain cycle. The pain from TPs can become overwhelming and trigger autonomic responses, which increase a person's overall stress level. This in turn increases chronic pain levels and can escalate the pain cycle.

Trigger point therapy—in which a practitioner applies at least seven seconds of direct, pointed pressure to a TP—is one of the most effective treatments for chronic myofascial pain. Faulty movement habits tend to create chronic muscular contractures that then develop TPs. Thus, the combination of TP therapy (generally known as *myotherapy* or *neuromuscular therapy*) and somatic patterning can be an effective treatment for releasing TPs and changing the muscle patterns that create them.

TPs often develop as compensation for other TPs, building in layers. Thus when one TP has been successfully eliminated, the pain may shift to a TP that developed

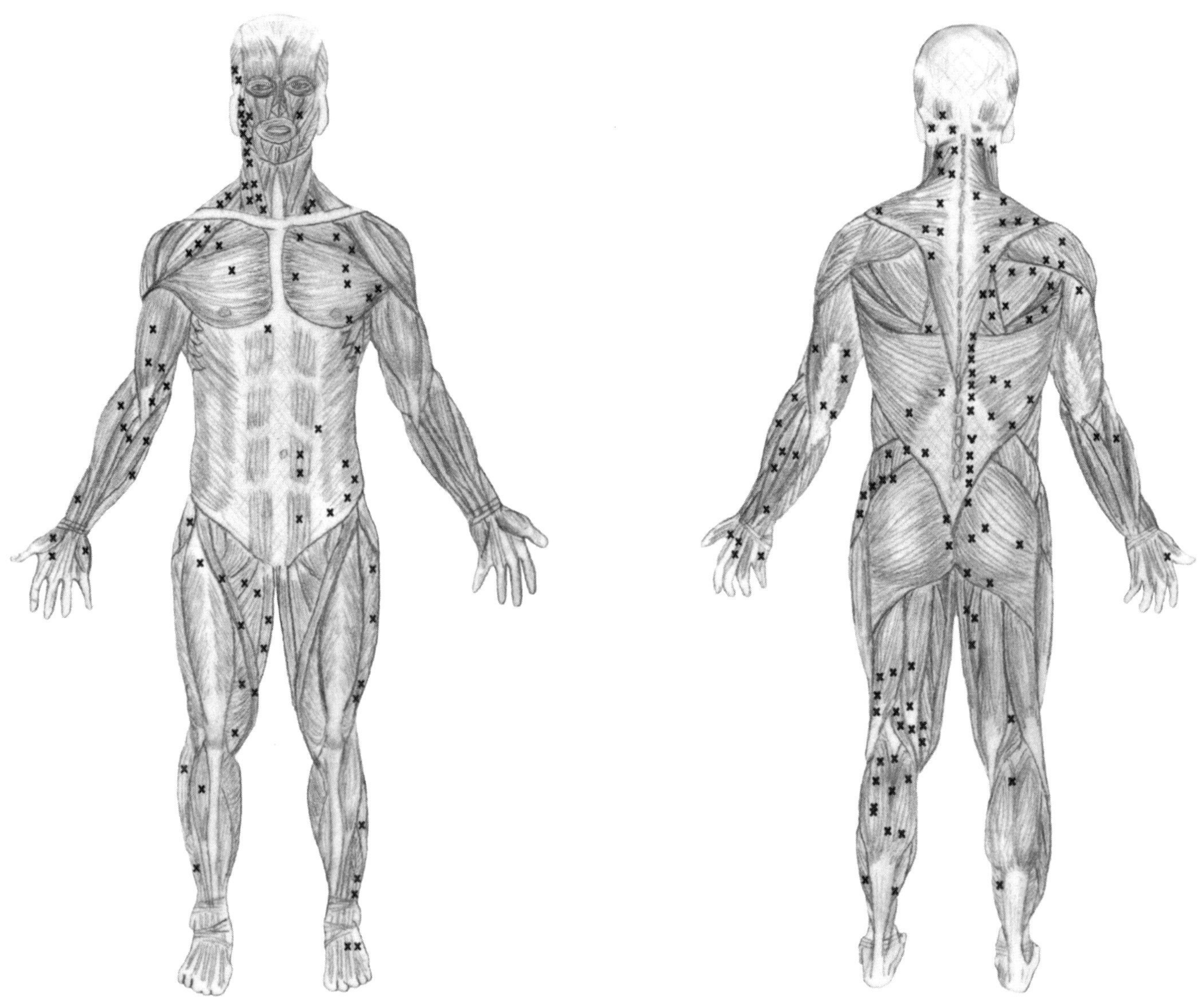

Figure 2.20 Although trigger points are bilateral, they are only represented on one side of the body in this general map of the common TPs.

earlier, so TP therapy often involves an unlayering process. Only when the initial, or primary, TP releases can the person recover without further treatment.[55] To uncover the initial TP, a person must first gain an increased sensory awareness of the area of pain or injury and be able to calm peripheral sites and tune into the source of the problem.

A person can release a TP by positioning his or her body on a golfball or using a theracane to put pressure on the point (Figure 2.21). To relax a muscle with a painful TP, a person can use an inhibitory stretch that turns off the neural signal triggering the contraction (see "Stretching Techniques" in Chapter 8).

Headaches

Many types of recurring headaches are considered chronic pain syndromes:

- *Migraine headaches* are marked by severe pain, nausea or vomiting, and intolerance to light, and generally have an unknown cause.
- *Tension headaches* stem from muscular tension in the jaw, neck, and upper back, which entraps nerves and restricts circulation.
- *Vascular headaches* arise from tension in the blood vessels of the head, which restricts circulation.
- *Cluster headaches* are occur in clusters, come and go within several hours, show up in severe, sharp painful patches on different parts of the skull, and have an unknown cause.

Headaches such as migraines and cluster headaches, whose source is unknown, may be caused by neurotransmitter disturbances that distort the transmission of pain signals to the brain. Treatment for them is difficult since the source is unknown. Many times these types of headaches are preceded by a series of warning signs such as nausea and tightening in the scalp. If people can learn to identify the signs by tracking body sensations that signal oncoming headaches, they can catch a headache at the onset and treat it before it escalates into a full-blown migraine or cluster headache.

Headaches caused by muscular tension can be reduced or eliminated by relaxing and stretching tight head and neck muscles, and by using trigger point therapy on chronically contracted muscles, especially at the base of the *occiput*. Also, most people are unaware of the range of movement they can make in the face, scalp, and neck muscles that can effectively reduce head pain. Stretching the *temporalis muscles* over the ears by pressing them straight up is very effective in alleviating headaches caused by jaw tension (Figure 2.22). Headaches caused by chronic contractions in extrinsic neck muscles can sometimes be alleviated by practicing micromovements at the base of the skull, which activates intrinsic muscular support while relaxing extrinsic muscular tension. (See Patterning Exercise #3 titled "Optical Support and Optical Righting" in Chapter 1 and Patterning Exercise #115 titled "Head Righting Reactions" in Chapter 11.)

Figure 2.21 Using a theracane to work trigger points in the shoulder

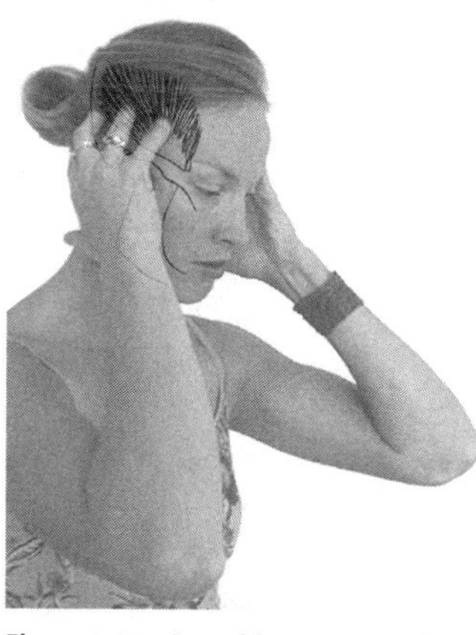

Figure 2.22 Stretching temporalis muscles to alleviate reduce jaw pain.

WORKING WITH PATTERNS THAT CAUSE PAIN

Many people tend to think of pain and holding patterns as things to get rid of, especially people who rely on surgery or drugs to solve their health problems. They also tend to view pain as something that invades the body from the outside, when in fact chronic pain often comes from internal processes. The orientation of people using Chinese medicine is exactly the opposite. Rather than being a negative force, they view illness as a cleansing. Likewise, we can view musculoskeletal pain and injury as the body's need for a mechanical tune-up, recognizing how pain caused by or aggravated by holding patterns tends to gradually dissipate when muscular balance and functional movement is restored.

Pain is nature's cry for help, it is a wake-up call from the tissues crying out for attention and pointing out that something needs to change. When using SP to address pain patterns, it is important for people who view pain as the enemy to reorient their attitude toward pain and view it as a healing beacon. Otherwise, people will reject the body part that hurts and be unable to work with sensations in it. Ironically, it is difficult to release a pattern if a person's energy is tied up in rejecting it.

Pain indicates an area in which something needs to be processed, where some sort of move-

Patterning Exercise #11: Engaging Intrinsic Neck Muscles to Relieve Tension

1. *Relaxing, then checking range:* Lie on your back in a comfortable position. Allow the weight of your head to sink into the underlying support. Turn your head side to side to check the range of movement in your neck (PE Fig. 11a-c).
2. Feel or visualize the place where your head meets your neck, an axis approximated behind the ears at the first cervical vertebra's *lateral processes* (PE Fig. 11d). If you were to draw a ring around your neck, it would be approximately in the center of this ring.
3. *Random micromovements:* Move this area with subtle, intrinsic, random motions. Allow the movement to be so subtle that it does not even feel as if you are actually moving. This is to relax the extrinsic muscles and to wake up the intrinsic muscles near the top cervical joints. To monitor the extrinsic muscles, place your hands on the back of your neck as you move to feel whether or not you are relaxing or working them. Then move your hands to the front of your neck to track tension or relaxation in the muscles there.
4. *Subtle nodding:* Subtly nod your head up and down in the "yes" gesture using the least amount of effort possible. Then subtly nod your head side to side in the "no" gesture, again using the least amount of effort possible. Imagine the movement greasing the small joints between your top cervical vertebra and skull.
5. *Sitting or standing:* Explore steps 1–3 while sitting or standing with your back against a wall. Lift the top of your head toward the ceiling to elongate your spine as you subtly rock your head.

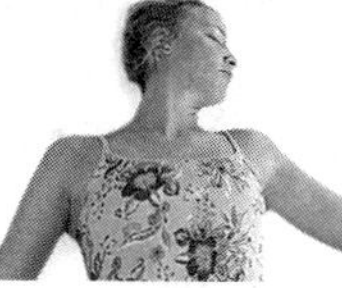

PE Fig. 11a

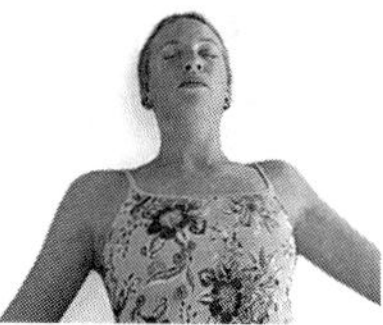

PE Fig. 11b

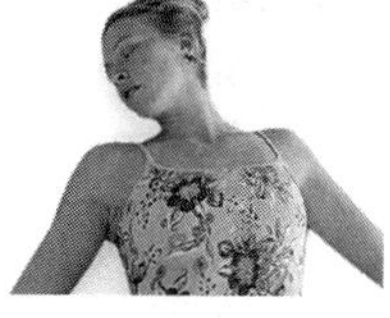

PE Fig. 11c

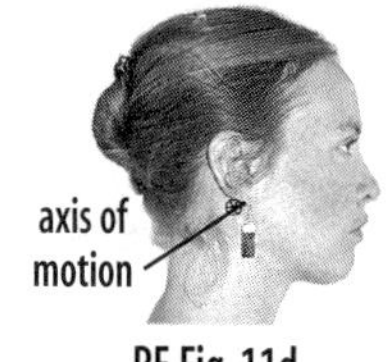

PE Fig. 11d

EMSPress.com

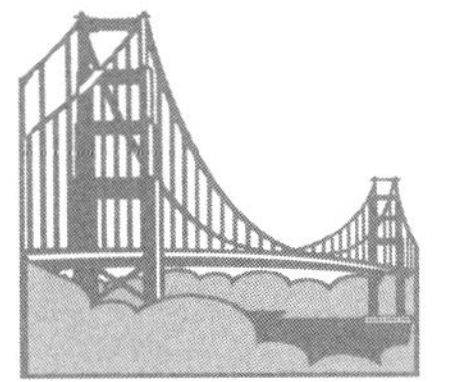

Helping Your Client to Relax Neck Tension with Micromovements

Have your client lie comfortably on her back and place your fingertips gently but firmly at the base of her skull where the head meets the neck. Explain how the extrinsic muscles can relax when the intrinsic muscles are working. Then have your client move with micromovements by subtly nodding her head, using the least amount of effort possible. As she moves, encourage her to use the intrinsic muscles by relaxing the extrinsic muscles that are under your fingertips. (When they relax, they will soften; if they are overworking, you will feel them pop out.) Give her feedback about whether her extrinsic muscles are relaxing or contracting.

Then have her turn her head very slowly right and left, again encouraging her to use the least amount of effort possible and allowing her head to be weighted as she moves it. Use your hands to guide her, gently nudging her to encourage her to let the weight of her head sink and her extrinsic neck muscles to relax.

ment needs to happen, from the energetic movement of healing awareness to the actual restoration of motion in chronically contracted tissues. If a person is able to feel chronic muscular holding around painful areas, then that person can also feel the potential circulation and movement that the holding inhibits. In this sense, a holding pattern is only one-half of a movement cycle: the areas that have become stuck point the way to where movement can be restored.

To begin processing pain, we must first feel the pained areas without becoming overwhelmed by the intense sensations in them. We have to find hope in the sensation because only by feeling pain can we eventually find relief from it. Therefore, getting the correct orientation toward pain is the first step toward healing. After this seemingly minor but crucially important step is taken, a person can then use sensorimotor education to identify and change the somatic patterns that cause pain and discomfort.

Current research by physiotherapist Michael Shacklock has shown that probably the most important element in determining whether or not chronic pain treatment will be successful is whether a patient is externally or internally focused. When asked what can relieve pain, an externally focused person will reply that the doctor, treatment, or drugs help them, all elements outside of that person's control. In contrast, the internally focused individual will reply that pain relief comes from stretching, getting enough rest, or maintaining good posture, all behavioral elements that are under that person's control.[56]

The Gate Theory of Pain

Exactly what causes pain remains elusive. In 1965, neuroscientists Ronald Melzack and Patrick Wall proposed the *counterirritant* theory, better known as the **gate theory of pain**.[57] According to their theory, two types of sensory neurons carry pain signals from the nociceptors (small peripheral nerve endings that respond to painful stimuli) to the brain. The larger, high-velocity *A fibers*, located in the skin and muscles, rapidly transmit sharp, sudden pain signals while the smaller, low-velocity *C fibers* transmit deeper, more constant pain signals. These signals enter the spinal cord where they are either relayed to the brain or blocked by a "closed gate" of inhibitory neurons (Figure 2.23). Both types of sensory nerves transmit pain signals. Yet when A fibers are stimulated, they flood the spinal cord with signals that cannot all pass through the gate. This causes the gate to close to incoming signals from the C fibers.

The A fibers can be stimulated by rubbing the skin, something people instinctively do to reduce pain, putting the gate theory into action. This may explain why touch can have a soothing, analgesic effect on painful areas, and why massaging one area of the body helps reduce the sensation of pain in another.

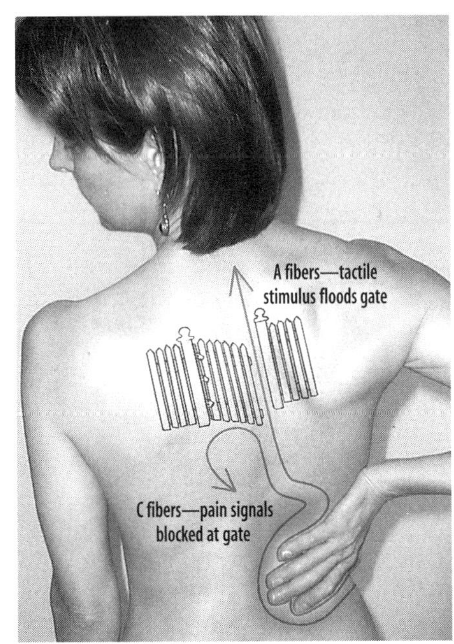

Figure 2.23 A schematic of the gate theory

Problems with Pain-Relieving Movement Habits

Many people who have chronic pain develop nervous habits, such as cracking the back, popping the jaw, or digging on muscles, in an attempt to relieve pain. The relief is usually only temporary because the nervous habit initially stimulates nociceptors in the skin or stretch receptors in the moving muscles or joints, creating new sensations that momentarily override pain sensations.

Moreover, habitually popping joints is likely to loosen and weaken already unstable joints, causing muscle spasms around them and tightening adjacent joints, while digging on painful tissues or habitually rubbing them overstimulates the tissue. This may actually increase the pain sensation and irritate already inflamed tissues. Plus, halfhearted adjust-

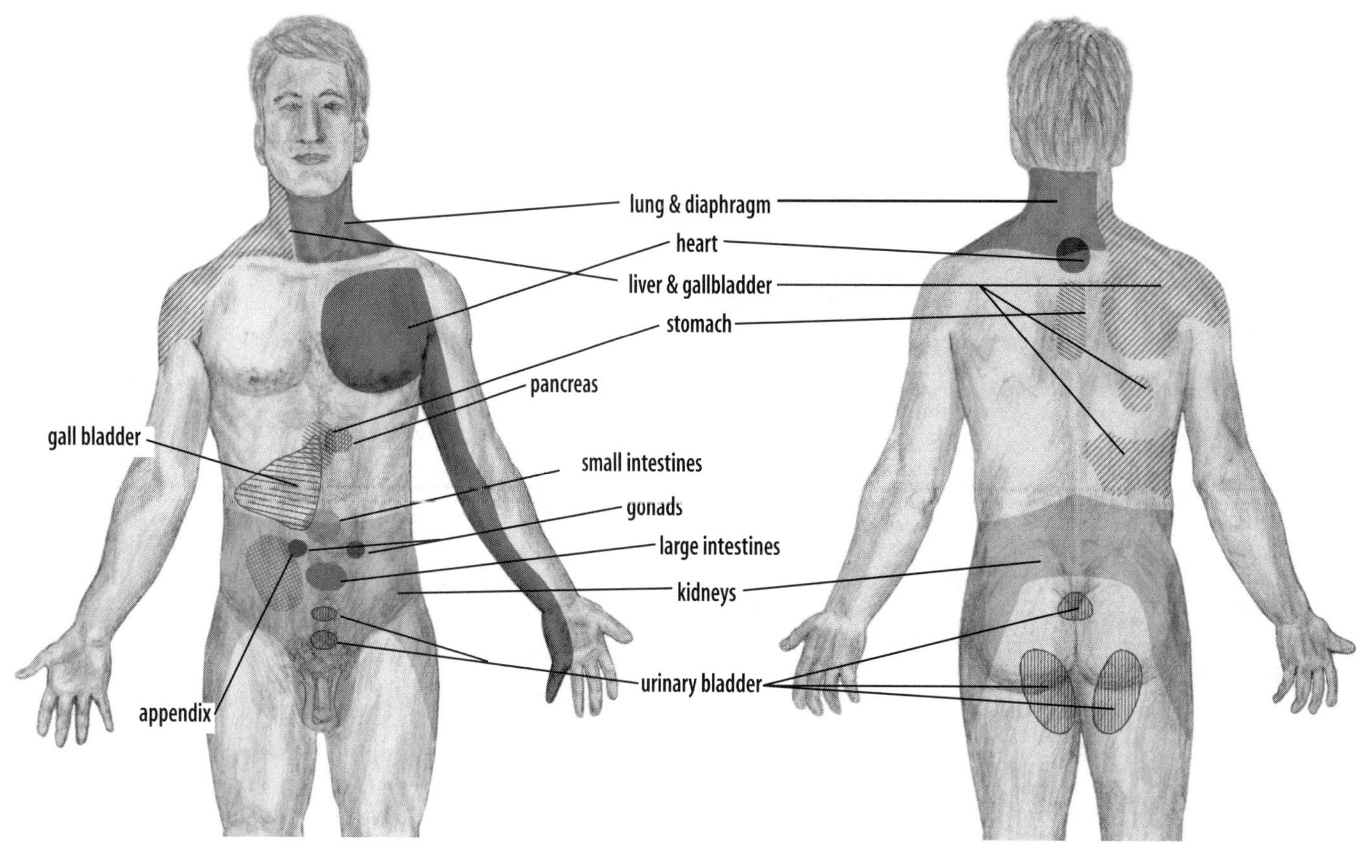

Figure 2.24 Organ pain referral

ments to reposition painful areas actually strengthen the neuromuscular pathways for the faulty movement habits that create pain in the first place.

An important step in changing chronic pain patterns is to learn to inhibit unconscious, reflexive habits used to temporarily relieve pain. Once people become aware of how the habitual adjustments actually increase pain, they can learn to inhibit these faulty actions.

Assessing Pain

Regardless of its psychosomatic nature, pain is a very physical problem. As discussed previously, it occurs when nociceptors become irritated or overstimulated. This can be caused by physical trauma, chronic muscular contraction, faulty posture, the stress of faulty movements, or by disease. Pain is exacerbated by its duration, by the level of nervous tension a person carries, by negative attitudes, by stress, noise, and pollution, by toxic diets, and by temperament. To make an accurate assessment of the source of pain, all these factors must be considered.

There are several guidelines for assessing physical pain. Pain originates in two main areas: the viscera (organs) and the somatic system (muscles and joints). The deep, aching, constant sensations of visceral pain may create referred somatic pain in the skin, muscles, fascias, or joints. Because organs have fewer nociceptors than the muscles and joints in the somatic system, visceral pain may indicate a serious organ dysfunction, damage, or dis-

Patterning Exercise #12: Assessing Chronic Pain

Keep track of the following information about your pain during a treatment program to give yourself feedback about the effectiveness of the program. Also, use this feedback to figure out what reduces chronic pain. Keep a daily log of answers to the following questions:

1. *Scale.* On a scale of 1 to 10, what is your level of pain?
2. *Body location.* Where is your pain? Is it localized in one area? Does it refer to another area? Does it radiate out from a central location?
3. *Time duration.* How long have you had the pain? Is your pain intermittent, or is it a sustained sensation? Do you feel it all day, part of the day, or while you sleep?
4. *Quality of sensation.* Does your pain burn, itch, ache, or feel like pins and needles?
5. *Onset.* When did you first feel pain? What were the precipitating factors (an accident, a movement, an emotional response, etc.)? What activities make it better? What makes it worse? Do certain activities or postures (sitting, standing, lying) increase or decrease it?

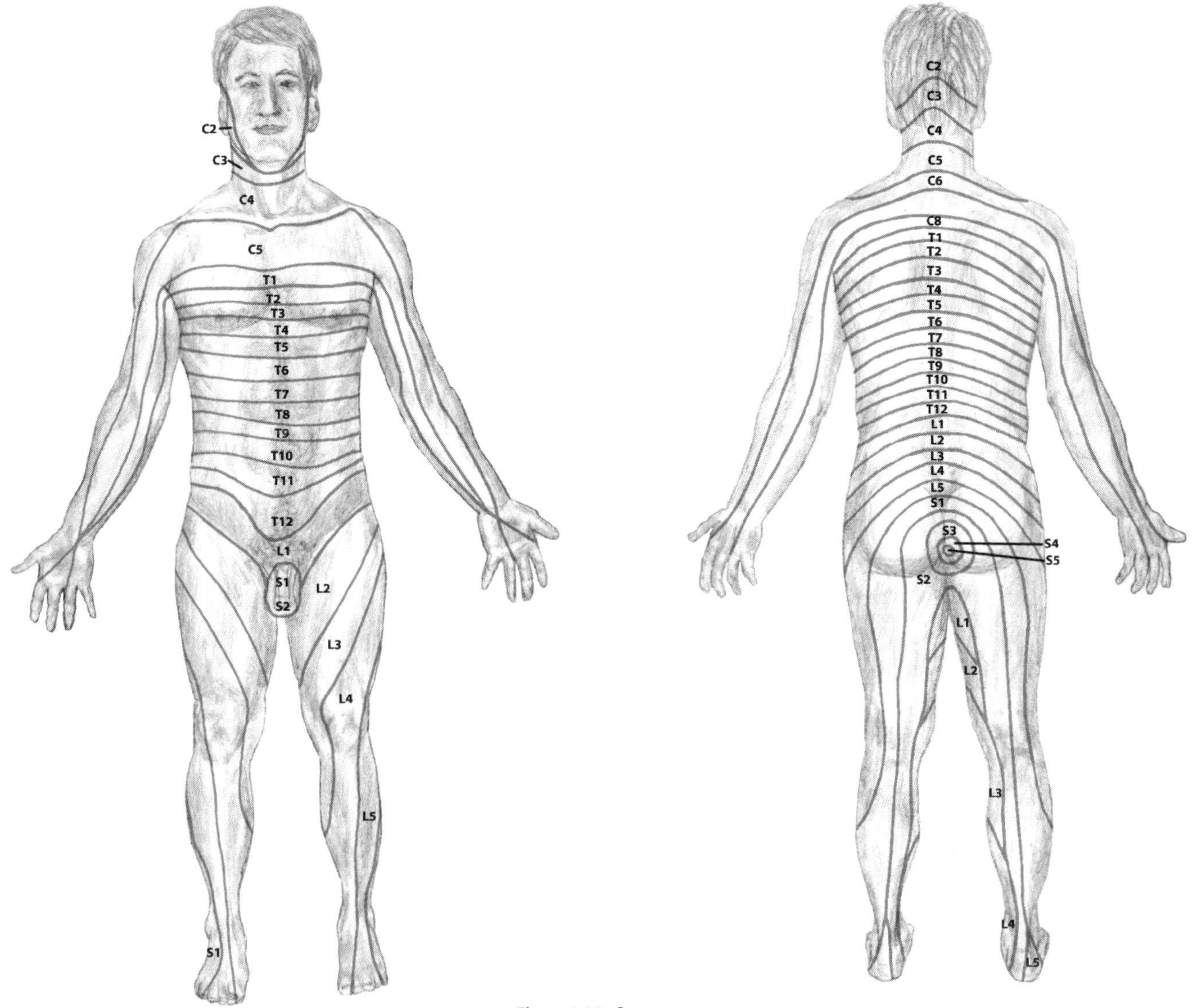

Figure 2.25 Dermatomes

ease. Organ or visceral pain may be more difficult to feel because the organs function below a level of conscious awareness. Because organ pain tends to refer, it can sneak up on a person, starting as a dim ache somewhere in the trunk, hips, or arms (Figure 2.24).

The musculoskeletal system has more sensory nerves and nociceptors than the organs; therefore, somatic pain caused by strained or damaged muscles, tendons, and joints is easily felt. Somatic pain is probably the most common source of minor or nagging aches and is usually not life threatening. The musculoskeletal system can undergo an enormous amount of abuse, including a long period of misuse, before it breaks down, although somatic pain increases as the damage becomes more serious.

The rich supply of sensory nerves to the skin makes it the largest tactile receptor in the body. Specific areas of the skin are innervated by a single spinal nerve, creating a topical segmented map on the skin called **dermatomes** (Figure 2.25). Although the dermatomes seem clearly delineated, overlap occurs between the nerve supply in adjacent areas. Still, the approximate location of pain coming from lesions in the spinal cord or nerves can be approximated through the dermatomes.

A variety of types of pain sensations can provide clues about where the pain might be coming from. Some general guidelines for assessing pain follow. *They are not given to diagnose a specific problem* but to provide general assessment guidelines and to alert the reader to conditions that may require medical evaluation.

1. Pain caused by muscles tends to be deep and aching in a general area.
2. Pain that occurs during active movement but subsides during inactivity is usually generated by strained or pulled contractile tissues, such as muscles and/or tendons.
3. Pain that occurs during passive movement is usually generated by non-contractile tissues, such as joint structures, ligaments, cartilage, or bursa.
4. Pain caused by spinal facet joint damage generally

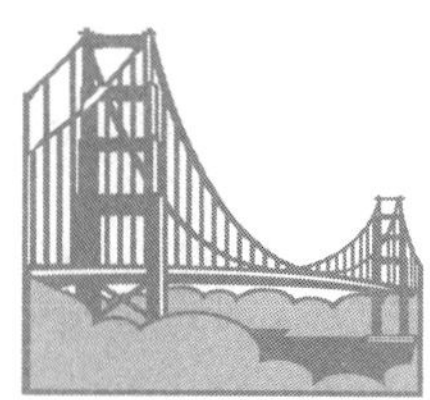

Bridge to Practice

Facilitating the Release of Painful Patterns

When working with clients whose pain signals overwhelm other body sensations, address their pain first. Collect information about your client's response to the pain by asking questions about the history of the pain and his attitude toward it. If your client has a history of letting the healthcare professional direct the work, it is particularly important to empower him to take charge of the session. Do this by asking him how he wants to work with his pain and mutually designing an appropriate SP program. (See Chapter 5 on "The Patterning Process.")

Explain the nature of opening pain (see "Opening Pain" on p. 68) during the release of holding patterns. Encourage him to breathe in or around painful areas, and through the entire body as well. When people release painful patterns, they often tighten and brace the body as new sensations arise. If this occurs, it is an opportunity to teach your client how not to brace around new sensations.

If a pattern is painful to release, proceed slowly. Small, manageable releases are more easily integrated than large, dramatic releases. Encourage your client to take small steps toward gradually releasing the chronic muscle tension by lightly contracting the tight muscles, then releasing it, then alternating between the two until he feels confident he can control the rate of release. (See Patterning Exercise #13.)

Encourage your client to feel his whole body rather than just focusing on a painful area. If need be, help him to consciously disassociate from overwhelming body pain by suggesting that he daydream about a particularly relaxing memory or imagine a fantasy environment that will induce deep relaxation.

Lastly, many people hold their breath or to breathe heavily when they feel pain. If breathing becomes work, suggest that your client stop trying to breathe and "let his body breathe itself." Also suggest that he sense or imagine easy breathing circulating oxygen throughout the painful areas. (See Patterning Exercise #34 on "Anatomical Imagery for Internal Respiration.")

feels pointed, like a nail, and strong and piercing (it can keep a person awake at night).

5. Unrelenting, constant bilateral (on both sides of the body) pain is very serious. It usually indicates a a damaged, prolapsed disc in the spine and requires medical attention.
6. Pain caused by nerve irritation may be sharp, stabbing, searing, burning, or itching. Compressed or pinched nerves radiate pain. When the body moves into a position that puts pressure on the nerves, pain shoot out at lightning speed along the nerve pathway. Nerve pain affects the tissues that a nerve innervates. The farther it radiates from the spine, the more serious the problem. A sign of healing is when the pain centralizes, that is, when peripheral pain gradually diminishes toward the spine.
7. Organ dysfunction can cause sharp, diffuse, and radiates over a large area. If all other causes of pain have been ruled out, the organs may be the cause and should be examined.

Unrelenting pain is constant, it never ceases. One indicator of unrelenting pain is discomfort so severe that it prevents sleep. When clients claim to have constant pain, it is helpful to ask if their discomfort interrupts sleep.

The more information a person can gather about chronic pain, the better equipped he or she will be to deal with it. Also, the information can be invaluable in helping a physician make an assessment about the cause of the pain. *It is important to realize that interventions done prior to an accurate assessment can mask the true cause of pain and may result in further damage and suffering.* Once the source of the pain has been identified, whether an illness, psychological problem, or physical injury, patterning can be an effective treatment or adjunct to other forms of treatment.

Patterning Exercise #13: Working with Holding Patterns

1. *Feeling the overall holding pattern:* You cannot release something you can't feel, therefore begin by sensing the overall shape and tension of your holding pattern. If you have trouble feeling it, tighten into your pattern a little bit. Sense the quality of tension in holding, feeling which areas you chronically tighten, what new sensation this creates, and how it affects the rest of your body.
2. *Identifying the purpose of the pattern:* Once you can sense the overall shape and tension of a holding pattern, sense the purpose of the pattern. If you were an performer in a play, what role would the holding pattern be playing? What function does it serve?
3. *Using awareness to release the pattern:* Just an awareness of a pattern can start to release it. Once you clearly feel your holding pattern, imagine or feel it slowly dissolving. Avoid making and muscular efforts to change it.
4. *Taking conscious control with exaggeration:* Sometimes the only way out is through. If you have trouble releasing your pattern, exaggerate it by tightening into it. Hold the exaggeration, sensing the energy and effort it takes to hold it. Then release the holding a little bit to free up some energy. Do this several times, exaggerating your pattern a little bit less each time, releasing it a little bit more each time. This contrast will deepen your awareness of the holding pattern plus teach you how to come out of it. (See the "Accordion Practice" in Chapter 15.)
5. *Release the holding while actively moving:* Explore micromovements, making the tiniest, most imperceptible movements you can. Move slowly enough to feel the release of chronic contractions and activation of more effective muscles. Also, as you move, breathe easily and sense your weight sinking into the ground as you exhale.

EMSPress.com

Building Healthy Patterns before Releasing Painful Ones

Janet had chronic pain in her pelvis, a weak pelvic floor, and difficulties with prolapsed organs. She feared that if she relaxed the tension she held in her pelvis, her reproductive organs would drop out the bottom. Before Janet could release these tensions, she first had to understand what purpose this tension served, which was to hold her organs up. The next step involved building tone in the pelvic floor muscles rather than locking peripheral muscles around the hips. Janet did this by slowly contracting and relaxing her pelvic muscles while lying on her back, trusting that her organs would not fall out in this position.

Janet toned her pelvic floor with kegal exercises and was able to gradually let go of tension in her extrinsic hip muscles. As she released, she felt anxiety and was able to recognize it as an "opening" fear that accompanied muscular relaxation. The fear actually became her cue that her pelvis was releasing tension and that she was beginning to trust her body. Janet practiced contracting and releasing her pelvic floor in small, manageable movements while lying down. With the new muscular control and the improved posture that Janet had developed, she felt secure enough to trust the support of her pelvic floor while standing. Her fear of having her organs drop out gradually diminished as her confidence increased.

Emotions and Thoughts that Restrict Motion

A lot of people feel overwhelming emotions when struggling with chronic pain. When emotions surface in a person used to repressing them, the tendency is to inhibit the flow of emotional response by contracting around uncomfortable or deep emotions. Emotions can be processed in the body through subtle movement, by simply giving their sensations some space and attention. If deep or overwhelming feelings restrict motion and trigger a freezing response, we need to give ourselves permission to move. To do this, we can ask ourselves, "How does this feeling want to move through my body?" For instance, people tend to choke back tears with tension in the neck and throat. An alternative would be to breathe gently into the neck, allowing the feelings and painful under the tears to sequence through breath, subtle movement, sound, or words.

Although the expression of emotions may seem negative to a person, it can be a healthy process if it helps resolve emotional issue related to pain patterns. Conversely, it is possible for feigned emotional expression to become habitual and perpetuate pain without resolving emotional issues. For example, a person might repeatedly express upset and anger with regular hostile outbursts that produce stress and elevate blood pressure yet fails to resolve the anger. For the sake of mental and physical health, it would be helpful for this person to inhibit the emotional response and examine the thought patterns that lead to the habitual outbursts. Then the person could work to transform negative, hostile thoughts patterns into positive thoughts that manifest through healthy responses and productive behaviors.

Habitual emotional responses tend to lack depth. For instance, a child becomes used to throwing a tantrum and crying to control his caretakers although the tears are shallow and lack real feeling. Likewise, emotional expression can be forced. Some people believe they need to express strong emotions like anger with screaming or punching. This can create more problems than it solves because fast or strong movements like kicking can actually raise sympathetic tone and spin a person into a tense state of high arousal. Such movements can also cause muscle spasms and tissue damage. For example, in the 1960s and 1970s "primal scream" was a popular therapy in which many participants actually damaged their vocal cords. Although expressive movement can release emotions that underlie holding patterns, the subtler the movement, the more intrinsic the release. Also, a subtler expression is more likely to release emotions in a healthy, safe manner.

Secondary Gain from Pain Patterns

A person with a chronic pain syndrome usually develops new behaviors to cope with the pain. These behaviors often have a secondary benefit, or **secondary gain**, which, surprisingly, can be either positive or negative. The psychological profile of patients diagnosed with chronic pain syndromes may help explain the nature of a secondary gain. For example, a chronic pain called reflexive sympathetic dystrophy (RSD) often develops in people who are extremely active and often in those involved in several sports at once. RSD typically begins with a minor injury that results in throbbing pain. Instead of dissipating, the pain signal grows louder, and eventually the pained tissues become swollen and disabling. Psychologists speculate that the secondary gain individuals with this profile may receive from RSD is being able to

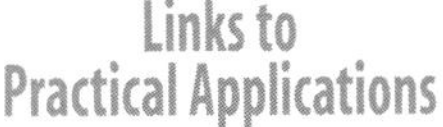

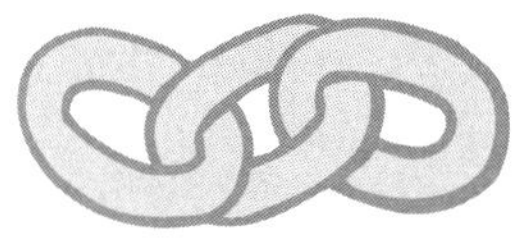

Assessing the Gain from Pain

What benefits, or secondary gains, do you get from being in pain? Although this may seem like an absurd question, consider the secondary benefits gained from sympathy, time off from work, or cash from an insurance settlement. Sometimes people banking on an insurance settlement from an injury or car accident, for example, may have trouble healing because once healed, they might not have evidence to present in court. Such secondary gain might not even be a conscious thought for the person, but the body can respond to the unconscious assessment of this gain.

Once you identify the secondary benefits of being in pain, you can figure out how to get the benefit without suffering the pain. For example, an overactive person can learn to reduce activities and rest without having to be injured or ill to do so, or a person can receive emotional support for a chronic pain syndrome without having to feel victimized.

decrease their activities and get plenty of rest with less guilt than they would experience without chronic pain.

The greatest benefit we receive from pain is that it forces us to become aware of our bodies. Pain leads many people into diverse forms of somatic education and/or therapy. Many people find somatic patterning after an injury or illness and begin to take better care of their bodies. Via this educational process, they often learn how to move more efficiently than they did before the injury and marvel that they not only reduce their pain, but come out of the experience better than they went into it. The rehabilitative benefits of somatic patterning can be far greater than expected. Holding patterns not only release, but the improvement in body awareness and movement efficiency leads to better mental health, more energy and body esteem, and an overall greater sense of well-being.

How can you tell the difference between pain from releasing and pain from holding?

The Unlayering Process and Opening Pain

Open a rusty door after a long period of immobility and there will be friction at the hinge. The same is true of the body. Release a chronic contraction to get an immobile area moving again and there will be new sensation, usually an **opening pain** emanating from tissues that are releasing tension and experiencing renewed circulation and sensation. To understand the nature of opening pain, imagine what would happen if a heavy object fell on a person's foot. Initially there is pain, but as circulation decreases the foot becomes numb. Then when the heavy object is lifted, fluids and sensation return to the tissues and the foot starts to throb. A person may even feel more pain when walking because movement stretches taut, fibrotic tissues.

Releasing the layers of compensatory contractions that build up over time around a holding pattern can trigger a journey back through a storage vault of old muscular tensions. As layers of pain unravel and resolve, obscure memories of long-forgotten injuries tend to resurface. It is important to discriminate between tension pain and releasing pain so a person does not tighten up when an opening pain surfaces. The sensation of opening pain can be viewed positively, as an indication that healing is taking place. But if misinterpreted negatively, the person may subconsciously or consciously contract around the opening and create another layer of holding. If healing is to occur, it is vital that circulation be restored without a person going into a new defensive contraction against the opening pain.

Most people can discriminate between opening pain and pain from chronic contractions if they understand the process and dynamics involved in releasing holding patterns. In general, the sensations caused by opening pain continue to change and eventually dissipate, whereas the sensations of pain from a holding pattern remain the same and often increase over time. For example, when the chronic contractions guarding neck and shoulder pain release and the shoulder muscles relax, the initial pain may subside, but new discomfort may arise because the arms are now hanging instead of being held up. Their weight now pulls on and stretches taut tissues, creating new pain. It takes a certain amount of time for the tissues to fully stretch to accommodate the weight of the arms, and until then the pull from the arms will be uncomfortable.

Links to Practical Applications

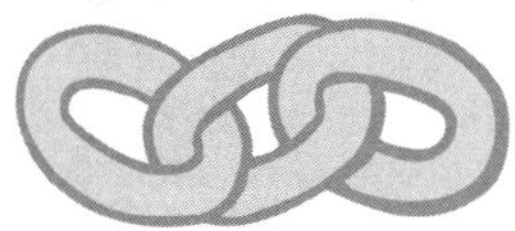

What Purpose Does the Holding Pattern Serve?

All holding patterns develop to serve a particular function, often to prevent or cope with pain or discomfort. This pain can be physical or emotional. A pattern will usually not release until the reason it developed is uncovered and addressed. If you have a stubborn pattern you want to release, first ask yourself what purpose the pattern initially served? Can that purpose now be served by less stressful means? If the pattern developed for protection, ask yourself if the danger still exists. If it is not a defensive pattern, it may release with awareness alone. If it is, can you come up with a more effective defense response that does not involve chronic muscular tension?

Dealing with Overwhelming Pain

When physical pain feels overwhelming, a hypersensitive person can learn to detach from it by thinking of it as sensation. This is important because sometimes a person's thought processes exaggerate how severe the situation actually is. For example, one client had a common pain pattern in the arm caused by a tight *pectoralis minor muscle* pinching the nerves of the *brachial plexus* in his shoulder. Instead, his was a common body problem that can be easily remedied with stretching, deep tissue massage, and postural corrections. (See Chapter 9 for more information on scapular stabilization and stretching for the pectoralis muscles.) However, not knowing the cause of his pain, he continually worried that he might need to have his arm surgically repaired.

Once he understood how minor his problem was and what caused it, he learned to disassociate from the pain to cope with it, to stretch his arm to relieve the pain, and to take his shoulder through its range of motion to reduce the restrictions that caused it. This meant staying conscious of his attitudes toward pain, being aware of his postural habits that chronically contracted the muscle, doing thorough stretches daily, and making postural adjustments each time he felt the area tightening.

Eventually, this client not only relieved his shoulder and arm pain, but he began improving his overall health by increasing his physical activity. With the combination of his new awareness, his stretching routines, and his newly found exercise regimen, he actually began to enjoy the benefits of his budding somatic awareness.

Patterning Exercise #14: Inhibiting a Holding Pattern Where It Starts

Every holding pattern has a point of initiation, a place where the neuromuscular chain of tension begins. This is akin to the seed of a holding pattern. By sensing where the pattern begins, you begin to regain control over it.

1. Sense your entire body, then tune into your holding pattern. See if you can sense the center of the pattern. Where does it initiate in your body? What muscles contract to maintain it?
2. Once you are able to locate the place where you feel it begins, tighten that area even more. This will help you feel more clearly exactly how the pattern starts. Also, by actively tightening into your holding pattern, you take conscious control over the pattern. Contract and relax the pattern several times.
3. Once able to control how your pattern begins, relax and gently breathe into that area. Visualize your breath melting the area. Then broaden your focus and relax the surrounding tissues. If you are unable to relax, sense the pattern as deeply as you can with a healing intention.

EMSPress.com

As discussed earlier, the initial pain of an injury or holding pattern becomes buried under many layers of adaptive, compensatory patterns. Therefore, it is helpful to determine exactly where in the body the pain started. To do this, a person needs to become quiet and sense the compensatory patterns until awareness can drop under them to the original pain center. This is a gradual process in which a person first learns to relax, and then to track subtle pain sensations in a slow, systematic manner. During this process, awareness alone serves as the healing agent, helping a person drop under the chaos of compensatory patterns, allowing them to slowly release in an unlayering process.

Accurately assessing the cause of pain is a crucial step toward effectively alleviating it. Once the source is understood, there are some basic guidelines for dealing with pain. A general rule of thumb in dealing with painful symptoms is to *never mobilize a symptom*. It is more important to stabilize a place that hurts, particularly if there has been a recent injury. Some general patterning strategies for working with pain follow:

1. *If pain is caused by injury*: After an injury, damaged tissues need at least three days to begin healing. Avoid stretching tight muscles immediately after an injury and allow the protective contractions to run their course. Wait at least three days after an injury before getting joint manipulation or massage because mobilization or deep tissue massage may irritate and re-injure already damaged tissues. During this time, usually no amount of bodywork or manipulation will take away the pain and may even make it worse. The tissues need to begin healing first.
2. *If pain is caused by inhibited postural muscles and unstable joints*: Explore micromovements. This will engage the deeper postural muscles and release contractions in superficial muscles. Also, learn stabilization exercises (see Chapter 9). This involves relaxing the large, extrinsic muscles, then isolating and contracting the postural stabilizers.
3. *If pain is caused by nerve irritation*: Breathe into the painful area to improve cellular respiration in symptomatic tissues. Stretch tight muscles that may be irritating nerves. If unstable joints cause the nerve irritation, learn stabilization exercises for that area. If rigid, immobile spinal joints cause the pain, go to a specialist (chiropractor, physical therapist, or osteopath) for spinal manipulation, then stretch the muscles around the area and practice gentle range of motion exercises to keep the joints mobilized. (See "Peripheral Nerves and Stretching" in Chapter 8.)
4. *If pain is caused by muscle spasms*: Put the spasmed muscle on a slow stretch. To increase the stretch, first contract the muscle, then relax it, then stretch it again. The contraction will stimulate the stretch reflex

Patterning Exercise #15: Shifting the Focus from Pain to Progress

Often pain creates a louder and more noticeable signal than our therapeutic achievements. Although we need to pay attention to pain, becoming overly focused on it can actually increase the pain. Being overly focused on pain can also drown out an awareness of your progress toward pain reduction, healing, and growth. To counter this tendency, keep track of your progress with the following exercise:

1. Keep a daily log of the degree of pain you feel (on a scale of 1 to 10), the location of the pain, and the type of pain.
2. Keep a daily log of your activities that precede pain and that reduce it.
3. Study the log to identify which activities cause pain and which relieve it.
4. Create a plan to modify your activities accordingly to reduce your pain.

EMSPress.com

Patterning Exercise #16: Exploring Micromovements to Reduce Pain

Exploring micromovements can help you interrupt chronic contractions in a pained area, get in touch with an area that you do not feel, and increase your awareness of a part of the body you are out of touch with.

1. Sit or lie in a comfortable position. Begin making subtle movements in any joint of your body. Make the movement as small as you can and still perceive it. Sense or imagine the movement lubricating that joint (it actually does lubricate by spreading synovial fluid in that joint).
2. Allow the micromovement to spread to adjacent body parts as though it were a ripple passing through water.
3. Notice any sensations that the micromovement generates. (Micromovements can be so small that they are imperceptible; therefore, be sure to make the movement large enough that you can feel it.) The sensations it creates will provide you with feedback that you are, indeed, moving. Slowly let the movement spread in or around areas where you feel pain
4. Breathe into the area you are moving. Sense or imagine the breath and movement either enlivening and energizing or relaxing the cells within the tissues you are moving.
5. When you finish, rest for a minute, then get up slowly.

EMSPress.com

and make the subsequent stretch stronger. (Also, feeling a muscle contract, relax, and stretch builds a proprioceptive awareness of dysfunctional muscle patterns, which can then be monitored and changed.) Then explore slow, conscious patterning exercises in that area to release excessive effort and to reorganize the recruitment order of your muscles.

5. *If pain is caused by asymmetry in movement*: Practice slow, conscious homologous patterns. Focus on feeling simultaneous and symmetrical movement of the right and left side. Sense the asymmetry while moving with the intention of relaxing the muscles that overwork and prevent symmetry, then engage the muscles that are not working.
6. *If pain is caused by rigidity*: Stretch. Practice joint mobilization exercises. Practice progressive muscle relaxation exercises. Practice slow movements that require minimal effort, such as rolling the head or body from side to side. Relax the body as much as possible while moving.
7. *If pain is exacerbated by emotional problems*: Practice relaxation exercises, such as lying quietly and sensing weight sink through the body on each exhalation. Slow, relaxing movement exercises also work well, such as the sensory awareness exercises of lying on the floor and slowly rolling, rocking gently, or practicing organic movement. Sense the emotional charge while moving, allowing the charge to dissipate with each exhalation.
8. *If pain is exacerbated by stressful thoughts*: Use breathing exercises to calm the body and mind (see Chapter 6). Then identify the stressful thought pattern or underlying belief system that is negative or self-defeating. Counter it with positive thoughts. (See Patterning Exercise #127 titled "Transforming Negative Thoughts into Productive Ones" in Chapter 14.) Strengthen your body with regular exercise and brisk walks. Ask a nonjudgmental friend to listen for 10 minutes while you unload your problems.

Importance of Movement after an Injury

After an injury has healed, it is common for a person who has become inactive due to pain to remain inactive. Inactivity contributes to feelings of helplessness, which many chronic pain sufferers experience. Immobility can also heighten pain sensations. A person needs to move after an injury has healed even if it is painful because movement restores normal function to previously immobilized areas. Movement, especially exercise, can stimulate the production of endorphins, which may even reduce pain, although exercise needs to be moderate at first so that a person does not overdo it and become discouraged.

Exercise can be balanced with patterning exercises in order to release holding patterns that develop around painful areas. This will also help to restore balance to movement in areas compromised by protective spasms after the injury. Many people find that after using patterning to release adaptive muscular holding from an injury, when they return to their previous exercise routine, their movement is more efficient and coordinated. Also, the new awareness they gained during the healing process may actually increase and improve their overall awareness of movement.

The human body is a perceptual organ designed to sense movement. People who do not sense their bodies or cultivate an awareness of movement lack a valuable kinesthetic sense. It is not possible to develop a proprioceptive awareness of the body by just sensing or visualizing it. A proprioceptive sense grows only with the direct experience of feeling muscles work and feeling the body in motion.

Movement restores a healthy awareness of the body, which often diminishes during immobility. The proprioceptive awareness we gain from movement is so primary, so fundamental, so constantly with us that describing it is like trying to describe grounding (see Chapter 15). Grounding is much more than merely having our feet in contact with the ground. It can be an energetic and dynamic experience that occurs when we connect with the exchange that always goes on between the ground and our body. This connection keeps the body linked to something much larger than itself. Likewise, movement maintains an energetic flow throughout the body connecting a person to a proprioceptive awareness of his living body and to the very process of life. When movement stops, energy stops flowing, circulation slows, proprioceptive awareness fades, and vitality diminishes. Inactivity slowly, cumulatively extinguishes the part of the self that is the moving body.

The importance of being active after the initial acute stage of an injury cannot be emphasized enough. Simply getting up and walking will increas circulation, loosen the joints, and tone the muscles. If a person is unable to walk, then simple exercises can be done in place. Even subtle micromovements will begin to restore circulation and awareness to a held and injured area.

SUMMARY

The natural responses to either physical or psychological injuries—protective muscular contractions—often remain long after an injury has healed. These contractions can tighten into holding patterns that affect both structure and function, and need to be addressed on both levels. There are many underlying reasons that holding patterns develop, including poor postural habits, gaps in early motor development, and even low self-esteem. Environmental influences such as tight clothing, nonsupportive furniture, and ill-fitting shoes also cause chronic muscular contractions that limit movement and underlie chronic holding patterns.

When chronic contractions restrict movement in one area of the body, another area usually becomes overly loose in response. For this reason, holding patterns usually involve a combination of rigidity and instability. The combination results in inefficient movement patterns that, because of tissue restrictions, often lead to pain. The process is circular: pain results in new holding patterns, and holding patterns lead to new pain.

Holding patterns reduce the efficiency of movement by disorganizing the recruitment order of contracting muscles. Efficiency is compromised even more when there is pain because pain triggers both the inhibition of postural muscles and spasms in the larger mobilizing muscles, which then contract to both guard against pain and to take over the job of postural stabilization. The chronic muscular contractions inherent in holding patterns tend to limit motion in one area while leading to excessive joint play in another area. With this muscular imbalance, even a small movement can strain an unstable joint; thus holding patterns make a person more susceptible to injuries that seem to arise out of nowhere. Such unfortunate injuries can at least have the positive effect. They force a person to pay attention to poor body-use habits and may even motivate a person to take active steps toward changing abusive postures and faulty movement patterns.

Holding patterns create stress in the autonomic nervous system, which shows up as both physiological and emotional pain. Pain signals come from sensory nerves called nociceptors. How we perceive these signals affects what type of pain we feel, leading some people to have low pain tolerance while others can tolerate a lot of pain. The process of pain is not well understood, and many of the chronic pain syndromes, such as myofascial pain syndrome or fibromyalgia, have unknown causes that make them difficult to treat. Psychological factors can also reduce or exacerbate pain. For this reason, a holistic approach to pain management is recommended, one in which a person works with the thoughts, emotions, and physical activities associated with pain patterns.

Since most pain results in chronic holding patterns, SP approaches to releasing holding patterns and changing faulty body-use habits can help people reduce or alleviate pain-inducing patterns and cultivate a more friendly relationship with their bodies, which is the essence of SP.

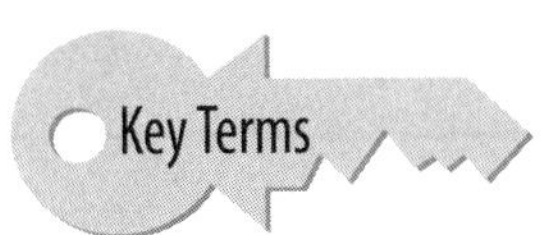

adaptive pattern
agonist
antagonist
autonomic nervous system (ANS)
axial compression
bracing
central nervous system (CNS)
centrally mediated pain
closed kinematic chain
concentric contraction
coupled pairs
dermatomes
dynamic system
eccentric contraction
extension
fascia
fibromyalgia
flexlon
gate theory of pain
hinging
hyperextension
inhibited
ischemia
kinematic chain
line of force
lordosis
mobilizers
myofascial pain syndrome (MFS)
neutral position of the spine
neutral zone
nociceptors
open kinematic chain
opening pain
over-facilitated
parasympathetic
peripheral nervous system (PNS)
phasic
position of mechanical advantage
prime mover
propping
proprioceptive feedback
recruitment order
repetitive stress injury (RSI)
scoliosis
secondary gain
skeletal nervous system (SNS)
splinting
stability dysfunction
stabilizers
stretch weakness
sympathetic
tonic
tonic function
trigger point (TP)

OVERVIEW OF CHAPTER 3

DISCOVERING SOMATIC CONCEPTS AND METHODS
- Roots of Somatic Patterning
- Somatic Patterning Applications

SIX BASIC CONCEPTS AND METHODS
- Holism
- Somatic Awareness
  - *Perception*
  - *Sensory Awareness*
  - *The Problem with the Perception of Pain*
- Core Movement
  - *Core Movement Patterns*
  - *Psychosomatic Patterns and the Core*
- Process Orientation
- Somatic Resonance
  - *Putting Somatic Resonance into Practice*
  - *Resonance and Intuition*
  - *Feedback and Objectivity*
- Oscillation between Dualities

3

Somatic Patterning Roots, Concepts, and Methods

The mind is like the wind and the body like sand; if you want to know which way the wind is blowing, you can look at the sand.

—Bonnie Bainbridge Cohen

Every field has a set of principles that establishes its foundation. The field of somatic patterning has many different approaches and techniques, yet there are a number of fundamental principles and concepts that underlie all of them. This chapter is a summary of the concepts that are found in so many patterning systems that they can be said to constitute the basic tenets of somatic patterning. They provide a language for understanding and conceptualizing somatic patterning.

This chapter provides an overview of the foundation of SP drawn from the review of somatic patterning modalities outlined in Part 3 of this text. In this chapter, we will examine the history, concepts, and methods of somatic patterning and its underlying roots within six major themes:

- holism
- somatic awareness
- core movement
- process orientation
- somatic resonance
- oscillation between dualities

Chapters 3 and 4 discuss the logic behind the various patterning approaches rather than the approaches themselves, which are introduced in Chapters 6 through 10 on taking theory into practice. The difference between the logic behind the approaches and the approaches themselves could be compared to eating. Anyone can eat food, but to provide the body with a supply of nourishing food, a person needs to understand some level of the inner working of the body and its metabolic needs. Similarly, many exercise or movement education programs provide people with a series of linear steps to follow. This chapter and the next present the logic behind picking and choosing the appropriate approach or exercise to meet a person's individual needs in somatic patterning.

DISCOVERING SOMATIC CONCEPTS AND METHODS

The concepts and methods presented in this chapter come out of a survey of the groundbreaking approaches to SP. This survey began in an effort to identify the overlapping concepts found in integrative movement and bodywork therapies (see Chapters 11 and 12). Upon looking at these therapies comparatively, it became clear that many of them use similar concepts and techniques but refer to them by different names. This brings up a number of questions, including: Are the various modalities actually using the same precepts and methods? And if so, what are these and where do they come from?

In looking for answers to these questions, it became apparent that many of the concepts and methods used in the movement and bodywork modalities overlap those found in other somatic fields, such as body-centered therapy, neurolinguistic programming, and biofeedback. In light of these overlaps, this study was expanded to include any modality that addresses body-mind patterns, adding physiological, cognitive and linguistic, and psychological approaches to the survey. Looked at in this way, the history of SP, which is presented in Part 3, covers five categories:

- integrative movement therapies
- integrative bodywork
- physiological patterning
- behavioral therapy and cognitive reorganization
- body-based psychotherapies

Several operational definitions need clarification before discussing the criteria used to include a modality in the history. Recall from Chapter 1 that movement is defined as physiological motion as well as kinesiological motion. In other words, movement encompasses both the intrinsic motility of bodily fluids and organs and the observable motion of the muscles and joints. A technique widely used in the somatic patterning modalities is **proprioceptive neuromuscular facilitation** (PNF), defined biologically as "a method to activate neuromuscular mechanisms by the stimulation of proprioception."[58] PNF is used here as a general term, not to be confused with the specific PNF patterns and techniques developed by Dr. Herman Kabat (see Chapter 12).[59] (Kabat developed a series of three-dimensional rotational patterns designed to take the body, specifically the joints, through a full range of physiological motion. In addition, he developed a series of hands-on techniques designed to maximize muscle function through a manipulation of muscle reflexes, such as the "contract-relax" technique.)

For the purposes of this study, there needed to be a similar term to identify the somatic modalities that use the proprioception of physiological movement to evoke change. Thus the term **autonomic proprioceptive facilitation** (APF) was coined. It is used in a context similar to PNF, except modalities that fall under APF work to effect changes in the autonomic nervous system rather than in neuromuscular mechanisms. APF is defined as any method of changing autonomic tone—the degree of relaxation or arousal in the autonomic nervous system—by the stimulation of proprioception of a person's psychophysiological state. This includes techniques that use a sensory awareness of physiological tone—such as an awareness of the heartbeat, breath rate, and skin temperature—to achieve the therapeutic goals of relaxation, stress management, and trauma resolution. The separation of PNF and APF is made to clarify therapeutic application. In PNF the practitioner's focus and intention are on musculoskeletal patterns tracked in movement of the joints and muscles, while APF is tracked through changes in autonomic tone, which indicate levels of stress or relaxation.

Because of the diversity of the broad field of somatic patterning and the fact that many of the original modalities have seeded succeeding generations of modalities, each system chosen for the survey had to meet three criteria:

1. It must have developed in the West.
2. It must use proprioceptive neuromuscular facilitation (PNF) and/or autonomic proprioceptive facilitation (APF) to improve body-mind patterns.
3. It must have introduced something original and innovative to its respective field.

Together, the common concepts and methods used across all of the modalities suggest a sensible protocol for the patterning process, one that is "rational, individualized, and comprehensive."[60] One way to look at this is to think of each of the many therapeutic approaches to SP as ways of entering the same room but through different doors. If the room is the body and the doors are mental, physical, and emotional entries, it seems only logical that an effective method of changing body-mind patterns would require access to all the doors and would be inclusive in the integration of diverse modalities.

This history does not include Eastern energy methods such as yoga, acupuncture, Jin Shin, or Reiki. According to the Academy of Traditional Chinese Medicine, energy is called "chi" or "qi" (vital energy); chi circulates through invisible channels distributed throughout the body called "meridians," which create both a topical and an internal map of how energy flows in the body.[61] A Chinese medical practitioner (Doctor of Oriental Medicine or acupuncturist) uses touch or needles to activate the flow of energy within the client's body along the meridians, which have been associated with pathways of movement (Figure 3.1). In contrast, energy is activated in somatic patterning by the perception of movement sensations in the body.

Energy is used here in its general sense to mean vitality and aliveness, as well as the body's capacity to do work. Most people can feel when they have more or less energy, though sometimes it is hard to verbalize what energy feels like. We usually notice when we lack it and feel fatigue. The feeling of energy flowing is heightened in the body after an intense workout, when the perception of increased tone and circulation is amplified. Blocks in the flow of energy through the body could be compared to stuck teeth in a zipper: they interrupt the natural flow of a movement sequence.

Roots of Somatic Patterning

All sciences develop out of a study of patterns. Somatic patterning developed out of the study of how movement serves as a healing agent for both body and mind. The alternative

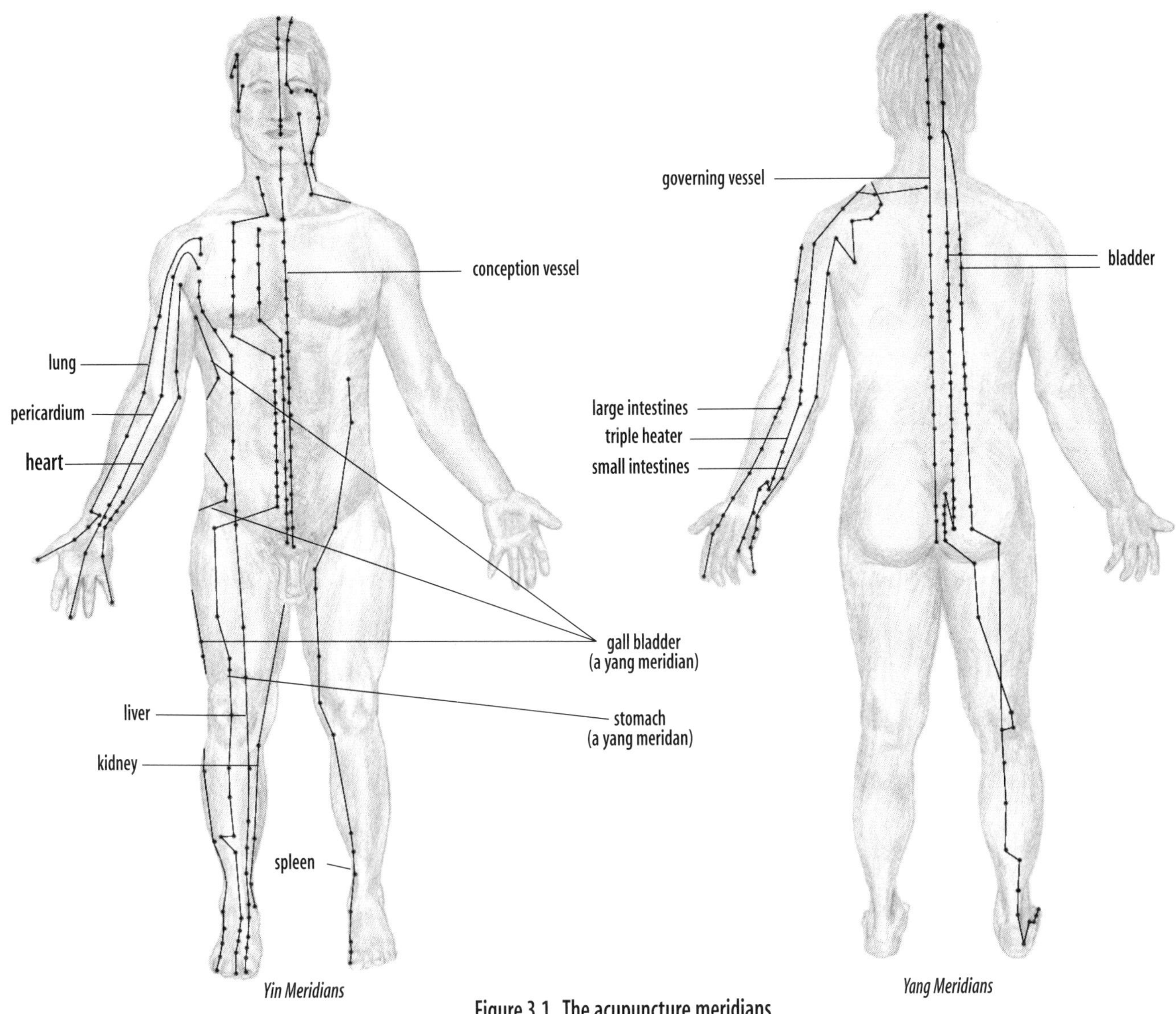

Figure 3.1 The acupuncture meridians

approaches to SP grew, in turn, out of a widespread desire by many somatic pioneers to understand how the fixations of the mind and emotions might underlie poor postural habits, faulty body mechanics, and psychosomatic stresses.

Initially, only nontraditional, alternative somatic therapies were included in the survey of somatic patterning conducted for this text. Upon further investigation, however, it became apparent that many of what are considered "alternative" therapies were actually created by scientists or medically trained therapists. Ida Rolf, for example, was a biochemist, Moshe Feldenkrais a physicist, Irmgaard Bartenieff a physical therapist, and Bonnie Cohen an occupational therapist. As a result, many of the somatic approaches have roots in traditional medical fields. Also, many alternative methods of SP overlap with many of the techniques that grew out of research conducted in the fields of physical therapy, biofeedback, neurolinguistics, and psychoneuroimmunology.

The primary difference between the nontraditional and traditional approaches to SP is that the alternative practitioners use an experiential method of application, themselves becoming adept at the somatic skills they are teaching; traditional practitioners use a more hands-off approach, teaching skills to patients that they may not have practiced themselves. The somatic pioneers who were trained in science used both their scientific and their experiential knowledge to develop their theories. Many of them felt that their methods had great value in helping people and relied on extensive anecdotal evidence to support the efficacy of their work. Wanting to make the work available as quickly and widely as possible, they launched their theories into practice without going through the traditional Western scientific method of research. Their experiential inquiries involved subjective, personal processes that are difficult to measure, a tendency that has been both a blessing and a curse to SP. Although it has made the somatic therapies readily accessible to the public, it has also created a huge body of work built largely upon personal experience, pseudoscientific theories, and overlapping and at times vague methods.

There is extensive anecdotal evidence that the somatic therapies effectively change body patterns. Due to the increasing popularity of somatic therapies among medical patients, who often introduce them to their doctors, many of the somatic modalities have come to the attention of the medical establishment. As a result, many of these methods are now grouped under the title of *complementary alternative medicine* (CAM), some are being studied at the National Institutes of Health. Also, references to alternative approaches can now be found in online medical database MedLine.[62] Numerous references are also made in the *Alternative Therapies in Health and Medicine Journal*,[63] and occasional references can even be found in the *Journal of the American Medical Association*.[64] As first mentioned in Chapter 1, references to alternative therapies from all these sources include yoga, martial arts, energy and spiritual healing, cognitive and behavioral therapy, acupuncture, Chinese medicine, exercise, and imagery, plus a vague, catch-all category of "mind-body."[65]

Many of the modalities discussed in the history chapters of Part 3 fall under the ambiguous body-mind classification. A reason for the ambiguity may be that this field is so broad that it defies definition. Also, many somatic practitioners are educated in various somatic techniques and do not present themselves as a practitioner of a single modality.[66] Hence, many of these modalities are remote to the mainstream population. In addition, there is so much overlap in these various fields that somatic practitioners tend to cross-train in several fields to be able to address somatic patterns through two or more channels. Consequently, somatic practitioners are usually generalists rather than specialists in holistic health, which may add to the nebulous mystique that many people comment about when describing the somatic modalities.

One point that most who study, practice, or receive SP agree about is that its various modalities prove to be remarkably effective, regardless of how vaguely they might be defined. The efficacy of many of the somatic therapies might be explained through the research findings that have led to therapies such as biofeedback and psychoneuroimmunology. For example, the psychiatrist Edmund Jacobson discovered that muscle activity accompanies all mental processes; the Viennese physician Hans Selye defined "stress" as a biological process that can be regulated from within; and Dr. John Basmajian found that it is possible to gain conscious control over a single motor neuron.

The implications of these discoveries are far-reaching. They prove that a person can change physiology with thought and change function with directed attention. These discoveries lend credibility to the power of the body-mind connection in healing and to the possibilities that exist for healing from within. Most psychiatrists choose to practice within the confines of allopathic pharmacology (treatments based currently on intervention with drugs) and do not put the nonpharmacological discoveries to practical use; however, many dedicated and compassionate physicians are changing this orientation and beginning to empower their patients to heal from within using body-mind approaches. While many Western psychiatrists in this century have overlooked the curative implications of the body-mind connection, holistic practitioners have not. As a result, huge bodies of alternative therapies and somatic modalities have sprung up in the counter-culture over the last half of the twentieth century and have steadily moved into mainstream applications.

A similar dynamic has occurred in other medical fields besides psychiatry. For example, most osteopaths have taken the allopathic route and dropped osteopathic techniques of realigning joints. But many of their hands-on modalities, such as cranialsacral therapy, are now being widely used by bodyworkers, massage therapists, and somatic practitioners. Likewise, physical therapists and occupational therapists are the allopathic experts on neuromuscular rehabilitation, being highly trained in biomechanical and neurological assessment and treatment of the body. A handful of innovators in the field of physical therapy, however, such as Dr. Herman Kabat and the therapists who have advanced the manual therapies, have collectively developed many thorough and practical science-based methods of rehabilitative neuromuscular education outside of the allopathic model.

Unfortunately, most physicians and physical therapists practicing in the United States today are limited by treatment specifications and codes often regulated by managed care organizations. They are also bogged down by the sea of paperwork required by insurance companies. As a result, few have time to learn, let alone practice, the sophisticated manual therapies developed by their associates, such as proprioceptive neuromuscular facilitation (Kabat's PNF system has more than 110 techniques). Thus, methods such as PNF, joint mobilization, and core movement training (an approach popularized by fitness programs like Pilates) are now being studied and widely used by somatic practitioners and bodyworkers.

Some medical practitioners contend that alternative practitioners are using watered-down or partial versions of the manual therapies, and are using them out of context. Many somatic practitioners argue that these approaches are too valuable not to put to practical use, so that some application is better than none. This has led many bodyworkers to search for science-based methods. Since most somatic practitioners are not trained to evaluate musculoskeletal problems, their application of the manual techniques is usually more generalized, for example, to improve proprioception, balance, and mobility, rather than to treat specific injuries or conditions.

To reiterate an important point here, many of the somatic therapies that will be described in the Part 3 survey of the field are ones that fall into the catch-all "body-mind" classification and are rarely included among the complementary alternative medicines (CAM). Why they are not included is unclear. Perhaps it is because their therapeutic efficacy is mostly anecdotal, although this effectiveness is increasingly being recognized by the public, evidenced by the growing number of people who use somatic modalities. Perhaps it is because the field of SP, as a whole, lacks definition. Somatic practitioners seek recognition by the medical establishment and are making attempts to establish a body of research to gain this.[67] Also, a large body of research-based information about somatic patterns is already available that explains how body-mind patterns work (see Chapters 12, 13, and 14 in Part 3). These findings could provide direction to somatics practitioners for how to establish credibility within the field of CAM.

Somatic Patterning Applications

What distinguishes a somatic patterning modality from a traditional one like physical therapy is that it is holistic, addressing both body and mind. (Some may argue that physical therapy addresses the whole person. Still, training in the field involves primarily a mechanical approach to joint and muscle function.) As discussed earlier, somatic practitioners believe that all body patterns have mental, emotional, and/or spiritual components. Because body patterns reflect so many aspects of a person, in order to change them, a person must view the body as a multifaceted whole and consider how all the facets relate. SP focuses on the relationships between posture and movement not only in specific parts of the body, but also as an outward manifestation of a person's thoughts, beliefs, emotions, and experiences. Whereas physical therapists typically work to help patients strengthen weak muscle groups and restore joint mobility, somatic patterners help clients feel how weak muscle groups affect the entire person, including the person's self-image, emotional states, and overall functional patterns.

Somatic patterning is an experiential educational process. In SP, movement and awareness are used to work with the deeper hidden patterns of the body and mind. Feedback coming from within a person—about the changing qualities of movement, changing tensions in moving muscles, changing sensations and emotions, and changing positions in space—guides the learning process. The primary educational tool of SP involves learning to track movement responses in the body, such as paying attention to when the body relaxes, contracts, or retracts. With this awareness, a person learns to direct movement and tone (such as muscle tone and physiological tone), to engage muscular support, and to encourage fluidity and integration so that a movement will flow with minimal effort through all parts of the body.

Somatic patterning uses methods that are built upon changing the perception of the body in three main areas: *psychophysiological patterning* (such as relaxation training or work with emotions), *behavioral* and *cognitive reorganization* (changing thought and speech patterns), and *movement education*. Relaxation training teaches people how to perceive physiological processes so that they can learn to slow their physiology down, resulting in a calmer system with reduced wear and tear. Cognitive reorganization teaches people how to change thoughts patterns that underlie stressful or unhealthy body patterns, and how to harness the power of positive thinking. Both use APF techniques such as sensory awareness and relaxation training to address stress-related problems that have a psychological component. Movement education uses primarily PNF techniques within the educational context to work with body problems that affect the mechanics of movement and posture.

When psychophysiological patterning, cognitive reorganization, and movement education are combined and integrated, a broader application surfaces. It is one that recognizes movement (mental, physiological, and physical) as the vital link among all somatic modalities, and as the key element to address health problems that are both physical and psychological.

SIX BASIC CONCEPTS AND METHODS

In an effort to flesh out the underlying precepts of the somatic modalities, the different principles and methods of each modality are discussed in Part 3. As these discussions show, a handful of concepts and techniques show up again and again in the different methods. Out of these, six overriding themes—*holism, somatic awareness, core movement, process orientation, somatic resonance,* and an *oscillation between dualities*—stand out. Each theme, to be discussed next, reflects an underlying concept of somatic patterning as well as a technique.

Holism

The first of the six common themes found in SP methods is the concept of **holism.** It is based on the theory that all living beings are far more than the sum of their parts. As patterns of posture and movement are the physical manifestations of the emotional, mental, and spiritual aspects of a person, so holistic health care is an approach that considers all parts of a health problem or a preventive program. In somatic patterning, the holistic approach is the same: the physical, emotional, and mental aspects of a body-mind configuration are all considered during the patterning process. A person takes into account what function a given pattern serves; when it started; how it feels; how it affects the body, posture, movement, and emotions; and what thoughts accompany it.

Holism naturally considers the context in which body-mind patterns develop and play out. When working with emotional and psychological patterns, the pattern is reflected upon in terms of the role it plays not only for the individual but in relationships and family dynamics as well.

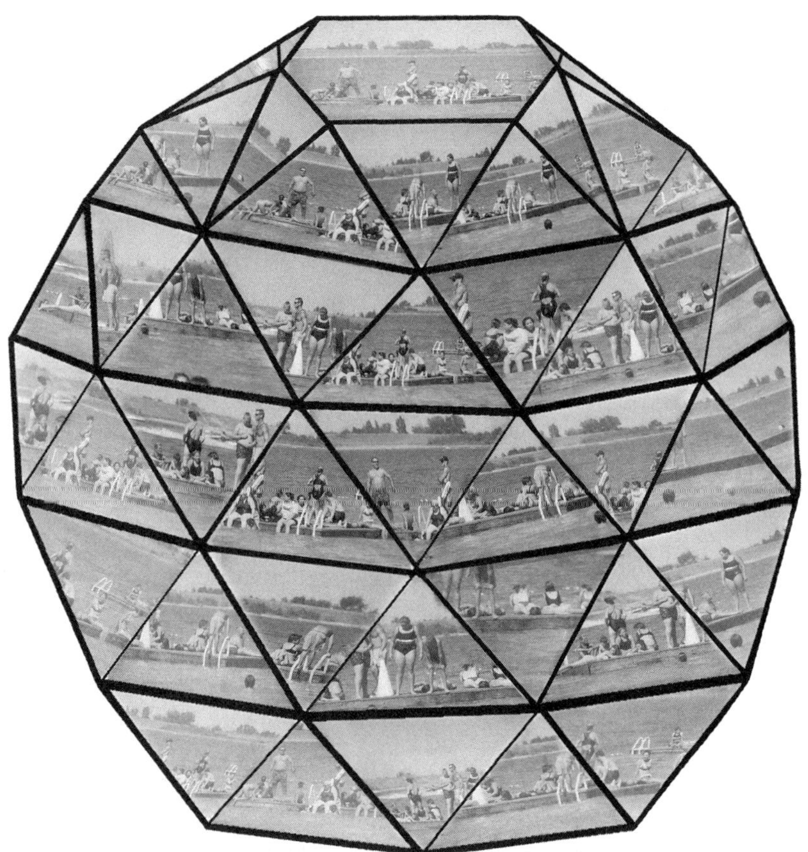

Figure 3.2 In a hologram, each part holds the entire form within it.

And in a holistic approach to working with physical problems, such as back pain or injury rehabilitation, a person pays attention to how an injured area affects the posture and economy of the entire body rather than attending to just one part.

As a technique, holism is applied by using a roving awareness of the different parts of a pattern. This involves intermittently scanning the relationships among various elements of a body-mind pattern during the patterning process. It includes both an awareness of what is presently occurring within the body and what new pattern is being learned. Awareness is used like a spotlight that continually moves among the parts of a pattern, seeking to illuminate all of its hidden elements. By doing this, a person expands awareness to include the relationship among parts of an existing pattern and the possibilities for growth. The purpose of an inclusive awareness is to integrate seemingly disparate or disconnected elements into a holistic totality. The more expansive and inclusive the approach and the more elements brought in, the more whole and integrated the end result. Holistic approaches have a synergistic effect. This means that a multifaceted awareness, combined with the efforts of multiple approaches, makes the effectiveness of the overall work far greater than the sum of its parts.

When people are oriented toward holism, they understand that the separation of body and mind is only an illusion. From a holistic perspective, each part of a pattern reflects the whole configuration in the same way that each fragment in a holographic image holds the entire picture of that hologram (Figure 3.2). On the simplest level, the process of the body at any given moment reflects exactly what is going on in the mind, and vice versa. Reading this process is complex. It is done largely through two channels: the language of the body, which manifests in sensorimotor processes, and the language of the mind, which manifests in thought and language.

Just by recognizing that mental and physical processes are inextricable, we achieve the orientation necessary for SP. A person who doubts this unity need only recall an embarrassing situation to exemplify the unity of the body-mind. What happens? Do the cheeks start to flush? Does the heart race? Is there, perhaps, a shriveling sensation, or a sickening feeling in the stomach? Although the memory seems mental, the response is obviously very physical.

Just recognizing the inherent nature of body-mind unity within us also brings a degree of integration and balance. The fundamental balancing takes place in SP by attending to the patterns of both the body and the mind within the same process. Some may argue that the body and mind cannot be separated, so that any activity constitutes an SP process. This is true. As was mentioned in Chapter 1, we are always training the soma—the living body in all its wholeness—with every activity. But an activity only becomes SP when the physical training is conscious and deliberate.

Somatic Awareness

A second major theme of somatic patterning is **somatic awareness**, which includes an awareness of all aspects of the body and mind, coming from both internal and external stimuli, including a sensory awareness of the body and all its perceptual mechanisms (Figure 3.3). When we speak of awareness, we need to keep in mind how broad and subjective this term is. Depending on what channel a person is tuned into, what constitutes awareness for one may be foreign to the next. Although meditation practices differ greatly, the most common practice is to gently center the awareness on a single focus, such as the breath, watching it without interference, without an agenda or goal. Many people who meditate have learned the curative value of a state of focused awareness, which tends to calm the body and mind. When awareness is focused on the body, it can be used as a therapeutic tool that brings attention to the parts of the body in need of a healing focus.

Somatic awareness entails not only body awareness, but a much larger awareness of the body-mind complex as it manifests in the movement of emotions, thoughts, and beliefs. Somatic awareness is holistic because it involves an awareness of multiple elements as they are occurring and as they interact. As a technique, somatic awareness is used to deepen and expand a person's perception of a present-moment experience in the body. To do this, a person learns how to track and observe thoughts, feelings, movements, and body sensations while they are occurring.

Pure awareness is the goal of many meditative practices undertaken to quiet the body and the mind, and to transcend habitual perception. A state of pure awareness is probably impossible to achieve because everything a person perceives is filtered through perceptual portals of the senses. Still, we cannot change a pattern until we can perceive it. The cornerstone of somatic learning is *awareness through movement*. When we move with awareness, we put a spotlight of attention on the natural, organic process of the body and uncover the thoughts, feelings, and attitudes that shape the health or unease of our bodies. We also bring into view the parts of ourselves that can move, the parts that are dysfunctional (rigid, unstable, taut, unbalanced, etc.), and the parts with which we have lost touch.

Perception

All the patterning modalities have the same intended outcome: *to change body-use patterns of behavior and movement to improve overall function*. The combined approaches of the diverse patterning modalities offer a wide array of tools and technologies for evoking healthy change, yet they are unified be a singular focus: *change follows perception*.

Perception is the result of sensory awareness; it is consciousness based on incoming sensory information. Perception is often based on **kinesthesia**—the sensory experience stimulated by changes in body positions and muscle tensions, which constitutes a large part of somatic awareness. Perception is colored by external stimuli such as what we touch, hear, see, and taste; and by internal stimuli such as thoughts, memories, belief systems, and body sensations. How we perceive our body complicates patterning because our perception is often a projection of what our mind believes. In this sense, perception is based on a point of view and a psychological process; it is the brain's interpretation of sensory information.

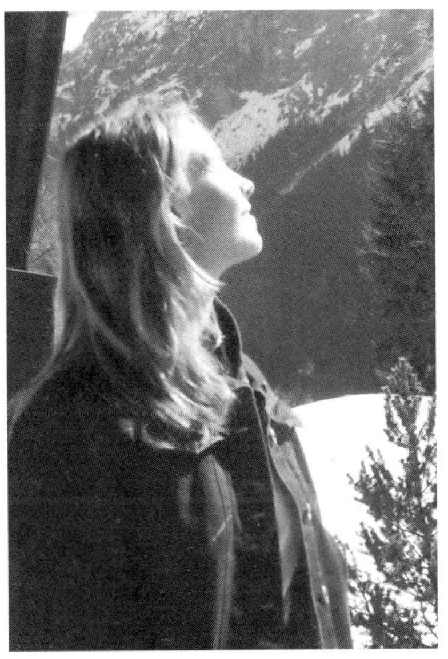

Figure 3.3 Somatic awareness (photo courtesy of A. Imboden).

Perception gained from sensory awareness is often distorted because it can be based on a habitual view rather than an actuality. For instance, many people posture by leaning slightly backward. When asked about the verticality of their alignment, people with off-center postures usually think that they are straight. Over time, their perception has become distorted by an inaccurate reading of sensory information. When posture is habitually off-center, the imbalance feels normal and the brain interprets it as normal. What actually occurs, though, is that the resting positions of the muscles become chronically shortened or overextended and remain unchanged over time. Since the posture is relatively constant, a person feels the distorted position is normal. And it is common for a person's range of perception to become habitual.

Changing a somatic pattern to improve function is not as important as being able to feel the change. Change is felt as a **perceptual shift**, a general feeling of a different state in such aspects as tone, position, well-being, or even in a person's state of mind. A perceptual shift accompanies any deep change; in fact, during somatic patterning change is inconsequential without a shift in perception. A person needs to be able to register a somatic shift within the perceptual field to recognize the difference between an old and new pattern. In other words, we cannot know where we are going unless we know where we have been. Many people receive bodywork and make profound shifts in body patterns only to slip back into the old pattern soon after the session ends. The reason is that they have not consciously recognized the change and have not actively made an effort to keep it, two vital elements that distinguish patterning from bodywork.

Sensory Awareness

Perception is based on the sensory information arriving through the sensory nerves, and on the motor responses that are felt as movement. **Sensory awareness** is the perception of sensations in the body as they are received through the sensory receptors of the skin, ears, eyes, nose, mouth, and musculoskeletal receptors (Figure 3.4). In addition, internal movements of physiological processes create sensations in a resting body, and the changing tensions generated by muscle activity create the dynamic sensations of the body moving through space. The musculoskeletal system has millions of joint and muscle proprioceptors that register changes in body position, in the speed at which the body is moving, and in the amount of force a motion generates or absorbs.

Sensory awareness is a primary tool for somatic learning. It is based on a self-awareness of the body at rest as well as during movement. Although

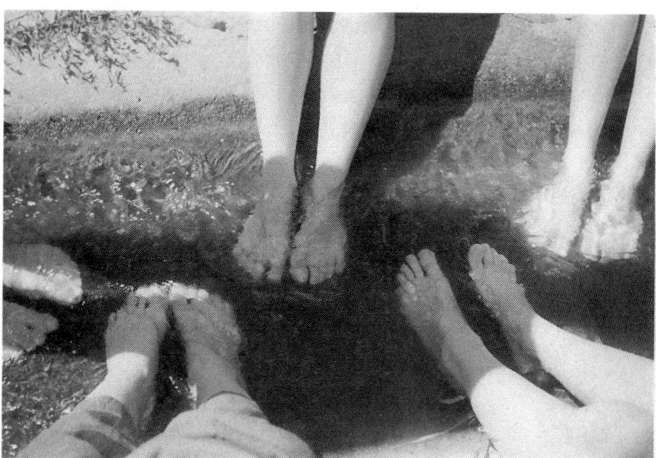

Figure 3.4 A sensory awareness experience

awareness is largely a sensory experience, the very act of pointing a sense organ toward incoming stimuli, such as turning the head toward a sound, is a motor process.

A person can explore many different activities to develop sensory awareness, such as scanning the body or taking note of the quality and locations of internal sensations within the resting body. Most people think of a stationary body as nonmoving, but it is still teeming with a myriad of intrinsic motions caused by interactive metabolic processes. The breath rises and falls, blood races through the veins, nerve impulses shoot down nerve tracts at lightning speed, muscle cells twitch, organs pump and churn, fluids press through cell membranes, and intercellular particles ebb and flow. For the novice, learning to be aware of intrinsic movements in the body at rest may seem an elusive task. It is similar to watching clouds moving quietly or watching the deeper currents of water through the surface of a calm lake.

The primary tool used to develop sensory awareness is the perception of movement. To explore this, a person can move in a slow, conscious manner, tracking the changing sensations generated by an improvisational movement. As a person becomes aware of movement sensations, she will begin to feel a kaleidoscope of sensations that she may have never noticed before. Sensation is generated from the movement of both internal and external processes, including compression in the joints, stretch in the myofascial tissues, pressure in the organs, expansion in the lungs, pain, or the changing points of contact on the underside of a moving body.

The Problem with the Perception of Pain

Somatic awareness is complicated by the perception of pain. The subjective and variable nature of perception is highlighted by the subjective nature of perceiving pain levels. The biggest problem with assessing what causes pain is that pain is a psychosomatic process. There are no actual pain receptors in the body. Small peripheral nociceptors (introduced in Chapter 2) found in the skin and throughout the body relay sensation to the brain for interpretation. This interpretation varies greatly from one person to the next and from one situation to the next. Despite many theories about the causes of pain and many treatments for different types of pain, overall, little is known about how sensations are transformed into the experience of pain. When sensations such as pressure, heat, and cold reach certain levels of intensity, they are felt as pain. It has been hypothesized that pain occurs when a flood of sensation overloads the sensory system and becomes too great for a person to process adequately.

Pain tolerance varies greatly because each person has a unique manner of perceiving sensation. What causes one person severe pain may cause minimal sensation in someone else, which makes figuring out the source of distress a difficult process. The implications of this are that the level of discomfort a person feels does not necessarily indicate the seriousness of a condition. Easily irritated individuals might interpret any unusual sensation as pain, while rugged individuals tend to minimize and ignore physical sensations.

The body tends to disappear when it is free of pain or noxious sensation. Because of this, perception of pain is usually much more highly developed than a perception of healthy function. In an effort to counter this tendency, a person can begin to sense what healthy postures and efficient movements feel and look like, and to build a body-based vocabulary for normal function rather than pathology.

Patterning Exercise #17: Cultivating Sensory Awareness

1. To build sensory awareness in your body, sit in a quiet, comfortable place, close your eyes, and relax.
2. Become aware of the parts of your body that have contact with the chair, supporting your weight. Start with you head and gradually scan your body mentally to feel these parts, one by one.
3. Follow the movement of your breath in and out of your body.
4. Slowly sway and track the subtle movements of the sway throughout your trunk, neck, and head.
5. Make a slow, subtle movement with a part of your body and pay attention to the changing shape of the movement. Then move another part, then another, continuing until you have moved the entire body.
6. During the course of your daily activities, take a minute to explore one or more of these sensory awareness exercises.

EMSPress.com

Core Movement

A third SP theme, **core movement**, is at once literal and figurative. Balanced movement initiates from or is supported through the core of a person. Full-body movements that initiate in the core tend to be powerful, stable, and coordinated. For example, a runner crouches to gather potential energy into the core, then springs forward through core movement from flexion into extension. Integrated core movement appears effortless (Figure 3.5). The absence of this integrated core connection shows up in heavy, uncoordinated, or weak movements that lack a stable center.

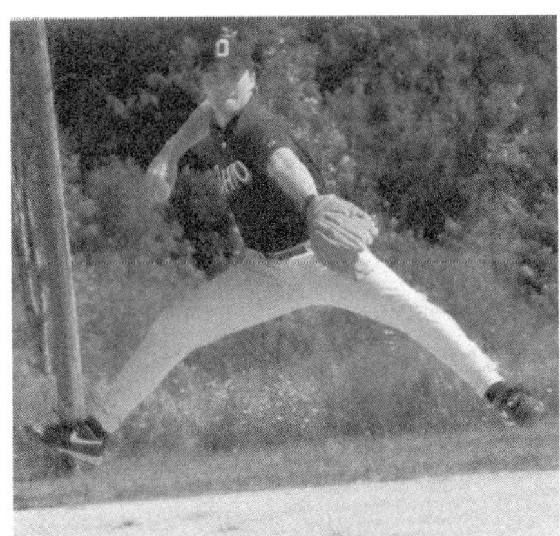

Figure 3.5 Core patterns show up in many different sports (photo courtesy of E. Foster).

Core integration and movement initiates within the center of the body and is reflected in a postural integrity of the spine. On a figurative level, core movement is behavior that initiates in and is carried out through a person's own volition, or will. This means that the idea or impulse to move arises from within a person, that the person generates the motivation and intention to move and then moves by the force of conscious effort. As a technique, core movement is used to organize movements that either initiate in the center of the body or are stabilized there.

Core Movement Patterns

The human fetus grows into a state of strong fetal flexion centered around the gut. The first patterns of flexion and extension organize the core of the body around the lifeline of the umbilical cord. As the size of the fetus increases, the space inside the womb gradually decreases; growing pressure from the shrinking space compresses the fetus into a deeper and deeper flexion, increasing flexor tone. Thus there is minimal extension in the body until birth. In a normal vaginal delivery, the newborn is pushed and squeezed out by the combined reflexes of both mother and baby into its first action of full-body extension.

The earliest movement patterns actually start at the navel and radiate out of the core of the body. Although an infant may seem to move only an arm or leg, it actually thrusts the limbs out in an action that initiates in the core, at the navel. First introduced in Chapter 1, this basic primitive pattern—expanding out and drawing back in from the center of the body— is called navel radiation. It underlies all subsequent movement patterns and is one of several core patterns. Other patterns organized around the core of the body include prespinal movement and mouthing patterns (see Chapter 7 on developmental patterning).

At the beginning of early motor development, core movement patterns initiate within the newborn in the soft tissues of the organs and the nervous system, when the neuromuscular system is still undeveloped; these earlier intrinsic core patterns underlie and shape subsequent musculoskeletal tone. Extensor tone builds as a newborn undergoes experiences that cause it to reach out, such as reaching out for food, listening to sounds, or visually tracking elements that draw attention. When hunger, thirst, or curiosity arise, the infant naturally extends out for food, drink, or interaction in a relaxed manner. Each one of these patterns develops at the same time that adaptive defense patterns form; therefore, core movement patterns reflect a person's deepest psychosomatic structure. Core patterns reveal the essence of a person's psychology and reflect a person's most primitive emotional responses. The startle reflex (discussed in Chapter 1) is, for example, a core defense reaction shaped by the development phase that an infant was in when the defenses were first rallied, often when full-body core patterns dominated motor development.

Many somatic methods focus on the center of the body as a place from which to control movement, to improve posture, and to integrate function. The Pilates system of exercise conditions the core with slow, strengthening movements initiated in and controlled by the muscles of the abdomen and waist (see "Pilates" in Chapter 11). Rolfing achieves structural integration by always stretching myofascia in relationship to the core, working to establish dimensional balance between the trunk and limbs (see "Rolfing" in Chapter 12). In Reichian models of body-based psychotherapy, the flow of energy along the core, between the head and the tail, reflects psychological health.

As discussed in Chapter 2, most of the muscles that stabilize the spine and ensure an aligned posture lie close to the spine, along the core of the body. Although their contractions are more subtle and difficult to feel, the stabilizers ensure a centered balance in the body in both posture and movement.

The core of the body, particularly the spine, is often associated with the state of being "centered." Many forms of yoga and meditation work on the premise that a centered body cultivates a calm mind (Figure 3.6). Although people usually speak of being centered as a metaphorical experience, it is also a physical experience that can be observed in the alignment of the spine.

Psychosomatic Patterns and the Core

Core movement has a strong psychological component. Many body-centered schools of psychotherapy equate the core of the body with the center of a person's physical and psychological self. As mentioned earlier, being centered is not only a psychological experience of self-control but an

Patterning Exercise #18: Core Movement and Navel Radiation

1. Lie on your back. Extend both arms and legs along diagonal pathways into a big X position (PE Fig. 18a). Keep your lower back connected to the floor. Avoid arching your lumbar spine or pulling it up from the floor.

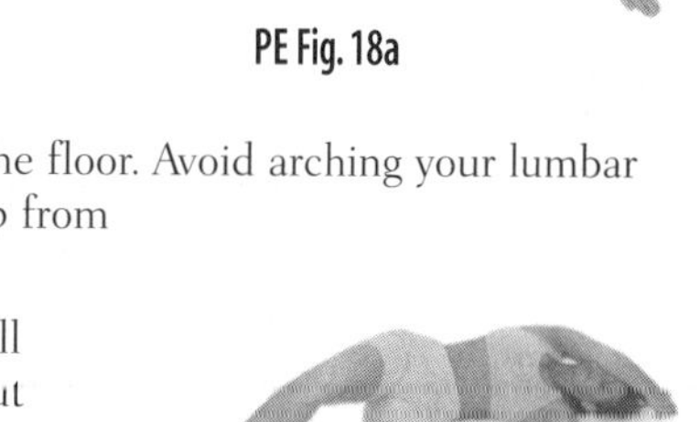

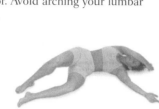

PE Fig. 18a

2. Reach out through all your limbs, taking out the slack between your fingers, toes, head, and tail, and your navel. Take a few deep breaths.

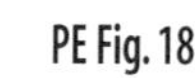

PE Fig. 18b

3. As you exhale, allow your abdomen to sink toward your lower back and draw all your limbs toward your navel (PE Fig. 18b). Simultaneously roll to your side, curling into full-body flexion (PE Fig. 18c).

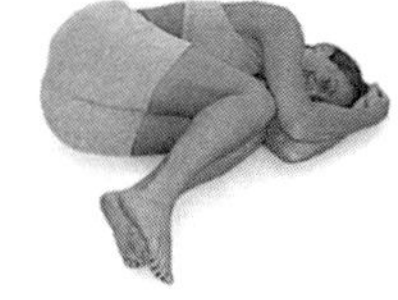

PE Fig. 18c

4. Inhale and extend your limbs back out while rolling onto your back, to your starting position. Extend all your limbs from your navel, keeping your abdominal wall pulled into your lower back.
5. Exhale again and repeat on the other side. Imagine your body like a starfish, extending all the limbs out as you breathe in, and curling to your side as you breathe out. Move slowly, in a relaxed manner, sensing weight sinking on your underside as you move.

actual physical posture centered around the core of the body. In the process of maturation, a person grows from the core out. Developmental psychologist Daniel Stern discusses the "core self" as the psychic structure from which psychological and emotional expression stem.[68] A psychologically healthy person identifies with an inner locus of experience rooted in the torso. In contrast, a person with narcissistic tendencies denies inner feelings for the sake of an outer image of self, building a sense of self based on what other people see and think rather than on inner feelings. The narcissistic body type is, in a sense, "shallow," lacking integration between the inner and outer layers, between the core and the periphery. Bioenergetic psychiatrist Alexander Lowen describes the narcissistic body as one with "heavy musculature" on the outside but with reduced spontaneity and aliveness on the inside (see Chapter 15).[69]

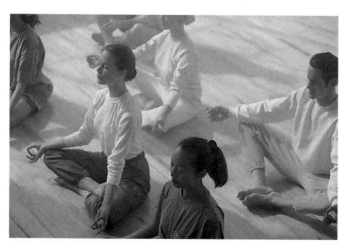

Figure 3.6 Yoga and meditation help many people to center themselves.

Conversely, emotions create autonomic responses, which change the visceral sensations that arise from the trunk. Many schools of body-centered psychotherapy cultivate the tracking of physical sensation in the organs as a tool for processing emotions. They are generally described as "knots" or "butterflies" in the stomach, or "gut feelings" or "pains in the heart." Stanley Keleman, a pioneering somatic psychologist, describes an emotion-based, "pulsatory" continuum that builds an energetic charge (build-up of energy in one place) in the core and finds expression through the limbs (see Chapter 15). Healthy expression occurs when a person can sequence feelings from the trunk through the limbs, bridging the core and the periphery, the inner life with the outer life, and self with other in relationship. The continuity between feelings and expression takes place as movement sequences from the core to the limbs.

In this model, emotional holding patterns are described as emotions that do not fully develop in the core or are unable to sequence between the inner and outer layers. They are either not given the time or attention they need to incubate in the trunk, or a person is unable to allow emotions to sequence between the core and periphery and express them. As an example, a person unable to speak about his feelings might block the energetic flow in a tightly held jaw or pursed lips. Or an angry person might block the full expression of anger midstream in a weak kicking or stamping gesture that does not adequately sequence from the core to the foot.

The spine reflects the "backbone" of personality and is often associated with integrity, strength, and conviction. Wilhelm Reich, who is often referred to as the "grandfather of somatic psychology," recognized how emotional experiences moved along the core in pulsations between the head

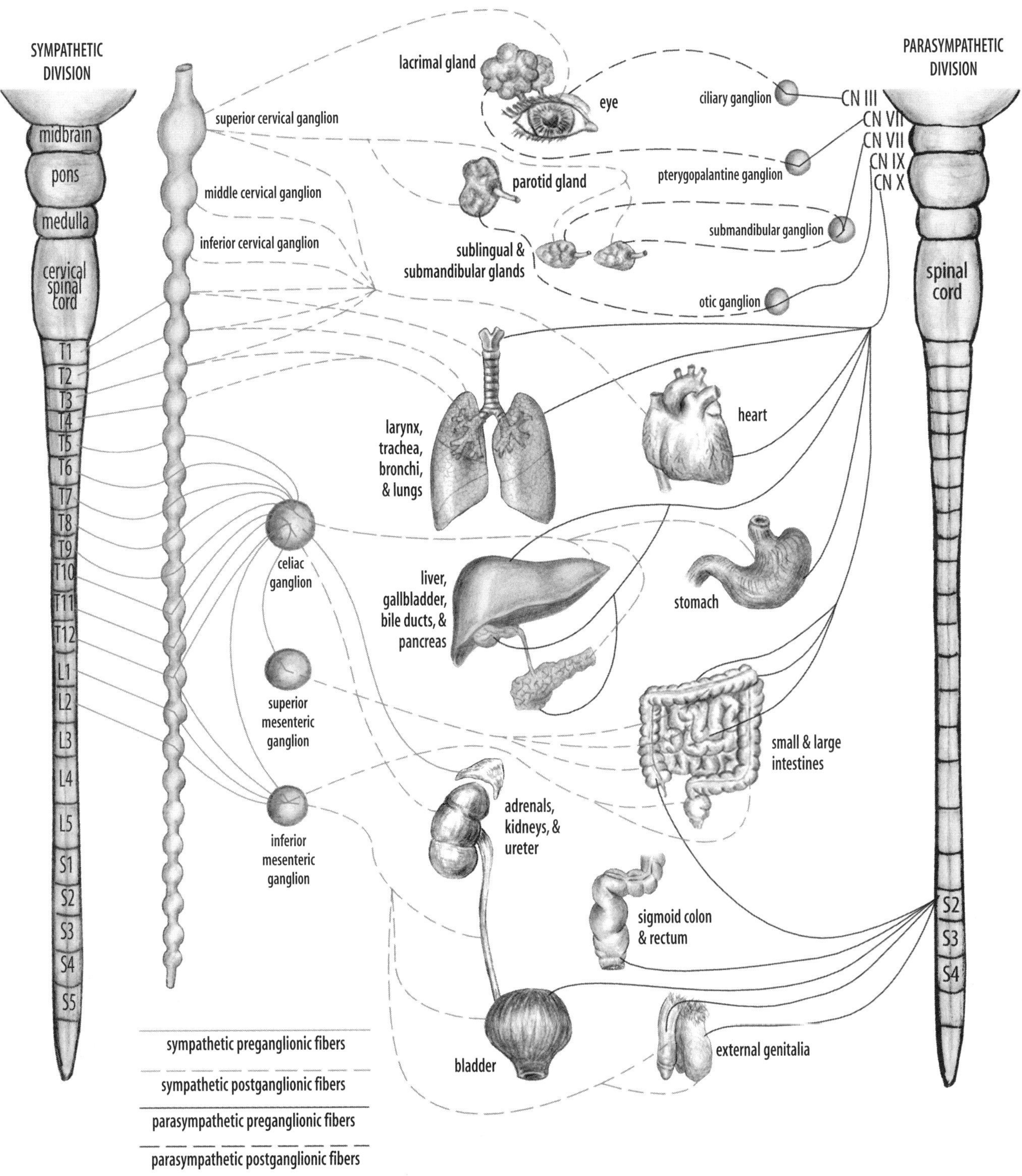

Figure 3.7 A schematic of the autonomic nervous system

and tail. He developed a system of character analysis that correlated muscular armor with the blockage of energy flow along the spine. He describes the movement of energy as both a psychological and a biological experience, one we feel in the mind and the body. Rings of armor that block this flow relate to a segmental arrangement of *autonomic ganglia*—groups of nerve cells arranged like beads along the front of the spine that regulate organ and glandular function (Figure 3.7; also see Figure 15.3).[70] According to Reich, the autonomic nervous system regulates both organ responses and emotional responses; therefore, the organ health and psychological health have a synonymous relationship. (In these models, core and organs are used synonymously.)

Since the core of the body is integral to the core of emotional patterns, any somatic patterning done in the organs has the potential of stirring up deep psychological issues, a topic that will be revisited in Chapter 6. To develop integration between the core and the limbs, we can cultivate pathways between them for emotional expression. This entails allowing feeling to flow through the trunk and make a full movement sequence through the limbs. The sequence can be actual physical movement or flow of energy.

Stubborn psychological issues tend to resist change when somatic patterning is approached solely on a physical level. If the core of the body resists change, it is likely that there is a holding pattern present related to a deep psychological issue. For this reason, the emotional and psychological implications of core issues must be taken into account when working with the mechanics of core movement. When profound somatic shifts occur within the core, they usually affect the person's entire outlook on life and tend to be deep and lasting.

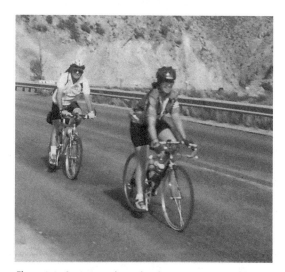

Figure 3.8 A process orientation focuses on the journey rather than the destination (photo courtesy of L. Bright).

Process Orientation

Every SP theme so far has been described as both a concept and a method. As a method, each theme involves a somatic process, which leads us to the fourth theme—**process orientation**. This theme is probably the one that most distinguishes somatic patterning from traditional movement therapies. *During somatic patterning, the focus on the process of change overrides goal orientation.* A person can still have an overall goal and purpose for practicing SP, but during the practice, the primary attention is put on a direct awareness of sensorimotor processes. Most of the SP modalities value a present-moment awareness of the ongoing process of somatic learning as the primary healing agent, a "be here now" philosophy, so to speak (Figure 3.8). Since learning in SP is based on sensorimotor processes, the patterning process is a body-centered sequence of changing experience.

The tricky part about working in a model of process orientation is in knowing where to begin. Since process is an ongoing experience, it could be thought of as a movement sequence, or even a continuum of changes in shape, tone, and effort. Familiarity with the many continuums of movement that exist assists a person in identifying where along the sequence he or she is and indicating in which direction to move to make an integrated sequence of movement.

The survey of primary SP approaches conducted for this book highlighted many continuums of movement patterns in the body. They include the developmental movement continuum of yield-push-reach-pull patterns; the continuum of changing tone from deep relaxation to full-blown exertion; and the continuum of neurological centers that coordinate movement, from spinal and brain stem through hindbrain, midbrain, and forebrain. One continuum that many believe links energy-based models such as Healing Touch (formerly called "Therapeutic Touch") with autonomic models that work to reduce stress is found in the tiers of composition of matter.[71] Energy work meets bodywork on a tactile, cellular level. The movement of millions of molecules and atoms within cells enlivens them. Energy practitioners believe they can positively manipulate this activity by projecting energy from their hands into the client's body, either using direct hands-on contact, or by holding the hands close to the client. SP modalities that address cellular patterning work on an energetic level. This level changes with physiological tone using relaxation exercises, breathing explorations, unstructured organic movement improvisations, techniques that address fluid balance and improve circulation, and energy techniques.

Cells become specialized according to their function; for example, we have muscle, liver, kidney, skeletal, and nerve cells. Each tissue is made up of a specific type of cells, plus varying amounts of fluid and fibers. The tissues are clustered in organs and groups to make up the various body systems, such as the digestive, circulatory, respiratory, nervous, muscular, skeletal, and endocrine systems. In addition, a muscle cell can be considered the "organ" of the muscle system, a neuron (nerve cell) the "organ" of the nervous system, and so on. The combination of these many body systems culminates in the structure of a single organism, that is, in one body.

The relevance of these continuums in regard to process orientation is that during SP, a person can actively focus on the ongoing body processes as they occur on many levels—energetic, cellular and systemic, tissues within various body systems (fluids, muscles, bones, nerves, etc.), and the whole person. Imbalance on any level provides relevant clues about what level and dimension the patterning process needs to occur on. For instance, a person who has physical pain rooted in deep stress (a systemic problem) may feel that the pain is coming from tight muscles, but may work to stretch and reorganize the muscles to no avail because the source of the problem actually lies at a deeper level. Conversely, a person with a lot of stress may work on learning how to relax, yet if the stress is caused by muscle weakness or a lack of coordinated movement, again, the source of the problem exists in a different realm than that being addressed.

Somatic Resonance

Everyone feels **somatic resonance,** the fifth SP theme, on some level, and most people are far more sensitive to it than they realize. Everybody has gut feelings about other people and picks up energetic vibrations upon meeting someone. These subconscious feelings are often rich in an array of intuitive knowledge. The average person can even sense another person in a nearby car, actually sensing through many layers of steel and glass. And people instinctively communicate through the use of body language, resonating with each other's gestures and movements in an intuitive and often incredibly truthful manner. The innate language of the body transmits information on a somatic level via a contraction or expansion of the body, and these natural responses often communicate on a level that goes much deeper than words.

How might a person develop a positive resonance and release dissonance within his or her own body?

Somatic resonance could be compared to a type of body intuition, or intelligence, that manifests through body sensations and subtle responses that can affect the entire body. (People often refer to resonance as "tuning in" or "being in sync," which points to the depth of somatic awareness in common language usage.) Somatic learning can be tracked in levels of resonance, by observing retraction or expansion in one body or between two people. Most if not all of the SP modalities use some form of somatic resonance as a primary form of feedback to guide the patterning process.

Most people can hear resonance in the tone of a person's voice or feel resonance in the sensation of energy flowing through their own bodies. A positive somatic resonance can be seen in two people who move in synchrony, matching or complementing each other's patterns of movement, breath, speech, thought, and vibration. This type of resonance creates deep connections between people.

It has been said that the body never lies because a positive resonance, or rapport, usually creates expansion and relaxation whereas a negative resonance, or dissonance, usually leads to subconscious guarding and holding. The two most basic movement responses, moving toward or drawing away from, reflect a resonance or dissonance between two people. All movement—body language, gestures, and innate unconscious responses to another person—is some combination of these two responses.

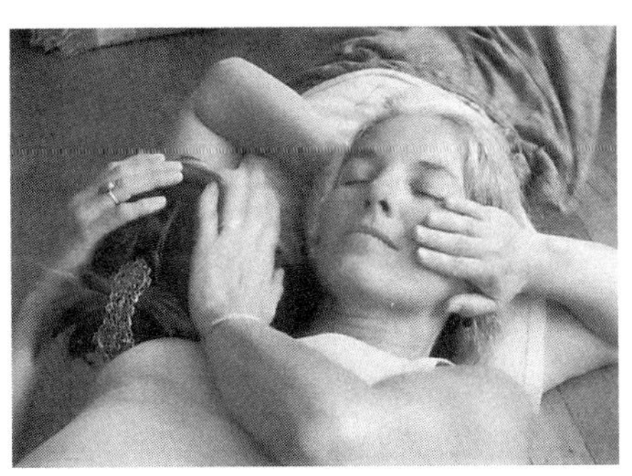

Figure 3.9 Sensing somatic resonance (photo courtesy of M. Seereiter).

Somatic resonance and dissonance show up in many physical and energetic sensations that span a continuum from positive to negative, from bonding to repulsion, from magnetism to revulsion. These innate responses can be felt in a wide range of systemic responses and autonomic symptoms such as chills, goose bumps, sweating, gut feelings, a rush of feelings, nausea, or muscular bracing triggered by a defensive reaction.

Putting Somatic Resonance into Practice

As a technique, a person can use an awareness of somatic resonance or dissonance to guide a hands-on or movement exercise. Noticing whether the tissues relax or retract provides a patterning participant and practitioner with valuable information about whether a patterning activity is working or not. Resonance is used as feedback to direct a patterning process, to deepen somatic awareness to a cellular and vibrational level, and to monitor the exchange of energies either between two aspects of one person or between two people.

A somatic practitioner can work with resonance within a client by identifying where her tissues have vitality and where they lack it. For example, some clients, in their exploration of somatic patterns, have found deep levels of somatic confusion in their bodies, such as reaching out while simultaneously drawing back. In one case, the client was simultaneously attracted and repulsed by what she was reaching for. This awareness helped her understand the tension pattern in her shoulders. She resolved the conflict by making a definite choice about which direction she wanted to reach.

To feel resonance with another, a person needs to make attentional and/or physical contact with another person (Figure 3.9). Practitioners often use deep pressure on the soft tissues to make an assessment, although the authors of *Outcome-Based Massage* point out that even noninvasive contact changes patterns. For example, the noninvasive, sustained tactile contact used to palpate and assess a client's body, if held too long, will begin to *vasodilate* the client's tissues, causing capillaries to relax and more blood to come into the area.[72]

Simply laying the hands on a client is a skill widely practiced in somatic patterning. It is used to bring awareness to the client's body and to calm the client (see Patterning Exercise #117 titled "Cellular Holding" in Chapter 11). Although this type of "listening" touch seems simple, it is often overlooked when the practitioner has a goal or leaps into the application of some type of tissue manipulation. Simple contact, be it through touch or just focused attention, can build rapport between a practitioner and client. It can help a person bring awareness to the body without feeling the need to make an effort to change it. This is a valuable tool because we can become so busy trying to change patterns the we overlook the primary and simple step of first feeling the pattern.

Many types of healing arts practitioners feel that they can channel curative energy through their hands into the client's system to promote healing. Attempts have been made to study the energy emitted by healers and the effects of this energy. A curious study sponsored by the National Institute of Mental Health was done at the Menninger Foundation in the early 1990s.[73] In the Copper Wall Experiment, biofeedback researcher Elmer Green constructed a room with copper walls, floors, and ceilings. Copper was thought by practitioners of Eastern spiritual practices to enhance the link between the conscious and subconscious mind and magnify healing energy. Green measured the energetic changes with a super-sensitive voltmeter and found that healers specializing in energy work were able to produce surges of up to 200 volts, with a median of 8.3 volts.[74] Dr. Richard Gerber also discusses the possibilities of energetic healing in *Vibrational Medicine,* where he presents a wide array of evidence to show that humans can emit healing energies. Gerber feels that with proper training, every person has the ability to change energetic frequencies to affect cellular metabolism in both the self and others.[75]

In respect to SP, the relevance of energetic healing is in the question of who heals whom. In the laying on of hands, a healer believes she is transmitting healing energy to a client through her hands, whereas in somatic patterning, the healing energy or thought is believed to be primarily generated within a client by his own volition. When a person works with a somatic patterner, change occurs as the result of a combination of the efforts and energies of both the client and practitioner, and a resonance of somatic energies. Each party generates energy to effect change within his or her own system, yet the combined energy is exponentially greater than the sum of two single energies. Although the SP practitioner's energy may thus contribute to healing, ultimately, a person must generate his or her own energy to heal from within.

Resonance and Intuition

The psychologist Eugene Gendlin discovered that successful psychotherapy depends on somatic shifts that occur inside the client. He coined the term "felt sense" to describe what happens within the client's body when the gut feelings, thoughts, and emotions align into a moment of healing clarity and insight (see "Focusing" in Chapter 15). Gendlin describes this intuitive experience as a body gestalt in which a person has a profound felt sense of knowing, one grounded in a simultaneous body-based

Patterning Exercise #19: Somatic Exploration with a Partner

During this exploration, notice how your body expands or retracts when it relaxes or tightens up, and where this occurs in your body.

1. *Spatial resonance:* With a partner, explore moving toward and away from each other. As you do this, answer the following questions in your own mind: What happens in your body when you move toward the other person? When that person moves toward you? When you move away from that person? When that person moves away from you? When you turn your back on the other? When the other person turns his/her back on you?
2. *Touch resonance:* Now explore touching each other (PE Fig. 19a). One person touches while the other receives the touch. As you do this, answer the following questions in your own mind: What happens in your body when you receive touch from the other person? When that person touches you? When the touch is at a certain location? When that touch has a specific quality?

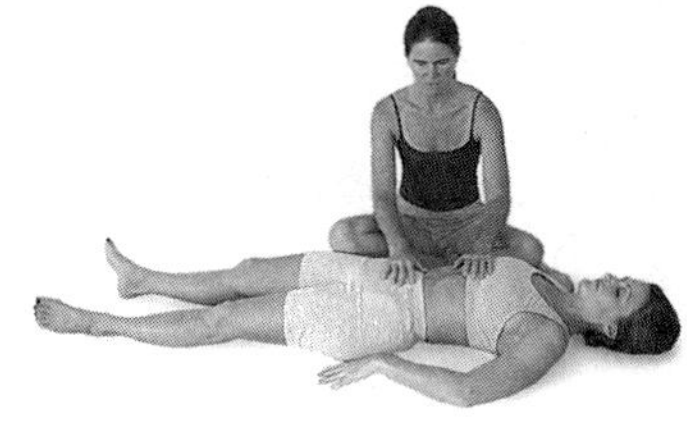
PE Fig. 19a

3. Explore different qualities of touch, such as strong, light, direct, indirect, moving, nonmoving, general, specific, sensitive, rocking, or squeezing. Notice your responses while giving and receiving each type.
4. *Trust exploration:* Stand back to back and sense each other (PE Fig. 19b). Then one of you slowly bend forward and the other one follow by arching over your partner's back, allowing your weight to sink into your partner (PE Fig. 19c). Slowly reverse roles, taking turns yielding your weight into your partner's support. Do you trust that your partner will support you? What quality of your partner promotes this trust?
5. Discuss the exploration with each other.

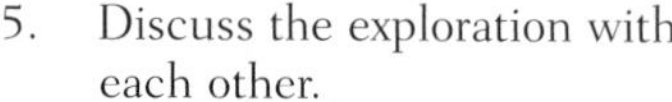

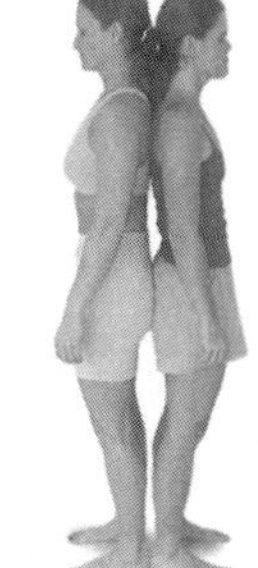
PE Fig. 19b

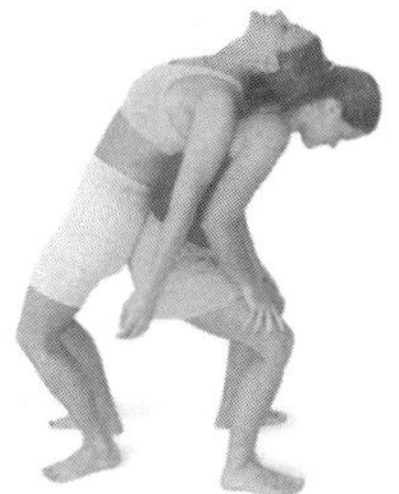
PE Fig. 19c

EMSPress.com

knowing and mental clarity about a troubling issue. The felt sense involves a feeling of somatic resonance that has been described as a type of "body intuition."

It is common for massage therapists, bodyworkers, and somatic practitioners to rely heavily or solely on intuition when practicing hands-on work with clients. **Intuition** is defined as a direct perception of truth, a keen and quick insight not based on cognitive processes and independent of any reasoning process. To integrate intuition with hands-on work, we need to ask what intuition in this realm really means. When a practitioner gets an intuitive feeling about something, is it or is it not accompanied by a body sensation, in either practitioner or client, or both? Without the body level of experience, it seems the intuition could easily be wishful or imaginative thinking. Since many somatic practitioners use imagery as a tool, if we also rely heavily on intuition to guide our work, then we need to ask, "What differentiates intuitive knowing from imagery or mental projection?"

Although everyone gets intuitive hunches now and then, how do we measure the accuracy of true intuition? There are medical intuitives, usually women, with unusual abilities to diagnose serious medical problems through intuitive channels. Obviously, their viability is measured by the accuracy of their diagnoses, which is amazingly high, often more accurate than an average physician's accuracy. Neurosurgeon and medical intuitive Mona Lisa Schulz describes how intuitive knowing comes through a different channel in every person, such as imagery, tone, impression, and physiological symptoms. Schulz also distinguishes her practice as a medical intuitive from her medical practice, describing it as a process of helping a client get in touch with health problems that manifest in emotional issues.[76]

But for some practitioners and SP participants, relying on intuition rather than body-based feedback to make somatic decisions can create problems because the mind can be lightning quick in interpreting the meaning of a hunch, vision, or sensation. Like our movement responses, perceptual channels can also easily become habitual. Thus, what we habitually interpret as intuitive knowing may actually only be the mind's tendency to jump to premature conclusions; what we judge as experiential knowing may actually only be wishful thinking. But there is a certain amount of general physiological feedback coming from the body that can be measured and assessed with a fair degree of accuracy by a person with training and experience in tracking somatic responses. If we rely on accurate feedback from the body to guide somatic patterning, we can keep a handle on what is actually occurring in the body and avoid the shortcomings of intuitive methods. Identifying the difference between what is genuinely intuitive, what is body-based response, and what is the mind's projection can help in making real and lasting positive changes in any somatic modality.

Feedback and Objectivity

We have to know where we are coming from to know where we are going; therefore, working with body patterns requires accurate feedback. Somatic resonance provides basic sensorimotor feedback about how a patterning process is going. When it is going well, the body generally feels open and resonant; when it is not going well, we often experience dissonance.

Another important feedback mechanism in changing body patterns is feeling the difference between the old and the new pattern. Feeling this difference may be more important than actually making changes because this feeling will always be available to remind us whether we are slipping into an old pattern or continuing with the new. Also, without contrast, there is no measure of what learning has occurred. And just recalling the image or sensation of a healthy pattern can help a person recreate it.

Positive feedback provides motivation and makes progress more evident. If a person takes the time to remember

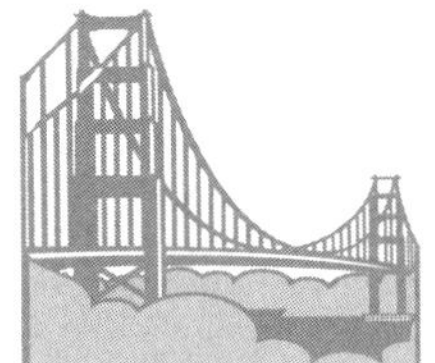

Bridge to Practice

Giving Helpful Feedback

Most people are oriented toward getting rid of all the "bad" things about their bodies rather than building the good. In addition, the eye is more easily drawn to distortion than to integration, and it is easy to be critical of body patterns, especially one's own. To respect the somatic sensitivity of other people, especially in a learning or therapeutic environment, and even cultivate it, you need to balance critical evaluation with objective, positive feedback. Here are some parameters to help you do so:

- Give objective feedback. To be objective, state what you see as if you were describing movement to a blind person. Avoid using interpretive language. For example, rather than saying, "You look depressed," you could describe what you see and say, "Your shoulders look heavy and pulled, your ribcage sunken, and your breathing shallow."
- Be compassionate. Use kind, gentle words to identify the strengths and positive changes about a pattern. This will counterbalance seemingly negative feedback about faulty patterns. Even negative feedback can become positive when it identifies what works along with what doesn't.
- Look for integration. Identify the integrated aspects of movement and posture.
- Preface critical remarks. When giving challenging or critical feedback, start with this statement: "This is what I see, and it may not be accurate." Then ask the person receiving the feedback if it fits.
- Couch negative feedback with consequences. For example, you might say, "If you keep slouching, your back pain will probably get worse." With an awareness of consequences, a person can make informed choices.
- Limit the amount of feedback to digestible portions. The less feedback given, the easier it is to process.
- Pause after giving feedback. This gives a person time to hear it, take it in, digest it, and respond to it. If you sense your recipient is confused, offer clarification.

Patterning Exercise #20: Setting Up a Feedback Loop

Before each patterning exercise, set up a feedback loop so that you can track positive changes and motivate yourself.

1. To set up a feedback loop, walk around the room. Notice how your pelvis moves as you walk. What jumps out when you begin noticing your body, a body part, a feeling or sensation, a quality or shape, etc.? Take note of your first impression.
2. Then ask what pathway or shape your movement takes or makes. How does your foot contact the floor? What kind of flow or restrictions do you feel as you walk? Do you feel any pain, tension, or uncomfortable sensations? If so, where? What is your breathing like? Make a mental or written note of whatever you find.

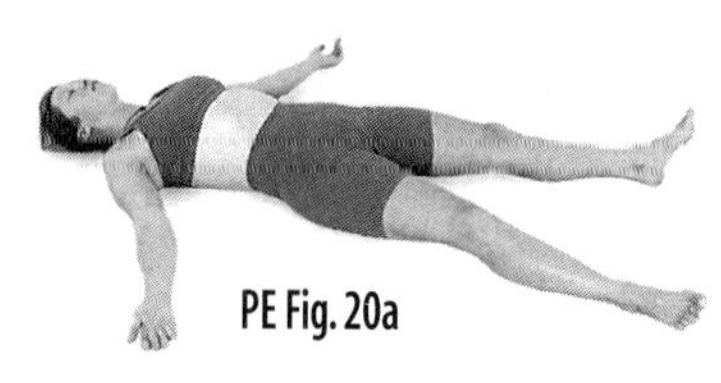
PE Fig. 20a

3. Now lie down on your back, preferably on soft carpet or an exercise mat, with both legs straight (PE Fig. 20a). Which parts of your body and/or spine touch the floor? Which parts move with your breath and which do not?
4. Next, practice a patterning exercise (which you choose at random and can be any of the movement exercises in this text). For example, take leg flexion and extension. To do this exercise, bend one leg and slide your heel along the floor toward your pelvis. As you move, monitor and release any excessive tension or effort you feel in your body. Use as little effort as possible, keeping your back relaxed and trunk stable, your abdomen dropped toward your lower back, and your spine long.

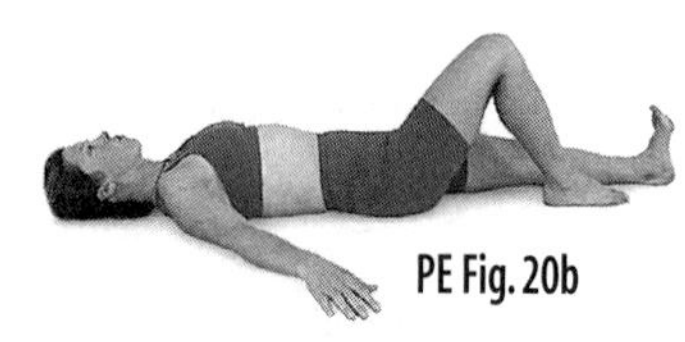
PE Fig. 20b

5. Rest your leg for a moment in the bent knee position, again scanning your body for tension and releasing it (PE Fig. 20b). Then extend your leg by sliding your heel along the floor until your knee and hip are straight.
6. Repeat the flexion and extension cycle several times. Move slowly, monitoring the rest of your body and releasing excess tension and effort, but also finding how to contract the right muscles to keep your body stable.
7. Rest for a minute and compare the two sides. Are they different? You could even get up and walk around to compare the two sides at this point.
8. Lie back down and repeat the exercise on the other side.

Closing the feedback loop: Pause, then stand up slowly and walk around. How is walking different from when you first started?

EMSPress.com

where he or she started, then comparing now to then makes progress more recognizable. Yet one major problem with feedback is that somatic processes are highly subjective so that objective feedback can be difficult to obtain. Recall the tendency for perceptual distortion in familiar feedback, for example, the tendency to believe that we are standing up straight when in fact we may be habitually leaning forward or backward. This was an issue for the developer of the Alexander Technique. Alexander was an actor with chronic laryngitis who found that he could not rely on his senses for accurate feedback. Alexander set up a system of three-way mirrors to watch how he was moving his head and neck to understand what was causing his problem. He discovered that he had the bad habit of depressing his throat in preparation to speak. He was able to inhibit this habit only with the help of mirrors. He not only cured his laryngitis but was inspired to develop what is now one of the oldest systems of postural education based on head righting responses (see Chapter 11).

Recall from Chapter 1 that we all have tendencies toward some degree of sensorimotor amnesia that distorts an accurate perception of body processes. The mind's ability to quickly interpret sensation complicates somatic learning processes. This is why children learn more readily: their thought processes are not mature enough to run interference.

Patterning is often complicated by the influence of the perceptions and beliefs held by the practitioner or the participant. A look at the dynamics of quantum physics highlights how perception and beliefs affect therapeutic exchange. Most physicists accept the Copenhagen interpretation of quantum mechanics, which maintains that the behavior of what is being observed depends, according to Heinz Pagels, "as much on how an object is observed, as on what we elect to see."[77]

Physicists found that even on an atomic level, the observer influences the movement of atoms simply by observing them. This implies that internal body processes are greatly influenced by the attitude a person takes toward the body. Likewise, a teacher or practitioner influences the client or student by mere observation. Therefore, any preconceived ideas about posture or movement have a great influence on the patterning process and on therapeutic exchanges. Although we need an image of integration to guide the patterning process, to initially observe our body-mind patterns as objectively as possible, we must suspend any ideals or images of how we *should*

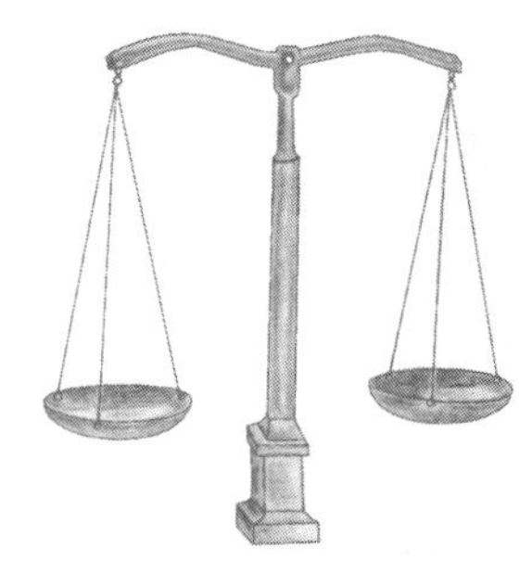
Figure 3.10 An oscillation between dualities balances somatic process

move while at the same time realizing that pure objectivity is impossible. The lens through which we choose to observe will always tint our observations.

Oscillation between Dualities

Movement is what happens between two points. Therefore, it seems only natural that oscillating one's attention between two elements will generate a third factor: a new possibility, a healing element. The body exists in a field of dualities, thus providing endless possibilities of elements to focus on.

The sixth and last SP theme is this basic but important **oscillation between dualities** (Figure 3.10). The concept of oscillation shows up in many of the somatic modalities—on various levels and in numerous ways. In essence, it involves the intentional movement of attention or focus between two elements of a duality to restore a balanced and working relationship between them. In its application as a technique, oscillation requires a person to volley attention between two balancing elements, such as thought and action, thought and feeling, or thought and movement. The oscillation of attention can also be used more mechanically. For example, during a patterning exercise, a person can volley attention between what is moving in the body and what is not, or can notice where muscle tone needs to be relaxed and where it needs to be increased. Or a person can oscillate focus between flexion and extension cycles, or between contractions of an agonist and the extension of its antagonist muscle. Probably the most fundamental tool with which to oscillate between dualities is the practice of following the **breath cycle** in and out of the body with a focused awareness.

Since this theme includes many topics that are addressed in more detail throughout the rest of the book, the discussion on this concept will be briefer than the other concepts. Several dualities will be discussed in the next chapter (establishing support before movement, balancing motility with mobility, and balancing organic with mechanical movement, to name a few) and will be evident throughout the rest of the text as well.

SUMMARY

In the survey of SP modalities conducted for this text (see Part 3), six primary elements were found in common among all the major somatic patterning modalities. The modalities were chosen for review based on two criteria: that they work to change patterns of movement in the body, mind, or physiology, and that they use techniques of either proprioceptive neuromuscular facilitation (changing neuromuscular patterns with awareness), or autonomic proprioceptive facilitation (changing physiological tone with awareness). Each of the six elements—holism, somatic awareness, core movement, somatic resonance, process orientation, and an oscillation between dualities—is applied as an underlying concept for a modality and/or a technique.

Holism is a theory based on an inseparable connection among all the parts of a living being. It is applied in SP by taking into account all aspects of a person's pattern and treating them in the context of the whole. Somatic awareness is based on a sensory awareness of physical processes, as well as an awareness of how perceptions and thoughts relate to physical patterns. Core movement is both physical and psychological, including any movement that initiates within the center of the body, or an experience that initiates as a result of a person's active volition and choice.

Process orientation involves a commitment to maintaining an awareness during SP of what is happening in the present moment regardless of the goals a person has set for patterning. Somatic resonance is a phenomenon in which tissues resonate at a vibrational and energetic frequency that ranges from expansive to compressed, manifesting in either a positive or dissonant response. This phenomenon can be tracked and used as feedback to guide the patterning process because positive changes usually manifest in an expansion of a person's energy and a relaxation of tissues, whereas negative changes usually involve somatic retraction and contraction. Finally, the oscillation between dualities balances the modulating elements in any somatic patterns such as body and mind, organic and mechanical processes, or sensory and motor processes.

The reader is encouraged to look for these elements in the following chapters and within Part 2 of the text to deepen an understanding of how these elements constitute the underlying concepts and methods in somatic patterning. In Chapter 4, we will look at how a single pattern can be approached through a number of different body-mind channels. We'll also consider the various approaches to SP, how to balance them within a single session, and how to choose the best approach for different types of problems.

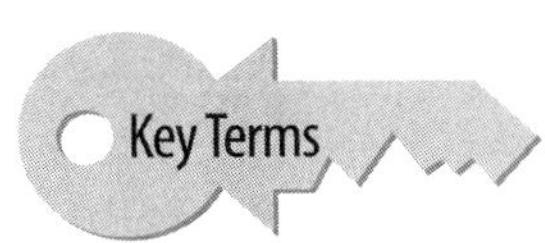

autonomic proprioceptive facilitation (APF)
breath cycle
core movement
energy
holism
intuition
kinesthesia
oscillation between dualities
perception
perceptual shift
process orientation
proprioceptive neuromuscular facilitation (PNF)
sensory awareness
somatic resonance

OVERVIEW OF CHAPTER 4

A COLLECTION OF APPROACHES

PSYCHOSOMATIC APPROACHES
- Cognitive Therapy and Behavioral Approaches
  - *Neurolinguistic Programming*
  - *Visualization in Healing Illness and Trauma*
- Brain Centers and Their Associated Patterns
  - *Forebrain, Midbrain, and Hindbrain*
  - *The Cellular "Brain"*
  - *Emotional Intelligence: The Brain as an Organ*
- The Body-Mind Dilemma: Patterning or Psychotherapy

A NEUROLOGICAL APPROACH
- Autonomic Patterning
  - *The Relaxation Response*
  - *Organic Movement Practices*
- Neuromuscular Patterning
  - *Reflexes*
  - *Developmental Patterning*

MODULATING DUALITIES
- Balancing Experiential, Body-Based Learning with Cognitive Learning
- Reflexive and Reflective Movement Coordination
- Integrating Facilitation and Inhibition
- Sensory and Motor Balance
- Establishing Support before Movement

INNER AND OUTER BALANCE BETWEEN ANS AND SNS
- Motility and Mobility
- Balancing Organic and Mechanical Approaches
  - *Organic Movement*
  - *The Workings of Mechanical Movement*

Balancing Patterning Approaches

4

When the only tool you have is a hammer, every problem looks like a nail.

—Abraham Maslow

In the last chapter, the six themes that make up the underlying concepts and methods found in somatic patterning modalities—holism, somatic awareness, core movement, process orientation, somatic resonance, and the oscillation between dualities—were introduced. Now the topic turns to the question of how to balance these various themes and their complex elements within the patterning process. In this chapter, various approaches to somatic patterning will be discussed, as well as how different methods of patterning can address the same problem. Also discussed will be how the approach a person chooses—be it the practitioner, client, or anyone practicing patterning—depends on that person's perception of what is causing the problem.

There are a handful of overriding approaches to SP; among them are movement education, sensory awareness training, cognitive restructuring, biofeedback, and body-based psychotherapies. What all these approaches have in common is that they are experiential: they are based on the perception of movement processes (both physiological and physical), and they strive to reintegrate the body and mind through both cognitive and sensorimotor learning. This chapter presents a theoretical overview of the individual patterning methods that will be developed in greater detail in Part 2.

This group of approaches can seem confusing and may bring up questions about what type of patterning to use when. Basically, any work with body-mind patterns proceeds along two basic tracks—the experiential, body-based *process* of sensorimotor function, and the mind-based perceptual *practice* of awareness. Together they establish the ground upon which SP is built.

The purpose of this chapter is to shed some light on how a person can weave many diverse elements into a simple process in order to make it as useful as possible for a particular somatic problem. The chapter will focus on the primary patterning choices we need to consider when attempting to balance the many modulating dualities inherent in somatic processes. The primary dualities covered here make up the operating precepts of SP. They include mental and physical approaches, mechanical and organic approaches, attention and intention, and reflexive movement and reflective thinking. We will also consider the necessity of establishing support before movement and of balancing autonomic with neuromuscular processes.

To balance patterning approaches, a person first needs to be aware of the many different approaches available and then must be able to discern which approach to use when and how best to proceed. A person usually chooses an approach congruent with the channel of awareness through which he perceives the problem. To illustrate this point, we'll look at a variety of approaches that a fictitious man struggling with a bent-over posture could take.

A COLLECTION OF APPROACHES

Meet Henry, a middle-aged man who suffers from a hunched, stooped posture (Figure 4.1). Henry has weak muscles on the back of his body and tight muscles on the front—his flexor tone overpowers his extensor tone, pulling his body in a chronic C-curve. Naturally, anyone stuck in chronic flexion has to lift the head to see where he or she is going; hence, the spine takes on a shape that, when viewed from the side, resembles an up-side down question mark.

If four different somatic practitioners worked with Henry, each might offer a different solution. The body-worker would probably massage and stretch Henry's tight muscles. The physical therapist would probably release the joint restrictions and teach Henry exercises to strengthen his weak muscles. The psychotherapist would probably work with Henry to resolve his burdened and bent outlook on life. Lastly, the developmental patterner would stimulate Henry's extensor reflexes to increase tone on the back of his body. (These are just a few of the options available; many more are presented in Part 2.)

Ultimately, the patterning solution would depend on Henry's own perception of the problem, the symptoms he feels, and whether his physical or emotional pain is overriding. Henry may feel damaged by his postural aberration, he may have obsessive thoughts about being stuck in this position, or he may even ruminate over unresolved emotions from a trauma, pathology, or painful events that led to his condition. The lens through which Henry perceives his pattern determines the approach he will probably take. (We'll assume, for the sake of discussion, that Henry's doctor has ruled out diseases such as osteoarthritis.)

If our fictitious man discerns that his problem comes from tight muscles, he might take a purely structural approach, one in which he attempts to change his structure without changing his neurological pathways, without actively reorganizing how he moves. To do this, Henry might actively stretch over backwards to elongate the front of his body, or passively lie backwards over a large ball, or even have a massage therapist stretch his muscles for him.

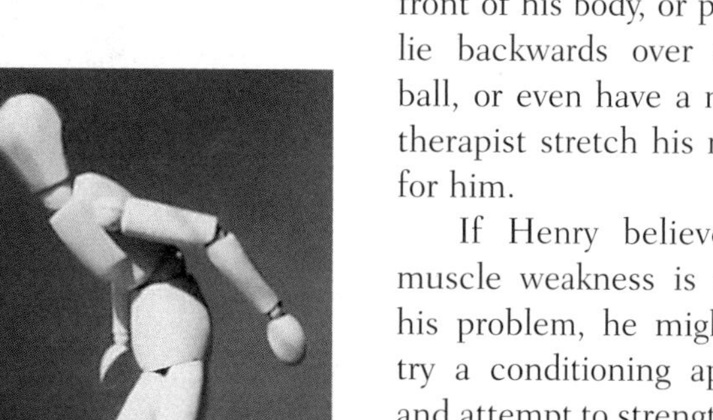
Figure 4.1 The fictitious Henry

If Henry believes that muscle weakness is causing his problem, he might even try a conditioning approach and attempt to strengthen his back muscles. Most people are familiar with the value of stretching and conditioning to correct muscle imbalances. They can both be done with a minimal awareness or understanding of anatomy. But in Henry's case, stretching and conditioning will only be effective if his stooped posture is caused by a combination of weak and overworked muscles. Yet, if he practices only sit-ups, his condition could worsen because it will increase his already too strong flexor tone.

Although muscle imbalances certainly sustain Henry's problem, they may not be at the root of the problem. Our fictitious character may be walking under the oppression of his negative self-image or struggling with a general psychological malaise that burdens him. He may even be a socially inept person who uses his posture to shy away from facing people, or he may be gripped with an obsessive fear of falling or of making a mistake. If Henry feels any of these things, he might choose a psychosomatic approach and begin to figure out what thoughts, memories, and emotions underlie his chronically flexed posture. He may even seek body-centered psychotherapy to learn how to deal with his fears, resolve his self-esteem issues, learn to relax, and as a result, begin to stand up straight.

Some would argue that a psychosomatic approach is imperative since every body pattern has a related psychological pattern. This is undeniable, but the situation is circular. Which came first—the posture or the effects associated with it? Perhaps Henry fell down a flight of stairs at age four and severely damaged his spine, and over time grew into his crippling posture. Or perhaps Henry gradually bent over while under a long-term situation of emotional duress and eventually found security in his psychological armor. In the last case, straightening his posture might only exacerbate his vulnerability.

Or perhaps Henry just learned bad habits from his parents, who might have considered a stooped posture normal. In this case, changing his habits might only require a cognitive and mechanical process of correction, one absent of emotional charge. In a purely cognitive, top-down approach, our model would begin to examine which activities take him into flexion and which take him into extension, and then change them accordingly. Or he might work on self-image, figuring out what images he associates with the bent posture and then starting to build new ones. He could learn to replace negative activities and images with positive ones, slowly reshaping his posture with deliberate thought and action.

If Henry took a neurological approach—which basically all patterning is on some level because the nervous system regulates all body function—he would learn to reorganize how his nervous system sets tone and coordinates movement. To do this, Henry might learn to lower the high autonomic tone that underlies his physical stress by consciously relaxing his body, or he might work to change his neuromuscular habits. By learning to activate and contract the weak muscles on his back side while relaxing the overworking muscles on his front side, in time Henry would gain control over his muscle patterns and would gradually build the muscular balance and coordination needed to pull his spine up straight.

Neuromuscular patterning requires a number of skills, such as being able to feel the difference between contraction, relaxation, and stretch within a muscle, and to control the rate, order, and duration of contraction among a group of muscles. Add to this the many forms a person can use to guide the *style* of movement (such as dance, sports, martial arts, and yoga), or the paradigms a person can use to guide the *mechanics* of movement (such as joint physiology, early motor development, and a study of reflexes), and the complexity of choices in neuromuscular patterning becomes evident.

If Henry chose to work with reflexes, he would need to identify which reflexes were overpowering and which were weak, then develop the weak reflexes. In this case, Henry's flexor reflexes are shortening the front of his body much like a taught string bends a bow. The flexor reflexes on the front are overpowering the extensor reflexes along his back. Working with reflexes is probably the most obscure approach to neuromuscular patterning because it requires not only an understanding of reflexes (which most practitioners lack), but also the ability to let go of mental control over the body in order to explore the spontaneous, automatic movement qualities inherent in reflexes. The paradox of working with reflexes is that they are automatic and cannot be elicited through controlled movement. They can only be elicited through the spontaneous, automatic movement responses that people make in activities like play and sports. A trained eye can spot a steady stream of reflexes in a group of young children hard at play, and conversely, can identify the missing reflexes in a group of stiff, clumsy adults struggling with coordination in an exercise class. Good athletes develop strong reflexes because participating in sports forces a person to respond to environmental challenges with quick and reflexive turns, jumps, and leaps.

The fun part about working with reflexes is that they are playful and challenging, surprising and energetic. In light of this, it seems highly unlikely that the stooped Henry would gravitate toward working with reflexes since his posture is so limited in energy and perspective—literally! Imagine the perspective of a person in a bent-over posture, looking at the ground, struggling just to lift the head. It has to be depressing, even oppressive. Yet surprisingly, working with the reflexes would probably help Henry the most because without the underlying extensor reflexes, no amount of muscle stretching, strengthening, or mental control will create neurological balance in his spine.

There is also a simple approach that Henry could use to work with his postural problem, so simple that it is often overlooked. It is based on the use of awareness and intention to correct muscle imbalance. This approach is crucial to any effective patterning program. To do it, Henry would simply learn how to stand up straight, then would need to monitor his posture all day long and regularly correct himself whenever he found himself stooping. Although this approach sounds simple—who can't just stand up straight?—it is not easy. It requires diligence and a clear image of upright posture (Figure 4.2). What makes this approach difficult is that a person needs to make the correction more often than he does the faulty pattern, which, depending on the severity of the posture, could be every few minutes or every few seconds. To use awareness and intention effectively to change posture, Henry would need to replace his faulty habit with a better posture every single time he felt himself stooping. Whether or not anyone is willing to put in this type of commitment to change a body pattern is questionable. It requires working at an edge, using extreme willpower that borders on obsession.

This discussion of Henry's options makes evident the numerous approaches a person can take to changing a single pattern. No one approach is better than another. The more levels of the pattern that are addressed, the more likely that positive changes will occur. It is, however, crucial for effective SP that the muscle patterns always be addressed. Muscles hold us up and move us. We have to actively change *how* we use our muscles to effect changes in how we posture and move. Passive stretching and conditioning will not directly reorganize neuromuscular patterns, but they are preferable to doing nothing at all to address a faulty body pattern.

If a pattern is rooted in psychological issues, this must also be addressed. Psychosomatic approaches to changing body patterns are probably the most common methods used to supplement somatic patterning. However, even if a person does not receive psychotherapy, the effects of psychological issues on the body need to be addressed, specifically when they affect autonomic tone and manifest as physiological symptoms of stress. The importance of balancing work with muscle patterns and with autonomic patterns is expanded upon later in this chapter.

Henry, like all of us, has numerous options for solving his postural problem. They include stretching and conditioning as well as different types of SP. A brief discussion of these methods—psychosomatic, cognitive, and autonomic approaches, neuromuscular patterning, working

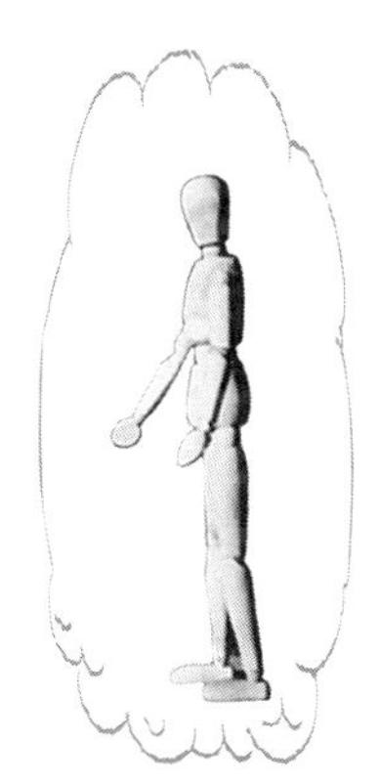

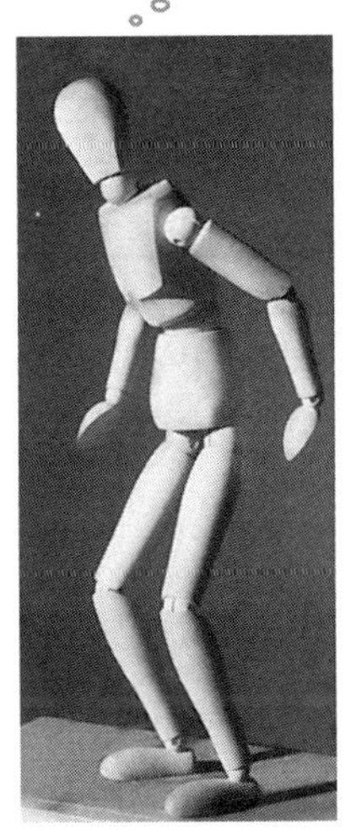

Figure 4.2 Henry holding the image of standing up straight to guide him

with reflexes, and using awareness and intention to make postural corrections—follows.

PSYCHOSOMATIC APPROACHES

The essence of SP is actively changing tone. Tone, which will be discussed in Chapter 5, manifests in the shape of a person's posture and the quality of the body's movement. Most people are familiar with muscle tone and the tone of voice; for now, think of the body's tone as its personality or attitude. A psychosomatic approach requires an oscillation of attention between a person's psychological issues and attitudes and their effects on the tone of the body.

Often when a person resolves psychological issues, the posture that supported that issue changes. Still, changing one's psychological outlook does not necessarily change muscle patterns. Therefore, if a person chooses a psychosomatic approach to changing faulty posture and movement patterns, this approach needs to be accompanied by some kind of neuromuscular patterning. This can involve many different types of neuromuscular education or can be as simple as monitoring a muscle pattern and making periodic corrections.

Some somatic practitioners feel that the emotions provide the crucial link between body and mind processes. They define emotion as, literally, "e-motion"—the motion of energy through the body. A person's quality of movement and posture can have, at any given time, an emotional tone to it, or it can seem to be devoid of emotion. In this view, movement that expresses emotions can provide an integrating link between the body and mind. Reichian and bioenergetic psychotherapists view emotional responses carried out in movement as the primary elements shaping posture and character, both literally and figuratively. In short, they believe that people block the sensations of painful emotions by chronically holding specific muscle groups. Reichian psychotherapists work with psychological patterns by promoting the flow of emotion through the body via expressive movement, thereby resolving the psychological issues that underlie postural fixations (see Chapter 15).

Cognitive Therapy and Behavioral Approaches

As mentioned in the case of Henry, a simple patterning technique is to become aware of maladaptive body-use habits or thoughts and replace them with balanced patterns every time they occur. Although the process is simple, many people find it difficult to have the discipline to do it whenever a maladaptive pattern shows up. Still, the number of repetitions needed to make a positive change depends upon the strength and duration of the faulty patterns. When successful, the outcome is that, with repetition, a balanced muscular pattern becomes stronger than a faulty pattern, and positive thought patterns gradually replace negative thought patterns.

Cognitive therapy is a form of psychotherapy in which a person learns to change maladaptive thought patterns associated with psychological problems. Behavioral approaches address the behaviors that then carry out these thought patterns. In an example of a cognitive therapy, psychologist Martin Seligman developed "learned optimism" in which clients learn to become aware of their dualistic thought patterns, where they view the world through a black-and-white filter, seeing everything as either right or wrong, good or bad. People then work with dualities in order to replace negative thoughts with positive thoughts and, with practice, are able to emphasize the positive side of dualistic thinking or even stop thinking dualistically.[78]

In SP, this process is helpful particularly when used in conjunction with an awareness of body patterns. To apply this same principle to muscular patterns, let's look at how postural muscles are trained. It is recommended that to restore normal function, a person isometrically contract and hold a particular postural muscle for at least ten seconds, then relax it completely. It is not enough to just hold a muscle contracted because oscillating between contraction and relaxation helps us learn to tell the difference between when the muscles are on and off. This type of isometric contraction and relaxation is done 30 times each, three times a day (for a total of 90 times). Most people are just not willing to put in that kind of time. Yet, if people can begin to understand that working postural muscles is easy because it requires only light isometric contractions in postural muscles that can be practiced anywhere—in a car, on an airplane, and even while waiting in line at the bank—the task is not so daunting.

A person can use the same technique to change maladaptive behavioral patterns. For example, suppose a person has a habit of becoming angry at the slightest provocation. This pattern not only creates conflicts with other people, but it causes this person an enormous amount of internal tension as well. To change the pattern, the person needs to address the anger anytime it flares up. This means calming the body, inhibiting the urge to act on it, and detaching from thoughts that come along with the feeling of anger.

Healthy detachment from the content or meaning of a habitual behavior is an extremely important part of changing that behavior. This is the basis of neurolinguistic programming (NLP), a method for change that evolved out of a study of the dynamics, rather than content, of effective psychotherapy (see Chapter 14).

Neurolinguistic Programming

The founders of NLP watched tapes of psychotherapists and their clients, noting which gestures and language patterns resulted in effective outcomes and which did

Patterning Exercise #21: Rewriting Stressful or Traumatic Memories

1. Recall a stressful or traumatic situation that you could not cope with at the time.
2. Sense the effect the memory of this situation has on you; feel the physical sensations it creates.
3. Now embellish your memory with a positive ending by visualizing a different outcome. Imagine you are in the original situation, then visualize the outcome you want. Do your physical sensations change from before?
4. Visualize the new outcome again and again and again, in one session and over days and weeks, until it becomes automatic and dissipates the stress of the event you are working to resolve.

Application: Every time you have this stressful memory during the course of your days, counter it with the positive outcome you have imagined, or with a healing or relaxing visualization, such as your ideal vacation or the memory of a time you felt really happy and secure.

EMSPress.com

not, while essentially ignoring the actual content of the sessions. They found that we communicate through channels—primarily visual, auditory, and kinesthetic—which are obvious in the verbs a person chooses. For example, three women might describe the same situation through different channels, one person describing what she *saw*, another what she *heard*, and another what she *felt*. The various channels also occur in sequences, for example, someone might say, "I saw (visual) that she felt overwhelmed (kinesthetic) when she raised her voice (auditory) to explain the problem."

In essence, the channels we habitually use determine how we experience life. The premise of NLP is that by reorganizing our channels and changing our sequences of thought, we can change our behaviors, improve our communication styles, and, basically, have more success in our lives. Although NLP came out of a study of psychotherapy, it is not psychotherapy. It addresses *how* we experience while bypassing *what* we experience.

Visualization in Healing Illness and Trauma

Visualization can be another powerful mental or cortical tool for changing somatic patterns. Healing visualizations are widely used in the field of psychoneuroimmunology (see Chapter 12), where images such as immune system cells vacuuming up cancer cells, white healing light entering with each breath to burn out toxins, or wounds shrinking and closing are employed. These cortically controlled images have been proven to help the body heal itself from disease and to improve skeletal alignment.[79]

Visualization is also used in the healing of emotional trauma. Memory is, in a sense, a visualization of a past event. Memories work in a similar manner to defenses: they fade over time or become embellished with more details and grow stronger. As mentioned in Chapter 1, repeatedly recalling a traumatic memory can increase the physiological charge of the memory.

What makes events traumatic or stressful is not so much the events themselves, but our response to them. The trauma specialist Lenore Tarr highlights this essential component of trauma in her study of the long-term effects on a group of 26 children who were kidnapped and imprisoned in an underground chamber for thirty hours. Most of the children remained frozen in fear, but one enterprising youngster actually dug a small tunnel through the ceiling of the vault that eventually led to the group's escape. Tarr found in her follow-up study that all the children suffered post traumatic stress syndrome (PTSD) except the child who dug his way out. She concludes that since this child was able to successfully move through the experience, he resolved his trauma more readily.[80]

Tarr's study suggests that the response a person has to trauma determines the long-term effects of the trauma. It also suggests that if a person is unable to move out of the trauma in the actual situation, she can do it later by rewriting her memories, a process that seems to fool the brain. It is only natural to embellish memories; thus by visualizing a positive response to a stressful situation enough times, eventually the brain adapts to the new image, and the adaptation response, over time, diminishes and eventually dissipates the physiological stress related to the trauma.

Brain Centers and Their Associated Patterns

It is beyond the scope of this book to describe specific and complex brain centers and their associated movement patterns in detail. Yet a basic understanding of the relationships among four brain centers can shed some useful light on different approaches to patterning. To understand the quality of movement coordinated at different neurological levels, we can think of the movement responses coordinated by the human brain as having four primary divisions based on embryonic anatomy. The first three centers, the forebrain, midbrain, and hindbrain, are familiar parts of the brain's anatomy, whereas the fourth, the "cellular brain," is a relatively new somatic concept that is not part of the generally accepted anatomy of the nervous system. This concept stems from the view that the nervous system permeates every minute part of the body, manifesting in the ability of each tissue and cell to effect changes in local processes generally thought to be under the control of the brain alone.

Forebrain, Midbrain, and Hindbrain

The **forebrain** is a general area of the brain made up of the *cerebrum* and *cerebral cortex*. The cerebral cortex has a coordinating role in the organization of neuromuscular pathways that can be compared to a project manager or overseer of movement patterns. The cortex coordinates reflective, or self-aware, thought patterns, including creative, analytical, and rational thinking. It also registers and records the movement patterns coordinated on all other neurological levels, whether conscious, subconscious, or habitual. Movements coordinated by the cerebral cortex tend to be measured and deliberate. In contrast, movements coordinated by the lower brain centers and the spinal cord are reflexive and spontaneous. Consider the difference between a person dancing freely in an uninhibited style and one dancing slowly, controlling the placement of the body on each step. The first is reflexive movement, the second, more cortically controlled movement. Each has a unique quality, and each reflects a quality of a different part of the nervous system.

The **midbrain** is a small area of the brain that serves as a conduit for information to pass between the forebrain and the hindbrain. This area includes the *diencephalon,* or *"ancient forebrain,"* made up of the thalamus and hypothalamus, an area often referred to as the **limbic system**. Many people refer to this area of the brain as the "emotional brain" because it regulates emotional and glandular responses.

At each neurological level, movement patterns take another evolutionary step. With each step come more complex movement pathways and more elaborate adaptive structures. The movement of marine creatures onto land required new anatomical structures to adapt from water to air. These adaptations include lungs for breathing, limbs and muscles for locomotion on land, and sense organs. When aquatic animals evolved and migrated to land, the limbic system of the midbrain started developing and first appeared in the amphibian frog brain. Developmental movement specialist Cohen associates the midbrain with reach patterns of movement and head righting reactions. This is interesting to note because the movement from water to land was an evolutionary reach up and out of the ocean.

Movement initiated by the limbic system has emotional overtones. Movements governed by emotional reactions often tend to have reactive or defensive qualities; they are the body's "call to arms." Breathing rate and heart rate quicken, the skeletal muscles become poised for action, and the senses sharpen and become more alert when the limbic system is involved. These changes prepare the body for an active response to an emotional state that involves a fight-or-flight reaction.

The bulk of our movement patterns are coordinated in the hindbrain. The **hindbrain** is made up of the *pons*, *cerebellum*, and *medulla oblongata* within the brain stem, which is continuous with the *spinal cord*. This part of the brain coordinates reflexive and autonomic functions such as digestion, breathing, and metabolism. The cerebellum coordinates 90 percent of neuromuscular patterns as well as controlling balance when the body is off-center. A part of the brain stem called the pons is associated with the scanning motion of the eyes following the horizon. Primitive flexor and extensor reflexes are also coordinated at a spinal cord level. These lower brain centers, often referred to as "reptilian," developed in species that live primarily in water.

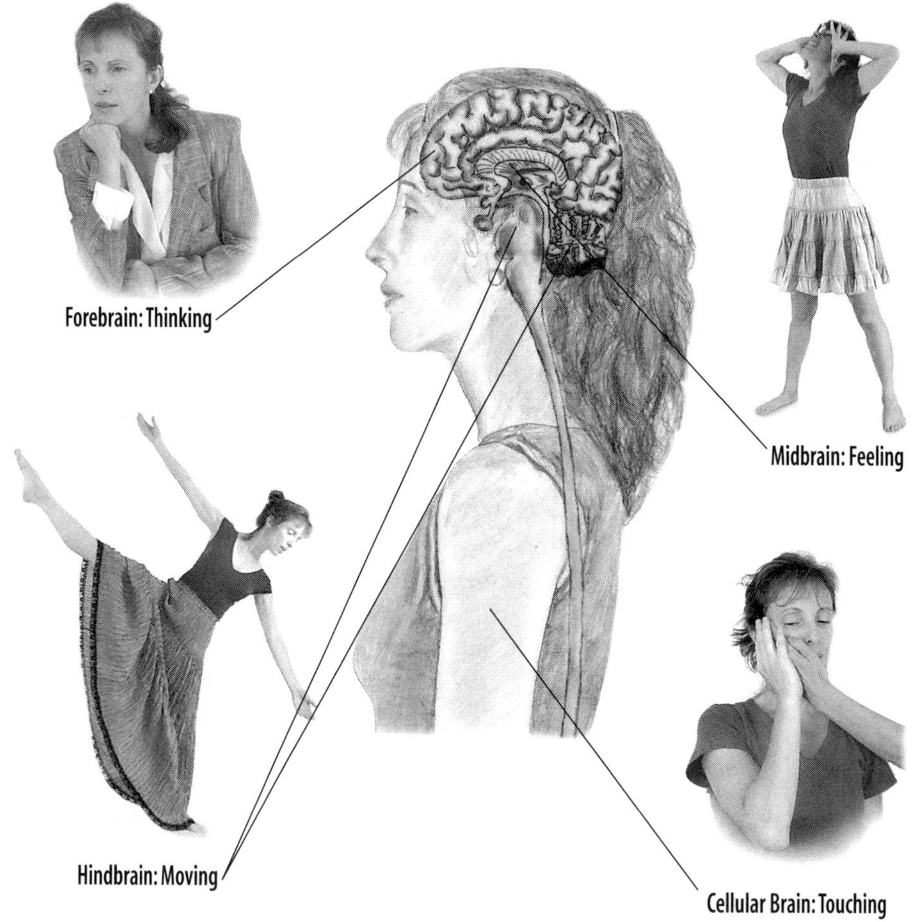

Figure 4.3 A schematic of the behaviors associated with our "quadripartite brain" functions

Patterning Exercise #22: Releasing the Brain as an Organ

Developmental movement specialist Bonnie Bainbridge Cohen believes that sensing weight through the brain, particularly during flexion, releases tension in the central nervous system. She designed this exercise. Mini-versions of it can be done at anytime during the day to release not only tension, but to relax an overactive mind.

1. Sit or stand in a comfortable position. Place one or both hands on your forehead. Let your head sink into your hands (PE Fig. 22a). Sense or visualize the weight of your brain sinking and settling into your forehead.

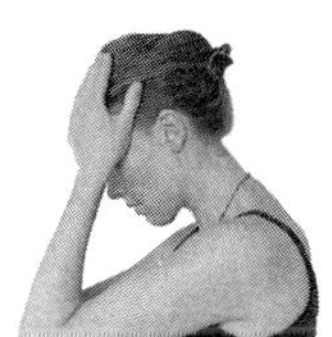

PE Fig. 22a

2. Continue to sense weight in your head-while gradually flexing your spine. Sense one vertebra at a time flexing. Imagine your neck curling like the shape of a sea horse as you sink through your forehead. You may feel a stretch in your neck through around the spine from the dura around the spine stretching. Sense or visualize your spinal cord like a tail on the brain, pulling through the dural tube.
3. Continue to sink forward until you have stretched all the way to your hips and coccyx (PE Fig. 22b). Remain in this position and sense the weight in your head.

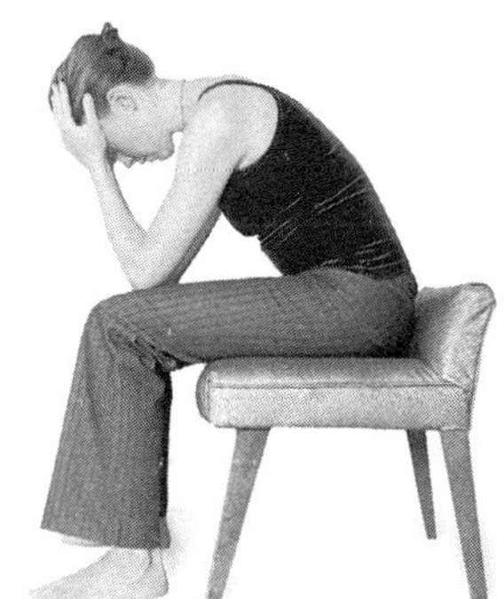

PE Fig. 22b

4. To end, you have two choices: Either lie down and relax, or reverse the movement and sit back up in one action. To lie down and relax, let your body slowly melt into the floor. To reverse the movement, reach your feet and coccyx down into the floor while rolling up in reverse. Come up in one smooth, fluid motion, slow enough to roll through each vertebra yet fast enough to be a single action.

Cohen generally associates the hindbrain with push patterns of movement as opposed to the reach patterns of the midbrain.

The Cellular "Brain"

Systemic cellular processes occur at the bottom of the neurological hierarchy. The primary cellular movements are the metabolic processes that go on within each cell's organelles such as the *cell nucleus*, *mitochondria*, and *ribosomes*. Each organelle can be compared to an organ system in the larger body; each cell basically functions as a body unto itself. For example, each cell has a respiratory system, meaning that it literally breathes by taking in oxygen and eliminating metabolic waste products. Each cell also has a rudimentary nervous system, a "**cellular brain**," so to speak, that makes choices about which substances pass through its membranes and which do not. And each cell has a primitive motor system with two elementary responses that can be observed in an amoeboid-like movement toward or retracting away from tactile stimuli.

Cellular movement is reflected in the earliest patterns identified by developmental specialist Bonnie Cohen—cellular breathing and navel radiation. Both show up in a healthy newborn who has minimal development in the other three centers. Also, one of the primary channels through which a newborn receives stimuli is tactile. Touch elicits systemic responses that are generally reflexive and resonate throughout the infant's body. For example, stroke a baby's foot or hand or cheek and his entire body will move in response. Most mothers soothe their newborns by rocking and singing gently to them, influencing the babies with a comforting quality of touch and a soothing vibration in the voice that communicates on a systemic level.

The view of a "cellular brain" is taking hold in the somatic world. Its most widely accepted application is found in the field of psychoneuroimmunology (see Chapter 13). It is based on many discoveries that the nervous system, immune system, and endocrine system, once thought to function in isolation, actually communicate with each other through an extensive cellular network. People practice PNI with efforts to influence cellular physiology in ways that will promote healing, using such activities as positive thinking and healing visualizations.

The cellular brain is included with the other brain centers that coordinate movement in order to expand our understanding of movement patterns to include the more primitive responses. Every movement is a complex coordination of all neurological levels. Although the nervous system is far too complex to conclude accurately that certain brain centers either initiate or inhibit specific movement patterns, our movement responses could be thought of as reflecting a "quadripartite" brain. The first three levels, the forebrain, midbrain, and hindbrain, are associated with the behaviors of *moving*, *feeling*, and *thinking*. The fourth and most primitive level of cellular processes is associated with primitive responses to tactile stimuli and the behavior of *touching* (Figure 4.3).

Emotional Intelligence: The Brain as an Organ

Why do highly successful, seemingly stable people sometimes fly off the handle and commit crimes of passion without presenting any warning signs of their violent tendencies? Psychologist Daniel Goleman addresses this question in his hypothesis of **emotional intelligence**—a term he coined to describe the qualities of the average person with a stable and thriving life.[81]

Goleman's ideas draw on the work of Joseph LeDoux, a neuroscientist who researched the neural connections between the *amygdala*, the emotional brain center, and the cortex, the rational brain center.[82] LeDoux found that the amygdala has more synapses to the cortex than the cortex has to the amygdala. What this suggests is that a person can experience strong emotions in the amygdala before the cortex can send the message to inhibit irrational responses. Goleman likens the amygdala to an "emotional tripwire" because it sets off irrational and impulsive emotional reactions without input from the cortex. This explains why a seemingly rational and intelligent person can commit acts of violence in a heated moment of passion.

Goleman believes this neural link provides a key to understanding and changing the violent behaviors that are increasing in our culture and our world. If we can individually and collectively learn to practice emotional intelligence skills, then we could strengthen the neural pathways running from the emotional brain centers to the rational brain centers and learn to inhibit and control damaging emotional reactions. These skills involve self-awareness, self-control, empathy, and skills for listening, cooperating, and resolving conflicts, with the primary skill being the ability to think before reacting.

Also, we tend to think of the mind as the brain, yet the brain is an organ whose actual physical health can be influenced. Like any other bodily organ, the brain undergoes changes that occur with aging, such as becoming less hydrated and more fibrous, and having physiological reactions that change its chemistry. We get direct feedback from other organs because they have sensory nerves and their functions generate body sensations. What makes the brain a unique organ is that it is impossible to feel sensations in it because it lacks sensory nerves; we receive feedback about changes in the brain via changes in the body's functions, such as shifts in tone, behavior, and movement. For example, any alteration in brain chemistry can lead to senility or mental illness such as mania or depression, and brain injuries such as strokes can lead to paralysis.

Somatic practitioners generally view the brain as an organ that can be influenced by actively changing the different states of consciousness that the various brain centers produce and the movement patterns that its various parts control. Many somatic practitioners work toward an end similar to what are considered emotional intelligence skills, helping their clients develop a more healthy integration between higher and lower brain centers by helping them learn to control when and how they act upon body sensations and emotional feelings.

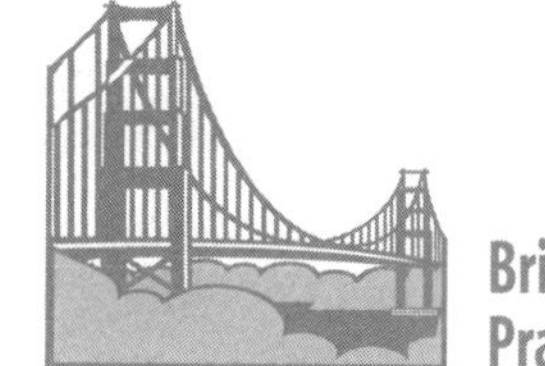

Bridge to Practice

Does Talking Support Healing?

Most people have habits of being overly mental and as a result, tighten up or lose awareness of their bodies during a discussion. Use this type of response as a therapeutic tool. If your client is describing a problem, ask her to notice what is happening in her body as she talks. If talking helps her to relax, then it can be therapeutic. If talking causes her to tighten the body, it may be interfering with the therapeutic process.

Track body-mind integration by noticing when talking helps a client relax and make body-mind connections. Conversation that causes a client to become detached from the body or tense should be discouraged. If this occurs, you might say to your client, "I notice that as you talk, your body tightens up. If you focus on your body and become aware of when you are tightening and when you are relaxing, you will probably get more out of this process." Then encourage your client to sense her body without having to discuss it.

On the other hand, talking about a body experience after it occurs, to reflect on what happened, is a helpful way to integrate the body and mind. People need to understand their experiences, and talking about body changes helps them to put the experiences into context.

The Body-Mind Dilemma: Patterning or Psychotherapy?

All somatic patterns have a psychological component, which creates a dilemma for bodyworkers and somatic practitioners. How can we work with body-mind patterns, yet still maintain boundaries between somatic therapy and psychotherapy? Elliot Greene and Barbara Goodrich-Dunn identify a clear boundary between psychotherapy and massage therapy in their text *The Psychology of the Body.* They encourage massage therapists to refrain from any dialogue that would probe the client for psychological material and would assist the client in processing emotional issues when they arise.[83]

Even though SP practitioners invite the whole person to emerge during a session, patterning is not psychotherapy. Analyzing a psychological process crosses into the arena of psychotherapy, which requires extensive training and experience. SP focuses on psychology as it manifests in physiology and body patterns. By staying focused on working with body patterns, we create a boundary between somatic work and psychotherapy. This does not mean a person should ignore emotional responses. Psychological issues and emotions naturally arise when working with body patterns. In fact, they indicate the degree of connection and integration a person has between the body, mind, and emotions. People often need to be reminded of this when they discount their feelings as extraneous to patterning processes. The practitioner can ask about the psychological reasons for patterns in her own mind to help make better choices, but discussing the "why" is not always useful with clients, for two reasons. It may take the client into

Patterning Exercise #23: Physical and Psychological Movement Sequences

Since each body pattern has a corresponding mental and emotional pattern, you can understand more about your somatic temperament by examining movement sequences on behavioral and physical levels.

1. *Behavioral*: Are you better at planning a task, beginning the task, carrying out the task, finishing the task, or resting afterward? What do your answers to each questions say about your personality?
2. *Physical*: With which type of qualities do you tend to move: quick and impulsive, slow and sustained, deliberate and planned, fluid and relaxed. Are your movements strong or weak? Do you put your whole body into an activity or just move parts?
3. *Psychological:* What do your patterns tell you about your temperament? If you were an actor in a play, what part would your behavioral and physical patterns be playing?

EMSPress.com

psychological content and cross over into psychotherapy, and it may take the client into mental processes and away from body-centered processes.

A person usually undertakes SP with the intention of restoring efficient movement, reducing stress responses, and/or changing bad habits. The essential tools that facilitate somatic processes are awareness, movement, and touch, yet techniques from cognitive therapy, biofeedback, and neurolinguistics are used to address the thoughts and emotions that maintain specific body movement patterns. In fact, many people come to patterning to change the body patterns associated with issues they have already worked through in psychotherapy.

Cognitive therapy and behavioral approaches supplement somatic patterning in two primary ways:

1. by working with the cognitive and behavioral patterns that somatic patterning illuminates;
2. by using cognitive and behavioral patterns to change body patterns.

To stay focused on the body-centered experience, a somatic patterner generally asks *how* questions rather than *why* questions. As patterning participants and practitioners, we address how movement is organized rather than why we move a certain way. The why questions can lead into the content of experience, into the mental realm, which can easily derail a body-based process. Underneath each story lies the meaning that the person's experience has for him or her. The meaning of a pattern often arises organically once the multifaceted details of the pattern are illuminated; it is not something a patterner needs to spend time or energy uncovering during SP. This is the role of psychotherapist.

A person can stay centered on the body by focusing on physical sensations as they occur in each moment. Comments and questions that a practitioner can offer a client to help integrate body awareness with cognitive processes include:

- Feel any sensations you have in your body as you speak.
- Can you describe the sensations? Where do you feel them? What are they like?
- Continue to notice sensations as you describe them.
- Be aware of what you are doing in your body as you talk.
- Can you think, talk, and sense your body at the same time?
- Can you sense your body while you are moving?
- Can you stay relaxed yet fluid in your body as you speak?

During SP, it is far more important to be able to feel what is happening in the body than to be able to describe it. When describing or thinking about a body sensation takes a person away from a direct experience of the body, thinking or talking interferes with the patterning process. Ultimately, we must learn to think and communicate without abandoning our awareness of the body. Being able to think or talk about what we are feeling while we are actually experiencing the feeling, experiencing both its sensation and its movement, indicates true body and mind integration.

A NEUROLOGICAL APPROACH

Every patterning approach considered earlier by our fictitious character Henry became progressively more sophisticated, requiring both a deeper understanding of how the body works and a deeper experience of the soma. Although stretching and strengthening can be part of a patterning program, somatic patterning works more directly on a neurological level. This means that patterning redirects how the nervous system organizes autonomic tone and neuromuscular coordination. A person evokes neurological changes by actively participating in the process, making changes from the inside through active awareness and body movement. For example, to reorganize muscle patterns, a person must actively change the way he moves or postures. Some people feel that an active approach, in which a person consciously directs the process of change, is the basis of self-healing.

A person can exercise, stretch, or even receive bodywork without actively working to change a pattern, which would not be taking a neurological approach. For example, when a person receives bodywork to change a pattern, whether or not a neurological approach is taken directly affects the level of change. If the client actively participates in the bodywork, releasing autonomic stress and actively relaxing or contracting specific muscles, and continues to work on these patterns in between sessions, neurological pathways will change. However, many clients receive bodywork for pain relief, to release chronic tensions that perpetuate the pain patterns, without actively participating in the process of change, and thus return session after session with the same body problem.

A neurological approach addresses the body functions regulated by the ANS and SNS. Somatic patterning emphasizes change in both the autonomic and the somatic nervous systems, which each have many subdivisions and overlapping functions. Tone in one affects the other; therefore, isolating patterning to one part of the nervous system is impossible, although each part can be addressed in accordance with its function. **Autonomic patterning** addresses changing tone in the autonomic nervous system, which can be done with relaxation exercises for a person who has high sympathetic tone, and with stimulating exercises for a person who has low sympathetic tone. **Neuromuscular patterning** addresses muscle tone and coordination, a complex and multi-layered process. Neuromuscular pathways can be organized with many different approaches, such as those presented in Chapters 7 through 10.

Autonomic Patterning

As discussed in Chapter 1, the autonomic nervous system (ANS) is the oldest part of the nervous system. It regulates our most primitive biological responses and controls the vegetative functions we need for survival, including defense responses. Since the ANS controls both metabolic and emotional responses, autonomic patterns manifest in both our physiology and our psychology. This psychophysiological relationship underlies the practice of psychiatry, which is biologically based. Psychiatry is a relatively new field that was founded by Sigmund Freud less than 100 years ago. Although people typically think of psychiatrists as analysts who do talk therapy to bring patients' unresolved emotions under control, the bulk of modern psychiatry is based on pharmacology (drug therapy) to balance physiological processes that underlie psychosomatic pathologies.

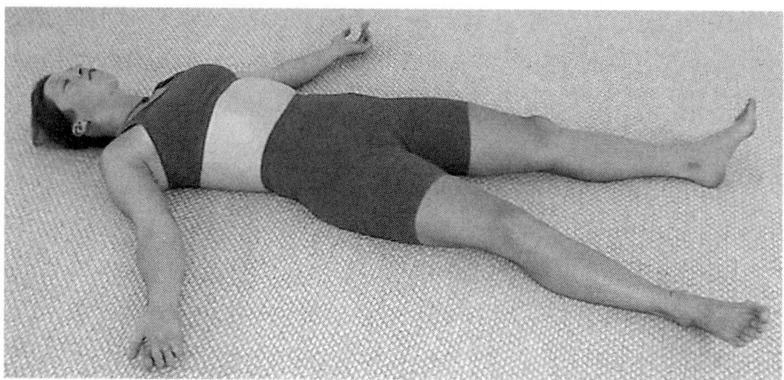

Figure 4.4 This yoga pose, called the "corpse," is ideal to practice relaxing.

A common and widespread imbalance in the ANS today is the condition of elevated stress. When a person experiences stress, autonomic tone goes up. Prolonged physiological stress occurs when the baseline of autonomic tone is set too high and the metabolic engine runs in a revved mode, putting undue psychosomatic strain on a person. This deteriorates not only the body's functions and its tissues, but also affects a person's psychology, which can create nervousness and anxiety. The broad effects of stress on both the body and the mind have spawned numerous therapies that work to change autonomic tone and promote psychophysiological relaxation.

The Relaxation Response

A physician named Herbert Benson studied the physiological states of seasoned meditators and found that two elements were commonly present when they could consciously evoke deep relaxation: being able to disregard external distractions, and repeating a word or phrase over and over again like a mantra.[84] Benson coined the term **relaxation response** to describe this physiological state and pinpoint the physiological skills involved in attaining it.

There are many different techniques used to evoke the relaxation response, all based on controlling and changing physiological responses. A person can actively relax by learning to release tension in the muscles, by slowing the breathing down, by controlling states of consciousness and thereby changing brain-wave patterns, and by allowing circulation to increase in the periphery of the body (Figure 4.4).

Since nearly all of us have the ability to consciously control the skeletal muscles, muscular relaxation is probably the easiest and most accessible method of lowering autonomic tone and calming nervous tension. Hence the popularity of **progressive relaxation,** a simple technique in which a person systematically contracts then relaxes each muscle in the body, starting at the head and working down. In short, progressive relaxation uses the ability we have to control the SNS to relax the ANS. This simple method is widely used in stress management because any willing person can easily learn it and practice it anywhere.

Progressive relaxation slows the physiological engine, relaxing both the body and the mind, thereby lowering autonomic tone and improving **autonomic flexibility**, the ability to move between a state of stress to one of relaxation. Because it is more important to be able to shift from a tense to a relaxed state than it is to try and stay relaxed, autonomic flexibility is a primary goal of most stress management programs.

Basic skills for working with autonomic patterns are:

- learning to track autonomic tone through sensation;
- learning to reduce autonomic tone through relaxation skills—slowed breathing, progressive relaxation,

autogenic suggestion, or other mental and visualization skills—or through organic movement (discussed below);
- improving autonomic flexibility by becoming fluid in moving from a tense state to a relaxed state.

Organic Movement Practices

All of the metabolic and homeostatic processes within our body systems generate some kind of organic movement. This includes physiological rhythms of various body systems, for example heart rate, digestion, breathing, lymph flow, and the movement of the cerebrospinal fluid throughout the brain, spinal cord, peripheral nerves, and myofascial webbing.

Most relaxation techniques involve stationary techniques like mild hypnotic, visualization, or breathing exercises that calm the body and mind. These types of internal approaches lack active movement through space. A novel approach to relaxation and an excellent way to integrate relaxation into daily activities is to learn to use a subtle yet expressive organic movement to unwind tension and calm the body. In this context, the term "organic movement" describes a quality of fluid, nondirected improvisational movement. The **organic movement practice**, a loosely structured, improvisational movement meditation, relaxes the body and releases autonomic tension while simultaneously increasing fluidity and restoring the body's natural and reflexive movement responses (see Chapter 6). Several types of organic movement practices described in Part 3—automatic movement, Continuum, and Authentic Movement—seem to cultivate autonomic flexibility and fluidity, as well as improve intrinsic motility and flexibility, elicit reflexes, and expand neuromuscular pathways.

Neuromuscular Patterning

Neuromuscular (NM) patterning changes how and when the muscles work. Coordinating the actions of more than 600 skeletal muscles (as opposed to smooth muscles in organs or cardiac muscle in the heart) into efficient sequences makes NM patterning a refined, detailed process. It requires a focused awareness of the muscles on many levels. First, a person must be able to differentiate between the feeling of when a single skeletal muscle is contracting, relaxing, and stretching. Then, a person needs to be able to sense the co-contractions of groups of muscles and control the sequence and duration of a chain of muscular contractions. Given the large number of skeletal muscles in the body, using NM patterning effectively requires some understanding of muscle anatomy and physiology or some accurate anatomical imagery. NM patterning is one of the most accessible forms of somatic patterning because most people can control their skeletal muscles to some extent.

There are many approaches to working with NM patterns. They involve varying combinations of a handful of basic techniques that increase a proprioceptive awareness of muscle activity. The general goal of NM patterning is to coordinate the recruitment order of muscles so that agonist and antagonist pairs of muscles become more balanced, neuromuscular pathways reorganize along more orderly and coordinated kinematic chains of action, and postural muscles work in harmony with prime movers.

Chapters 7 through 10 present the theories underlying the NM approaches as well as practical methods for application. Most people who are familiar with somatic patterning are probably most familiar with NM methods. The most obscure of the NM approaches involve working with reflexes and with patterns of early motor development. Both of these approaching are very effective in organizing pathways along more efficient kinematic chains.

Reflexes

Elaborate neuromuscular circuits of reflexes coordinate the automatic movements that we carry out so often and so effectively we rarely appreciate their complexity. As mentioned before, anyone who has had to relearn simple movements after an injury such as walking or brushing the teeth can appreciate the role of reflexes in coordinating the bulk of our actions. When the reflexes are intact, the body moves with incredible spring and agility, and impeccable timing. For instance, the extensor thrust reflex causes an arm or leg to thrust out and catch us when we fall, and the flexor withdrawal reflex pulls our limbs away from dangers such as scalding heat or cutting edges. Without the protective action of reflexes, movement becomes stiff and guarded, clumsy and awkward.

Reflexes strengthen with use and weaken when dormant. Agile athletes such as rock climbers, kayakers and team sports players, who navigate varying physical challenges in often unpredictable terrains or interactions, tend to develop a broad range of diverse and sophisticated reflexes. Conversely, sedentary people who lack movement challenges, particularly seniors, tend to lack strong reflexes. As a result, seniors often seriously injure themselves in falls that could have been minor had protective reflexes engaged to catch them.

It is never too late to strengthen reflexes. The stronger the reflexes are, the less tense and guarded the body will become to avoid falls. Reflexes can be developed by practicing simple balancing exercises, such as standing on one leg, or balancing while sitting or standing on an unstable surface such as a physioball or a balance board. Practicing a range of reflexive movements, particularly those that catch us when we stumble, can help us to age with confidence that our bodies will catch us if we fall.

Developmental Patterning

Developmental patterning entails relearning the series of early motor patterns that each person goes through from conception to walking. This approach provides a direct

Patterning Exercise #24: Developing Simple Reflexes

Caution: If your balance is tipsy, start these explorations with your eyes open. Also, if you have a fear of falling, move slowly and with caution. Make sure there are no sharp corners or glass objects nearby that you might fall into. As you gain more confidence, you can explore these exercises with your eyes closed.

1. Practice standing on one leg. Reach your arms out for balance and pick a point on a nearby wall to look at for optical support. Hold until you lose your balance. Notice how your free leg naturally extends to the floor to catch you when you fall (PE Fig. 24a). Switch legs and repeat on the other side.
2. Sit on a physioball with both feet on the floor. Slowly shift the weight on your hips from front to back, side to side.
3. Now explore balancing with your eyes closed and your feet flat on the floor. Notice the reflex mechanisms that extend your arms and head to keep you upright (PE Fig. 24b).
4. Sit on a physioball with both feet on the floor. For optical support, pick a point on a nearby wall and look at it. Raise both feet and balance your body for as long as you can (PE Fig. 24c). When you fall off balance, your legs will reflexively extend to catch you, just let it happen With practice, you'll be able to balance for longer intervals. These exercises strengthen head righting and protective extension reflexes.
5. Lie over a physioball on your belly with your hands and feet on the floor. Explore leaning side to side (PE Fig. 24d-e).
6. Lie over a physioball with your knees bent and toes on the floor behind you. Reach with both hands and extend your arms (PE Fig. 24f). Alternate pushing off with your feet and catching yourself with your hands (PE Fig. 24g). Then push off with your hands and catch yourself with your feet. This exercise will strengthen flexor withdrawal and extensor thrust reflexes.

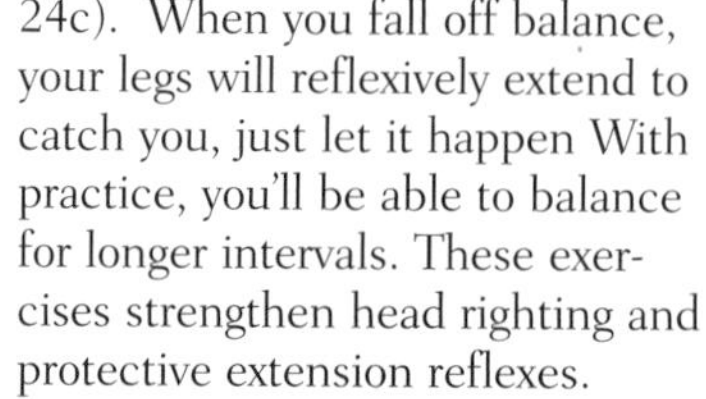

PE Fig. 24a

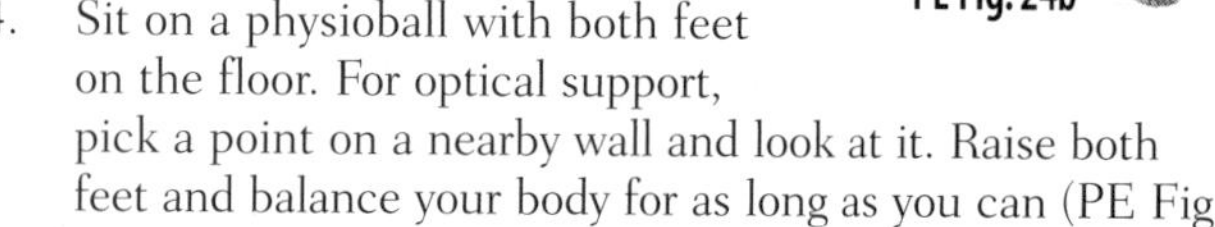

PE Fig. 24b

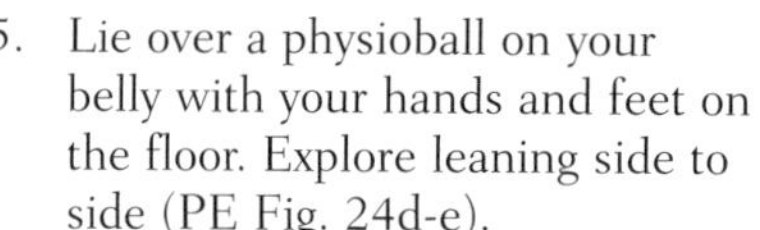

PE Fig. 24c

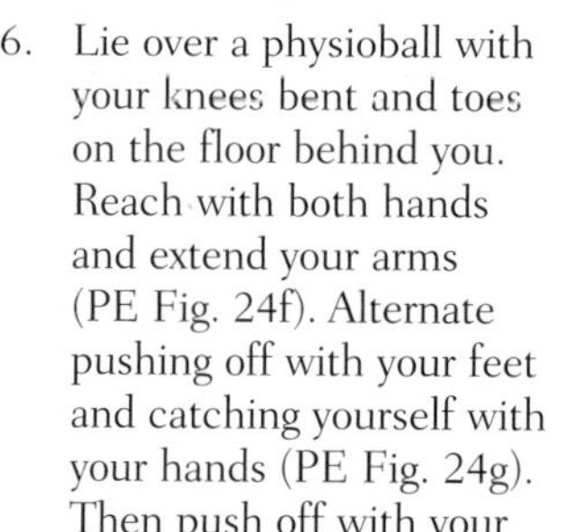

PE Fig. 24d

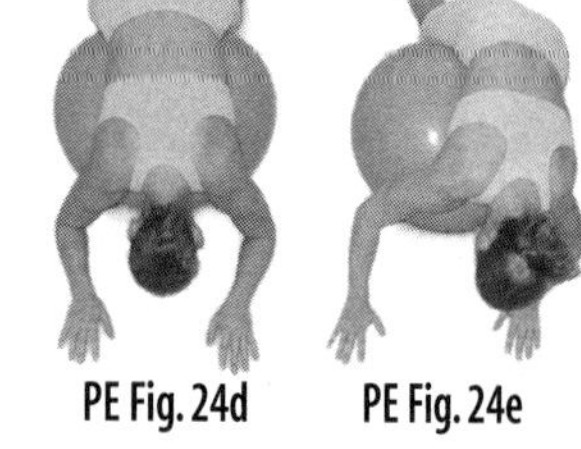

PE Fig. 24e

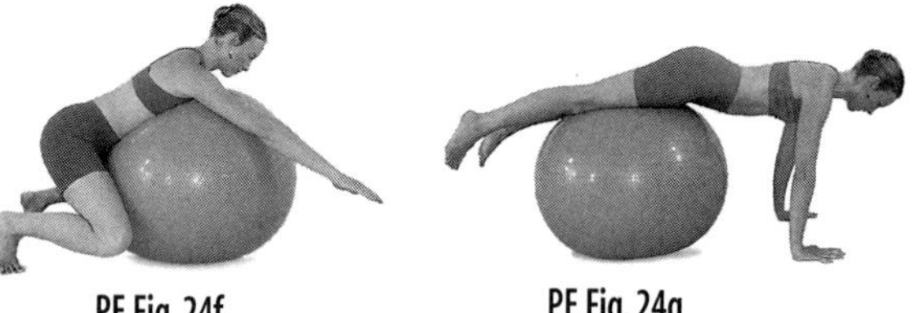

PE Fig. 24f PE Fig. 24g

EMSPress.com

route to working with movement problems rooted in a person's psychology because the structure of the psyche forms during early motor development. Every discovery, feeling, or frustration that we went through in infancy and early childhood is reflected in the body patterns laid down during early motor development and carried into adulthood.

Each developmental pattern carries a dynamic and tone that embody specific psychological strengths and weaknesses, both literally and figuratively. The four most basic patterns (usually referred to as *actions* because they describe the quality and direction of movement rather than define a pathway) are *yield*, *push*, *reach* and *pull*. Yield relates to trust and bonding, push to boundaries and an ability to contain oneself, reach to having connections with others, and pull to the ability to grasp something and take it in.

Although the developmental process appears complex, the developmental movement patterns are easily identifiable markers of the stage of personal development a person might be in, evident in which states are strong and which are underdeveloped. No single pattern or stage is preferable to another. What is important is that a person has gone through most of the general stages and has a balance between modulating stages. This balance builds a neuromotor foundation for psychological and cognitive development, as well as physical development.

Each developmental pattern (Cohen identifies 14 major patterns and about 100 underlying reflexes) has a modulating pattern. The balance between patterns can be roughly assessed in a person's movement preferences. Push balances reach because pushing movements compress joints and establish concentric (shortening) tone in muscles, whereas reaching movements pull joints open and establish eccentric (elongating) tone in muscles. Without the modulating forces of reach patterns, joint compression from overly strong push patterns can stress joints. Without the modulating forces of push patterns, the joints lack connection and become unstable. Joint extension from overly dominant reach patterns can underlie joint patterns that lack axial compression and overall patterns of postural instability.

Developmental patterning is generally approached in two ways:

1. By learning the series of early motor patterns in a linear fashion. This is the format used most com-

monly in teaching developmental patterns to groups. Although this format is thorough and inclusive, it can be mechanical and risks imposing an external pattern on people rather than having them find their internal motivation for change.

2. By approaching patterning through developmental process, which occurs when students move from their current stage on the developmental continuum to their next level of development. (This will be explained more fully in Chapter 7.) This approach is more likely to access a person's intrinsic motivation to change and thus yield deeper, more internally integrated changes.

Can you integrate top-down (cognitive) and bottom-up (sensorimotor) activities, being able to think or talk and move at the same time? Or do you stop moving to think or talk? How can you coordinate these functions?

MODULATING DUALITIES

The topic of modulating dualities is an overriding theme in SP because the body functions in a field of dualities. For balance, experiential learning needs to be balanced with cognitive learning, reflexive processes with reflective processes, and internal support with external movement.

To **modulate dualities** is to counterbalance two opposing elements. This is done in the patterning process by determining which element in a polarity dominates and which element tends to lie dormant, identifying the nature of the imbalance, then targeting the element that needs expression. This does not mean addressing both elements at the same time because, like light and darkness, when one element comes forward, the other recedes. For example, during sleep conscious wakefulness lies dormant and vice versa.

In this discussion of body-mind dualities, it is important to remember that the body and mind are not separate; they are merely two halves seamlessly joined in an ongoing continuum of human experience. Every continuum has its relative center. What integrates and balances the body and mind represents the modern quest for the Holy Grail. Some believe the body-mind link resides in the emotional body, others believe it is spiritual, and still others feel it is physiological. In the SP paradigm, we view movement as an integrating link between body and mind. Movement takes place along many continuums between dual elements, having numerous degrees, dimensions, and qualities of tone.

Many terms to denote the body-mind continuum have been used in this discussion to reflect the varying degrees of separation and unity between the two: "body and mind," "body-mind," and "somatic." The last term, somatic, implies the ultimate unity, transcending the body-mind split entirely to denote holism. The body and mind have obviously different functions that make them appear separate. Still, the brain and nervous system work as organs of the invisible overseer of the body that we call mind. Although body and mind functions differ in many respects, they ultimately function toward the same end. In the same way the heart pumps blood, the brain could be considered a pump of consciousness.

Just as thoughts can become limited by dualistic thinking, so bodies can become locked into chronic fixations that restrict normal flexion-and-extension cycles. This results in an imbalance between modulating forces in the body. These modulating forces manifest in a balance between muscles contracting or extending , breathe cycles flowing in and out, the movement of joints flexing or extending, and nerve impulses traveling up and down sensory or motor pathways. When the therapeutic goal is to balance these modulating forces in the body, every movement problem presents an opportunity for growth. Integration becomes attainable when imbalances are identified, pointing to how the scale has tipped and which end needs to be balanced. For example, if the spine is stuck in flexion, extension will balance it.

Any body pattern perceived as negative actually holds the key to its resolution, evident in its opposite. If a muscle can contract, it can also relax. If we can think negative thoughts, we can also think positive thoughts. From this perspective, each body problem holds within it a solution. The solution lies in the element, or pathway, that is not being expressed, that is stuck in the background and needs to be brought to the foreground.

We have spoken of many dualities in the soma throughout this text: the body and the mind, flexion and extension, agonist and antagonist, breathing in and breathing out, moving toward or moving away, push and reach, stability and mobility, and inner and outer processes. This seemingly endless list of dualities in fact forms a backbone for understanding SP (Figure 4.5).

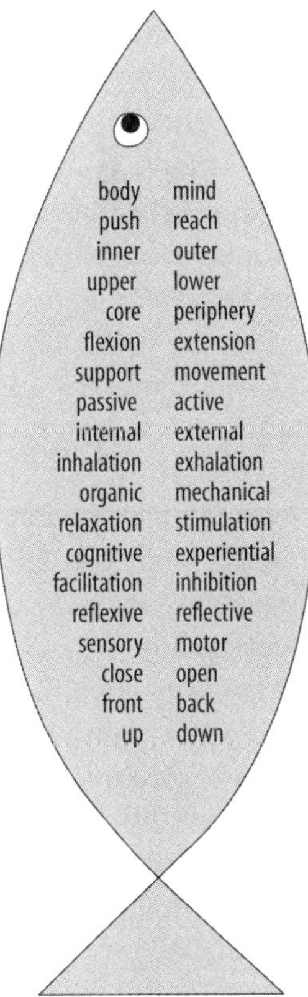

Figure 4.5 Balancing somatic dualities as the backbone of SP

Intrinsic Motivation in Patterning

An example of the problem that occurs when patterning is attempted without the client's active participation follows:

Roger was a toddler who was developmentally delayed and unable to crawl. His concerned mother took Roger to a group of patterning specialists. In a number of sessions, each of four practitioners held one of Roger's four limbs and mechanically moved him through the crawling action. Under these circumstances, the child was fussy and unable to learn how to move from an internal motivation. The mother, upon seeing that the work was not helping her son, eventually terminated the sessions. She felt that since her son was not actively participating or moving in a natural manner, he was not making internal changes.

The mother sought out a more process-oriented practitioner who played with Roger, placing toys and food treats just out of his reach. Eventually Roger, in his efforts to reach the toys, spontaneously crawled. Once he did this of his own accord, the practitioner and mother were able to gently nudge and pull his hands and feet to stimulate reflexes and guide him through complete and successful movement sequences.

Balancing Experiential, Body-Based Learning with Cognitive Learning

As a child matures into an adult, the attributes of the body and the mind become more and more differentiated. The body functions in a tangible, spatial world, the mind in an invisible, temporal world. The body speaks through the language of fluctuating sensations and pulsations, the mind through an ongoing parade of images, words, and ideas. One operates in the sensorimotor world while the other functions in the largely abstract realm of thought.

In somatic education, the nature of body-mind duality requires an approach that balances feeling with thinking, moving with perceptual awareness, and organic with mechanical aspects of somatic function. To this end, SP can be initiated in body-based or mind-based processes. The two are markedly different. Physical, **experiential learning** is tangible; it can be directed through movement processes and it progresses through the accumulation of physical experience. **Cognitive learning** is abstract, it progresses through linear processes, and although it is not directly observable, we see the outcome of thought in the body via fluctuations in tone, posture, and activities.

The SP methods summarized in Part 3 work with somatic learning initiated both through cognitive processes and sensorimotor activities. In a cognitive, top-down approach to SP, mental processes are tracked through body responses. The hidden landscape of a person's attitudes and beliefs becomes apparent through gestures, postures, and movement patterns that outwardly express thought patterns. In a body-based, bottom-up approach to SP, changing postures and movement patterns are viewed as an ongoing expression of the mind in the body. Experiential learning builds a broad ground in which the mind can express through bodily experience.

The beauty of an experiential, body-based approach is that by tuning into the body, we tune into the present moment. This act alone has a quieting effect on the mind because physical experience occurs in the present moment, suspending the tendency of the mind to project into the past or future, into memory or desire. Although reading this book takes a mental approach to SP, do not be fooled by the illusion of body-mind separation. It would be virtually impossible to read about these concepts without absorbing some of the ideas and feelings this information arouses in the body. Simply reading about movement cultivates a greater awareness of where the body does or does not move. A person would have to be pretty detached from the body not to feel a chord of resonance strummed by some of these topics, especially if a particular topic rings true for the individual.

Taking a physical approach to SP is perhaps the easiest because it is the most direct. It does not involve much planning or thinking. Plus, the body is immediate, always accessible. To feel something, we simply need to tune into the sensations that are occurring in our bodies at any given moment. A cognitive approach to SP, on the other hand, requires more focus because habitual or random thoughts shoot through the mind so rapidly that we have to concentrate to quiet mental chatter and order our thoughts. This process is akin to tuning radio static into a clear channel: it requires deliberation and focus to be effective.

All patterning process involves some kind of balancing act between physical and cognitive learning, a volley between thinking and feeling, sensing and moving. We tune the mental station to bring in a deliberate, clear signal to send to the body. At the same time, we remain receptive to any information the body provides, via sensations, about the SP process. In SP, a person simultaneously practices moving while being aware of the changing perceptions created by movement, and growth occurs as a result of this state of body-mind attention.

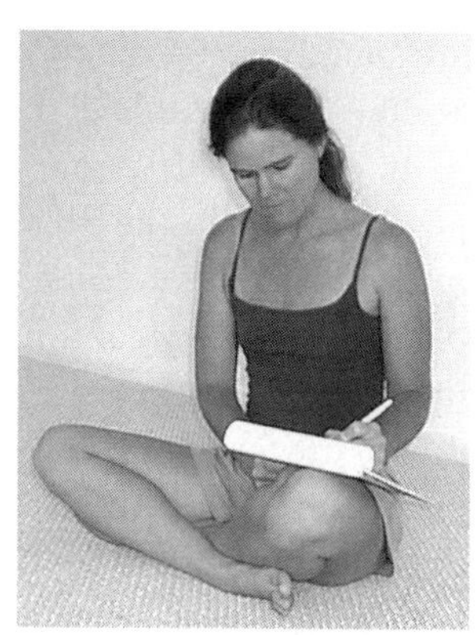

Figure 4.6 Writing about an experience is an excellent form of reflective thinking.

Reflexive and Reflective Movement Coordination

Thinking about moving can and often does lead to action. As mentioned in Chapter 1, thoughts that initiate movement occur at lightning speed, usually below conscious awareness. Thoughts also initiate a commitment to action. Just thinking the thought "I'm going to the store" can start a chain of actions that could lead a hungry person into a grocery-shopping spree. After a period of time, which can range from a moment to many hours, reflective thinking, if acted upon, can lead to incredibly creative actions. If not acted on, however, reflective thinking can lead to tension, frustration, and even physical distress (imagine the frustration of a person growing hungrier while thinking about food).

A top-down approach requires reflective thinking. By making a logical assessment of a somatic pattern, a person can establish an effective plan about how best to proceed (Figure 4.6). Reflective planning underlies the evolution of our intelligence because we are able to build on a preexisting knowledge base rather than having to go each time through lengthy trials of discovery. It is as though we stand on the shoulders of all the minds that preceded us, which enables us to take learning and personal development to new heights. This is the nature of human evolution: our learning extends beyond our teachers'.

Have you ever known someone who moves predominantly with control, slowly and deliberately, measuring each action? What was this person's body like? What was the personality like?

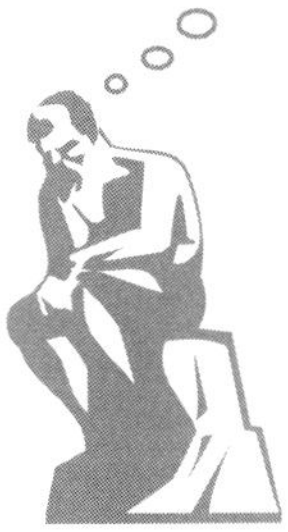

In Western cultures, most adults tend to favor top-down learning (an approach focused on book learning) and view experiential learning as child's play or recreational activity. Given this tendency, most adults would become more balanced by adopting a bottom-up approach to patterning, one based more on experiential learning and less on reflective thinking and mental planning. Mental processes can still be integrated into experiential learning, setting a framework within which to make intelligent choices, yet once the body is moving, the mind needs to let go of control to allow movement to be coordinated at lower, more subconscious neurological levels.

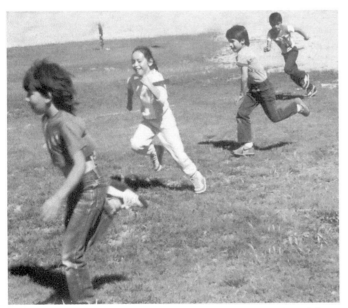

Figure 4.7 Diverse play activities are crucial for children to develop a full range of reflexes (photo courtesy of L. Bright).

The downside of a top-down approach is that the cerebral cortex does not coordinate movement very well. To understand why, imagine the "painfully shy" person who measures every action and every word. This style of self-consciousness most likely stirs the sympathy of a compassionate observer. It also brings up the question: Why does the average person move so awkwardly when he or she knows that someone is watching? Probably because when we know someone is observing us, we become self-conscious and start controlling the movement. But whenever we consciously control motor responses, we use a part of the brain that evolved for reflective thinking. Movement coordinated by the cortical centers tends to be less efficient, resulting in movement that often has a clumsy quality.

The spinal cord, brain stem, and hindbrain evolved to coordinate the broad array of movements we do on an automatic, largely subconscious level. These subcortical neurological centers are far more efficient than the cortex for the overall coordination of movement. Because of this, volitional control directed by cortical thinking is not recommended as a primary coordinator of movement. However, it is possible to improve the economy of an inefficient pattern by slowing it down far enough to identify where along the chain of action a movement is faulty. Just feeling the rocky part of a movement sequence is usually enough to change the pattern.

Because of the sophisticated function of the human cortex, children require a long period of reflexive, spontaneous, bottom-up learning to build a strong neurological foundation for cortical development. Hence, a child goes through years of play before reaching maturity. Play builds a wide range of automatic patterns, ultimately leaving the cortex free for creative thinking. If cortically based movement tendencies dominate the motor pathways at too early an age and play is interrupted by overly external and visual cerebral activities (such as electronic games or television), the neurological foundation for subsequent cognitive development and creative thought is weakened. In other words, natural and effortless movement abilities like the spontaneous actions of a child running and jumping can decline in direct proportion to how often a child consciously controls movement with reflective thinking (Figure 4.7).

Patterning can be approached from either end of this reflexive-reflective continuum, at either a subcortical or cortical level, from the bottom-up or top-down. The very nature of intellectual study, such as reading this book, is a top-down approach. At the very bottom, the goal is to develop automatic movements that elicit reflexes and spontaneous responses. As mentioned in the first chapter, both reflexes and reflex-

Patterning Exercise #25: Cortical Patterning with the Arms

To release excessive effort and make a movement more efficient, pick any movement that you have difficulty with and slow it down, sensing each tiny increment of motion. For now, we will focus on arm movement.

1. Lie on your back in a comfortable position. Bend your knees to keep your lower back relaxed. Put both arms out to the sides, palms up (PE Fig. 25a).

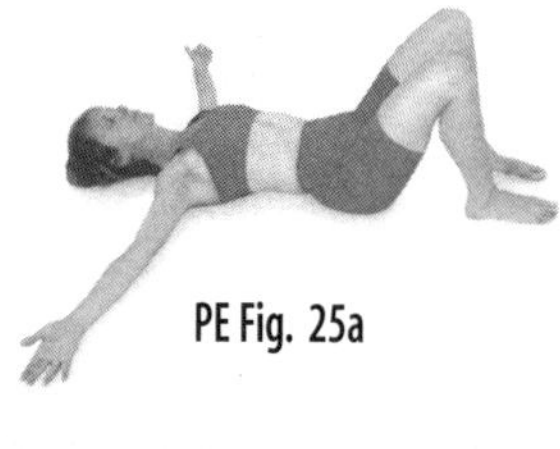

PE Fig. 25a

2. Keeping your arms straight, bring your palms together directly above you (PE Fig. 25b). Then return your arms to their original position.

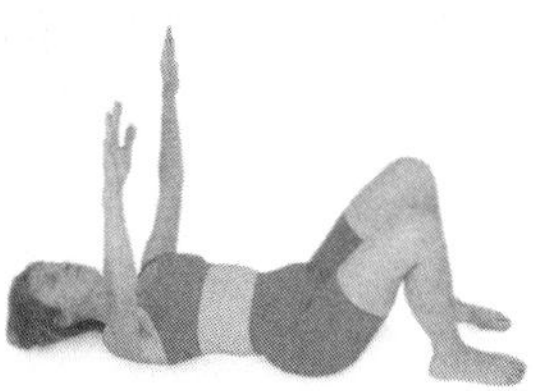

PE Fig. 25b

3. Do the movement again and notice how your shoulders move. Are they symmetrical? Is there any stress in the action? What happens between your shoulder blades?

4. Repeat the movement very slowly (PE Fig. 25c). Reach through your fingers as you raise your arms. Keeping your shoulders on the ground, sense the upper arm gradually turning in the socket. Widen the space between your shoulder blades. Breathe deeply into this space as you move. Relax any tension you feel in your neck, spine, or hips as you move your arms.

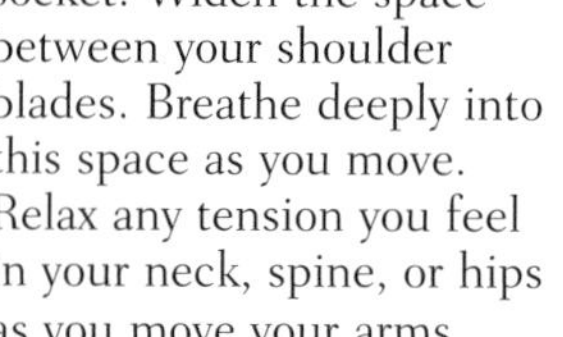

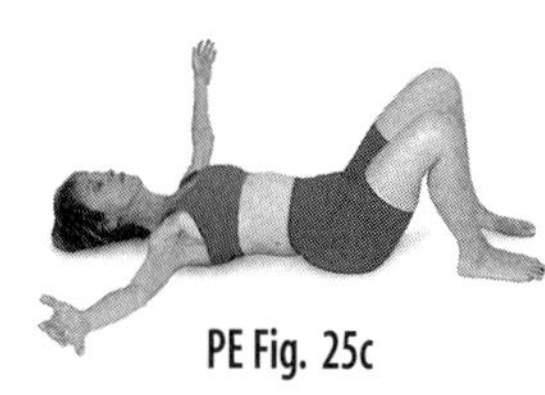

PE Fig. 25c

5. Slowly reverse the motion and return your arms to the original position. Again, keep breathing. Keep the space between your shoulder blades wide. Open and widen your chest. Relax any tension you feel anywhere in your body.
6. Repeat the movement one more time, this time visualizing that your arm moves on your shoulder like a door on a hinge. Then rest.

Feedback: Could you feel how doing the movement slowly allows you to make subtle changes? If so, great. Use this approach with other movements that you might have difficulty with. If not, then this style of patterning may not be suited for your needs.

EMSPress.com

ive movements are automatic, coordinated mostly on a subconscious level. Evoking reflexes involves activities that trigger reflexive responses, such as standing on a balancing board or playing on a physioball. It can also include non-structured, improvisational movement practiced to cultivate fluidity and to release autonomic tension. A bottom-up approach typically involves some kind of improvisational movement exploration marked by the absence of control.

It is important to note that this discussion of top-down and bottom-up approaches creates a false dichotomy for the purpose of clarity, much as our looking at the body and mind as separate entities in order to study their primary functions does. In fact, these approaches are the extremes of a continuum. A number of patterning approaches incorporate both aspects of learning, cognitive and experiential. Also, by oscillating between thought and action, exploring a wide range of movement exercises, and embodying a broad array of movement qualities, a person will inevitably access many gradations of both reflective and reflexive movement coordination along the body-mind continuum.

Integrating Facilitation and Inhibition

One of the most basic patterning skills, found in every patterning technique, is the **facilitation** of desired movement and the **inhibition** of faulty movement. In short, this means mobilizing what is stuck and quieting or stabilizing what is overactive. Any patterning process involves a combination of facilitation and inhibition. Facilitation is the process of eliciting movement. One method of facilitation used to elicit a muscular contraction is the PNF technique of pushing against resistance. Inhibition is the process of stopping a movement, getting a contracted muscle to relax or an over-facilitated muscle to quit firing, or, in a more general application, suspending a habitual response or faulty pattern.

Facilitation and inhibition are two skills fundamental to the process of patterning because they arise out of and reflect the basic function of the nerves. Nerves are capable of either excitation or inhibition. They relay impulses between the brain and body that result in either a response or the inhibition of response. The nervous system expends most of its energy processing sensory information. Although the coordination of a single action occurs in a wink, every small movement we make is actually a flood of neural impulses that simultaneously signals hundreds of muscles, directing some

Links to Practical Applications

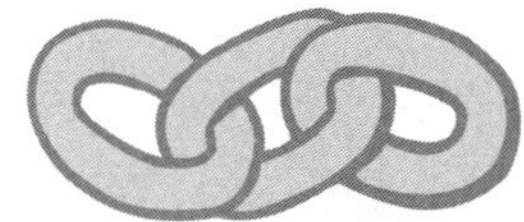

Inhibiting and Facilitating Muscular Responses

To inhibit an overworked muscle, place your hand on it as you do a particular movement and consciously relax it. If you are successful, you will feel the bulge of the contracted muscle soften under your hands. To facilitate an inhibited muscle, place your hand on it and consciously contract it. You should feel the muscle bulge under your hand. If you cannot feel whether a muscle is contracted or relaxed, actively contract it and relax it several times until you can sense the difference.

to contract and others to relax. In a fraction of a second, a single bit of sensory information relays through millions of synapses in every direction, opening some channels and closing others, either facilitating or inhibiting sensory and motor signals.

The nervous system is the only body system capable of inhibition—of putting a "brake" on action. Because of this ability, the nervous system can dominate the other systems; in other words, *the mind can stop movement in the body*. People often attempt to control the orchestra of simultaneous body functions occurring within the body. Thoughts about how our body should look, or move, or even posture often facilitate or inhibit movement inappropriately, resulting in faulty habits or holding patterns. Thoughts can also repress biological or emotional needs. For instance, a woman may need rest, yet her overactive mind may drive her body to perform until she breaks down from fatigue. Fortunately, the nervous system can also inhibit its own errant impulses. Inhibition can even be used to facilitate a process—a person can learn how to stop stopping.

Facilitation of a new pattern involves first identifying what movement or behavior needs to occur to organize an efficient neuromuscular pathway. Once initiated, the movement must be carried out along a specific pathway in the body, which is determined by a clear image of the desired movement or behavior, and/or a precise understanding of an efficient physiological response or a muscular chain of action. For instance, part of the relaxation response is the vasodilation (opening) of the peripheral capillaries; therefore, a person who wants to learn how to relax might visualize warmth soaking into the arms and legs.

Whenever something is inhibited, or taken away, something else needs to be added to take its place. It is not enough to learn how to stop doing an undesired behavior or movement; it needs to be replaced with something new. As the old adage goes, nature abhors a vacuum; if we don't choose a positive replacement, our body might substitute a random pattern and develop another faulty habit. People put this concept into action whenever they decide what they want to change and begin to replace the faulty patterns by visualizing something new—a new job, a new level of health, or a desired weight, for example.

Oscillating between the old and new has deep physiological effects on a person. Trauma specialist Peter Levine discovered the profound effects of this patterning principle. He applied it in his treatment protocol with people plagued with recurring symptoms of post-traumatic stress caused by the shocking memory of such victimizing experiences as a violent crime, serious accident, or war memory. Levine began by having his clients feel the physical sensation of trauma as deeply as they could. Then, to get a conversation going between the primitive and conscious areas of the brain, he has his clients oscillate their attention between a visualization of the traumatic event(s) and a peaceful and relaxing setting, such as lying on a tropical beach soaking up the sun. He found that bumping the thoughts between these two extremes, which he calls the "trauma vortex" and "healing vortex," produces a third element that results in a deep physiological resolution of the trauma. This resolution involves not only a deep relaxation coupled with discharge of held energy, but a release from the tendency to ruminate over the traumatic memory.

The oscillation of attention between old and new patterns is found in all effective patterning techniques. In an intricate example of muscle patterning that uses both inhibition and facilitation, a person with a tendency to hike her shoulders goes through the following steps: she starts by becoming aware of the pattern, making contact with the shape and sensation of hiking the shoulders. Next, she senses the muscles in which the hiking initiates and inhibits them by consciously relaxing them. Then she facilitates a new pattern by learning a more efficient arm movement, for example, a push pattern with the arms (efficient arm movement rarely initiates in the shoulders, which are the middle of a neuromuscular pathway). She does this by pushing her hands into the floor and sensing a concentric contraction traveling up the muscles of both arms, into the muscles of the shoulder cuff, then down the back through her *trapezius* and *latissimus dorsi muscles*. During the new action, she actively inhibits the tendency to hike her shoulders.

Sensory and Motor Balance

Every action we undertake involves a complex, synchronous organization of many overlapping sensory and motor processes. Since sensorimotor learning distinguishes somatic patterning from other forms of learning, during SP, all channels of awareness are grounded in sensory awareness. We focus on **sensory processes** by becoming actively aware of sensory stimuli. This awareness can include focusing on one element (such as a body part or a physical sensation), oscillating between two or more elements, or having a roving awareness of many elements. From

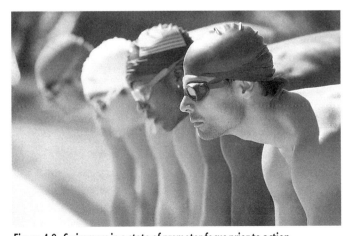

Figure 4.8 Swimmers in a state of premotor focus prior to action

Balancing Sensory and Motor Input

To exemplify how important it is for a bodyworker or somatic practitioner to balance sensory and motor processes, look at the following case:

A patterning practitioner was working with a client, whom we'll call Mic. Mic arrived for his SP session with a severe headache associated with overworking. Mic had originally planned to practice movement exercises with the practitioner, but his headache was so bad that he was tired and wanted to rest. So Mic asked his practitioner to place her hands on his head to help him relax. The earnest practitioner, in her misguided efforts to help, placed her hands on Mic's head, but rather than just helping him rest, gave him a steady stream of suggestions, such as "breathe into here, relax here, let this part sink, let this area go."

In Mic's effort to follow each directive, he tried harder and harder, using more and more effort. He was getting farther away from his goal to relax and calm his headache and consequently left the session feeling worse than when he came in.

a more holistic perspective, rather than just sensing physical sensations, the elements can include feelings and thoughts.

By focusing on the responses we make to sensory input we become aware of **motor processes**, which range from initiation of an action to the full response in a movement sequence. Motor processes can be seen in observable actions although even focusing a sense organ on a sight or sound, or getting ready to move (which Cohen describes as "pre-motor" focus) is a motor process (Figure 4.8).

Most SP methods balance sensory and motor processes by using techniques that involve sensing the body while actually moving it, although the definition of movement is broad because it includes subtle motor processes such as active relaxation.

The case study above, titled "Balancing Sensory and Motor Input," describes a clear example of a practitioner giving a stressed client so much input that the client, in his effort to follow the directives, worked too hard to be able to relax. The practitioner was asking for too many motor responses, and the client went on sensory overload in his inability to process the practitioner's seeming demands. To understand this process, realize that although relaxing is an active process in the nervous system, it is generally a passive process in which a person focuses on slowing down and resting. Relaxing takes minimal effort. It requires a state of **passive volition**, of "allowing" rather than "doing" (see "Autogenics" in Chapter 13), a state of relaxed awareness, with just enough focus to feel the body and just enough effort to allow change to occur naturally at its own rate. In the case described in the box to the left, the client was so tired he had barely enough energy to focus on letting go. The practitioner's directives compounded the situation by interrupting the client's state of relaxation to ask for more effort, which required a response. This example illustrates the importance of a practitioner finding that delicate balance between directing the client to do something and supporting a sensory experience to achieve balance between the sensory and motor systems.

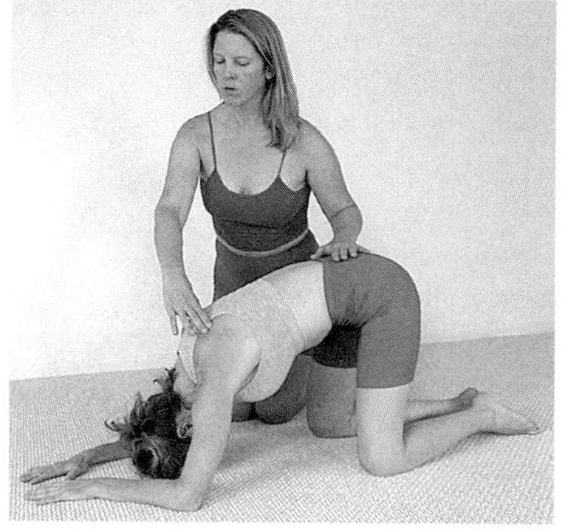

Figure 4.9 Using track and bump, the practitioner guides the client to relax in one area and move in another.

Finding this balance also applies to an individual practicing patterning exercises alone. Each of us has a client and a practitioner within, a part of ourselves that needs something from patterning and a part that has many ideas about how to get these needs met. For example, if we undertake a patterning exercise with the intention to relax, yet are busy trying a number of different ways to relax, we may be so busy "trying" that we will be unable to simply feel the body relaxing.

On the flip side, a person can become so focused on using minimal effort that he or she does not have enough tone to exert enough effort to adequately carry out an action. Low tone can become a real problem when patterning methods rely heavily on sensing the body because there must be a muscular action to build tone. Also, recall from Chapter 1 that movement precedes an awareness of movement. This naturally implies the importance of weighing a patterning process or exercise more heavily on the movement it inspires rather than sensing what makes it possible. Plus, movement increases sensory awareness whereas inactivity tends to diminish sensory awareness.

It is important to integrate sensory and motor aspects of patterning exercises by balancing input with output, sensing with moving. This does not necessarily mean that the amount of sensory input needs to be the same as the motor output, but that the person practicing patterning is able to adequately process any incoming information and make appropriate motor responses. Awareness builds the sensory ground of the patterning processes; intention directs the motor responses.

We can achieve sensorimotor balance during the patterning process by oscillating our attention between observing the process and directing it through the use of a technique called **track and bump**.[85] Dog trainers use track and bump techniques when teaching a dog how to heel. The leash provides the feedback: as long as it is slack, the trainer observes the dog's path with-

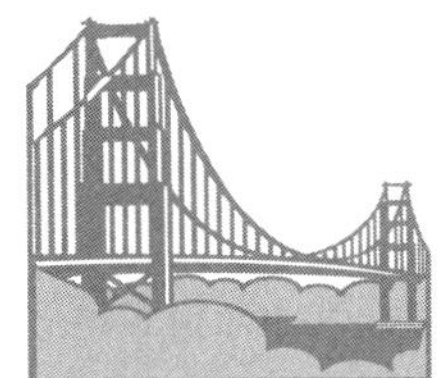

Bridge to Practice

Track and Bump

Simultaneously help your clients relax one area while facilitating movement in another area with a simple technique called "track and bump." To do this, place one hand on an area you want to help the client relax and the other on an area where you want the client to move. Then provide your client with verbal cues to support the intention of your hands, such as suggesting that your client "relax here, now move here; now relax here, now move here." You can also use bumping to bring attention to excessive muscular tension in areas adjacent to where your client is actually moving, or for keeping your client's attention from getting fixed on one point.

Sometimes patterns are not ready to shift; therefore, the bump needs to be gentle so that the client has the option to follow it without being forced into it. It is important that your bump is light and easy so that you are not pushing your client to move a certain way; rather, you are leaving your client room to choose whether or not to move in the direction or manner your touch suggests.

Track and bump is also a helpful technique to guide a client through a new movement pathway. It is especially beneficial for clients who work so hard "trying" to learn a new pattern that excessive effort increases muscular tension or neurological confusion and blocks the organization of a new pathway. When this occurs, bump the overworking muscle with a light tap to signal that your client needs to relax it. Then track your client's movement as it occurs. Whenever the client uses too much effort, gently bump the overworking area with a light nudge to give him feedback to relax that area.

out correction. When the dog pulls the leash, the pathway is off track, so the trainer bumps the dog back on track by nudging it gently to avoid choking it, which would only create more tension. The nudge is gentle at first, to give the dog the opportunity for self-correction, then stronger to make the undesirable behavior unpleasant.

During patterning exercises, awareness is the "leash" and intention the bump. To track a pattern, a person observes its direction of movement, the rate or quality of movement, and/or the shape of a pattern, using touch or attention to highlight specific aspects of a pattern. To bump or move a pattern in a certain direction or manner, a person does something to change the pattern, gently nudging the body with the intention of providing direction for movement. The bump has to be gentle to allow the system plenty of room to either follow it or not. If the bump pushes too hard, it could elicit resistance in the form of autonomic stress or muscular contraction. The bump can be a light directive or a tactile nudge applied and released numerous times during the patterning process to keep the process on track.

A person can use track and bump to oscillate the awareness back and forth between a place that needs to relax and another place that needs to move (Figure 4.9). This simple technique can also be used to oscillate between the elements of support and movement by feeling stability or relaxation in the supporting part of the body, then feeling the moving part move while sensing the underlying support. Track and bump can also occur between moving and feeling, or between moving and thinking.

Track and bump can be practiced between two body parts as well. A person can move one part while sensing what is happening in other parts of the body to either monitor or relax tension in the peripheral areas, or to monitor and actively stabilize peripheral areas that are too loose. For example, a person might want to focus on relaxing the shoulders and neck while doing a pelvic tilt, or on keeping the pelvis stable while moving the legs.

Establishing Support before Movement

One of the most basic principles of movement efficiency is that *the body must be supported before it can move*. This is a basic physiological truth: without support, the body loses its capacity for mobility. The more support the body has prior to moving, the more efficient the subsequent movement will be. The movement patterns of a cat exemplifies this fundamental principle of **support before movement**. Our feline companion spends hours motionless while sleeping. But if he hears a sound, his ears perk up; the perception of the sound causes an increase in muscle tone, causing the cat to instinctively gather support to ready itself for a chase. When a cat senses danger, his tone jumps up a notch as he rises to attention. A sniff of the air brings more evidence of approaching danger, and the cat jumps another notch in tone as he prepares to flee.

Like the cat's, our NM system also changes tone in order to have the support we need to move. If the tone is too low, a person might drag the body through an action that lacks adequate tone for, say, lifting something heavy.

Support in the body is intrinsic. It comes from the combined functions of many different systems. For example, support comes from the tonic contractions of postural

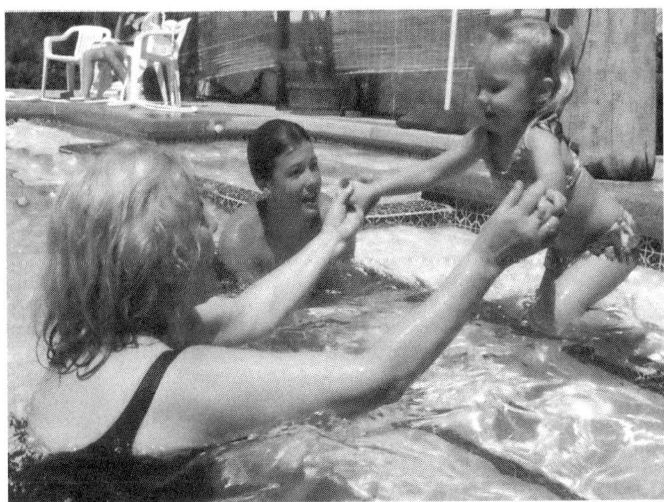

Figure 4.10 Having support before moving is crucial for effective action (photo courtesy of M. Seereiter).

Patterning Exercise #26: "Toning Up" while Sitting

If you have a desk job, be forewarned: standing up without raising your tone first can be like lifting a sack of dead weight, putting you at risk for injury. To avoid this, keep your muscles active with these simple exercises. Repeat each exercise at least five times; run through the whole set once an hour.

1. Breathe deeply and expand your lower ribs and chest, then relax as you exhale. Repeat several times.
2. Pull your lower abdominal wall in and hold it for ten seconds, then release. Repeat several times.
3. Rock back and forth on your sit bones (those bony protuberances on the bottom of your pelvis). Repeat several times.
4. Push your feet into the floor and contract your leg muscles, then relax. Repeat several times.
5. Stretch your arms behind you while you bend over. Then stretch one arm overhead and sidebend toward the other side. Repeat with the other arm.
6. Nod your head forward and back several times, then nod right and left several times, all without shortening your neck. Alternate nodding with lifting the top of your head up and holding it there for ten seconds, then relaxing it.
7. Pull your shoulders forward, then back, then up, then down while keeping your shoulder blades wide (do not pinch them together).
8. Opening your eyes as wide as you can, next scrunch them shut, then relax them. Roll your eyes around in a circle in one direction several times, then the other.
9. Twist your spine to the right, then to the left. Repeat several times. Then sidebend your spine right, then left, repeating several times both ways.
10. Alternate arching your spine backward and looking up, then flexing it and looking at your navel. Repeat several times.
11. Make fists with both hands, then open them and stretch your fingers. Repeat several times.
12. Extend both your arms in front of you and push your palms away while pulling your fingers back. Hold one minute.
13. Roll your ankles one way several times, then the other.
14. Straighten your knees and point your toes, then bend your knees and flex your toes and ankles several times.
15. With your feet on the floor, raise and lower your heels, then your toes. Then alternate feet as though you were walking in place.
16. Alternate pulling one hip backward as the other goes forward.
17. If you have a rolling chair, hold the edge of your desk and roll back as far as you can go, stretching your arms and spine. Undulate your spine several times in this position, then relax.

muscles, coordination and balance between opposing and working muscles, the tensional network of myofascias, the rigidity of the bones, the turgidity of organs and fluids, the pumping action of the heart and the lungs, and moving from a position of mechanical advantage.

On a psychological level, support comes from trust, both inner and outer. Children build self-trust when their surrounding environment is secure and they are free to act from their intrinsic motivations. Early somatic interactions with caretakers imprint a child with a sense of trust and support that can be observed in a child's posture and movement (Figure 4.10).

The respiratory system supports posture and movement in a number of ways. Breathing provides oxygen to fuel the metabolic processes. Deep breathing provides mechanical support by filling and lifting the thorax on each inhalation, and by mechanically pumping lymphatic fluids. Respiration also keeps the spine mobile by moving it through a slight physiological flexion and extension on each breath cycle. The *respiratory diaphragm* also provides support as both a prime mover and a postural stabilizer. It generates movement that both expands the ribcage and stabilizes the spine by increasing intra-abdominal pressure, stiffening the torso in a manner similar to the way water pressure stiffens a tube.

Another important physiological support is the ability to move from a relaxed state. The resting state of the body is carried into action. For instance, a person who sits with the shoulders drawn up around the ears is likely to carry that postural tension into standing and walking. This is why it is important to initiate action from a relaxed state. Relaxation allows us to move into action with the support of the parasympathetic nervous system. Granted, the body needs to increase tone for action, but this differs from carrying chronic tension from one activity to the next.

It is also important to set adequate muscle tone for an action. Before moving, the postural muscles need to be active to ensure maximal support and stability in the joints, particularly the spine. Once in motion, the ability of our neuromuscular system to gauge the precise tone needed for a movement is uncanny. This coordination occurs largely on a subconscious level, with only a fraction of conscious input. For instance, when stepping down a step, the body adjusts tone to make the downward motion. But if a person fails to see the step, the neuromuscular mechanism sets tone for walking on flat ground and the foot slams down into the unexpected step. The missing moment of perceptual input—the sight of the step—would have been just enough input to initiate a subconscious adjustment in tone.

In other words, had the person been watching where she was going, her NM system would have adjusted accordingly. A similar thing happens when picking up a light object that was expected to be heavy: the body is sent flying backward because the tone for action was set too high.

The opposite is also true. If a person lifts a heavy object and does not set enough support or tone for the action, the soft tissues are susceptible to injury. For example, if the tone is too low to lift a heavy garage door, instead of the door moving up, the shoulder and arm get pulled down. People injure themselves all the time this way, tearing soft tissues or straining joints. The appropriate tone can be set before lifting by accurately estimating the weight of the object and the strength needed for the job, and adjusting the muscle tone accordingly.

We have the unique ability to override the neuromuscular mechanisms that set adequate tone for a movement and to move from an unsupported position, one without intrinsic postural support. This phenomenon occurs in the person who habitually slouches, leans backward, or holds the body in a rigid pose, then carries the shape of the slouch or lean or rigid pose into the gait pattern. But we do have choices. We can take a moment before moving to gather postural support and increase tone for the ensuing movement or risk injury by habitually lifting the body like a sack of dead weight. By taking a moment to gather support before moving, using simple actions such as pushing the feet down, straightening the spine, and contracting the abdominal muscles, transitions from one position to another can be made with more ease, efficiency, and safety.

INNER AND OUTER BALANCE BETWEEN ANS AND SNS

The autonomic nervous system (ANS) regulates metabolic processes that affect a person's physiological responses. We can perceive ANS functions not only through changes in autonomic tone, but also through metabolic processes such as the intrinsic movements in organs and the circulation of bodily fluids. The skeletal nervous system (SNS), on the other hand, regulates movement generated by the neuromuscular system. We perceive SNS function in the neuromuscular system through actual changes in the tension of working muscles and joint motion. Somatic patterning addresses these two primary divisions of the nervous system, the ANS through autonomic patterning, and the SNS through neuromuscular patterning.

Working with the relationship between the ANS and SNS is analogous to working with the inner and outer layers of the organ and muscular systems. When a person is relaxed and in a parasympathetic state, the activities of the inner layer, the vegetative functions of the organs and resting metabolism, dominate while the outer layers relax. When a person is active and in a sympathetic state, the ANS draws energy from the inner layers, increasing respiration and circulation so that skeletal muscles in the outer layers have enough fuel for action.

The relationship between ANS and SNS function is important to consider in patterning to understand which part of the nervous system needs to be addressed first. The ANS transfers neural signals between the brain and organs; the SNS transfers neural signals between the brain and the skeletal muscles. If a person has pain exacerbated by high autonomic tone, neuromuscular patterning will not be effective until the ANS has been calmed down. Conversely, muscular imbalances cannot be addressed effectively through autonomic patterning.

Although these two aspects of the nervous system are being discussed as separate parts, keep in mind that, as with all the dualistic systems we've discussed, their functions are mutual. The ANS is in parasympathetic mode during slow, vegetative organ functions; it is in sympathetic mode during activity to fuel the metabolic needs of the muscles. The more efficient the ANS functions, the less stress there will be in the SNS and vice versa. Since the ANS is the older part of the nervous system with more primal functions, its functions build an underlying support for the SNS and should probably be considered first in somatic patterning.

Links to Practical Applications

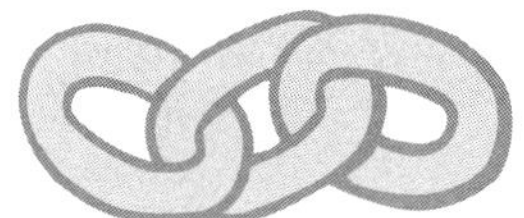

Getting into a Supported Posture before Lifting

Before lifting something, get into a supported position by putting your spine in a position of mechanical advantage in which the head is over the thorax, the thorax over the pelvis, and the pelvis over the feet. If you can, use a mirror to check your position. Stoop down or bend over with a straight back; actively contract your postural muscles along your spine, hinging only at the hips and bending your knees. Then put your hands under the object you are going to lift. Once you feel stable and ready, particularly in your core, maintain this aligned posture while you push your feet down and simultaneously lift the object up. Use your whole body, particularly your legs and back, to support the weight. Make sure your shoulders stay down to effectively transfer the weight from your arms into your trunk and legs, evenly distributing the load throughout your spine.

Motility and Mobility

In the same way that healthy ANS functions provide an underlying support for SNS functions, organ and fluid motility underlies full-body mobility. **Motility** describes the intrinsic, physiological movements that occur within the body all the time, whether it is actually moving or not. **Mobility** describes the movement of the body through space. The internal motility of metabolic processes such as digestion and breathing underlies the external, observable mobility carried out by the musculoskeletal system.

This relationship is most obvious in the movement patterns of an infant. A newborn moves with deep undercurrents of organic motility. Although the infant is

Links to Practical Applications

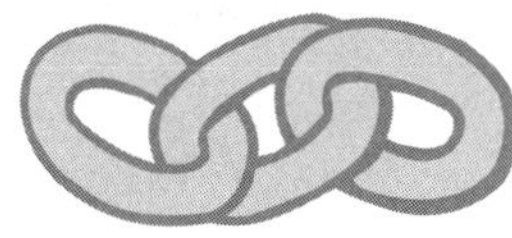

Inner Motility during the Workday

You can support motility and fullness in your organs and fluids during the course of your day in many ways. Some simple methods involve tuning into the rhythm and changing shape of your breathing, quietly pulsing to the rhythm of your heartbeat, or slowly swaying while sensing your fluids and organs shifting within your body like pouring sand.

unable to move his body through space, his body moves in a gel-like state, ebbing and flowing with subtle rhythms of an inner motility generated by biological functions. His inner motility is evident in the churning and squeezing movements of sucking, digestion, and elimination; in the rapid pumping of his heart; in the slow tides of his cerebrospinal and lymphatic fluids; in the quick circuitry of his roving senses; and in the oscillating winds of his respiratory pump.

Over time, the infant's musculoskeletal system starts to develop as he begins moving through space, although the intrinsic motility of the organs and fluids is still evident. This is why toddlers and small children seem to have such naturally plump bodies. The volume and fullness of their organs and fluids fill out their musculoskeletal packaging. Also, their lack of cognitive maturity makes their movement impulses more spontaneous and effortless. Babies have yet to learn the mental control that many adults use to repress intrinsic impulses and hold the body in rigid postures.

Deep physiological movements are always going on inside the body, even while a person is sleeping, only stopped by death. Adults, particularly adults in more rigid societies, are adept at repressing spontaneous movement, especially intrinsic organic and fluid movements. In fact, unless a person is involved in some kind of sporting event or dance, any movement other than the most pedestrian (sitting down, standing up, walking, and gesturing) is generally considered out of place.

This brings up the dilemma of how to maintain an intrinsic fluidity in the body as we go through the course of the day. How do we not sacrifice the inner motility of organs and fluids to the potential rigidity of the musculoskeletal system?

An integrated body has balance between muscular tone and inner fullness. The inner motility of the fluids and organs balances the strength and flexibility of the musculoskeletal system. Inner motility reflects adequately hydrated tissues, healthy circulation, a lack of tension in smooth muscles, and a vitality and health in the body's metabolic functions.

Balancing Organic and Mechanical Approaches

The balance between organic and mechanical approaches to patterning becomes clear when contrasting movement dominated by a quality of inner fluidity and movement dominated by mechanical motion. In an organic approach to patterning, a person focuses on fluid rhythms, organic motility, and even emotional expression. In a mechanical approach, a person focuses on muscle and joint actions in patterned movements. Although the mechanical principles of muscle and joint physiology guide musculoskeletal patterning, the organic nature of muscle patterns must also be considered in order to integrate organic and mechanical approaches.

Typically, when there is pain in the body, we first suspect mechanical causes and look for a muscle or joint injury. In doing so, we relate to the mechanical part of the problem. However, organic aspects of the body may also be involved and consciousness may also plays a role in body problems. In fact, muscle patterns always have a psychological component, not only in creating problems but also in alleviating them. Recall from Chapter 1 how, during early development, the template for psychophysiological tone is patterned in early defense responses, which affect both the autonomic nervous system tone and the patterning of neuromuscular pathways. In short, a person's psychology underlies both organ and muscle tone.

Therefore, to change somatic patterns, we must simultaneously address both the organic and mechanical patterns of the body. Addressing mechanical patterns involves focusing on muscle and joint action by improving the efficiency of their organization along neuromuscular pathways. Addressing organic patterns means reducing autonomic tension and improving autonomic flexibility by allowing organic and fluid movement impulses to flow through the body. Since most faulty patterns have corresponding thoughts and emotions, it is also important to address the negative thought patterns and process unresolved emotions that accompany faulty organic or mechanical patterns. This is what makes psychotherapy and SP complementary.

This brings up a primary question about approaching patterning: How does a person work simultaneously with organic and mechanical patterns, and when is it best to direct the focus on one or the other? Organic movement, which has the inherent protoplasmic characteristics of an organism, can address ANS imbalances as effectively as mechanical movement addresses musculoskeletal imbalances. To decide which approach to take, a person can assess tone in both the autonomic and neuromuscular system, decide in which the pattern manifests with the most strength, and then address that system first with either organic or mechanical approaches.

The organic movement of the organs and fluids creates an intrinsic support for the mechanical movement of the muscles and bones. **Mechanical movement** is used in this text to describe an approach a person takes to patterning. Although the muscles are inherently organic because they are living tissues, movements practiced with a focus on the mechanical aspects of muscle and joint function constitute mechanical movement. Of course, any patterning done to improve musculoskeletal balance stems from organic, living processes, so the more we can establish organic movement in the body, the more support the mechanical processes of the musculoskeletal system will have. Organic movement can be developed alone or in conjunction with mechanical patterning exercises to establish a biological foundation for the mechanical. Also, since somatic patterns always affect all levels, ultimately, both mechanical and organic aspects of a pattern need to be addressed. At the very least, a person practicing neuromuscular patterning needs to attend to organic processes in the background in order to cultivate a balance between autonomic and skeletal nervous systems.

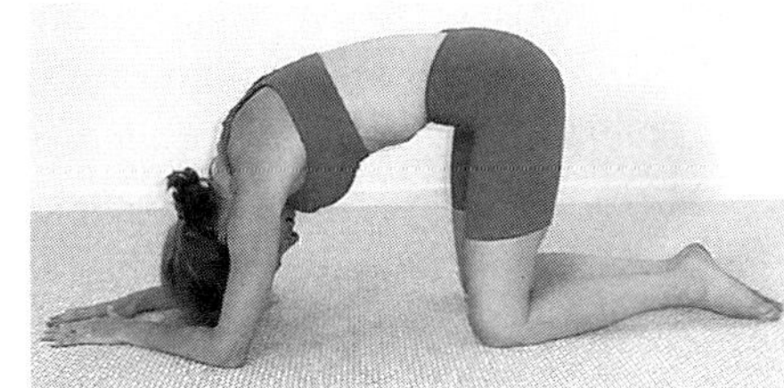

a.

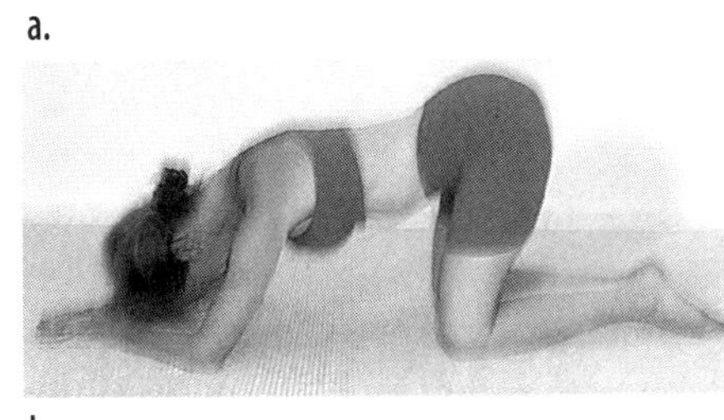

b.

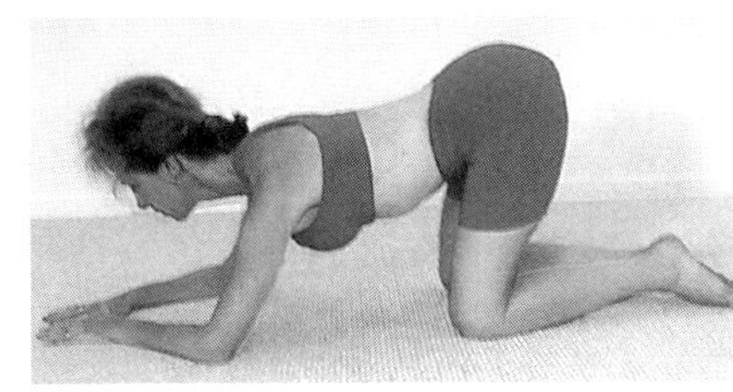

c.

Figure 4.11a-c Spinal undulation for loosening

and the myofascia unwinding will come into awareness.

In Chapter 6, an organic movement practice is briefly described in which a person uses unstructured, improvisational, fluid movement to relax the body and release autonomic tension. What is unique about this type of moving relaxation practice is that it tones the body while at the same time relaxing it. The physiological rhythms slow down and become more efficient as the body becomes more energized and moves at a quicker pace. This is what happens to Emilie Conrad during Continuum Movement, a fluid movement and breathing practice that she developed (see Chapter 11). Researchers found that after 20 minutes of strenuous yet fluid Continuum practice, Conrad's heart rate actually decreased and her blood pressure went down.

Patterning can proceed progressively from organic to mechanical processes, from inner support to outward movement, to allow a person enough time and focus to gather the underlying support of the intrinsic processes. Motility can be cultivated through organic movement practices. These practices are found in many of the movement modalities and in freestyle movement improvisations practiced to release tension, increase fluidity, improve reflexes, and process emotion.

Still, many body problems are perpetuated by mechanical imbalances in the musculoskeletal system that may or may not be addressed by organic processes. For this reason it is helpful to differentiate organic and mechanical approaches to patterning, and then to integrate the two within one process. Organic movement combined with mechanical movement balances release with form and flow with structure. For example, spinal undulations cultivate a quality of organic fluidity and flexibility along the spinal pathway (Figure 4.11a-c), while symmetrical spinal movements in each plane cultivate joint symmetry. A person can using

Organic Movement

Organic movement describes the quality of movement in the organs and bodily fluids initiated by generally unconscious biological and physiological processes of the body. These processes are often hidden but may initiate observable movements that are usually subconscious and spontaneous, marked by nonlinear motion along largely unpredictable and often convoluted pathways. Organic movements carry out and work through the body's unconscious processes, an example being the unpredictable movements a person goes through while asleep, or the continual flow of movement that can be observed in a fussy infant.

A buzzing hive of simultaneous physiological processes is found in the constant organic movements ebbing and flowing through the bodily tissues at any given moment. A symphony of biological movements can be felt in many systems at any given time, including the rise and fall of the breath, the convoluted unwinding of organs, the humming of an adrenal rush, and the miniscule muscular fluctuations of postural sway.

Organic movement impulses occur below a level of conscious awareness, yet it is possible to feel them by tracking the subtle impulses and currents initiated by metabolic processes. Since organic movements are constantly occurring within the body, one need not actually move to feel them. A person can lie down, relax, and pay attention to the intrinsic movements of the body, and eventually a chorus of organic impulses such as the guts gurgling, the lungs pumping, the fluids flowing, the muscles twitching,

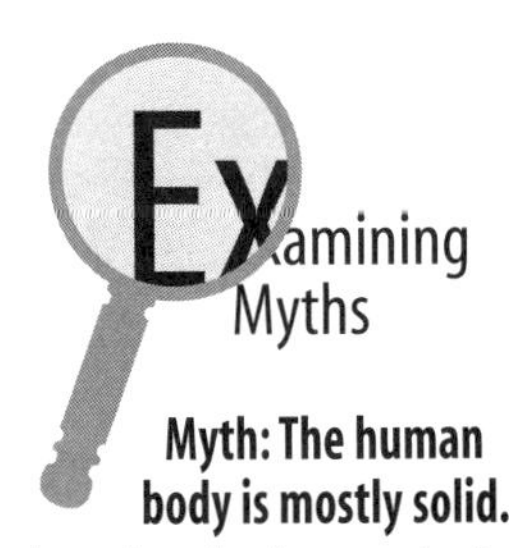

Myth: The human body is mostly solid.

Actually, the human body is far more liquid than solid; it is composed of anywhere from 60 to 80 percent fluid. The body is not only composed of mostly fluids, it is also a dynamic form in a state of constant motion. A living body teems with diverse intrinsic organic rhythms that churn, fire, spray, shoot, erupt, gurgitate, pump, and pulsate in continual metabolic processes that go on within.

clear, linear joint movement during patterning exercises while still allowing subtle organic impulses, such as fluid and unwinding micromovements, to surface and sequence.

The Workings of Mechanical Movement

Mechanical movements are generated by the phasic contractions of muscles, which act as pulleys to lever bones and move them through space. As discussed earlier, musculoskeletal coordination, though affected by ANS tone, is regulated by the somatic nervous system (SNS). Mechanical approaches to patterning work with the structured movements of the muscles and joints. In a broader sense, mechanical patterning is any type of modality that imposes structure on the body, providing direction, timing, and control to the manner in which we contract muscles and move joints.

Myofascias (muscles and their associated fascias) wraps the body like a form-fitting suit, which needs symmetry and balance in rest and motion to fit well, lest it become puckered and snagged in some areas while being overstretched in others. Mechanical patterning works to establish geometric balance in the muscle function and joint movement. The organized spatial pulls of muscular fibers maintain tensional balance in the body. For instance, it is important to stretch muscles after an injury to provide a linear stress and pathway along which the random, cross-hatched fibers in scar tissue can organize.

The underlying fullness and motility of the organs and fluids can also lend an intrinsic support to the extrinsic myofascial sleeve wrapping the outer layers of the body. Without this inner fullness, this myofascial suit feels flat and lifeless. With inner support, a person can maintain a buoyant equilibrium in the body as it moves through space. This support is cultivated through a sensory awareness of the organs and fluids. Cohen differentiates between a movement dominated by the organ, glandular, and fluid systems and a movement dominated by the musculoskeletal system by using a "contents-container" analogy. Of course, all movement of the body in space or through space is carried out by the musculoskeletal system, yet a person can focus on the organs and fluids during patterning to give the motion a fuller, more dimensional quality. This creates a communication between the contents and the container, which in turn allows the autonomic responses of the organs and the emotions to be carried out through muscular action.

Links to Practical Applications

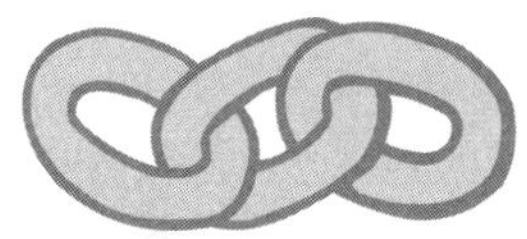

Patterning in an Upright Position or while Lying Down

Somatic patterning exercises can be practiced in either an upright posture or while lying down. Whether or not a person wants to pattern postural muscles will help determine which position is better for practicing an exercise. Generally, all upright postures require the support of postural muscles. Although you can pattern postural muscles while lying down, the horizontal position is favored when a person wants to release chronic tension without having to tend to supporting the body or working with postural tone.

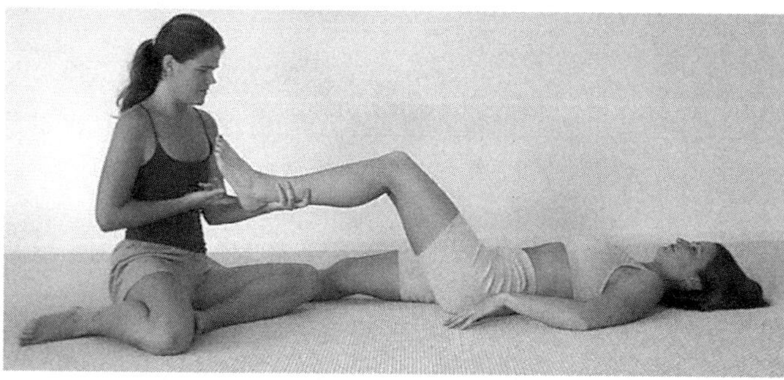

a.

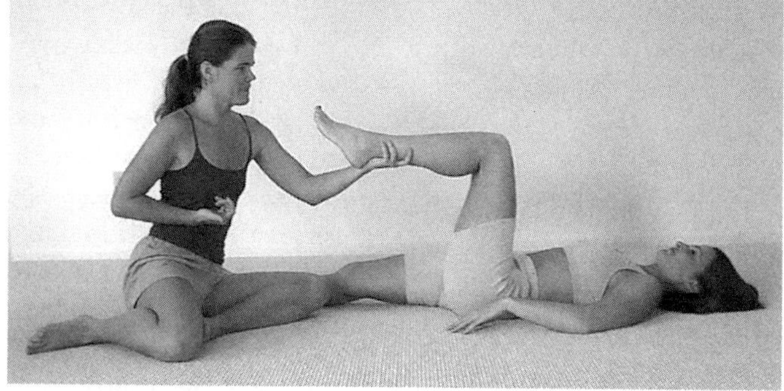

b.

Figure 4.12a-b A practitioner stimulates the flexor withdrawal reflex with light stroking on the sole of the client's foot.

Also important for coordinated neuromuscular actions are intact reflexes. The simple act of rising from a lying position to sitting, for example, requires a coordination of many reflexive movements, including head righting and tonic reflexes (reflexes that maintain position as opposed to phasic reflexes); balanced extensor and flexor reflexes; and the coordination of numerous other reflexes underlying push, reach, and pull patterns. Eliciting reflexes can effortlessly organize a chain of muscular action with minimal mental effort. For instance, a practitioner working with a client who has a habit of locking her knees can elicit the flexor withdrawal reflex and extensor thrust by lightly brushing the soles of the client's feet (Figure 4.12a-b). By doing so, the practitioner gets the client to extend the legs in a manner that reflexively sequences from the foot *through* the knee to the hip.

SUMMARY

There are a number of approaches to somatic patterning, the primary ones being those that involve one or more of the neuromuscular, autonomic, developmental, and cognitive channels of experience. Which approach people choose depends largely on the perception they have of their body or their problem. With this in mind, it is helpful to have a broad understanding of the choices available so that the perceptual field is inclusive of all the possibilities.

Movement patterns have qualities that reflect the brain centers that are the primary coordinators of each type of pattern, with the forebrain associated with thinking, the midbrain with feeling, with the hindbrain with moving, and the cellular brain with patterns of systemic resonance and touch. Any patterning experience can be targeted toward a specific part of the brain by focusing on one of these behaviors.

Somatic patterning works with psychological patterns as they show up in the physical body, although it differs from psychotherapy in that the primary focus of SP is on changing body patterns. Thus, when speech and thought patterns have a negative effect on body patterns, somatic patterners often draw on techniques from modalities such as neurolinguistic programming and cognitive therapy to change mental patterns.

Since developmental movement processes lay the foundation for all body patterns and sensorimotor learning is the primary channel through which developmental processes take place, both should be considered in any patterning process. A primary part of the SP process is working to balance modulating dualities, such as neuromuscular with autonomic patterning, cognitive with experiential approaches, and organic with mechanical approaches. Organic approaches work with nonstructured movement, cultivating spontaneous, fluid impulses as they arise to improve biological function. Mechanical approaches use structured exercises to improve neuromuscular coordination and the efficiency of muscle and joint function. Since all movement has both organic and mechanical aspects to it, to balance autonomic and neuromuscular systems, it is important to use a combination of both organic and mechanical approaches in SP.

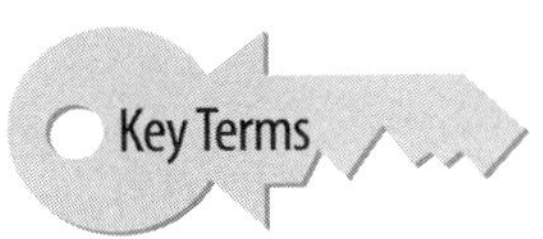

autonomic flexibility
autonomic patterning
"cellular brain"
cognitive learning
developmental patterning
emotional intelligence
experiential learning
facilitation
forebrain
hindbrain
inhibition
limbic system
mechanical movement
midbrain
mobility
modulate dualities
motility
motor processes
neuromuscular patterning
organic movement
organic movement practice
passive volition
progressive relaxation
relaxation response
sensory processes
support before movement
track and bump

OVERVIEW OF CHAPTER 5

TYPES OF PATTERNING EXERCISES

STARTING THE PATTERNING PROCESS

EFFORT

- Relaxation
- Tone
- Responsiveness

INITIATION AND SEQUENCING MOVEMENT

BREATHING

- External versus Internal Respiration
- Respiratory Anatomy
  - *Ribcage Motion during Respiration*
  - *Breathing Cycles*
- The Respiratory Diaphragm as a Postural Stabilizer
- Psychosomatic Patterns of Breathing
  - *Paradoxical Breathing*
  - *Breathing as a Body-Centered Practice*

MOVEMENT INITIATED BY SENSE ORGANS

- The Temporomandibular Joint
- Eye Movement
- Equilibrium, Hearing, and the Ears

INTEGRATION AND APPLICATION

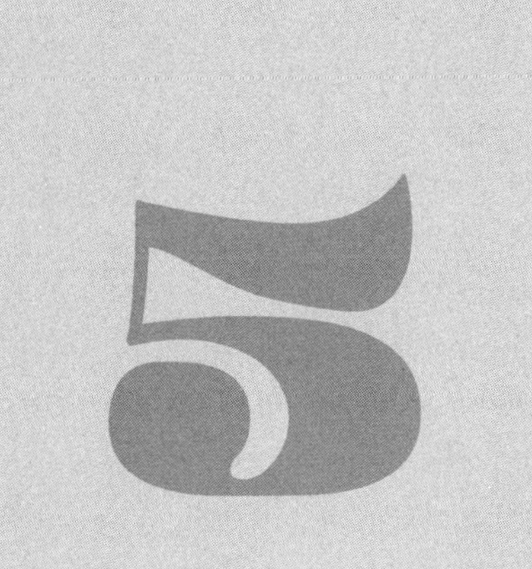

The Patterning Process

> **You cannot increase your sensitivity without simultaneously reducing your effort.**
>
> ***—Moshe Feldenkrais***

This chapter focuses on the transition from theory into practice. It begins with an introduction to the steps in the patterning process and follows with fundamental skills that can be integrated into and will support any of the patterning exercises. These skills include gauging effort and tone, starting an action and following it through a complete sequence, establishing breath support, and exploring movements initiated by the sense organs. All of these skills develop an underlying support for efficient and coordinated movement.

Due to individual differences and needs, it would be impossible to describe one SP program suited for everyone. Programs need to be tailored to each individual. Also, in a book this size, it would be impossible to present the hundreds of patterning exercises that exist and the diverse ways in which each might be practiced. This chapter introduces preparatory exercises to somatic patterning. Part 2, in turn, takes a closer look at how the human body works and moves into practice by presenting SP exercises designed specifically for working to change somatic patterns.

Somatic patterning can be thought of as a brain gym: the mind can direct the way we move through the gym with cognitive skills. In SP, a fundamental basic cognitive skill is that of using sensory awareness to monitor attention and intention. Attention provides feedback and develops the ground for sensorimotor awareness; intention provides direction and initiates action. A volley between the two creates a third force—the element of change.

A person must also be able to trust the body enough to let the body breathe and move independently of mental control. Developing trust involves not only an attitude of passive volition but also the willingness to release mental control and excessive effort. This may be the most important SP skill a person can learn because, as has been thoroughly discussed previously, the mind's tyrannical control over the body often restricts natural movement. Occasionally the SP process needs to be drawn in and directed by cortical control, but generally, the mind needs to relax while body responses drive the process. The importance of practicing what appear to be relatively easy skills such as breathing, relaxing, gauging effort, and setting tone should not be underestimated or overlooked as they are the foundation of somatic patterning.

TYPES OF PATTERNING EXERCISES

In Chapter 4, the numerous approaches to patterning were presented. Many of these approaches are often combined within a holistic framework. Holistic patterning requires diversity. The more diverse the approaches to patterning, the greater the likelihood of improving overall function and coordination. Most

SP exercises in this text can be categorized in one or more of the following approaches:

- sensory awareness
- relaxation
- breathing
- organic movement
- reflexes
- developmental patterns
- tonic development and postural stability
- phasic development and movement fundamentals
- cognitive skills

This list seems daunting, yet most of these elements are simultaneously present during a patterning exercise. Differentiating them helps ensure that the primary somatic elements are considered in the patterning process, which is important because leaving out any one may leave a gap in the overall process. A patterning exercise usually only focuses on one element, although as skills build, a person is able to tend to more than one element at a time.

Think of each element as a door to a complex bio-neural network. Entering the process through many different "doors" or pathways, a person is more likely to balance the functions of diverse parts of the nervous system.

STARTING THE PATTERNING PROCESS

When beginning patterning, many people think they need to know exactly how to change a pattern or how a muscle contracts to enact change. There are many theories about how a muscle actually contracts, such as the sliding filament theory, but even scientists do not know exactly how the nervous system coordinates this multifaceted process. The good news is that we don't need to understand exactly how each anatomical part or metabolic process within the body works to change a pattern. We simply need to have a basic understanding of functional anatomy to provide the right image for a new movement pattern and the nervous system will coordinate the rest.

Links to Practical Applications

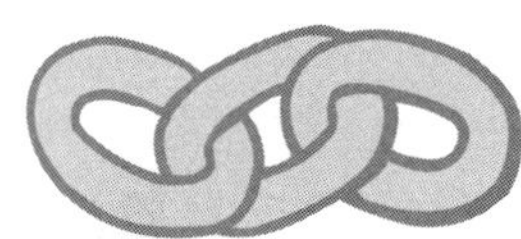

Keeping an Open Mind

To keep all doors open and possibilities available, begin patterning by assuming that what you do not know is greater than what you know. This orientation will help you to maintain a holistic, inclusive attitude, one that expands your awareness to include the parts of a pattern that you are unaware of. And it also elicits curiosity, a reach into unknown areas of experience that will keep your efforts open to new possibilities.

Patterning Exercise #27: Different Approaches to Patterning the Pelvic Tilt

This exercise is an example of how the same patterning exercise can be done with many different approaches.

1. *The basic tilt:* Lie on your back with your knees bent, feet on the floor, and legs parallel. Tilt your pelvis by lifting your tail (coccyx) and sacrum toward the backs of your knees, and pressing your lumbar spine into the floor (PE Fig. 27a). Then reverse the tilt, moving back to your original position, lengthening your tail toward your feet (PE Fig. 27b).

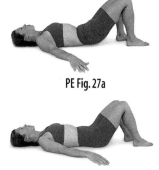

PE Fig. 27a

PE Fig. 27b

2. *Focus on weight:* Imagine your trunk filled with liquid sand. Slowly tilt your pelvis, sensing or imaging the sand sink and pour into your lower back. Slowly reverse the movement by pouring the imaginary sand toward your hips.
3. *Focus on organs:* Imagine your organs like a group of water balloons filling your torso. Slowly tilt, visualizing the balloons rolling into the part of your back where you feel weight. Sense movement in one balloon at a time, the back of the sacrum, then lumbar spine, then waist, then ribs. Reverse the tilt using the same imagery.
4. *Focus on fluidity:* Rock your pelvis back and forth with the movement quality of a rocking chair. Let the movement be fluid and spontaneous, using a easy rocking rhythm. Do not try to control the movement. Allow it to rock and loosen your entire trunk.
5. *Focus on emotions:* As you do several tilts, feel any emotions or emotional associations you have with pelvic motion. Does it bring up pleasure, anxiety? If so, notice if the feelings change as you move. (Many people develop holding patterns in the pelvis around puberty, when they are self-conscious about their budding sexuality.)
6. *Focus on the sequence of movement through the joints:* Visualize an imaginary string of pearls between your coccyx and your lower ribs. Slowly tilt your pelvis by lifting one pearl at a time, moving up your spine until you have progressively transferred your body weight into your feet, and then into the back of your lower ribs. Then reverse the movement, lowering one pearl at a time.
7. *Focus on relaxation:* Explore tilting your pelvis in a slow, relaxing manner. Begin by placing your hands just above your pubic bone and start the tilt there, sinking back and widening above the pubic bone. Allow your body to become heavier as you tilt, feeling the weight of your sacrum and lower back gradually sinking and widening into the floor. Stay focused on the feeling of weight as you reverse the tilt and return to the starting position.

EMSPress.com

Each SP program needs to meet a person at his or her level of ability and proceed from there. For instance, a person with minimal body awareness can begin with sensory awareness exercises such as slow movements done with focused awareness, breathing exercises, or relaxation techniques. A tense person can explore subtle, safe movements to build a sense of trust and relaxation in the body. An uncoordinated and stiff person can explore playful improvisational movements to release tension, elicit reflexes, and organize coordinated neuromuscular pathways. In each of these cases, the patterning exercise offered would be only the first stage of the SP process with each additional stage building different skills. After gaining proficiency with one skill, a person can build on it and expand into other areas.

There are a number of stages in a patterning process. Although the stages are presented here in a logical progression, they can be explored in various orders, either one at a time, two or three at a time, or as a progression. A typical session might address only one or two stages, with the entire progression showing up eventually through a series of sessions. The most common steps in a process follow:

1. Setting goals or intention.
2. Setting up a feedback loop.
3. Tracking instrinic sensations.
4. Actively relaxing.
5. Establishing support before movement.
6. Moving with the least amount of effort possible.
7. Exploring fluid movement.
8. Exploring organic, automatic movement.
9. Stabilizing loose areas, then mobilizing tight areas.
10. Identifying and releasing holding patterns.
11. Learning new patterns.
12. Resting and recuperating after each exercise.
13. Closing the feedback loop.

A person can begin the patterning process at any stage, yet the best place to begin is where that person already has awareness and can have a successful experience. For example, a man may come to patterning with a history of mentally overworking at the office during weekdays, then physically overworking his body in weekend weight-lifting routines. This man suffers from "workaholic" syndrome with body pain associated with mental fatigue and overworking his body on the weekends.

This man would probably approach SP as he approaches his job and exercise routine, like a drill sergeant ruthlessly driving his tired muscles. The pitfalls of overworking for a hyperactive person with a type A personality is that he rarely gives his body a chance to rest and he overrides sensory feedback coming from the body. This individual would benefit most from SP exercises that help him consciously relax and learn to feel his body. Since he is a bodybuilder and familiar with the muscles, he would probably be more comfortable starting with progressive muscular relaxation rather than exploring subtle sensory awareness or improvisational movement exercises, both of which would probably be foreign to him.

There are many types of patterning exercises on the continuum between rest and action. Knowing exactly where to begin patterning is not as important as just experiencing a new way of sensing or moving the body. Each patterning exercise can be done in a variety of ways to access different centers. For example, the exercise called the pelvic tilt can be explored with a focus on bones, muscles, fluids, or organs; at different rates and rhythms; in different planes; and in different combinations with other patterns.

Patterning Exercise #28: Dealing with an Overactive Mind or Body

When your muscles are overworking:

1. Once you become aware of how much energy you waste using excessive effort, you can begin to gauge how much effort is actually needed for an action and release the excess. Move slowly. Sense the effort you use, then reduce it, moving with only one-tenth of the effort.
2. Take conscious control over an effort pattern by exaggerating the effort. Do so by going into the pattern, tightening more muscles than you need, and hold. Sense the extra energy you spend exaggerating pattern. Then release that effort. Exaggerate and release the pattern several times until increasing or decreasing your effort becomes as natural as changing the volume on a radio.
3. If you are unable to let go of excess tension, drop the exercise. Go do something else to take your mind off it.

When patterning exercises become too mental:

4. Every time you notice your mind becoming controlling, give your mind a job to distract it, such as monitoring your breathing or repeating a suggestive word, prayer, or mantra, over and over again, such as "relax, relax, relax . . . "
5. Change the quality of your movement to something easy and automatic. For example, do a repetitive exercise that does not require much thought, such as a fluid rocking or undulating movement.
6. Move in a slow, relaxed manner using the least amount of energy possible. As you move, focus on relaxing. Notice any areas where you feel tension and repeatedly pause your movement mid-sequence to consciously relax this area.

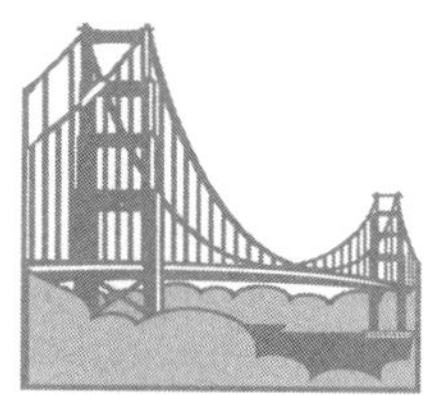

Working with a Client's Overactive Mind

There are clues that indicate a client has an overactive mind. She may have trouble concentrating because she is thinking about other things, may keep introducing peripheral topics, or may even have a nervous habit such as tapping her foot, biting her nails, or looking around. If she is lying with her eyes closed, you might notice her eyes rapidly moving under her eyelids or notice a crease in the middle of her forehead between her eyes.

If you see these signs, ask her if her mind is active. If so, suggest she become aware of how her thoughts are affecting her body. When asked to notice mental activity, many clients comment that their mind is busy elsewhere (working on their taxes or figuring out some problem) or that their mind is overly active trying to dictate what is going on in the body.

Next, ask her to focus her mind on a simple, repetitive task, such as breathing, or feeling where her body touches your massage table, or even wiggling her toes. If these body-based tasks fail to quiet her mind, suggest a mental task, such as visualizing a peaceful setting or repeating a word over and over again. (Recall from Chapter 4 that continually repeating a word evokes the relaxation response.)

The mind can also be put to work as the benevolent overseer of the body. Every time your client's attention wanders away from the body, ask her to scan the sensations within her body. These can be sensations of movement, of relaxation, or of breathing. Or suggest that your client occupy her mind with this question: "Is what I am doing right now, in this moment, helping me or hindering me to attain my goals?"

The mind can also be given the task of maintaining a global, full-body focus. Every time your client notices mind chatter or that her attention is becoming overly focused on one body part, have the client shift her focus to the entire body. This task uses the mind like a spotlight, first to highlight when the attention narrows, and second to illuminate more of the body with a broader focus. This task also oscillates a person's attention between the parts and the whole, which cultivates an awareness of full-body patterns and improves mind-body cooperation.

EFFORT

Efficient, fluid, and integrated movement is characterized by a quality of ease and minimal effort. During an efficient movement, **effort**—the amount of energy needed to carry out an action—is distributed throughout the body so that all the working parts contribute equally to the stability and mobility of the whole body. Too much work in one area and too little in another will imbalance the distribution of effort among the many parts involved in an action.

The process of setting the right tone and effort for a movement is so automatic that if we misjudge the distance we are moving or the load we are lifting, we get a surprise. Recall the example of a person walking on level ground who is jolted by an unexpected step. Since the muscles were unprepared for the level change and unable to set the muscle tone accordingly, one leg slammed down. Had this person actually seen the step, the neuromuscular circuits would have automatically set the tone to prepare the body to step down. This shift is mostly a subconscious process triggered by a quick sight of the step, a snapshot preview that allows us to gauge effort and coordinate the ensuing motion with ease. Likewise, effort can be monitored during a patterning exercise to gauge just the right amount.

It is also extremely important that each movement sequences through a full initiation-action-rest cycle. Generally, a thought or intention initiates a movement, and then the action is coordinated and enacted on a subconscious level. If the mind becomes overactive in directing a movement, it can interfere with the smooth coordination of a movement sequence. In addition, the mind will exhaust faster than the body because the

Links to
Practical Applications

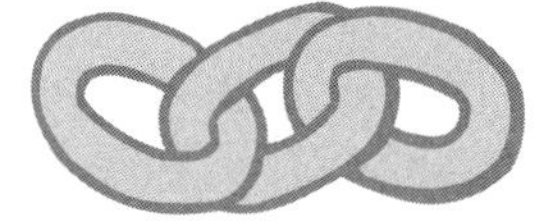

Relax before Going to Bed

Practicing relaxation exercises before going to bed or while you are waiting to fall asleep will usually improve the quality of your sleep.

Patterning Exercise #29: The "Sand-Bag" Brain and Body

This exercise teaches you how to relax during movement by moving with a heavy, slow quality of motion.

1. Lie on your back in a comfortable position. Imagine that your head and body are filled with sand.
2. Gently roll your head from side to side. Visualize sand sifting from side to side. Move very slowly, as though you could feel one grain of sand move at a time.
3. Next, imagine your whole body filled with sand. Then slowly roll your body to one side, then to the other, imagining the sand gradually pouring from one area to the next as you roll (PE Fig. 29a-c). Sense your body's weight sinking into the floor in the places where you feel contact. Roll back and forth several times until you feel heavier and more relaxed.

Variations: Repeat the exercise while sitting, or have a partner slowly roll your head from side to side while you use the visualization of sand slowly pouring. Can you yield the weight of your head into your partner's hands?

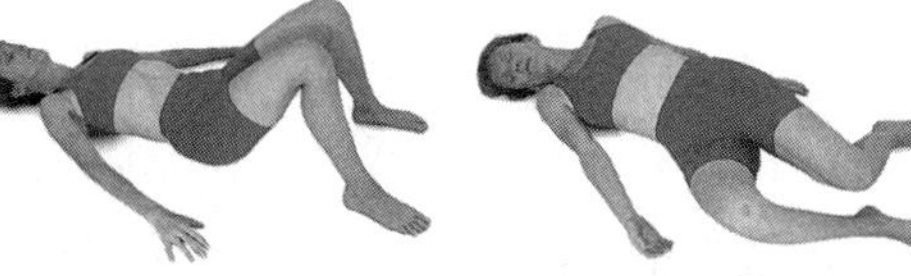

PE Fig. 29a PE Fig. 29b

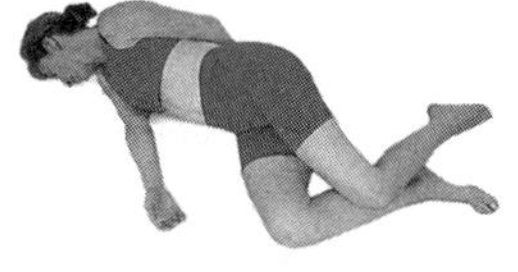

PE Fig. 29c

EMSPress.com

brain has evolved to coordinate movement at a subcortical level. Given this, overly controlled patterning interferes with the rest phase of a movement sequence and can be mentally taxing.

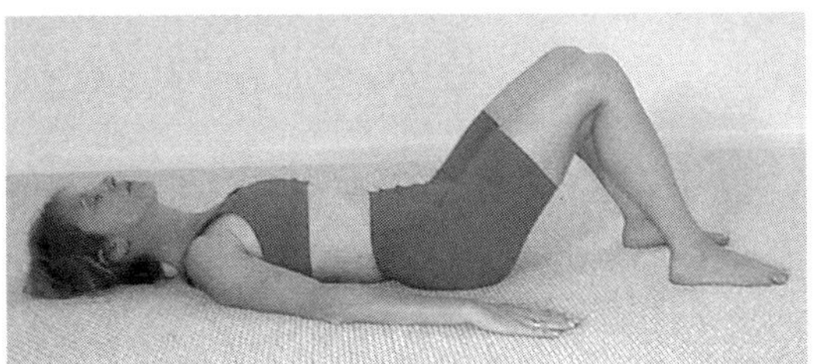

Figure 5.1 A woman relaxes her back in the constructive rest position (CRP) during the middle of a busy day.

Relaxation

Efficient movement begins in a relaxed state, and every efficient sequence has subtle, relaxing pauses within the chain of action. The more relaxed and rested the body is when it begins moving, the more effortless the subsequent movement will be. If patterning exercises are practiced from a tense, rigid state, they will drive stress deeper into the body. By learning how to relax and move from a relaxed state, we are able to reset the baseline of resting tone from which we initiate movement.

It is important to understand that *relaxation is an active process in the nervous system.* Some people think that becoming passive or limp relaxes the body, but that's not necessarily so. Relaxation creates deep physiological changes that do not automatically occur when a person stops moving. The relaxation response occurs only when the autonomic nervous system moves into a parasympathetic mode. To become adept at relaxing, a tense person needs practice it on a regular basis (Figure 5.1).

Can you maintain a state of relaxation that you reached in quiet position once you start moving again?

By cultivating relaxation and minimal effort during patterning exercises, we promote healthy action-and-rest cycles and allow for recuperation within a sequence. For instance, during a long walk, a person could focus on relaxing each time the foot hits the ground, or during each exhalation. (This may sound hard because there is so little time between repetitions, but since thought initiates action at a lightning speed, it is actually easier than it sounds.)

A person can be in a position of rest while remaining wound up inside. Unfortunately, lying down and resting does not ensure that autonomic tone will come down. Tension carries into activity, including sleep. A person who goes to bed tense will usually have a restless night of tossing, turning, and teeth grinding, and then wake up with a headache or muscle spasm and wonder why.

Relaxation can be achieved in many ways:

- Through progressive relaxation exercises.
- Through guided imagery.
- Through a sensory awareness of the body's weight sinking into its supporting surface.
- Through breathing exercises.
- Through slow, steady movement.
- Through fun, rhythmic movements like dance.
- Through unstructured fluid and organic movement improvisations in which a person releases mental control over body movement.

Tone

Tone is the overall state of neural excitability in the body prior to action. There are many kinds of tone in the body, though muscle tone is probably the one people are most familiar with. **Muscle tone** is the amount of contraction that occurs in a muscle at rest. When at rest, a number of muscle fibers within muscles still actively contract. Healthy muscles have good resting tone and the ability to relax. Muscle tone that is abnormally high will lead to spasticity, tone that is abnormally low can cause flaccidity.

Autonomic tone describes the level of relaxation of excitability in the autonomic nervous system, which fluctuates between parasympathetic and sympathetic tone. Parasympathetic tone occurs when the body is relaxed and vegetative functions such as digestion and tissue repair dominate. Sympathetic tone occurs when the body is active, at which time blood and metabolic energy is drawn away from the digestive organs and concentrated in the skeletal muscles.

All exercises, whether they are done for conditioning or for patterning, change tone on some level in some body system. For instance, the relaxation response lowers autonomic tone whereas stress elevates it; bodybuilding builds phasic tone in the muscles whereas isometric exercises builds tonic tone.

Every body system has its own tone quality, although good muscle tone improves tone in all other systems, especially in the lymphatic and cardiovascular sys-

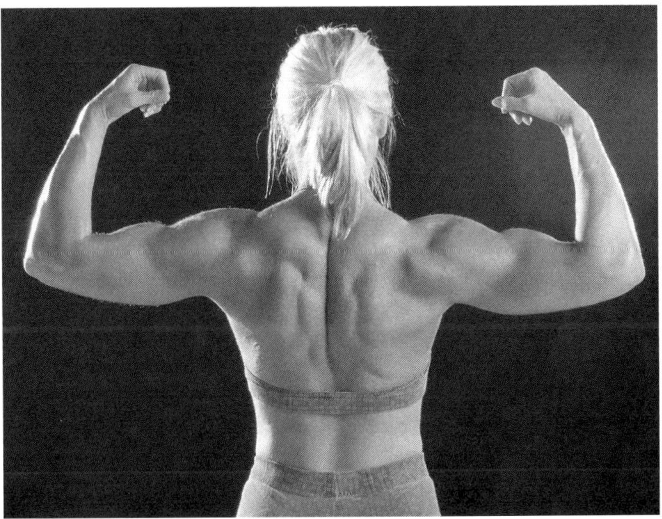

Figure 5.2 Note the continuity and symmetry of muscle tone in her back.

Patterning Exercise #30: Full-Body Flexion and Extension

(Adapted from Bonnie Cohen's exploration of physiological extension, the birthing pattern.)

1. Lie on your side in a fetal position with both feet against the baseboard of a wall. Preferably, lie on a wood or vinyl floor, a surface you can easily slide on.
2. Pull your entire body into as deep a flexion as you can manage (PE Fig. 30a). Rest there and feel the buildup of potential energy, as though holding yourself in full-body flexion was loading a spring.

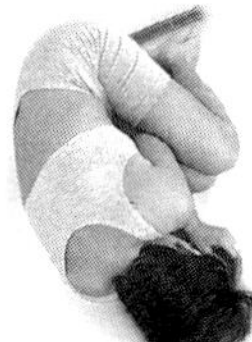

PE Fig. 30a

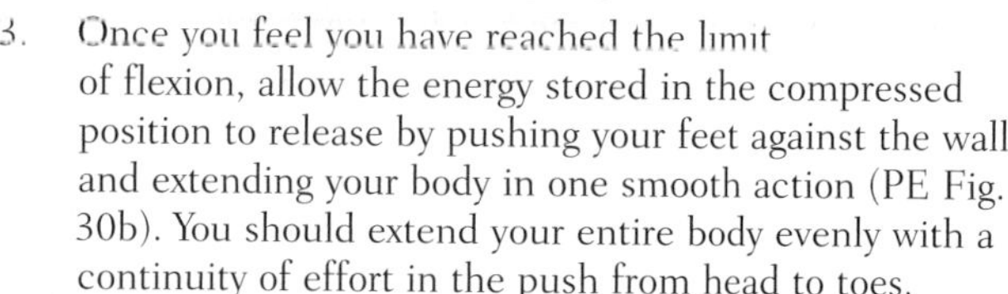

3. Once you feel you have reached the limit of flexion, allow the energy stored in the compressed position to release by pushing your feet against the wall and extending your body in one smooth action (PE Fig. 30b). You should extend your entire body evenly with a continuity of effort in the push from head to toes.
4. Once you have reached full extension, sense how your body naturally rebounds and is ready to curl again into flexion. Wait for the impulse to flex, then pull your body back into a flexed position.
5. Scoot over toward the wall and assume the starting position. Repeat the flexion/extension cycle several times until you feel a spontaneous, reflexive impulse to extend from a flexed position,then curl back into flexion from a hyperextended position.

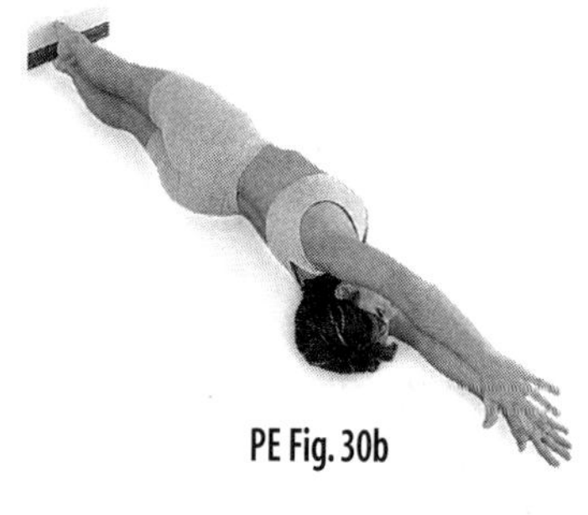

PE Fig. 30b

EMSPress.com

tems. Poor muscle tone will result in the sluggish circulation of all bodily fluids, especially lymph and blood.

All body patterns have corresponding mental, or emotional patterns and the tone quality of one aspect can affect the tone of another. Habitually negative emotions wear down the immune system and paranoid thoughts show up in a guarded quality of movement. Ideally, there is a **continuity of tone** among systems and throughout the skeletal muscle system (Figure 5.2). When the muscular system lacks continuity, some muscles chronically contract and hold while others become flaccid and overstretched, causing bilateral groups of muscles to lack symmetry.

A person might also lack an inner and outer continuity of tone. For example, a man filled with anxiety might have a reserved and quiet posture. On the surface his muscles seem relaxed, yet inside his nerves are racing with anxiety. Upon closer observation, his high autonomic tone becomes evident in clammy skin, halting speech patterns, and twitchy habits. High autonomic tone from a racing metabolic engine can either be spent in activity or lowered by rest. This high-strung man has several options. He can learn how to relax, release stress through rigorous physical activity, process physiological stress through organic movement, or restructure the thoughts, memories, and behaviors that create his anxiety in the first place. Once he is able to relax, his inner tone will match his outer countenance, creating inner/outer continuity.

A healthy posture is balanced between **flexor tone** and **extensor tone**. Flexor tone is the tone of the muscles along the front of the trunk and neck; extensor tone is the tone in the muscles along the back, from the head to the tail. If one overpowers the other, the result will be either a posture that is chronically flexed or one that is hyperextended.

Flexor tone begins developing before birth as the fetus grows into deeper flexion and the space within the womb becomes smaller. A newborn arrives curled in fetal flexion that is so strong that the baby stays curled like a snail when

Patterning Exercise #31: Improving Postural Tone while Traveling

Traveling is an excellent time to tone up postural muscles because they are developed with isometric contractions and subtle, intrinsic movements. Explore the following movements whenever you are sitting or driving for long periods.

1. As you press the gas pedal with your right foot, push your left leg into the floor to encourage symmetry in your pelvis.
2. Rock on your sit bones, alternating between turning your pelvis under and extending it. Then find the neutral place in between and stop there.
3. When in a neutral posture, lightly pull your lower abdomen in and hold it for the count of ten, then relax.
4. Contract your pelvic floor and hold it for the count of ten, then relax it.
5. Lift the top of your head toward the roof to elongate your neck. Then subtly nod your head to engage the intrinsic muscles in your neck.
6. Move your chin forward then back several times.
7. Push both feet into the floor and feel the push press your sacrum back into the seat behind you.
8. Push your steering wheel with both hands and feel the push open the back of your shoulder blades. Then release.

EMSPress.com

Patterning Exercise #32: Feeling Responsiveness with Rocking Motions

This movement exploration is to check the level of responsiveness in your body and to help you relax into rhythmic motion.

1. *Heel rock* (adapted from the Bartenieff Fundamentals): Lie on your back with your legs straight, relaxed, and as close to parallel as is comfortable. Take note of which parts of your back are touching the ground and which are not.
2. Rock your body form your ankles, flexing and extending them in a free-flow motion (PE Fig. 32a-b). It may be easier to do if you lie with your feet against a wall and rock by gently pumping your feet against the wall (PE Fig. 32c). Keep the back of your knees relaxed; isolate the movement in your ankles. Imagine digging a groove in the floor beneath your heels. Sense how the rocking motion moves your entire body. Allow it to gently rock your body from feet to head. Allow the movement to reverberate through all of your bones and joints, as though you were a bag of loose bones. As you rock, consciously relax tense areas.

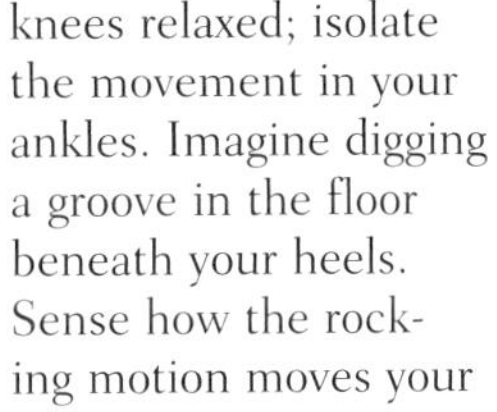

PE Fig. 32a-b

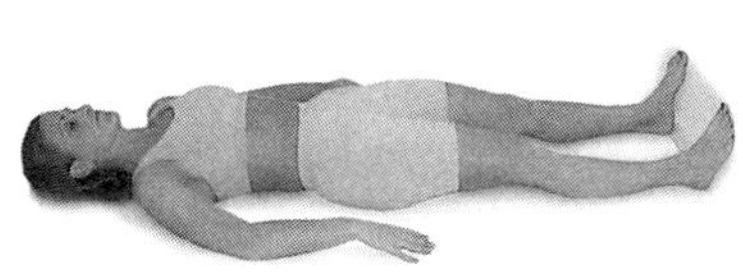

PE Fig. 32c

3. To loosen tight areas as your rock, tighten them up even more. Then release the tightening and let the movement surge through that area. Now rest. Check the contact your back makes with the floor. Has it increased?
4. *Pelvic rock:* Bend your knees, putting your feet flat on the floor and keeping your legs parallel (PE Fig. 32d). Push your feet into the floor in a rhythmic manner to rock your pelvis. As you rock, sense your organs shifting toward the back of your body, from head to tail, and let your abdominal wall sink toward your lower back.

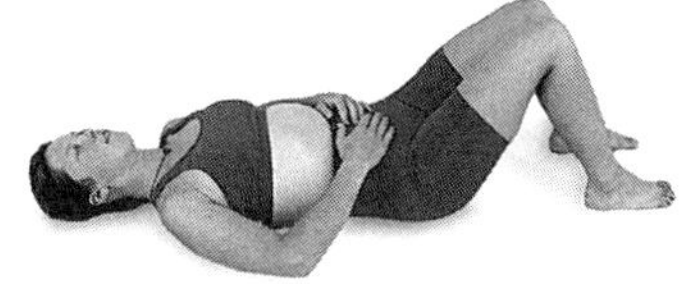

PE Fig. 32d

5. *Pelvic roll:* Bring your knees up to your chest and roll from side to side (PE Fig. 32e).

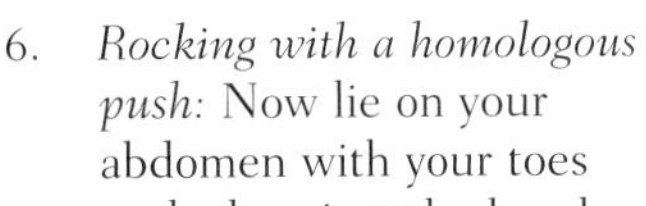

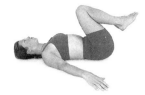

PE Fig. 32e

6. *Rocking with a homologous push:* Now lie on your abdomen with your toes tucked against the baseboard of a wall (PE Fig. 32f). Rock by pushing with your toes, keeping your thighs weighted and on the floor. As you rock, consciously release tension along the front of the body, letting your torso sink into the floor. Next, rock your entire body by rhythmically pushing your forearms against the floor.

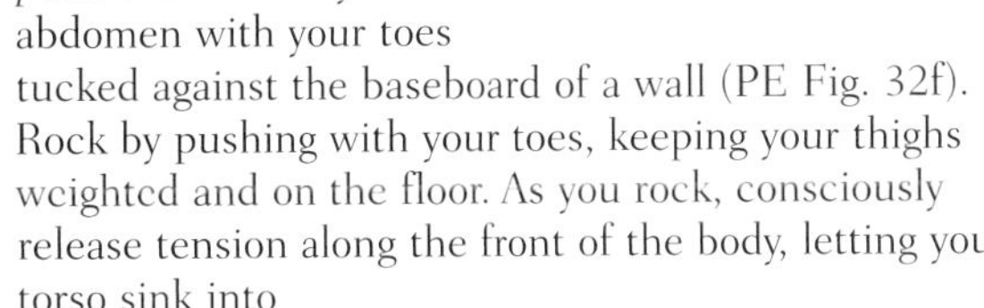

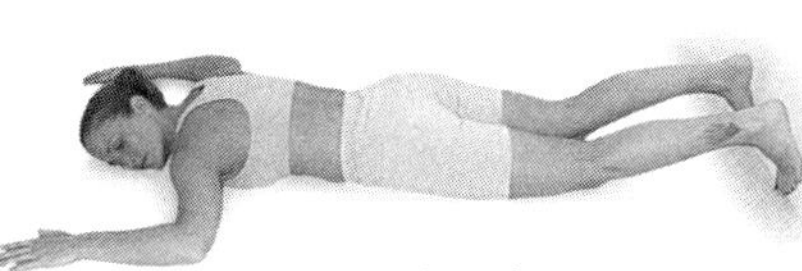

PE Fig. 32f

7. *Rocking a partner:* Get a partner and have her lie on her back. Have her describe how much of her back is in contact with the floor before you begin. Next, gently rock her body from her feet (PE Fig. 32g). Notice which parts of her body are responsive and moving and which are not. Suggest that your friend relax into the motion, letting her back sink into the floor.

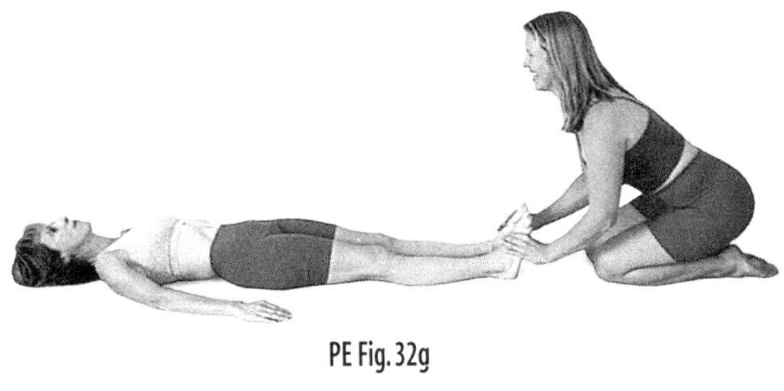

PE Fig. 32g

EMSPress.com

held up in the air with its belly down. This early pattern of full-body flexion is called **physiological flexion**. It develops during the last trimester when the rapid growth of the fetus pulls the walls of the uterus progressively more taut. Physiological flexion begins in the lower abdominal organs and feet, sequencing successively up to the head. The tight fetal curl creates rotation and deep flexion in both the arms and legs, folding them across the body.

Physiological flexion is modulated by **physiological extension**, a full-body pattern of extension that first appears at birth, when the newborn thrusts out the womb through the birth canal begin with a push from the feet that extends up the body. The concept of physiological flexion in developmental movement was first presented by Dr. Josephine Moore; Bonnie Cohen added the concept of physiological extension.[86]

Weak flexor or weak extensor tone will affect posture. When the muscles on the back of the body have higher resting tone than the muscles on the front, a person has weak flexor tone. This shows up in postures of chronic hyperextension in the spine and knees. Conversely, if flexor tone overpowers extensor tone, the muscles on the front of the body will have a higher resting tone than the muscles on the back. This pattern is obvious in postures of chronic flexion (like the example of Henry in Chapter 4), where the front of the body is held shorter than the back creating a tucked pelvis, a flat lumbar spine, a hunched-over thorax, and perhaps even a bent-knee posture. By practicing the modulating pattern, a person can begin to balance flexor and extensor tone.

Patterning should be practiced with gradual increases or decreases in tone rather than jumping between low and high tone. Abrupt changes cause stress. For instance, when a person wakes up in the morning, she usually stretches and slowly rouses the body to an awakened state. This gradual process brings the tone up slowly, giving each part of the body ample time to shift. In contrast, quickly jumping out of bed changes tone from low to high in one move, which can shock the body. This is similar to suddenly blasting the volume on a radio: it hurts the ears because they do not have time to acclimate to changes in volume. During any patterning exercise, when the tone changes too fast or the starting tone is not quite right, a person can begin the exercise over to reset tone. Also, by becoming aware of exactly where and how a pattern begins, we can reset the initiation of an action to change the direction and tone of the movement sequence that follows.

Responsiveness

Throw a rock into a pond, and ripples spread out across the water. The same is true for movement in a responsive body. **Responsiveness** describes the ability of a person to be fluid and open enough that organic movement impulses sequence through the entire body, no matter how small the impulse. Various degrees of responsiveness can be observed by how a movement flows through the body or is blocked by restrictions. Even the smallest impulse travels completely through a responsive body on an energetic level. A responsive body has good muscle tone yet is still flexible and fluid, making movement appear effortless rather than stiff. We will revisit this topic in Chapter 6.

What parts of a movement sequence are you best at: planning, getting started, carrying out the action, finishing, or resting afterwards? What steps do you need to focus on in order to make sure that you complete a full sequence?

INITIATING AND SEQUENCING MOVEMENT

Every movement has recognizable stages: the initiation, sequence of movement, completion, and rest-recuperation period. Some people are better at different parts of the sequence than others, both figuratively and literally. A hyperactive, type A personality tends to initiate an action quickly and impulsively rushing from one activity to the next without resting, whereas a slow, impassive personality might have trouble initiating a project. The traditional sensorimotor loop involves the following phases: "sensory input, perceptual interpretation, motor-planning, motor response, sensory feedback, [and] perceptual interpretation."[87] We have previously discussed all these phases except *motor planning*, the stage in which a person makes a preparation to move (Figure 5.3). For example, imagine the posture a diver assumes for a moment of mental preparation before springing off the board. This motor planning stage is also obvious in the moment of hesitation a cat takes prior to agile jump up to a seemingly out-of-reach ledge.

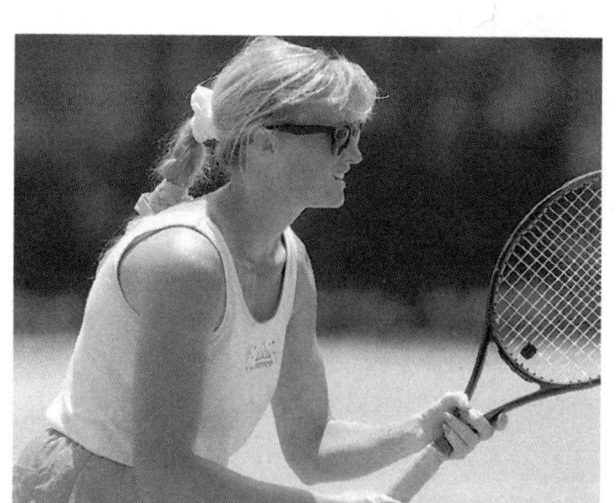

Figure 5.3 Motor planning during a pause in a movement sequence

Cohen points out that in a traditional sensorimotor sequence, two important phases that occur prior to sensory input are missing. The first phase is based on how preconceived expectations we have influence how we pay attention. Since experience is always colored by expectations we carry from our memories of similar experiences, these expectations influence the initiation of the movement we are about to make. For example, if a person has habitually fallen short when jumping across a ditch, her fear of falling short will probably be reflected in the posture she takes prior to jumping a ditch. The second missing phase is a *pre-motor focus*, the motor act of directing perception in a specific direction and manner.[88] For example, we turn our ears toward the direction of a sound, or turn our faces toward the direction in which we will speak.

The pathway of a movement can be observed between the place in the body where it begins and ends. The basic neurological pathways of movement in the body (spinal, homologous, homolateral, and contralateral) are wired to sequence along pathways between two endpoints—the hands and feet, and the head and tail. Each pattern passes from one endpoint to another along a contiguous kinematic chain of muscular action. Ideally, an action passes from one joint to the next through a series of linked joints and overlapping muscles without becoming stuck mid-sequence in a locked joint or skipping over a chronically contracted area.

The shape of the body between two endpoints while a person is in a neutral posture often reflects where a movement sequence is incomplete.

Links to Practical Applications

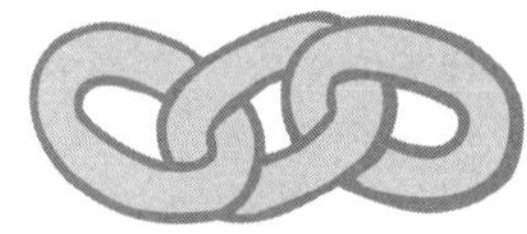

Starting Over

If, during any of the patterning exercises, you begin a movement that feels awkward or wrong, rather than trying to change it mid-sequence, simply start over.

Patterning Exercise #33: Movement Initiation

In the following exercise, explore how the pathway of movement is affected by where it initiates.

1. Sit or lie in a comfortable position.
2. *Hand:* Draw imaginary pathways of movement in the air with your elbow. Feel the quality of motion. Next, carve spatial pathways in the air with your hand and fingertips. Contrast initiating in the hand and the elbow. How is the sequence of movement different? Switch sides and repeat with the other elbow and hand.
3. *Foot:* Draw imaginary lines on the floor with the toes of one foot. Contrast this with movement initiated by drawing imaginary lines with your knee. How is the movement quality different when it initiates in the foot and the knee?
4. *Head:* Draw imaginary lines above you with the top of your head. Contrast this with initiating spinal movement in the middle of your neck. How are the two different?
5. *Tail:* Put your hand on the end of your coccyx, or tail. Draw imaginary circles below you with your tail. Contrast this with spinal movement initiating in your lower back. How are the two different?

For instance, a person with a forward head posture probably has a habit of initiating head movement by hinging in the middle of the neck rather than using the whole spine (Figure 5.4a). This incomplete action puts undue stress on the vertebral joints at the apex of the hinge and breaks the continuity of tone and movement along the spine. To break this habit, this person could practice sequencing movement through the whole spine by arching over forward or backward one vertebra at a time, starting at either the head or the tail (Figure 5.4a). (See Patterning Exercise #96 titled "Arcing: Flexing and Extending the Spine.") To encourage a full sequence of movement along a pathway such as the spine, a person needs to intentionally and specifically mobilize the held, restricted joints while at the same time stabilizing the typically loose or hypermobile joints. In the example just described, the woman would actively move stiff areas in the middle and lower spine while stabilizing the area where she tends to hinge and hyperextend the neck.

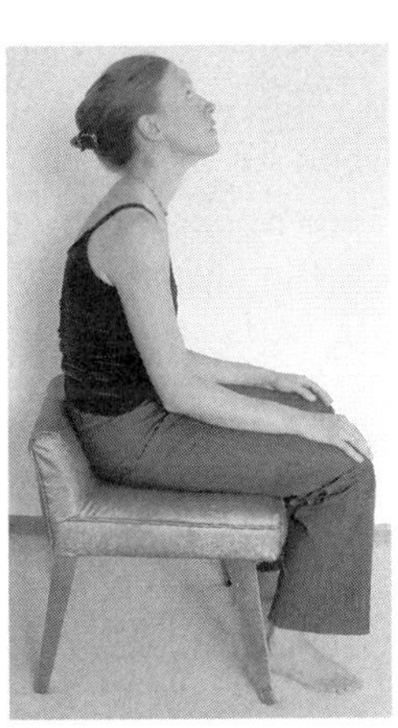

Figure 5.4a Hinging the neck stresses the spine at the point of collapse.

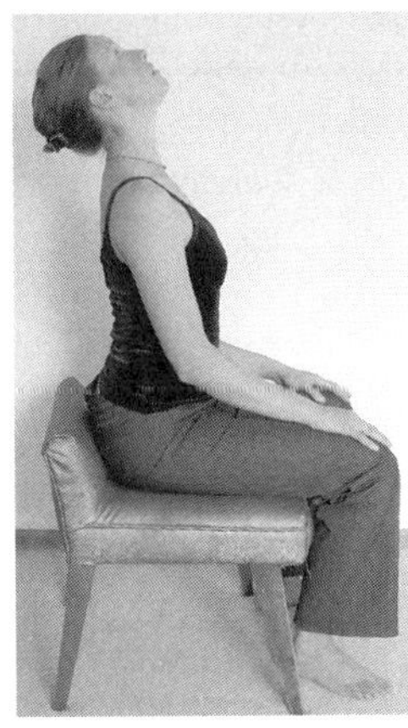

Figure 5.4b Extending the entire spine keeps the neck supported.

The initiation of a movement sequence determines the pathway of that movement. Integrated actions, especially push and reach patterns, generally initiate in the smaller muscles of the hands or feet, head or tail, where smaller, more articulate motor units (see p. 213) are concentrated, and then sequences through larger motor units along a pathway to another endpoint. The woman in our example could initiate movement between the head and first cervical vertebra to start a sequence that engages the whole spine.

When movement habitually initiates in the larger muscles between endpoints, sequencing is disturbed. This is particularly true of movement that begins in the elbows, knees, or middle of the spine. To illustrate this effect, imagine holding the end of a rope and whipping it so that the rope undulates. The undulating ripple will travel from your force to the other end of the rope. Now imagine holding it in the middle and performing the same action; the ripple only sequence along one half of the rope. Likewise, when we reach to touch something with our fingers, the movement travels up the arm and into the body. If we reach with the elbow or shoulder, we skip past the articulations of the hand. A similar dynamic occurs in the spine where responsive movement travels through many intervertebral segments to make a complete sequence.

Movement that initiates at the periphery is more likely to sequence through the whole body from one end to another. Compare a diver who pushes off the board from her feet and one who pushes off by locking her knees or swaying her back with a diver who pushes with the feet has a greater chance of having the motion sequence all the way through the legs and into the trunk than does the locked-kneed diver, who breaks the continuity of action in locked joints. Even the smallest gesture

Links to Practical Applications

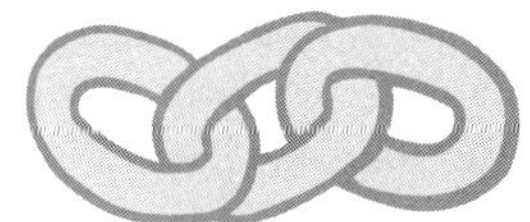

After Patterning

When patterning requires a lot of concentration, you may feel fatigue after going through a series of focused exercises. Even though they don't require physical exertion, shifts in neuromuscular pathways can consume a lot of energy, so you may need to rest. If you find yourself tired after a patterning session, spend some time in low-key activities to give your newly reorganized neural circuits time to settle. Avoid rigorous activities or any new type of sport or exercise for several hours.

can initiate a sequence that travels from one end of the body to another. By practicing responsive, full body movements, movement sequences through more muscles and joints, keeping the entire body supple and mobile.

BREATHING

Volumes have been written on how to breathe, and dozens of healing programs are devoted solely to breathing therapies and techniques. With the multitude of theories, schools, and opinions about how a person *should* breathe, there must be a "correct" way to do it. Yet there are many different ways to breathe.

Although there is no right or wrong way to breathe, breathing can be more or less efficient. *Efficient respiration* occurs when the air we take in is sufficient to meet the metabolic needs required by the body for its current activity. *Energizing and healing respiration* occurs when breathing continues to improve in efficiency and the bloodstream delivers a gradually increasing amount of oxygen to the tissues.

Many clients claim they "never breathe," yet respiration continues automatically regardless of what we do and whether or not we think about breathing. More than food or water, air is the most crucial element for survival, and respiration ensures the continuance of life by providing a constant supply of air. We can survive without food for one to two months, and we can survive without water for up to ten days, but we can only survive without air for about four minutes, six at most. To ensure a constant supply of air, our respiratory apparatus functions on automatic pilot, below a level of conscious awareness. Respiration is powered by the continuous pumping motion of the diaphragm muscle, which creates changes in air pressure and air volume.

How can you track external respiration in the body? How can you track internal respiration in the body? Can you track them with touch? If so, how?

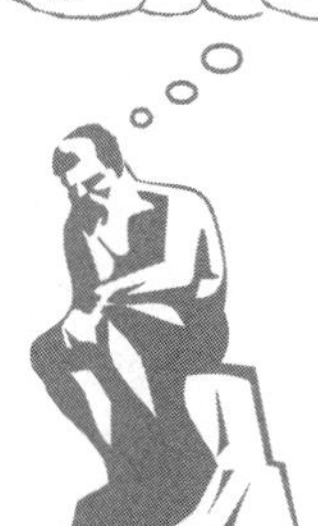

Breathing can be also consciously controlled, which can actually restrict respiration. During sleep, the body naturally breathes without interference from the mind so that patterns of control over breathing dissipate or disappear. It is common for a massage client's breathing to be restricted while awake, then to become opened and relaxed when the client falls asleep. To consciously release patterns that restrict breathing, it helps to understand the dynamics of normal respiration, which include both anatomical and physiological elements.

Links to Practical Applications

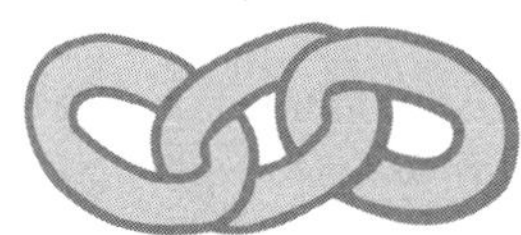

Breathing before Sleeping

Since you carry whatever state you are in—relaxation or stress—to sleep with you, if your breathing is restricted, it may become even more restricted during sleep. With this in mind, take several easy breaths after you lie down to sleep, relaxing your body with a focus on long, easy exhalations. Imagine any tensions or circular thoughts left over from your day washing out with each exhalation.

Patterning Exercise #34: Anatomical Imagery for Internal Respiration

(Adapted from an exercise called "cellular breathing" by Bonnie Cohen.) Use this exercise to induce deep states of relaxation. Read this script into a tape recorder, then listen to it while in a relaxed position. Pause after each sentence to visualize and/or sense its effects.

1. Breathe deeply yet quietly. Expand your lungs with each inhalation. Relax your body on each exhalation. As you inhale, sense air passing through your sinuses into your lungs; sense your diaphragm and chest expanding in all directions.
2. As you exhale, sense your lungs deflating and your body getting heavier. Relax at the end of each exhalation. Continue to take several more breaths, feeling the alternating expansion and deflation.
3. Now shift your focus from external to internal respiration. First imagine the millions of *alveoli* in your lungs as tiny elastic bubbles, bunched in grape-like clusters, each covered with a thin web of thousands of capillaries. Visualize or sense fresh, clean oxygen dissolving through the alveoli into your bloodstream. Also visualize freshly oxygenated blood nourishing your heart.
4. Switch your focus again. Imagine or sense your arterial tree. See the main arteries as large tubes, similar to garden hoses made turgid by fluid pressure, filled with surging blood that carries oxygen throughout the body. Each tube or artery divides into smaller and smaller vessels, branching down to the level of single-celled capillaries where oxygen passes into the cell membranes.
5. Next, visualize the cells in your various tissues. Visualize oxygen molecules like bubbles under water seeping out of the blood and permeating the cells in _______ (*fill in the blank with each of the following*): your brain, any organ in your body, your head, face, neck, shoulders, chest, right arm, left arm, abdomen, lower back, right hip, left hip, right leg, and left leg.
6. Continue breathing and focus on a specific area that you want to relax and revitalize.
7. After completing this exploration, relax and rest for a few minutes. Get up slowly. Give yourself time to reorient, particularly if you sank into the state of reverie that occurs between sleeping and waking states (see Chapter 13 for more information on this state).

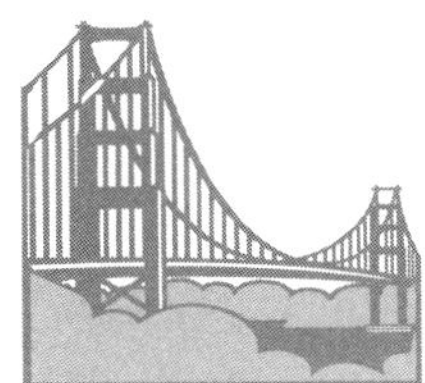

Bridge to Practice

Helping Clients Let Go of Labored Breathing

Sometimes people become so focused on breathing deeply or "correctly" that the muscular effort they contribute toward deep breathing actually blocks full and efficient respiration. If this is the case with your client, encourage him to get out of his own way and let his body breathe itself. This helps him release control over breathing so that it becomes more subconscious and automatic. To help him shift his focus from external respiration to internal respiration describe some anatomical imagery to him (see Patterning Exercise #34). Often just a focus on internal respiration is enough to help a client relax, release respiratory holding patterns, and breathe more easily.

External versus Internal Respiration

External respiration is the movement of air between the outside environment and the body. External respiration is powered by the movement of the *respiratory diaphragm*, a muscle that functions similarly to a bellows. It rhythmically contracts to pump air in and out of the lungs for the continuous exchange of gases between our internal and external environments. As the diaphragm contracts and pulls the lungs open, internal air pressure decreases creating a vacuum into which air rushes to equalize pressure. As the diaphragm relaxes, lung volume decreases causing air to drain out.

Most people think of breathing as only an expansion of the lungs and ribcage, yet **internal respiration,** which occurs within a fluid environment inside the body, is the exchange of oxygen and carbon dioxide between the bloodstream and the tissue cells. Internal respiration maintains health and vitality in the tissues by delivering nourishment to the cells and carrying wastes away from them.

The mechanical motion of the diaphragm during respiration also pumps lymphatic fluids. The lymph system is an essential part of immune system function because it filters bacteria and harmful debris from the interstitial fluid. Given this, deep and full breathing, even while in a resting position, is crucial for immune system health.

The link between external and internal respiration provides a key to integrating external and internal body processes. External respiration can be seen and sensed in the expansion and deflation of the ribcage and any other externally observable body movements caused by respiration. Internal respiration is a deeper physiological process that is more difficult to feel but can be somewhat sensed in the subtle, intrinsic sensations caused by the oxygenation of the tissues. People feel the energizing effect of increased internal respiration during a strenuous workout when the tissues receive more oxygen. Feeling internal respiration during a resting state requires a refined sense of body awareness and, at the very least, imagination. If people are

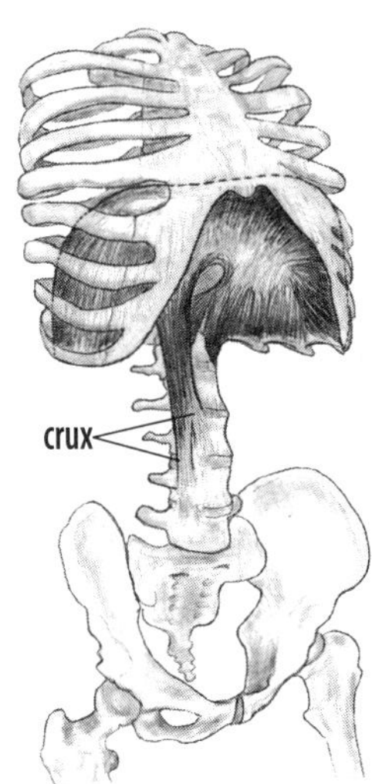

Figure 5.5 The respiratory diaphragm is a domed-shaped muscle attached to the lower ribs and the lumbar spine.

Patterning Exercise #35: Feeling and Stretching the Respiratory Diaphragm

Read this entire exercise before you begin because you will not be in a position to read it while doing it.

1. Sit in a chair with both feet flat on the floor. Place your fingertips up under the front of your lower ribs, directly below your *costal arch* to either side of your solar plexus (PE Fig. 35a). Gently press your fingertips in on either side, being careful not to press in the center, on either the *xiphoid process* (a small bony protuberance at the end of the sternum) or on the *linea alba* (along the center). You can also gently jimmy your fingers between the diaphragm and organs (liver and stomach).

PE Fig. 35a

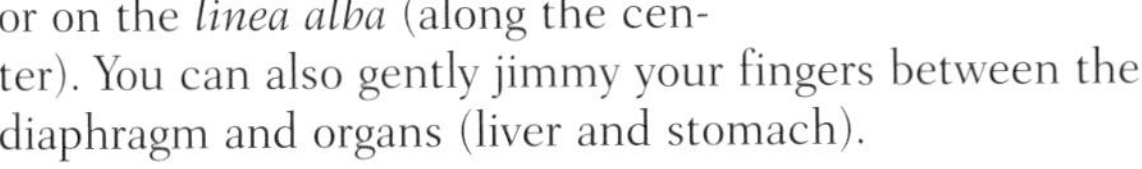

2. Bend over so that your upper body and head is hanging over your knees (PE Fig. 35b).
3. As you inhale, your diaphragm will push your fingers out.
4. As you exhale and your diaphragm relaxes, sink your fingers in farther to relax and stretch the diaphragm. As you inhale again, relax your fingers and let your diaphragm push them out. Follow several breath cycles. pushing in on the out breath, then relaxing.
5. Repeat step 4 with your fingers in several different positions along the costal arch.

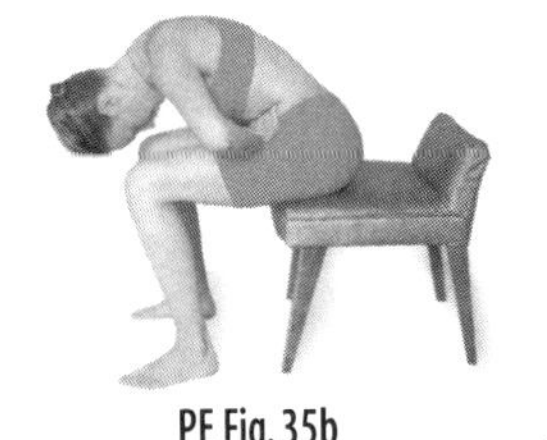
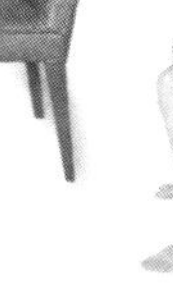

PE Fig. 35b

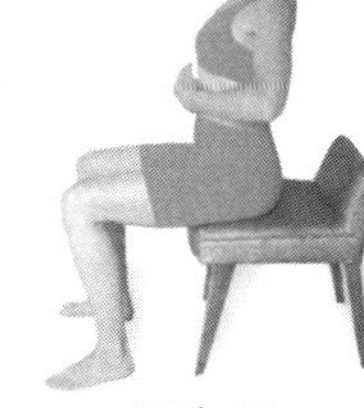

PE Fig. 35c

6. On a final inhalation, extend your spine and arch over backwards to stretch your diaphragm even further (PE Fig. 35c).

EMSPress.com

Patterning Exercise #36: Awareness of the Ribs and Lungs during Breathing

This exercise is designed to increase your awareness of the five lobes of the lungs and the movement of individual ribs during breathing, as well as to open the space between each pair of ribs.

1. *Expanding your lungs:* Place your hand on the sides of your lower ribs (PE Fig. 36a). Breathe in as deeply as you can, then breathe in again without exhaling, then again, expanding the lowest lobe of your lung into your hand. Then exhale and relax. Move your hand up to the middle of your ribcage and repeat the entire sequence, breathing into the middle lobes. Then move your hand under your armpit (PE Fig. 36b), and then on top of your shoulder to breathe into the upper lobe. Repeat the entire sequence on the other side.

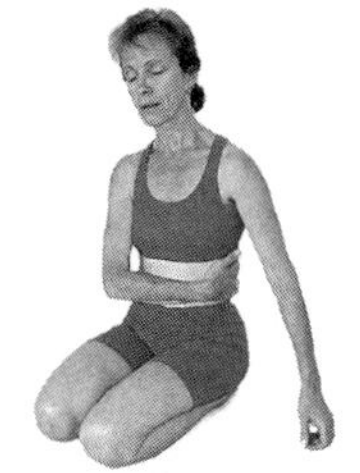

PE Fig. 36a

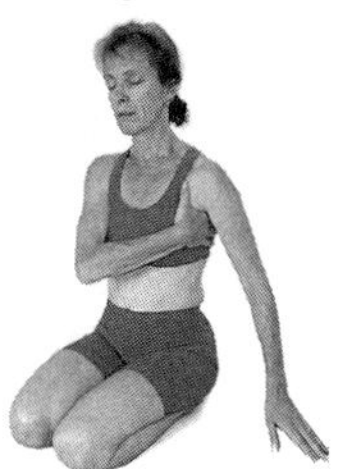

PE Fig. 36b

2. *Expanding individual ribs in a sitting position:* Sit in a comfortable position. Place your hands on the sides of your lower ribs (PE Fig. 36c). Breathe in (PE Fig. 36d). Without exhaling, breathe in again, then again to expand that area into your hands. Then exhale and relax. Gradually work your way up the sides of your rib cage, expanding one area of ribs at a time. Work all the way up into your armpits, where your top ribs can be palpated.

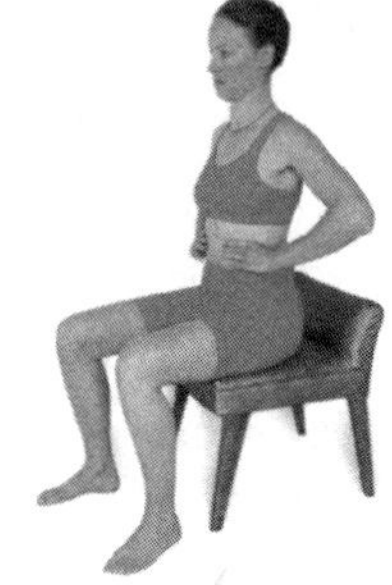

PE Fig. 36c

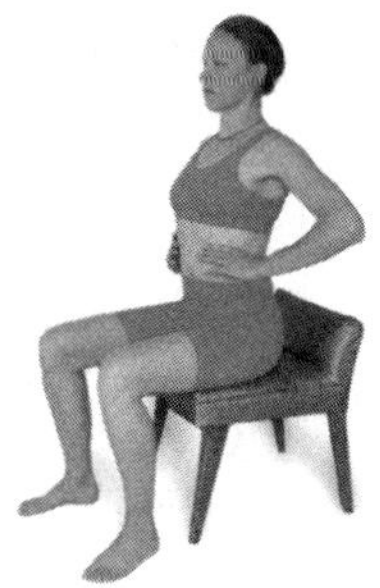

PE Fig. 36d

3. *Expanding the ribcage and lungs in a side-lying position:* Lie comfortably on your side on a soft surface like a mattress or foam pad. Put a pillow under your head and between your knees to make yourself more comfortable. Place one hand across your body under the lower third of your rib cage. Gently breathe, expanding this part of your ribcage into your hand. Sense or imagine weight sinking through your lung tissues as you exhale. Next place your hand in the middle of the rib cage and expand your breath into this area. Lastly, place your hand under your armpit at the top of your ribcage and expand your breath into this area.

4. Slowly roll onto your other side and repeat this process.

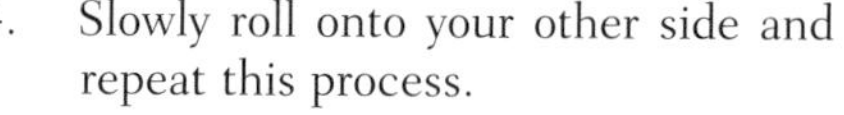

EMSPress.com

unable to sense internal respiration, they can visualize the processes using anatomical imagery, such as the bloodstream picking up oxygen in the lungs and delivering it throughout the various tissues to the cells.

Respiratory Anatomy

The respiratory diaphragm is a strong, dome-shaped muscle that separates the thoracic and abdominal cavities (Figure 5.5). It attaches along the rim of the lower ribs and has two tendons, called *crura,* which insert along the front of the lumbar vertebrae. The lungs and heart, which rest on top of the diaphragm, and the organs tucked up under it (the *liver, spleen, pancreas, stomach,* and *kidneys*) receive a mechanical massage on each breath cycle. In fact, during strenuous breathing the diaphragm moves up and down as much as four inches, which is why physicians have patients hold their breath to put injections in tissues near the diaphragm. When the diaphragm contracts, it flattens and moves down like a piston, pulling open more space in the rib cage into which the lungs can expand. Also, during inhalation the body expands in all directions, most noticeably in the ribcage but also along its longitudinal axis.

Links to Practical Applications

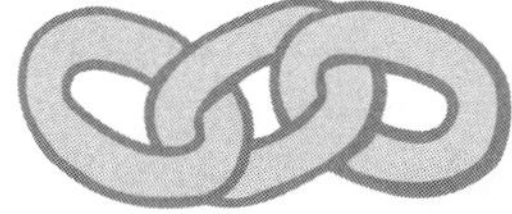

Relaxing or Energizing with Breathing

To relax your body with breathing exercises, make the exhalation longer than the inhalation. To wake up and energize your body with breathing, make the inhalation longer than the exhalation.

When a person breathes in, the expansion of the lungs is a mechanical process initiated by the muscular contractions of the respiratory diaphragm and *intercostal muscles* between the ribs. The lungs adhere to the inside of the thoracic cavity via the two thin fascial membranes that are suctioned together by a *serous fluid,* similar to how two glass slides stick together when wet. The contraction of the diaphragm and the intercostal muscles during inhalation literally pulls

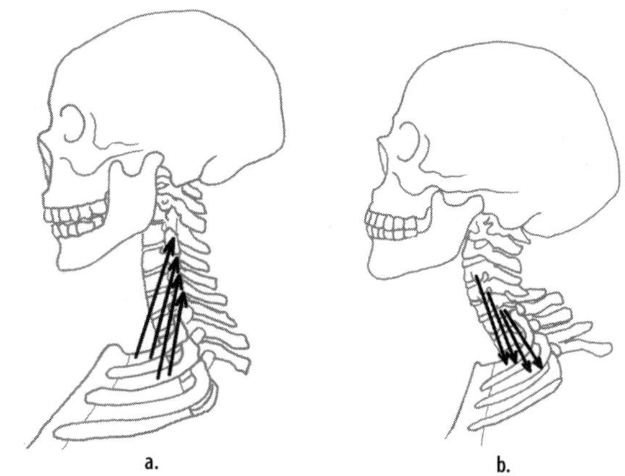

Figure 5.6a-b The arrows show the pull of the scalene muscles, either (a) pulling the ribs up, or (b) pulling the neck down.

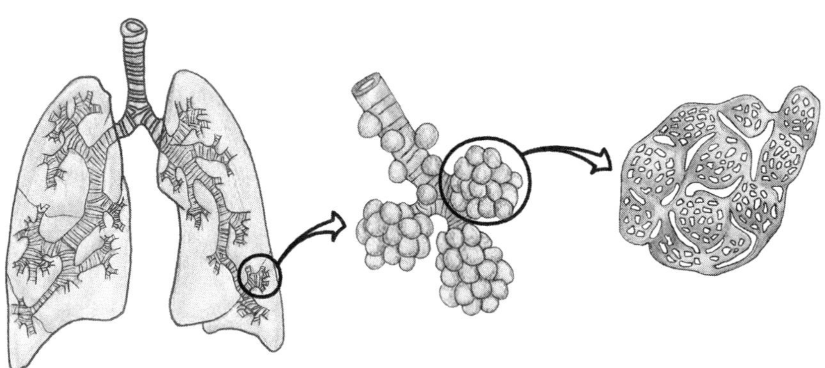

Figure 5.7 Lungs, bronchioles covered with alveoli, and capillaries surrounding alveoli

the ribs apart, which then pulls the lungs open, creating a low-pressure vacuum in the millions of hollow alveoli into which air rushes.

The ribcage expands by the contraction of the intercostal muscles, which turns each rib to pull the spaces between the ribs open. Also, the *scalene muscles*, auxiliary respiratory muscles that suspend the upper ribs from the cervical vertebrae, lift the upper ribs during normal respiration (Figure 5.6a). If the ribcage is depressed, a postural pattern common in people with collapsed postures and distended abdomens, the scalene muscles can become dysfunctional and fail to lift the ribs, instead pulling the neck forward and down (Figure 5.6b).

Each of the lungs is made up of a spongy, highly vascular tissue filled with millions of blood capillaries and elastic *alveoli sacs* (Figure 5.7). The lungs literally cup the heart. The right lung has three lobes and the left lung has two lobes, being shorter because it lies adjacent to the apex of the heart, which tips to the left against the lower portion of the left lung. The bulk of the lungs lie behind the midline of the body, where the lungs cradles the thoracic spine. Each lung is about 19 inches long and the apex (top) of the lungs extend slightly above the *clavicle* or collarbone (see Figure 5.10). As the lungs expand, they give not only the ribs, but also the shoulder girdle, a mechanical lift. A person can focus on lung and rib expansion to lift and widen the shoulders and chest. Lung capacity can also be expanded with inhalation after a forced exhalation, with a forced inhalation, and with regular cardiovascular exercise.

Ribcage Motion during Respiration

The ribs open and close like gills during each breath cycle (Figure 5.8a-b). Each rib pair of the floating ribs moves like calipers; each rib pair from ribs 4 through 10 turns like a bucket handle, rotating while it lifts; each rib pair in the first 3 ribs moves like a pump handle lifting straight up. The bulk of expansion occurs on the sides and in the front of the rib cage, elevating the very thin and light *sternum* (breastbone). On exhalation, each rib pair reverses its motion, rotating and sinking back down toward the one below it, closing like the slats of a venetian blind.

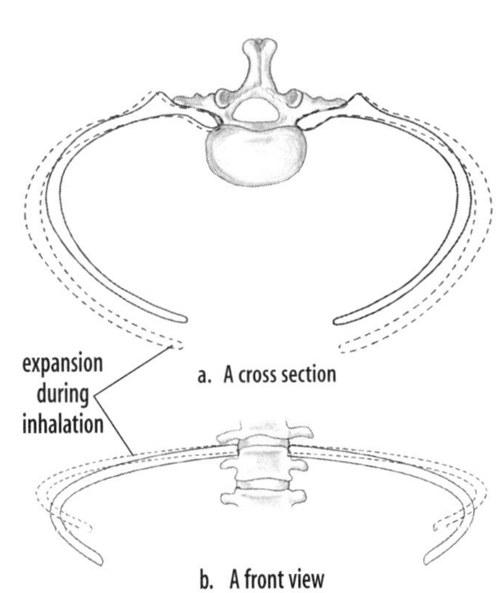

Figure 5.8a-b Rib motion during respiration

Ideally, the space between a pair of ribs opens and closes evenly. Restrictions occur when the intercostal tissues become tight and glue adjacent ribs together. Imagine pinching two slats of a Chinese lantern together: it distorts the shape of the entire lantern. A similar distortion occurs in the ribcage if rib motion becomes fixated in any way. Several common respiratory holding patterns are the depressed chest, in which the auxiliary breathing muscles in the neck, the *scalene*, *pectoralis minor,* and *sternocleidomastoid muscles*, overwork to try to lift the chest. A belly-breather tends to have an excessive kyphotic or "humpbacked" posture and a rigid and often depressed anterior chest.

Patterning Exercise #37: Focusing on Breathing Cycles

1. Pick one of the following four phases of the breathing cycle, and focus on it for a while: 1) inhalation 2) pause at the end of the inhalation 3) exhalation 4) pause at the end of the exhalation. Switch phases until you have focused on each of the four phases separately.

Feedback: Was one phase easier for your to focus on than others? Is one phase more difficult? It is common for one phase to be easier than another for different people due to their different types of holding patterns.

2. Focus on the whole sequence in a four-step series. Count the steps as you breathe, or name them, using the words as a breathing mantra. Repeat in your mind: "Inhale, pause, exhale, rest."
3. Practice focusing on your breathing as you walk. To synchronize breathing with walking, repeat a phrase in your mind, such as "Inhale–2–3–4, exhale–2–3–4." Coordinate your words with the speed of your steps.

Patterning Exercise #38: Mobilizing the Spine with Breathing

1. Lie on your back in a comfortable position. If your lower back is uncomfortable when your legs are straight, bend your knees and rest with both feet flat.
2. Inhale through your nose. Imagine or feel the inhalation filling first your pelvis, then your thorax, and then your head. Allow the front of your spine to open and lengthen as you inhale, expanding and filling your torso and head from bottom to top.
3. Relax your jaw and exhale through your mouth. Allow the breath to drain out of your mouth, then your thorax, then your pelvis. Allow the back of your spine to sink and elongate as you exhale.
4. Continue to breathe, inhaling from bottom to top, exhaling from top to bottom. Imagine the breath like mercury in a thermometer, first rising, then falling. Feel each breath filling and emptying your entire spine.

EMSPress.com

An upper-chest breather tends to have an inflated rigid ribcage that is difficult to relax during exhalation.

Breathing Cycles

The respiratory muscles contract during inhalation and relax during exhalation. Many people feel they need to squeeze air out of their lungs to exhale correctly, but this extra muscular effort is unnecessary. Each cycle of inhalation and exhalation moves the body through alternating states of levity and gravity. Inhalation inflates the hollow spaces of the lung's alveoli, literally floating the upper body and sinuses in a moment of buoyancy (Figure 5.9). Focusing on the inhalation can help a person feel expansion and levity through the body, particularly in the chest and head. As the respiratory muscles relax, the size of the ribcage shrinks, lung dimension decreases, and air rushes out. Focusing on the exhalation can help a person feel weight sinking through the body as the lungs deflate and muscles relax, improving relaxation skills. Focusing on the pause at the end of each breath cycle can help a person feel a moment of physiological rest.

The rhythm of respiration creates a constant pumping action that subtly expands the ribcage on each breath cycle (Figure 5.10). The respiratory pump also flexes and extends the spine. Each inhalation elongates the front of the body, opening and subtly extending the spine into a long, convex curve. Each exhalation elongates the back of the body, subtly flexing the spine into a concave curve. Focusing on breathing along the spine is one of the simplest methods of mobilizing the spine with the constant physiological rhythm of respiration.

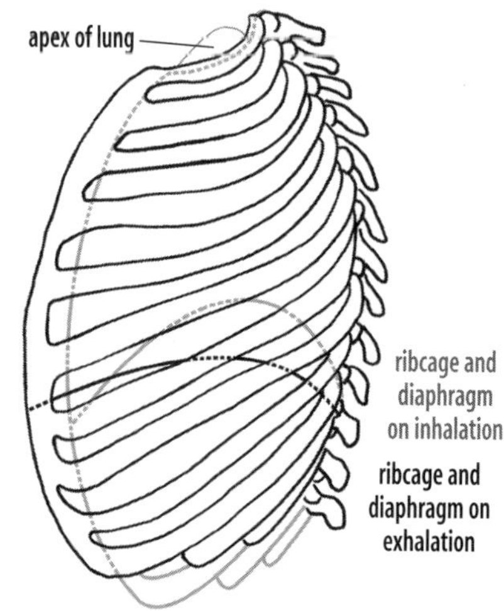

Figure 5.10 Thorax movement in respiration

Respiratory holding patterns can emphasize either the inhalation or exhalation phase. An **exhalation fixation** is marked by a posture weighed down with a depressed, sunken ribcage, and by difficulty taking a deep breath. A person with this pattern would benefit from practicing strong and focused inhalations that force expansion in both the dimension of the lungs and the ribcage.

Conversely, an **inhalation fixation** is marked by the rigid posture of an overly inflated and puffed-out chest, and difficulty fully exhaling. A person with this imbalance would benefit from sensing the respiratory muscles relax during the exhalation, as well as feeling the ribcage deflate and sink.

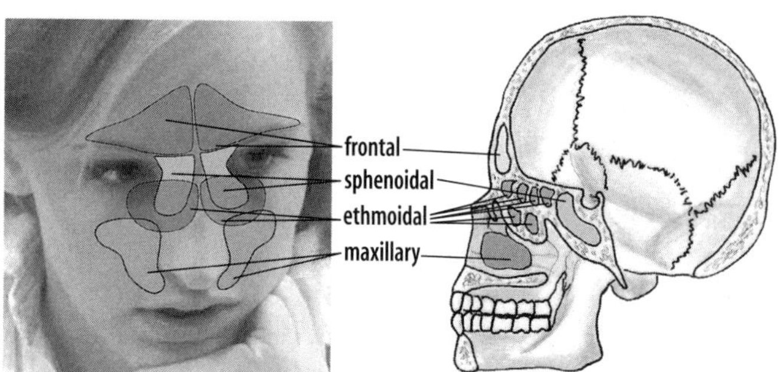

Figure 5.9 Location of the sinuses. Note how the ethmoidal and sphenoidal sinuses extend several inches into the skull.

The Respiratory Diaphragm as a Postural Stabilizer

The respiratory diaphragm functions as both a physiological pump and a postural stabilizer. Its stabilizing function is dependent on the **intra-abdominal pressure (IAP)** created by tonic contractions of deep postural muscles in the lower abdominal wall and pelvic floor. To understand how IAP works, visualize the diaphragm as a dome that rests in a convex shape during relaxation. As it contracts, the center of the dome descends, pushing down like a piston on the abdominal organs. If the lower abdominal wall and pelvic floor muscles are lightly contracted, they slightly compress the abdominal organs and make the torso a somewhat

Patterning Exercise #39: Feeling Intra-abdominal Pressure

1. In a sitting or standing position, let your abdominal muscles completely relax and hang out (PE Fig. 39a). Take several deep breaths. This will help you develop a kinesthetic sense of what breathing feels like without the lower abdominal support.

PE Fig. 39a

PE Fig. 39b

2. Now pull your lower abdominal wall straight back toward your spine, using one-third of the maximum effort you could use to contract it (PE Fig. 39b). Holding it there, take several deep breaths. Expand your lower ribs as you inhale.
3. If you have trouble feeling this while sitting or have a large belly, explore this exercise lying on your back. Bring your knees to your chest. Then lightly pull your lower abdomen into your lower back, sensing the hollow shape it creates (PE Fig. 39c). Breathe. Let the breath expand your back. On each exhalation, allow tight areas in your back become weighted and sink into the floor.

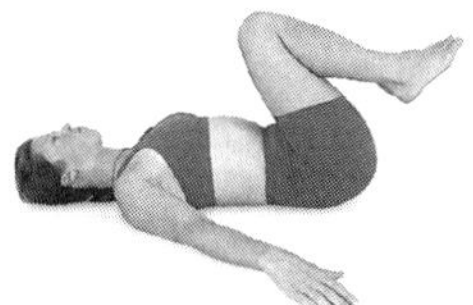

PE Fig. 39c

4. Put your hands on your lower abdomen to monitor the muscles there. Slowly lower your feet to the floor without changing position, without bulging your lower abdomen up, and without tightening your back.
5. Next, let your abdominal muscles completely relax and hang out. Take several deep breaths. Then gently contract the muscles above your pubic area, pulling your lower abdomen back into a hollowed-out shape (by the action of the *transversus abdominis muscle*) and holding it. Take several deep breaths. Sense your lower ribs expanding on each inhalation.
6. Move into the side-lying position and repeat step 5.
7. Move in the quadruped position (on your hands and knees) and repeat step 5.

Practical Application: During the course of the day, actively contract your lower abdominal wall and hold for ten seconds while you take several expansive breaths. Ideally, you'll get into the habit of slightly contracting your lower abdominal muscles all the time, which will not only improve your breathing, but will stabilize your lower back and sacroiliac joints.

EMSPress.com

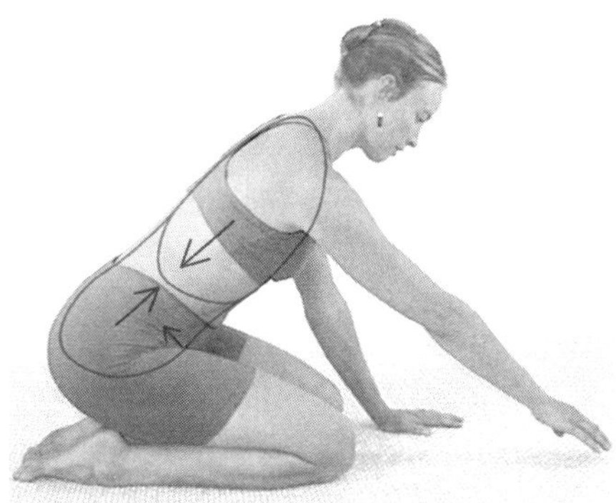

Figure 5.11 Intra-abdominal pressure requires a tonic contraction of the lower abdominal muscles.

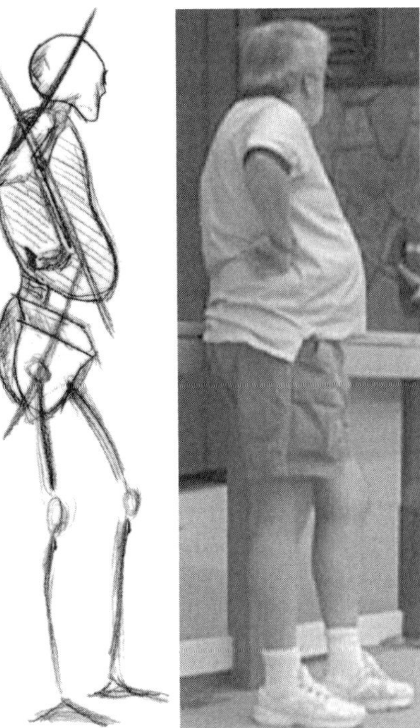

Figure 5.12 A distended belly puts a drag on the ribcage and restricts breathing.

stiff tube. The diaphragm can push down only so far because it meets the resistance of intra-abdominal pressure created by good muscle tone in the muscle wrapping the waist (Figure 5.11). When the diaphragmatic dome can no longer descend, its sides lift, expanding the lower ribs and triggering an expansion that sequences up the thorax. Given these dynamics, inhalation actually has two phases: first a downward motion, then an outward and upward motion. It is as though the downward pressure of the diaphragm bounces back up into the ribcage, but only if the postural muscles in the lower abdomen lightly contract to compress the viscera.

Weak lower abdominal muscles, particularly the *transversus abdominis muscle* (see Chapter 9 for more information about this muscle), interfere with the two-phase action of the respiratory muscles. If the transversus abdominis, an important postural stabilizer that wraps the waist and abdomen like a cummerbund, is too weak to counter the downward push of the diaphragm, the diaphragm keeps descending, distending the abdomen's contents. This condition not only interferes with the normal expansion of the lungs and ribcage, it puts mechanical stress on the entire spine, dragging it forward and down. For this reason, it is common for a person with a "potbelly" to have either a sunken chest and forward head posture or a rigid upper body held in a stiffened holding pattern to compensate for the muscular deficit below (Figure 5.12).

Psychosomatic Patterns of Breathing

All emotional responses create changes in breathing. Respiration speeds up to meet the sympathetic demands of a fight-or-flight response, shallow breathing usually accompanies depression, and rapid, upper-chest breathing usually accompanies anxiety. The process is also circular. For example, anxiety tends to increase the rate of breathing, and rapid breathing tends to increase anxiety.

Once an emotional process ends and the body starts to settle and relax, respiration usually returns to normal. But if an emotional process becomes fixated, a person's respiration also tends to fixate at some phase in the breathing cycle that corresponds to the emotional holding. The breath can get fixated at any phase, in a gasp, a sigh, or even in rapid breathing. If a person chronically holds the breath in a gasp, the chest is held in an inflated posture (an inhalation fixation) and exhalation is restricted. Then, on each inhalation, a small intake of air mixes with the stale air already held in the lungs. In the opposite pattern, the chest is chronically held in a sigh during the exhalation phase (an exhalation fixation), compressing the lungs and ribs and restricting inhalation. A person with this pattern might feel depressed or fatigued because of the reduced oxygen intake caused by not being able to adequately inflate the lungs.

Members of a group draw from the same supply of oxygen and have been known to be surprisingly sensitive to each others respiratory patterns, particularly if there is an emotional charge in the group. We hear references to this innate sensitivity to the air we share with expressions like "the air was so thick you could cut it with a knife" or "she blew into the room like a breath of fresh air." Groups of people even tend to synchronize breathing rhythms, which often reveals the level of harmony or conflict occurring within the group. People filling a tense courtroom might hold their breath in unison right before the verdict is delivered. After the verdict is read, those who are pleased with the decision let out a sigh of relief, while those who are not gasp for even more air.

In many schools of body-centered psychotherapy, the belief is that the amount of air people breathe in can reflect the amount of space and energy they feel they deserve. For example, the stooped posture commonly associated with low self-esteem literally compresses the lungs and prevents a full inhalation. This posture creates a physiological reinforcement of a belief that the person is undeserving. The script varies, yet the dynamics are the same. A shallow breather might subconsciously believe that he doesn't deserve air, or that if he takes too much air there will not be enough for others. Feelings of being smothered, either by an overprotective parent or in a relationship, can also underlie patterns of shallow breathing. Fortunately, air is freely available to most of us. A person can take up more space in the world simply by breathing more deeply and expanding the body.

Links to Practical Applications

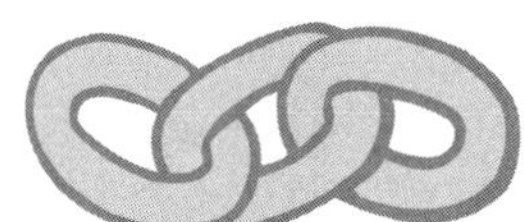

Feeling the Movement of the Diaphragm

Focus on the diaphragm muscle to pattern it during breathing. To do this, place your hands on the sides of your lower ribs and expand them into your hands during the inhalation. Make sure your lower abdominal wall is slightly contracted to maintain inter-abdominal pressure.

Examining Myths

Myth: A person should always breathe into the belly.

Is abdominal or belly breathing—pushing the abdomen out during inhalation—really the right way to breathe? It is okay for inducing relaxation while you are waiting to fall asleep, yet it is often encouraged by health professionals as a way to activate the diaphragm. This notion is a bit of a fallacy. First of all, control over a muscle is best achieved by focusing directly on that muscle; in this case the focus should be on the diaphragm, not the abdominal muscles. Second, abdominal breathing expands and bulges the abdomen rather than expanding the lungs. If a belly breather has tight lower back and a "potbelly," the viscera spills out even further, which pulls the lumbars forward, creating more tension in the lower back muscles that contract to support the distended visceral load.

Paradoxical Breathing

The pattern of **paradoxical breathing** often occurs during emotional distress. In a person with this pattern, the diaphragm moves backwards. It actually rises as it contracts, moving in the opposite direction of normal respiration. This decreases the amount of space that the lungs have to expand into, thereby decreasing lung capacity. This pattern tends to develop during extreme states of fear or trauma in which a person's respiration speeds up and moves into the upper chest. People with a paradoxical pattern breathe in fast, short cycles. They tend to gulp air as they breathe and talk. And often, the harder they try to get a deep breath, the stronger the pattern becomes. For this reason, paradoxical breathing can be self-perpetuating. This pattern reduces oxygen intake and may feel suffocating, causing a person to panic and gasp. During a gasp, the diaphragm lifts during inhalation, thus causing the pattern to become ingrained in a circular paradox.

Links to Practical Applications

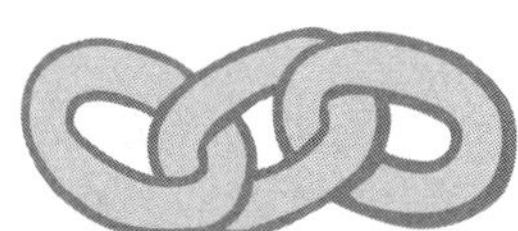

Handling Hyperventilation

If you tend to hyperventilate, slow your respiration. If it happens while you are doing a rigorous activity that requires a lot of oxygen, stop and relax. If a person around you hyperventilates, urge him/her to slow down and relax. In severe cases, breathe into a paper bag to take in more carbon dioxide and rebalance the blood gases.

Links to Practical Applications

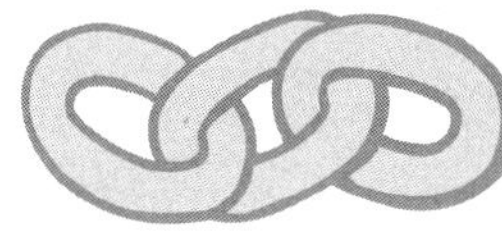

Letting Go of Effortful Breathing

If your breathing feels labored, you are probably using too much effort to breathe, and that effort may restrict easy and full respiration. If this is the case, let your subconscious processes take over. Reassure yourself that your body can breathe on its own. Or focus on internal respiration, sensing or visualizing your blood carrying oxygen to all of your cells. (See Patterning Exercise #34 on "Anatomical Imagery for Internal Respiration.")

Whenever people with restricted or shallow breathing begin to breathe deeper, they take in more oxygen. This can result in **hyperventilation,** an imbalance in lung gas exchange that occurs when the amount of oxygen coming in exceeds the amount of carbon dioxide going out. It causes a range of symptoms: dizziness, light-headedness, tingling, or fainting. A person may even go into *tetany*—a tonic muscle spasm that feels like paralysis in the hands and feet. Therefore, a person needs to be cautious with deep breathing exercises, to practice them in small doses, and to rest if any symptoms of hyperventilation such as dizziness show up.

Breathing as a Body-Centered Practice

Many practices of meditation use an awareness of breathing to focus the mind. One universal yet simple practice has the participant observe the breath moving in and out the body. Whenever the mind wanders, the meditator brings her awareness back to the breath. Other systems have the meditator observe how the breath changes the shape of the body, again returning to this observation each time the mind wanders.

Breathing is the most constant, audible, and obvious rhythm in the body. It is one of the easiest rhythms to match or entrain within another person. Couples, for example, often find that they unconsciously hold their breaths or sigh at the same time.

Focused breathing is a primary somatic patterning skill. When a person becomes aware of the breath, she establishes a body-based awareness of the present moment. This is the fundamental role and power of breathing in somatic patterning, which cannot be stressed enough. Breathing underlies the efficiency of all movement. It must be tended to in patterning as regularly as it is in meditation. Breathing can be an active meditation that we can practice no matter where we are or what we are doing. All it takes is awareness and intention. Meditative or focused breathing can be practiced during the day to center oneself, to increase body awareness, to relax the body and release tension, and to calm the mind. A person can also take a series of deep breaths to reduce fatigue and combat the drowsiness that tends to set in during sedentary work. Coordinating deep breathing with arm movements by raising the arms during inhalation and lowering them during exhalation will stretch respiratory muscles and open space in the lungs for more air.

MOVEMENT INITIATED BY SENSE ORGANS

The oscillation of breath in and out of the sinuses and airways perpetuates a deep physiological flexion and extension in the head and trunk. The sense organs also initiate constant movement sequences in the head, neck, and spine. The head is continually making subtle responses to a perpetual succession of sights, sounds, smells, and sensory stimuli coming in through the eyes, ears, nose, and mouth.

The sense organs have a dimensional balance in both their structure and function. The bulk of our head movement occurs in the *horizontal plane* as we turn to look around. The mouth, throat, and nose are oriented along the *sagittal plane,* and they initiate flexion and extension in the head and neck as a person speaks, swallows, and sniffs. The ears are oriented in the *frontal plane*; hence, a person tends to cock the head to one side or the other to point the ear toward a sound while listening. (See Figure 8.4 of the three planes.) The same way that each of the sense organs initiates movement of the head and neck, and even the entire spine, each sense can be explored in patterning the movement of the spine initiated in the head.

The Temporomandibular Joint

The jaw articulates with the skull at the *temporomandibular joint (TMJ),* a modified hinge-type joint connecting the *mandible* (jaw) to the *temporal bone* (Figure 5.13). The TMJ is unique in that we use it more than any other joint in the body, during eating and talking, and even in response to gravity's pull. If the antigravity muscles around the jaw did not continually contract to keep the mouth closed, the jaw would hang open. Since the mouth is the first limb to reach during oral rooting as the infant searches for the mother's nipple, the TMJ is the first joint to develop. It sets up a baseline of tone in the entire musculoskeletal system. Thus, it is imperative that the TMJs on each side of the

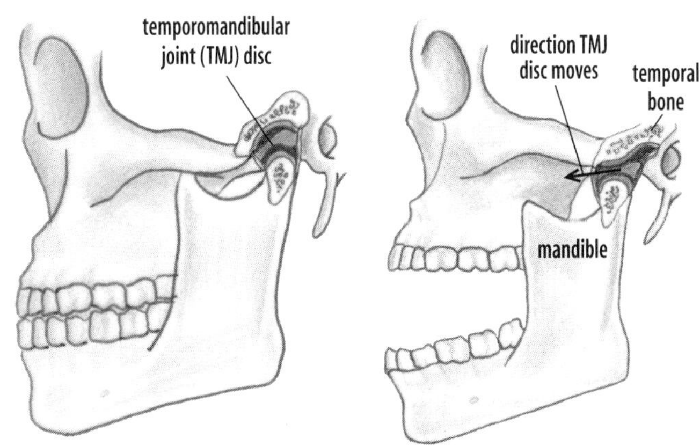

Figure 5.13 As the jaw (temporomandibular joint) opens, its disc slides forward; as the jaw closes, the disc slides back.

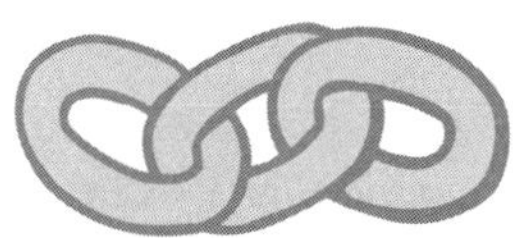

Links to Practical Applications

Relaxing Your Tongue and Jaw

When your tongue is resting, is it suctioned up against the roof of your mouth? If so, let it relax and rest on the bottom of your mouth. (Normally, the tip of the tongue naturally rests on the back of the front teeth, you do not need to hold it there.) To relax your jaw, keep a small space between your back molars. To feel this, press your teeth together, then slowly relax them and sense that space open.

jaw move with symmetry because their tone underlies bilateral symmetry in the entire body.

The TMJ has a complex range of motion: it opens and closes like a hinge, rolls like a ball-and-socket, and glides from side to side. It has the mobility of a ball-and-socket joint without the stability of the socket. As the mouth opens, the disc moves forward to cushion the joint. We use the muscles of the mouth, jaw, and nose whenever we talk, eat, and even breathe. The TMJ muscles are also often involved in stress responses in which a person clenches or grinds the teeth, a maladaptive habit that has a strong psychological component. Excessive grinding can wear the disc out, damage this highly mobile joint, grind the teeth down to stubs, and lead to *temporomandibular dysfunction (TMD)*. TMD usually involve a combination of muscle tension and joint damage; its symptoms include joint pain, muscle soreness, headaches, clicking, and/or locking in the TMJ, and perhaps even ringing in the ears. People with chronic neck pain and headaches often have some level of TMD.

Dentists diagnose TMD through motion testing and palpation, and often treat it with a splint that prevents the back teeth from touching. A person with TMD can also inhibit grinding by learning to relax muscles around the jaw using biofeedback therapy. Anyone with TMJ tension can reduce it by stretching mouth and tongue, by practicing rooting patterns to break up holding patterns around the jaw, and by learning to relax the TMJ muscles and the tongue. The tongue is a very strong and active muscle that attaches along the front of the upper cervical vertebrae; chronic contraction of the tongue can pull on these vertebrae and perpetuate chronic muscle

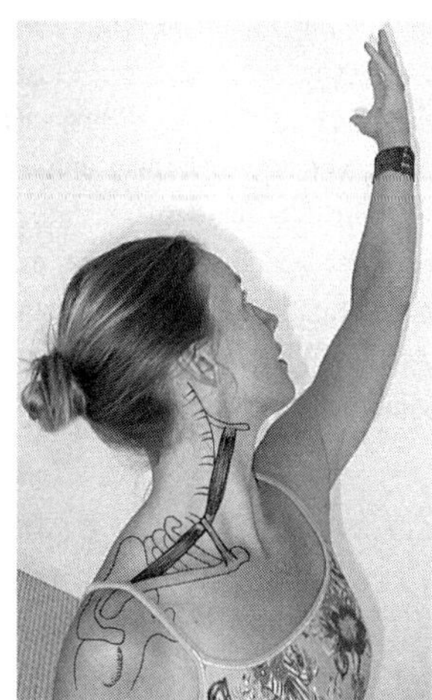

Figure 5.14 Omohyoid muscle

Patterning Exercise #40: Exploring Tongue and TMJ Movement

1. *Palate movement while breathing:* As you inhale, sense the space under your upper palate (the roof of your mouth) widening and lifting. To do this, you will need to relax your tongue and avoid pressing it up on the roof of your mouth.
2. *Tongue:* Press your tongue hard against the roof of your mouth and sense how this affects the muscle tone in your neck, throat, and jaw. Relax your tongue and notice the difference. With your mouth closed and tongue relaxed, breathe in and feel the space inside your mouth and throat expand.
3. *TMJ motion* (these TMJ exercises are from the School for Body-Mind Centering): Open and close your mouth several times. Sense how your cranium rocks on the first cervical vertebra as you move.
4. *Tracking the TMJ:* Now place your fingertips directly in front of your ears, over your temporomandibular joints. Open and close your mouth several times. You should feel movement in the TMJs. Notice whether your jaws move with symmetry or whether they pop open. If they move asymmetrically, focus on opening and closing with symmetry. If they pop open, the disc may be snapping forward; therefore, open them slowly and evenly to allow the disc time to slide forward with ease. Also, practice step 7 below to guide the disc as you open your mouth.
5. *Feeling three-dimensional TMJ motion:* Feel the difference between opening your mouth by reaching forward with your upper palate or by just lowering your lower jaw. Reaching with your palate initiates a three-dimensional action involving rotation and counter-rotation in the joints involved (PE Fig. 40a), whereas lowering the lower jaw initiates a flat, one-dimensional movement that lacks full rotational capacity.

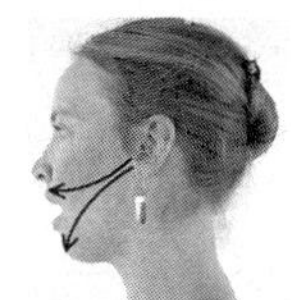

PE Fig. 40a

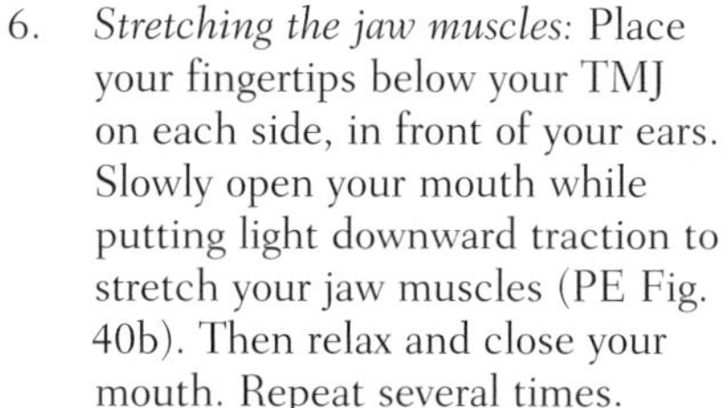

6. *Stretching the jaw muscles:* Place your fingertips below your TMJ on each side, in front of your ears. Slowly open your mouth while putting light downward traction to stretch your jaw muscles (PE Fig. 40b). Then relax and close your mouth. Repeat several times.

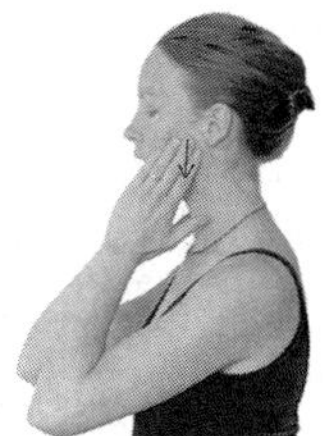

PE Fig. 40b

7. *Tracking the disc:* Move your fingertips up a bit so that they are directly over the joint. (You'll know you're there because you will feel a hollow as you open your mouth.) Again, slowly open your mouth, only this time put a light forward traction on your jaw to encourage the TMJ discs to glide forward with symmetry (PE Fig. 40c). Then relax and close your mouth. Repeat several times.

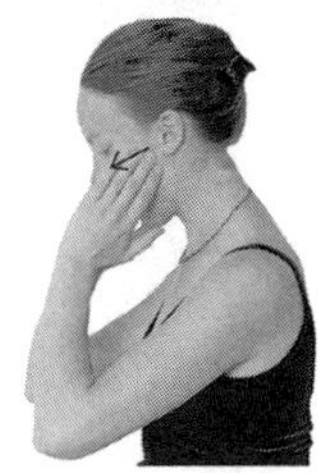

PE Fig. 40c

EMSPress.com

Patterning Exercise #41: Exploring Hyoid Movement

(This exercise was created by Body-Mind Centering teacher Sandy Jamrog.)

1. *Hyoid movement:* Palpate the front of your neck. Trace the edge of your jaw, then palpate the hyoid bone in the crease above your Adam's apple. Keep your fingers lightly on your hyoid bone to monitor muscle activity as you proceed (PE Fig. 41a).

PE Fig. 41a

2. Swallow and notice how the muscles around your hyoid bone are involved. Keeping your lips together, move your mouth as though you were chewing. Again, notice how the hyoid muscles are involved.
3. *Cervical flexion and stretching:* To stretch the deep muscles at the base of your skull and down your spine, begin by lifting your hyoid bone toward your ears. Then slowly curl your head forward, flexing at the top vertebra. Slowly roll down one vertebra at a time through all seven cervical vertebrae until your chin is resting on your chest. You should feel a deep stretch along your spine. Hold the stretch and breathe into it, then reverse the motion and roll back up.

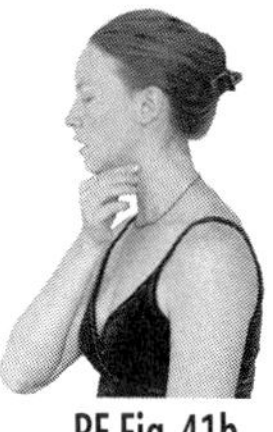

PE Fig. 41b

4. *Neck movement:* Slowly turn your head side to side, again noticing how the hyoid muscles work. Lead the motion with your hyoid bone (PE Fig. 41b-c). Does this feel different from how you are used to turning your head? How does it change the tone around your throat?

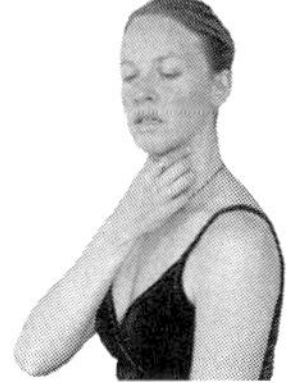

PE Fig. 41c

5. Contrast turning your head from the hyoid with turning your head by lifting the back of your skull and pointing it first to one side, then the other. Again, does this feel different from how you are used to turning your head?

EMSPress.com

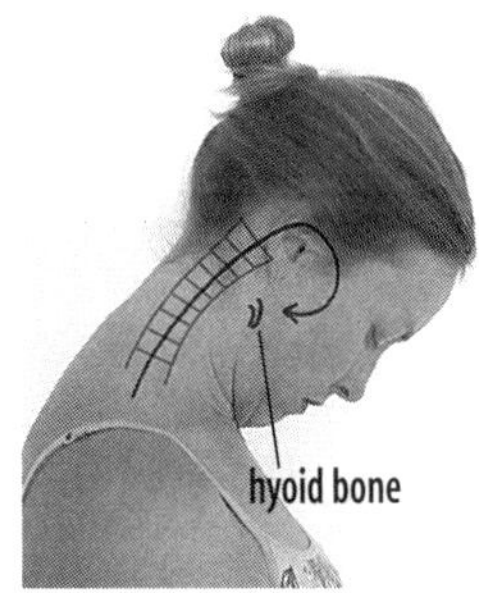

Figure 5.15 To begin flexion at the first vertebra, flex around the axis of the hyoid bone.

tension in the neck. The founder of the Alexander Method created an exercise called the "whispered 'ah'" to teach people how to relax their throat, jaw, and neck muscles (see Chapter 11).[89] TMJ muscles can also be manually stretched by specialists, often by bodyworkers who work inside the mouth directly on muscles like the *pterygoids.*

Many of the muscles of the lower jaw and throat attach to the *hyoid bone*, a small, horseshoe-shaped bone about an inch wide with half-inch wings on either side. The hyoid is nicknamed the "floating bone" because it is the only bone in the body not directly attached to another bone. It is suspended between many muscular and ligamentous attachments in the chin and the mouth. Two double-bellied muscles, the *digastric muscles* and *omohyoid muscles,* also connect the hyoid bone to the mastoid process of the temporal bone and to the scapula. Most people are unaware of this unusual connection between the hyoid and the scapula, which can be stretched during diagonal movements of the head (Figure 5.14).

The hyoid bone provides an attachment sight for muscles also attached to the mandible that form a horizontal muscular sling making up the floor of the mouth. Another group of small hyoid muscles descends from this small bone and covers the voice box ("Adam's apple") and trachea. Recall from earlier that other hyoid muscles (the digastic and omohyoid muscles) have attachments on the skull and scapula. Because of these vital connections around the mouth and throat, excessive muscular tension around the hyoid may restrict jaw mobility and even create tension in the throat, the base of the skull, and all the way down to the shoulders.

Since the hyoid provides such an intricate and central attachment site for so many muscles related to mastication, speech, breathing, and head movement, it provides an important bony landmark around which a person can pattern head and neck movement. For example, to get a deep stretch of tissues at the base of the skull and along the spine, a person can initiate cervical flexion around the hyoid, which will help mobilize the top cervical vertebra (Figure 5.15). Also, early developmental patterns such as rooting can be practiced with a focus on the hyoid to improve head, neck, and throat coordination.

Does your head turn where your eyes are looking? Or do your eyes roam while your head remains stationary?

Eye Movement

Like the TMJs, the eyes are in perpetual motion. We get an enormous amount of postural and perceptual support for the head and the entire body from our vision. Optical righting reactions level the head so that the eyes are horizontal. (See Chapter 1 Patterning Exercise #4 titled "Optical Support and Optical Righting.") Optical righting reactions also help an infant whose muscles are not yet strong enough to lift his relatively large head, which is much larger in proportion to the body than an adult's head. Visual scanning from side to side also initiates head, neck, and even spinal rotation, differentiating movement between the right and left sides of the body. Visual tracking patterns the hand to eye coordi-

Patterning Exercise #42: Visual Patterning

1. *Eye tracking:* Hold one index finger about two feet away from your face (PE Fig. 42a). Slowly move it from side to side, watching your finger the entire time. Let your head turn with your eyes. (It is common for people with holding patterns in the neck and head to move the eyes without moving the head.) Move slowly, with the least amount of effort possible. Relax the extrinsic muscles in your neck as you move so that you engage intrinsic muscles.

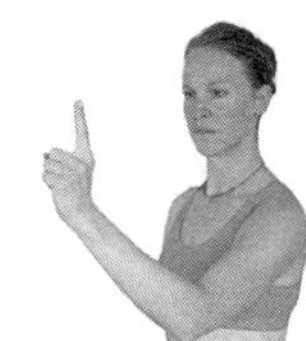

PE Fig. 42a

2. Now move your finger up and down and continue to watch it by moving your head as well as your eyes.

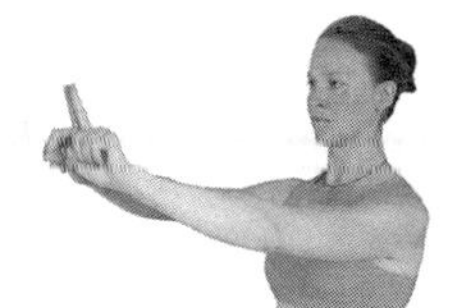

PE Fig. 42b

3. Then move your finger along random pathways. Keep watching it and following it with the movement of your head.
4. Hold both index fingers in front of your face (PE Fig. 42b). Gradually and simultaneously move both fingers out to opposite sides. Watch them both with your peripheral vision as long as you can (PE Fig. 42c), then bring them back together.

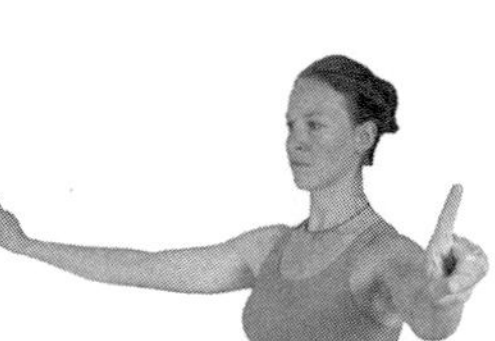

PE Fig. 42c

5. *Relaxing the eyes:* Lie down in a comfortable position and close your eyes. Allow them to sink toward the back of your head. Feel the weight of your eyelids. If you feel tension in your eyes, imagine them as two ponds and allow the ripples in the ponds to slowly settle. If you feel extreme tension in your eyes, place a towel or the palms of your hands gently over them until they relax.
6. Once your eyes feel relaxed, slowly open them. Rather than looking out, sense light slowly entering your eyes. Visualize the light traveling through your eyes to the back of your head until a visual field gradually forms.
7. *Exploring the sensory aspect of vision:* Look at something with texture or minute detail. Choose a patterned rug, textured wall, grass or trees, or even the pores in your skin. With a soft vision, look from one small detail to the next, allowing your eyes to slowly sequence from one tiny detail to the next.
8. Notice when your eyes tend to habitually jump across areas. Whenever this occurs, relax your eyes, then go back and look at the details in the place your eyes jumped over. Continue this exploration until your eyes relax and you break habits of jumping across certain areas of your visual field.

EMSPress.com

nation, organizing movement in the arms with movement of the head, neck, and spine (Figure 5.16).

People can have preferences for internally or externally focused vision, one seeming to look in, as though thinking, while the other looks out, as though focusing. People with poor vision tend to have eye strain and associated neck tension, and may even squint. Since the eyes are always roaming, people tend to develop spatial habits in the visual field, such as nervously darting the eyes between areas of visual preference or fixating on one point in a stare. Trauma and stress also affects the eyes, giving them a shocked or glassy look. A stressed person might even bulge the eyes and stare, or have poor coordination between head and eye motion, holding the head still while moving the eyes.

There are many ways to work with visual patterns. A person can learn how to relax the eye muscles. A person can also stretch and strengthen the eyes with calisthenics such as first looking all the way up, then down, then right, then left. Visual patterning can also be used to orient the head in space and to organize the intrinsic muscles at the base of the neck.

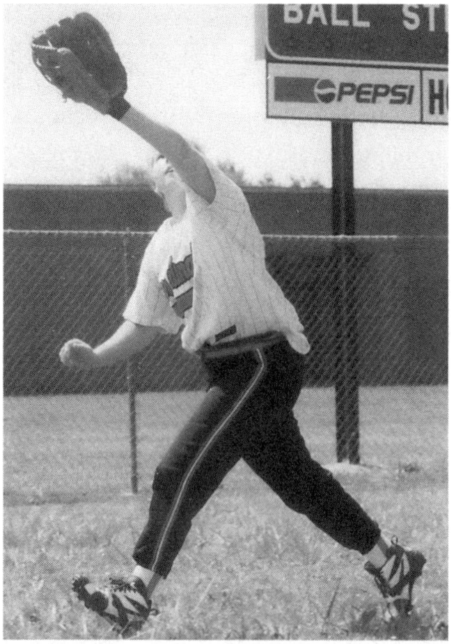

Figure 5.16 Hand to eye coordination (photo courtesy of E. Foster).

Tracking exercises can relieve stress in the eyes as well as the entire autonomic nervous system. For example, some psychotherapists use a therapy called "eye movement desensitization and reprocessing" (EMDR), which is based on the belief that trauma has associative sensorimotor components that become locked in visual holding patterns. Its developer, psychotherapist Francine Shapiro, describes EMDR as an accelerated learning process that accesses the rapid eye movement (REM) patterns that accompany negative psychological issues and processes the physical and emotional elements together to resolve stubborn traumas.[90] Although EMDR has many steps, the actual visual patterning occurs as the client simultaneously works on psychological issues while watching the therapist's hand or finger move from left to right in a series of short sets.

Patterning Exercise #43: Exploring the Planes in the Inner Ear

1. Sitting or standing, close your eyes and slowly move your head, sensing or imagining the subtle flow of the fluids within your inner ear. sensing or imagining the subtle flow of the fluids within your inner ear. Slowly tip your head along each axis, nodding, turning, and side-bending one ear toward a shoulder.
2. Open your eyes and slowly tip your head along the diagonal axis, looking down toward one knee, then looking up along the return diagonal path. Repeat on the other side.
3. Slowly roll your head forward and roll down your spine, allowing your head to be weighted (PE Fig. 42a). Sense the subtle adjustments in your spine and inner ear that keep you upright as you move your body off-center.
4. Slowly roll your head to one side and let your spine follow. Let your head be weighted as you move. Then reverse the movement and come back up. Again, sense the subtle adjustments that your body makes to stay upright as you move your head off center.

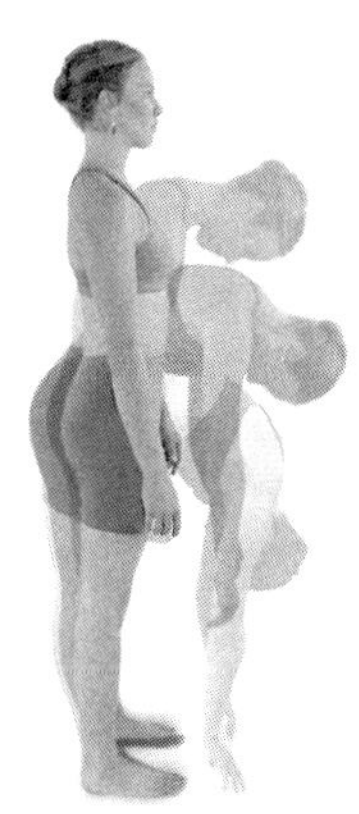

PE Fig. 43a

5. Slowly roll your head back and look up. Hyperextend your whole spine to support your neck.
6. Lie on your back or belly over a physioball and gradually roll your head side to side, releasing the weight of your head as you move. Then slowly roll the ball forward and back, again yielding the weight of your head as you move.
7. Sit on the ball with your eyes closed (PE Fig. 43b). Slowly explore movement of your head in all three planes (PE Fig. 42c-e). Sense or visualize fluid shifting within the inner ear as you move, and notice the subtle adjustments your body makes to keep your spine vertically oriented.

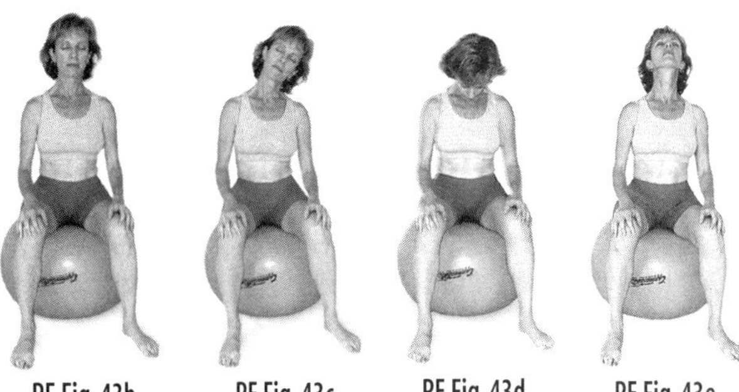

PE Fig. 43b PE Fig. 43c PE Fig. 43d PE Fig. 43e

EMSPress.com

Equilibrium, Hearing, and the Ears

The ears house intricate mechanisms both for maintaining equilibrium and spatial orientation, and for hearing. These mechanisms in the inner ear help us gauge where we are located in space, and where up and down are whenever the head and body move into an off-center position. If these mechanisms are dysfunctional, a person will have trouble with balance and may even experience a range of symptoms such as dizziness and nausea.

Sensory mechanisms in the *vestibule* of the inner ear adjust muscle tone in the body in response to changes in position and the pull of gravity. Changes in the position of the head trigger the tonic labyrinthine reflex (see Chapter 6), which increases flexor tone when the face faces down and increases extensor tone when the face faces up. Nerve fibers within the *saccule* and *utricle* of the vestibule also register linear changes in velocity, such as the linear acceleration and deceleration one feels when riding in a car that starts and stops along a straight road.

The *semicircular canals* register the angular movements of the head, such as the sensations one feels when riding in a car that tips right and left as it turns along a winding road. Each of the three semicircular canals is oriented in a different plane and helps us maintain a sense of spatial orientation when the head tips. The canals are filled with a thin, clear fluid that stimulates hair-like nerve cells with each change in angle or rotational direction.

Hearing is a more primitive sense and develops earlier than vision. A preborn hears and responds to sounds in the womb, which travel through vibration and the buffer of amniotic fluid; therefore, a newborn recognizes its mother's voice at birth.

The process of hearing takes place in a series of stages through different media from the outer ear into the brain (Figure 5.17):

1. *First stage:* The outer shell directs the vibration of sound waves traveling through the air into the tunnel of the auditory canal.
2. *Second stage:* The sound waves in the auditory canal cause the eardrum to vibrate, in turn causing the bones in the middle ear to vibrate.
3. *Third stage:* The vibrations of sound waves in the middle ear bones travel through the fluids of the inner ear.
4. *Fourth stage:* The nerve endings in the inner ear transform the fluid waves into electrochemical impulses that are transmitted to the brain, where the sound is perceived and interpreted.

The medium of each stage has a different capacity for transferring vibrations: one is a gas, one a solid, one a fluid, and one electrochemical. Listening through each medium can create different perceptions: some people are more sensitive to one medium than another. Depending on a person's

Patterning Exercise #44: Hearing through Different Media

Sit or lie in a comfortable position. Notice the mood changes that listening through each of the following media evokes.

1. *Air Currents:* Cup your hand around your ears and listen to the sound the air currents make. Turn your head slowly with your ears still cupped and notice how the reception changes depending on the position of your ears. Now put your ear to a conch shell and listen to the air currents within the shell.
2. *Bone Conduction:* Place your ear on a wooden table and lightly tap on it. Or gently knock on the top of your head and listen for the vibrations through your bones.
3. *Fluid Conduction:* Put your head under water in the bathtub, and tap on the tub. Or place your ear on a water bed or water balloon and scratch the surface of the bed or balloon.
4. *Electrochemical currents:* It is probably not possible, but some people feel they can hear the sounds of electrical impulses coming from computers or power lines. To get a vague sense of this level of hearing, focus on any internal dialogue or chatter that is running in your brain. Or you might explore humming various pitches and feel how it affects your inner ear.

EMSPress.com

auditory patterns, a sound that is pleasant to one person can irritate another; for example, music that soothes one person can be unnerving to the next. Likewise, a certain pitch of the voice or the repetitive sound of a machine can be either grating or relaxing. Many people vacation at the ocean to escape the cacophony of city life and to hear the soothing sounds of the wind and water.

By becoming aware of auditory patterns and preferences, a person can begin to sense how hearing affects not only head position, but also the psyche. For example, people with hearing loss may become depressed because they feel isolated from the world. Also, people with speech impediments might withdraw from relationships due to embarrassment or shame. To change speech patterns, a person needs to be able to first hear the patterns, then to learn muscular control over speech production. A person can explore hearing patterns to understand why specific sounds evoke pleasant sensations while others provoke irritable feelings (Figure 5.18). Lastly, we can seek out pleasant sounds, either in natural environments or on tape, such as a babbling brook or the sounds of birds chirping, to evoke the relaxation response.

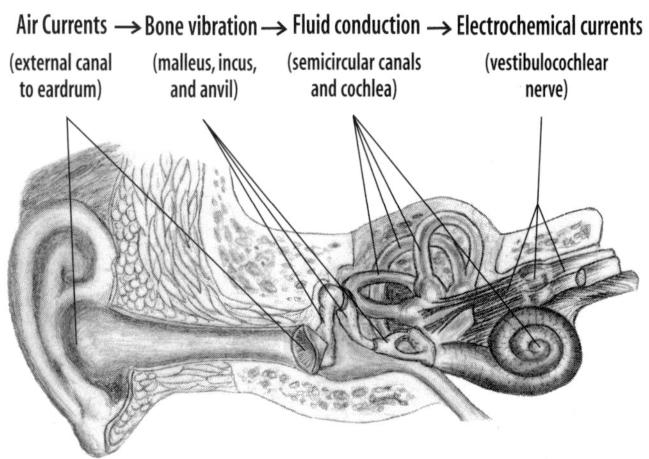

Figure 5.17 The anatomy and stages of hearing

INTEGRATION AND APPLICATION

The last phase of any patterning process or exercise involves integration. There are several elements to the process of integration. If a person has been practicing an exercise with one part of the body, she will need to integrate that part into the whole body, or at least into the center of the body or the spine. For example, say a person has a shoulder problem and has been practicing slow, precise movements with one arm. To integrate that arm back into the body, first she would need to move both arms together, with symmetry. This would not only integrate the changes into the spine, but also make a neurological connection between right and left sides. Next, this person would be advised to do some kind of spinal patterning to bring her back to midline and to the core of the body. (See "Midline" in Chapter 7.) Coming back to midline cannot be emphasized enough. If a person patterns new movements only on one side of the body or in one limb, she will probably feel lopsided if she ends without integrating the pattern into midline.

There is also a tendency to focus patterning on a problem area of the body, usually where there is excessive sensation such as pain or discomfort. It is important to remember that even though one area, say a hip or shoulder, may hurt, the other side also needs to go through the same kind of patterning exercise to establish symmetry of function between the sides.

Always ending with a movement along midline and always ending with a pattern that will integrate a part into a full-body or spinal movement will lead to integration of a new pattern. Also, it is helpful to end a patterning session with some kind of awareness or exercise in the feet to ground and center the body. This is particularly helpful if, during a patterning process, a person has become really relaxed and even slipped into an altered state (which often happens during organic, non-structured movement explorations practiced with the eyes closed). Grounding can be as simple as opening the eyes and looking around to orient oneself, then pressing both feet into the ground to renew awareness in the feet and establish lines of force from the feet into the trunk.

After a person has been exploring organic, fluid movements, it is also often helpful to do some kind of structured exercise to reconnect to an awareness of the muscles and bones. Fluid movements tend to dissolve a sense of boundaries; therefore, a structured pattern will help a person feel more bounded and grounded. The opposite is also true. If a person has been practicing a concentrated, controlled, mechanical movement, it will be best integrated by ending the patterning exercise with some kind of fluid, free-flow movement to loosen up and release any tension or stiffness from the concentration. A simple rocking or shaking movement will do the job.

Whenever a person becomes extremely relaxed during a patterning process, and especially if that person is lying on the floor, he will need to consciously bring up muscle tone before getting up. This involves getting up slowly, moving and stretching to bring up tone in the muscles, pushing down to sit or stand up, then reflecting on any changes that have occurred to integrate cognitive awareness with experiential process. Push patterns are helpful for simultaneously bringing up the tone and grounding the body. If a person jumps up from a very relaxed state without first bringing up the muscle tone, he may become dizzy and may even have a muscle spasm triggered by jumping from a low tone state.

It is also very integrating after a patterning session or exercise to take a moment to reflect on the difference between what a person felt like when starting the process and what he or she feels like afterward. Sometimes the changes in patterning are so subtle or deep that they might go unnoticed without feedback offering some kind of before-and-after comparison. This comparison will provide feedback about any positive changes that have occurred, will help a person realize if goals have been met, and will provide motivation (given that there have been positive changes) to continue patterning.

Some people like to keep a log of the changes they make during patterning. By periodically reviewing the log, people can chart their progress and may even recall exercises that they have forgotten. Other people like to take before-and-after pictures so that they can have visual feedback about any changes they made. Although this is not necessary for patterning, it can be motivating when the changes are obvious.

The final part of any patterning process is figuring out ways to apply the new patterns to daily living activities. Just carrying an awareness of a new pattern and a more balanced posture out of a patterning session is an important step toward application. Application takes personal commitment. After a patterning session, a person can make a promise to himself to actively apply what he learned to other activities. For instance, suppose a person worked on diaphragmatic breathing. He might want to make a commitment to practice his new breathing pattern at least once an hour, or perhaps every time he hears the phone ring, takes a bathroom break, or finds himself waiting in a line, in the car, or anywhere else.

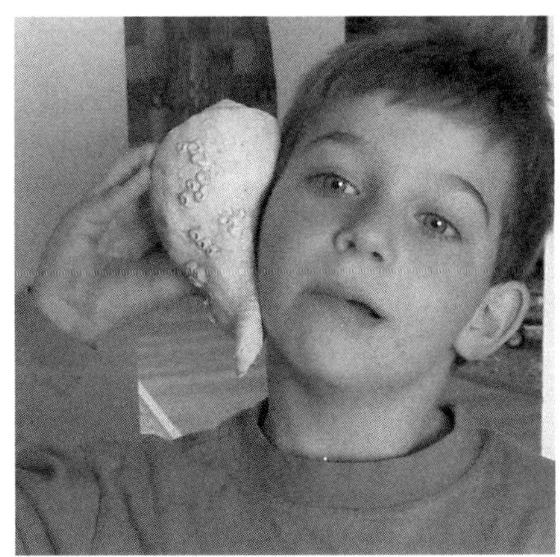

Figure 5.18 Listening to air currents in a sea shell

SUMMARY

This chapter on the patterning process provides a transition between the patterning theory presented in Part 1 and the patterning practice that makes up Part 2 of this text. Although the steps of the patterning process are presented in a linear fashion, it is important to realize that these steps can be addressed in many different ways. A patterning session might include just one step, a group of steps, or the entire process. Typically, as a person becomes proficient at patterning skills, such as being aware of the body, breathing, or gauging effort, the skills accumulate from session to session.

The patterning exercises outlined at the beginning of this chapter underlie many of the exercises found in Part 2. To review, the first four types of patterning exercise elements discussed—sensory awareness, relaxation, breathing, and organic movement—lay the foundation of all biological processes, so it makes sense to address them first. Just working with these four elements can take a person a long way in improving function, particularly balancing autonomic tone and building autonomic flexibility. Fluidity is a quality of relaxed and natural organic movement. It can be cultivated by moving in sync with the rhythms of the bodily fluids and is covered in Chapter 6 along with organic movement. The next four types of patterning exercises—reflexes, developmental patterns, tonic development and postural stability, and phasic development and movement fundamentals—are covered in Part 2 on practice, in Chapters 7 through 10. These chapters address the mechanical considerations innate to the neuromuscular system, such as skeletal architecture, joint function, and neuromuscular coordination.

The patterning skills presented in this chapter—setting up a feedback loop, moving through a full movement sequence, gauging effort and tone, breathing, and moving with the support of the sense organs—provide a foundation for the more complex skills that are presented next in Part 2.

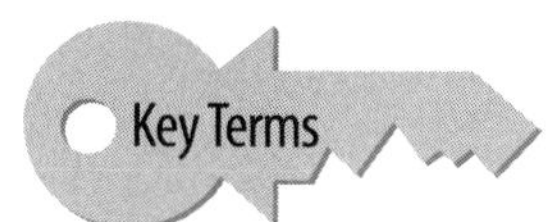

continuity of tone
effort
exhalation fixation
extensor tone
external respiration
flexor tone
hyperventilation
inhalation fixation
internal respiration
intra-abdominal pressure (IAP)
motor planning
paradoxical breathing
physiological extension
physiological flexion
responsiveness
tone

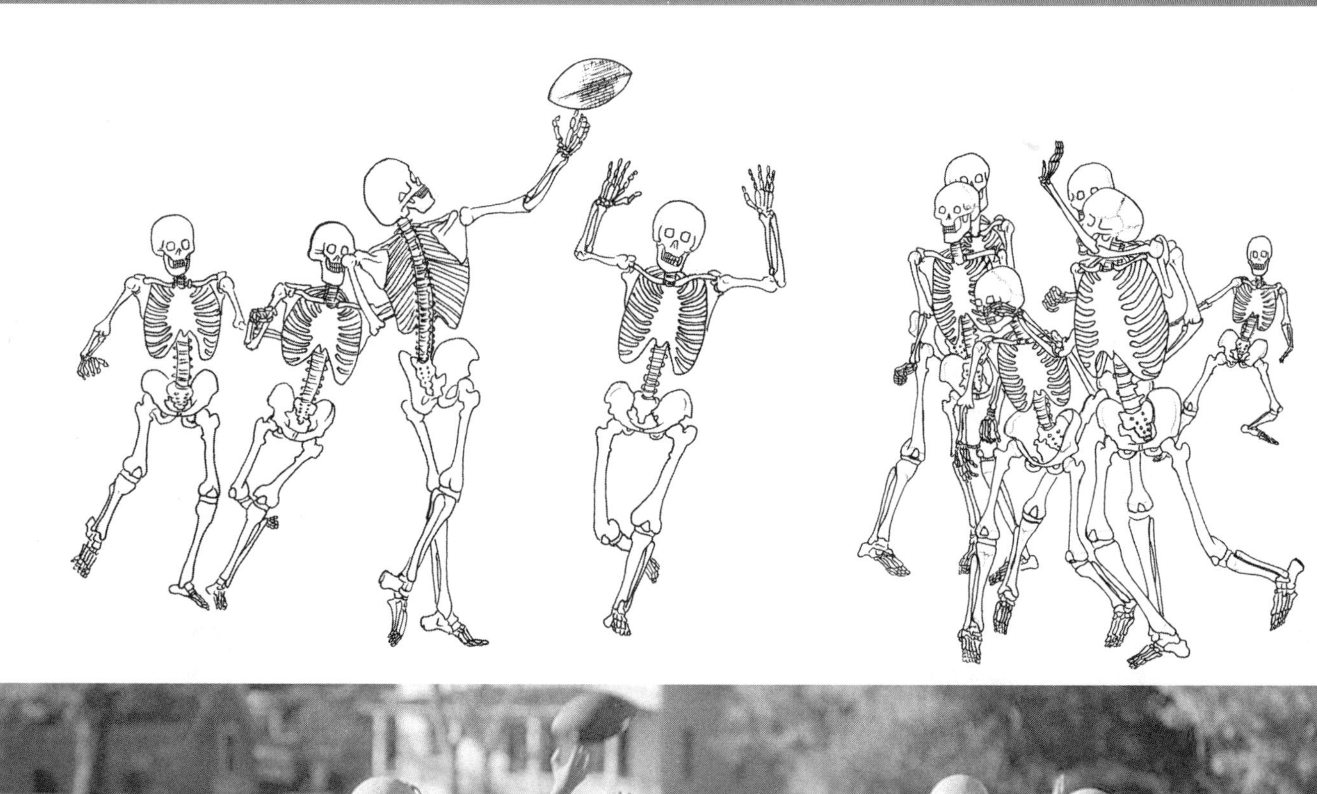

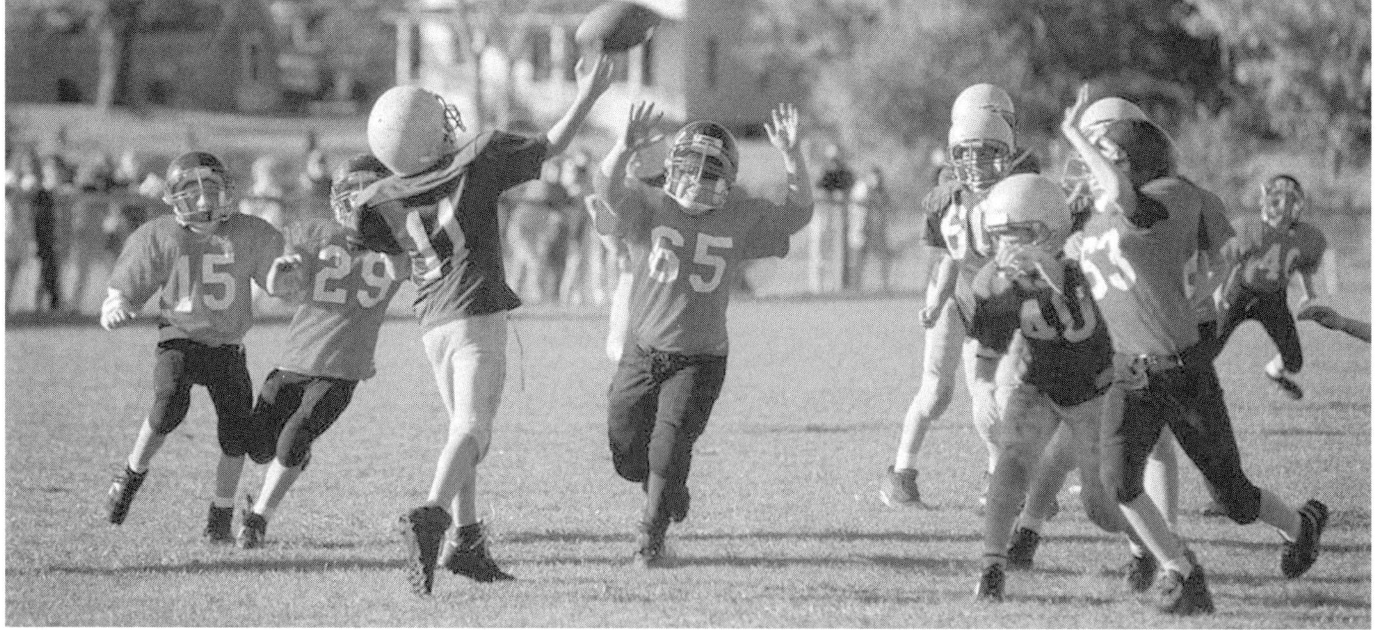

Part 2: Practice

As any reader who has explored any of the somatic patterning (SP) exercises presented so far knows, SP does not involve sweat. Yet while the SP exercises are easier than working out, they can be much more mentally challenging because the proprioceptive feedback a person gets from vigorous exercise is much stronger than the subtle sensations generated by patterning exercises. Unlike training for strength and endurance, SP trains for coordination, balance, and efficiency through the refinement of posture and movement. This refinement naturally enhances exercise and sports performance because it improves the economy of all body movements.

The refinement of movement patterns is made necessary by the immense functional changes that the human body has had to adapt to in recent history. Consider that in only the past hundred years, work-related demands on the human soma have evolved through three major transitions: from the physical labor of agriculture, to the mechanical exertions of industry, to the mental tasks of technology. Unless a person comes from a strong gene pool that breeds sturdy, resilient bodies, these changes have occurred much faster than the average body has been able to adapt to. Maladaptations are rampant as evidenced by the prevalence of structural and functional breakdowns in the body that the average person has to deal with, the most obvious being poor posture, which tends to accelerate the normal changes associated with aging.

Increasingly complex challenges call for comprehensive methods of postural education. The most popular method, ergonomics, is extremely helpful for the correct positioning of the body in relation to chairs and desks, yet it overlooks the intrinsic postural adaptations that people can carry with them into any activity. A comprehensive somatic patterning program can fill this gap because it is inclusive of mechanical, neuromuscular, and organic, biologically based approaches.

Although it will become obvious in Part 3 on the history of somatic patterning that a person can take numerous approaches to changing body-mind patterns, this section focuses primarily on patterning methods that involve actual body movement and muscular control. Because it would be impossible to source every single movement exercise, credits are given in this section only for exercises that are unique and have a clear source. However, whenever possible, the source of a specific theory or approach is provided.

OVERVIEW OF CHAPTER 6

THE MOTILITY OF ORGANS AND FLUIDS

THE ORGANS
- Organs and Emotional Processing
- Feeling Organ Sensations as a Therapeutic Tool
- The Gastrointestinal (GI) Tract
- The Heart and Lungs
- The Urinary and Reproductive Systems

FLUID SYSTEMS
- Fluid Forces
- Circulation and Physiological Rhythms
  - *Flow*
  - *Accessing the Fluids' Rhythms*
- Water
- Intercellular and Extracellular Fluids
- The Heart
  - *Blood Distribution*
  - *Cardiac Health and Heart Rate*
  - *Circulatory Rhythms*
- Interstitial Fluid and Fascia
- Lymph
- Cerebrospinal Fluid (CSF)
- Lubricating Joints

RESPONSIVENESS AND ORGANIC MOVEMENT

6

Organic and Fluid Movement

> **A [hu]man is obliged to live by the constant dissolution of form.**
>
> ***—Baird Spalding***

All too often in our society, people strive for a physique based on images of glamorous models and movie stars rather than an actual understanding of the body. To understand what this means in terms of body image versus body knowledge, let's look at the following example. Because of their different views of the body, two women walking behind a young, athletic man, when asked for feedback, saw two completely different things. The first woman commented that the runner had great "gastrocs," the double-bellied muscle on the back of the calf (Figure 6.1). The second woman commented, "They may look good to you, but they're frozen. They aren't moving." The first woman was taken aback. As though the other's comment had popped scales off the first woman's eyes, she commented, "Oh, my gosh, you're right; they aren't moving. I can't believe I didn't see that. I was just looking at the shape, but now I can see the lack of motion. His calves may look great, but they're stiff and held."

This contrast in perception is common between an average person and a somatic practitioner. Trained in organic and improvisational fluid movement form, the latter can spot a frozen muscle from its lack of intrinsic motion and its static shape. Movement is, basically, changing shape. The movement of muscles involves a pumping action—not just a mechanical, up-and-down pumping, but the swelling and shrinking of the round, shape-shifting, primarily liquid form of the working muscles (the average body is 60 to 85 percent fluid). A functional muscle pumps through obvious and alternating cycles of shortening and elongating. When a muscle is fixated in a chronic contraction, it lacks intrinsic motility. It may look good in a photo, but it is nonfunctional when it's rigid.

Although the action of working muscles is in some ways analogous to a pump, it is much more complex and organic than a mechanical pump. Even if the mechanical pump has an elastic bladder that stretches and shrinks on each cycle of motion, the movement is still restricted to solely a change in position, like a piston going up and down. A muscle is living tissue, made up of plasmatic fluids, minerals, charged particles, and fibers. Each muscle cell is a fluid-filled sac teeming with biochemical changes that alter its intrinsic shape on each contraction cycle. The intrinsic motion fueled by metabolic process, whether of a muscle, an organ, or any other tissue, is referred to as *motility.*

THE MOTILITY OF ORGANS AND FLUIDS

Recall from Chapter 4 that motility denotes the subtle, intrinsic movements of the fluids and organs, and mobility denotes externally observable movements that change the position of the body in space. Inner motility has an ebbing and flowing quality through plasmatic currents that a person might observe in the ripples under the skin of a sleeping snake. In humans, the intrinsic patterns of

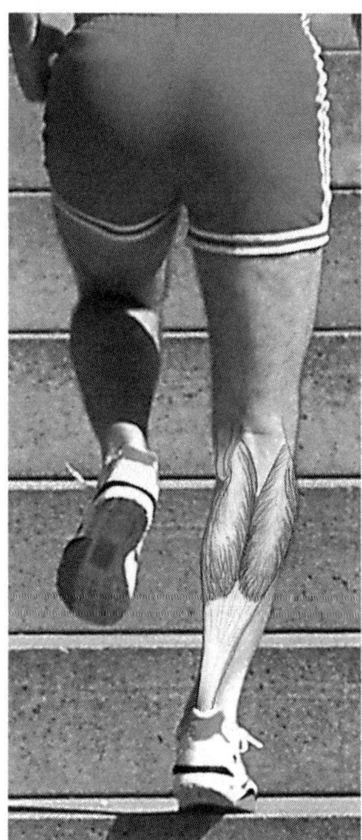
Figure 6.1 The gastrocnemius muscle

motility provide an underlying support, fullness, and ease to the seemingly mechanical movements of the body changing positions in space. Motility can be clearly seen in a newborn who arrives in a seemingly jelly-like state and whose movements, prior to muscular development, are generated by biological impulses that sequence in an incredibly organic and fluid manner. The question is, as adults, how can we recognize, embody, and rediscover this innate quality of movement that is found in all living organisms? And why would we want to?

Most people think of fluidity in a figurative sense, as an overall quality of grace, ease, and flow in the body, but fluidity also reflects the quality of movement inherent in the circulation of bodily fluids. Fluidity has an actual basis in our anatomy and physiology; it is a visible reflection of a level of circulation among body systems. Circulation is usually associated with the bloodstream, but all bodily fluids have distinct patterns and pathways of circulation, each in a specific physiological rhythm.

Fluidity is also an outward manifestation of physiological rhythms. For example, African dance embodies the arterial blood-pulse rhythm, Tai Chi embodies the flow of cerebrospinal fluid, and even blowing up a balloon follows the rhythm of the breath. Fluidity is both figurative and tangible. It is a somatic experience and a physical state of being, as well as a type of body consciousness that encompasses flexibility, effortlessness, fullness, and an openness of mind.

Many people have the habit of holding the body very still as they think, talk, or work, or whenever they are involved in mental activity. At these times, they lose the dynamic and interactive quality of fluidity and become stiff. Given that the bodily fluids are always circulating within us, the dampening and stifling of organic fluid rhythms is a learned habit ingrained by the dominance of the mind over the body. All too often the fluid and organic qualities of movement inherent in human beings are sacrificed to the learned stiffness that we become adept at carrying from one activity to the next.

A lack of inner motility is not only caused by muscular tension; it is also a reflection of deep tensions in the organs and restrictions of fluid circulation, which, in turn, can trigger chronic muscular holding. The cycle perpetuates itself because the chronic holding of skeletal muscles rapidly becomes habit, creating a rigidity that affects the tone of the organs and circulation of the fluids, which in turn triggers more muscular holding. Conversely, cultivating healthy patterns of motility in the organs and the circulation of the fluids can only improve musculoskeletal patterns.

Sometimes, organic processes in somatic patterning are approached on energetic levels or with therapies such as emotional processing or expressive movement. On a more tangible level, organic processes have a substantial ground in the patterns of motility in the organ systems and bodily fluids. Therefore, we can actually work with organic processes and improve inner motility by exploring patterns of circulation in the movement of our organs and fluids. To do this, we need to be able to actually move in sync with our physiological rhythms in an improvisational manner that will increase organ motility and fluid circulation. Internal motility can be improved by practicing movements that shift the organs, compressing, rotating, and stretching them to improve their tone and increase a feeling of inner vitality. The practice of organic movement (introduced in Chapter 4) can also be used to release autonomic tension.

THE ORGANS

Every cell is an organ unto itself. Muscle cells are the organs of the muscular systems, bone cells the organs of the skeletal system, liver cells the organs of the liver, and the brain, which is made up of many nerve cells, the main organ of the nervous system.

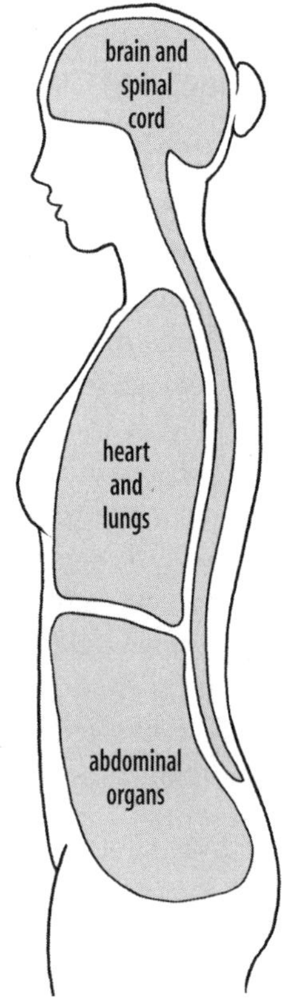

Figure 6.2 The organ compartments

Although each cell is a self-contained organ, in a general context the word "organ" is used to refer to organs of the various body systems, such as the brain, heart, lungs, and intestines. The organs carry out the body's fundamental metabolic processes—breathing, circulation, reproduction, digestion, absorption, and elimination. A group of organs that serves a common function makes up a body system.

The organs that fill the skull and the torso are separated by fascial membranes into three protective compartments: the skull and vertebral column around the brain and spinal cord, the thorax around the heart and lungs, and the abdomen and pelvis around the abdominal viscera, which include the digestive, reproductive, and urinary organs as well as the liver, pancreas, and spleen (Figure 6.2). Each compartment is packed tightly with organ tissue and fluids. All the organs except the brain are either vascular beds of capillaries (lungs, liver, pancreas, and kidneys), or hollow muscular tubes, pouches, and sacs (stomach, urinary bladder, esophagus, heart, and intestines). Individual organs often function in systems as trios, such as the heart and lungs, or the kidneys and urinary bladder. They also have coordinated functions with endocrine glands, such as the kidneys and the adrenal glands, the uterus and ovaries, the penis and testes, and the brain and hypothalamus.

The quality of motility in each body system has a distinct personality, much like the members of an extended family. For example, muscles are the workhorses of body movement, fluids the transport network that links all systems, the nervous system the body's master coordinator, bones the stiffening struts and levers, and organs the processors of our inner workings.

Organs and Emotional Processing

Since the organs carry out deep and often quiet metabolic processes, they are the body system most associated with deep emotional processing. Many somatic disciplines convey the belief that sensations of the deeper emotions center in the heart, lungs, and abdominal organs and are processed through "gut" feelings and "heartfelt" experiences. Difficulties often arise with cathartic psychotherapy techniques such as beating pillows or screaming because the excessive activity in the skeletal muscles may drown out the quieter, slower sensations in the organs. We also know that prolonged states of cathartic emotionality tend to stress the organs by revving the autonomic tone too high, thereby disturbing their optimal environment—a relaxed, parasympathetic state. With this in mind, emotional processing that is slow and gentle will more likely promote the optimal state in which deep psychophysiological shifts can occur. This is particularly important when working with psychological issues rooted in traumas and shock that become locked in the body via states of high sympathetic tone.

What is the difference between the quality of emotional processes expressed through the parasympathetic and sympathetic nervous systems? How does this relate to working with trauma or shock?

Each organ system has disease processes associated with specific emotional processes. For example, the gastrointestinal system could be viewed as a physical counterpart for emotional processing. We take in our experiences like food; they can be either nourishing or upsetting. Negative emotions are like toxic food: they are difficult to process and quietly eat away at our insides. Conversely, positive emotions, like nourishing food, permeate and energize us with healthy feelings.

Dysfunctional tendencies in each organ system are often treated using a range of patterning modalities. For example, irritable bowel syndrome is a psychosomatic condition in which stress manifests stress in a number of symptoms that include gas, cramping and bloating, abdominal pain and distension, diarrhea or constipation, nausea, and a general loss of appetite. Treatments range from digestive aids and dietary changes to cognitive therapies that help a person change maladaptive thought that triggers gastrointestinal (GI) tract tension. People also learn how to relax GI tract muscles using biofeedback therapy (with electrodes placed on the abdominal wall over chronic contractures), relaxation training, breathing, and a combination of imagery and hypnotherapy. Although a thorough discussion of the psychological correlates to organ systems is beyond the scope of this text, the reader is still encouraged to consider these relationships while working with patterns in the organ systems.

Feeling Organ Sensations as a Therapeutic Tool

Organ needs drive our behavior, particularly those that ensure survival, such as hunger, thirst, or fear. The intermittent sensations of normal organ needs are always with us. These sensations occur as a kind of background noise that tends to go unnoticed until they become abnormal and grow constant or nagging. Emotional reactions can rise from the gut on a hair trigger. The sensations generated by organs become exaggerated during movements that displace their weight. The distinct sensation of the viscera rising up, then dropping with a thud after an elevator ride is unmistakable. Or we feel them slide to the side while making a sharp turn in a car, or sloshing and swaying in sync with waves while boating. More commonly, when two people are together, it is often hard to distinguish from which body the rumbling and gurgling of the digestive processes is coming.

Although the physiological processes that take place within the organs are involuntary, it is possible to develop some voluntary control over them. Relaxation skills are just as important for organ tone as they are for muscle tone. Relaxation shifts the body from sympathetic tone to the parasympathetic state, pulling blood away from the skeletal muscles and sending it to the GI tract to aid digestive processes. This is why abdominal viscera tend to gurgle and growl when a person relaxes and why it is not good to eat while on the run or while highly stressed: most of the blood is in the muscles, making digestion difficult. It's surprising how many people become embarrassed

Patterning Exercise #45: Organ Awareness through Touch and Movement

(Adapted from Body-Mind Centering.)

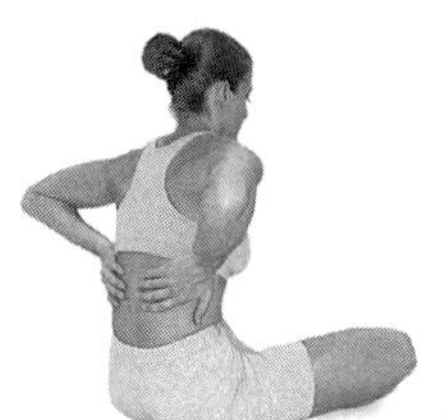

PE Fig. 45a

1. *Feeling and moving individual organs:* Sit in a comfortable position and place your hands over any organ. For example, place your hands on your back over the kidneys, at the level of the lower ribs (PE Fig. 45a). Then begin to slowly move your spine back and forth and side to side, sensing or visualizing your kidneys shifting toward or away from your hands as you move.
2. Now place your hands over your heart, on your sternum (PE Fig.45b, upper hand). Once again, slowly shift your sternum forward and backwards, sensing or visualizing your heart moving toward or away from your hands.

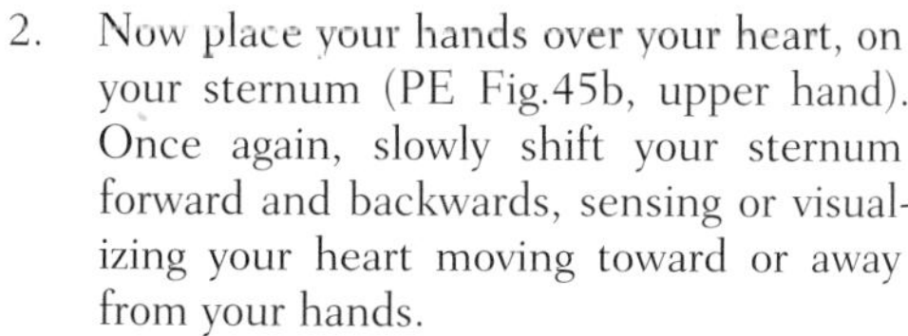

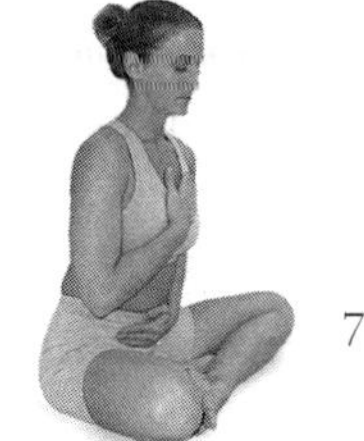

PE Fig. 45b

3. Then place your hands on your abdomen, over your lower intestines (PE Fig.45b, lower hand). And again, slowly shift your waist forward and backwards, sensing or visualizing your intestines moving under your hands.
4. Practice sensing and moving any organ of your choice, such as your lungs, bladder, liver, stomach, trachea, and even your brain.

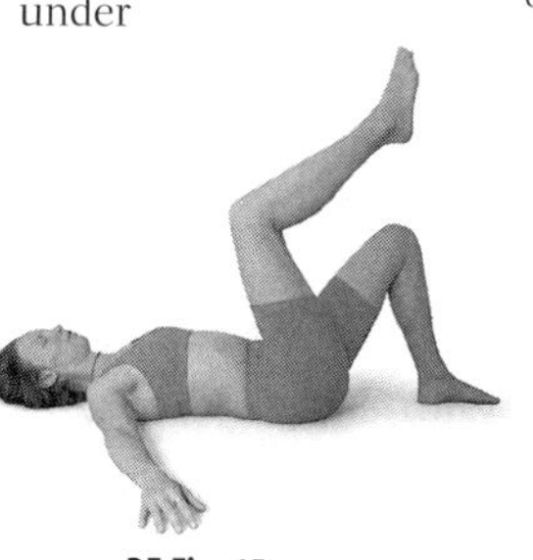

PE Fig. 45c

5. *Moving a limb with organ awareness:* Lie on your back with your knees bent and feet flat. Slowly raise one leg and sense the kidney on that side sink back, as though your kidney were a sandbag attached to your leg (PE Fig. 45c). Then slowly lower your leg, sensing or visualizing weight sinking through the kidney the entire time. Repeat on the other side. Slowly move each leg in any direction, sensing weight sinking through another organ, such as the back of your lungs, liver, intestines, even your heart and brain.
6. Roll to your side and lift your arm toward the ceiling. Move your arm slowly while sensing weight sink into the lung on the underside of your body (PE Fig. 45d). Roll over and repeat on the other side.

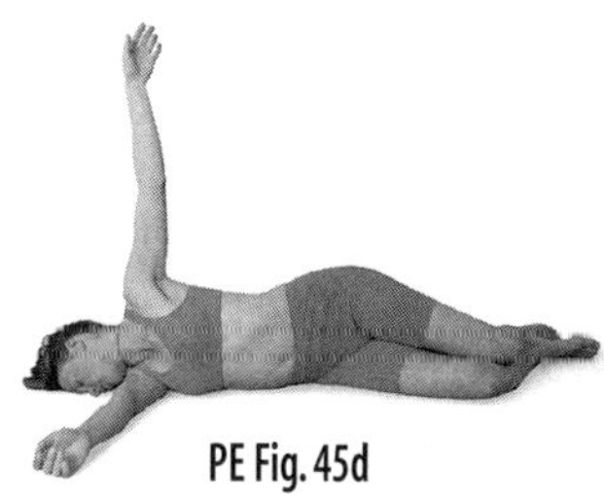

PE Fig. 45d

7. Slowly roll your knees to one side, sensing weight sinking into the viscera on that side (PE Fig. 45e). Go both directions.

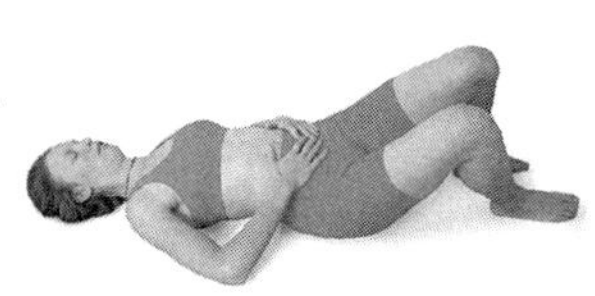

PE Fig. 45e

8. *Yielding organ weight:* Lie on your belly (PE Fig. 45f). Sense your organs sinking through the front of your trunk into the floor. Focus on one organ at time, make subtle intrinsic movements to shimmy and sink each organ into the floor, starting at your head and progressively moving toward your pelvis.

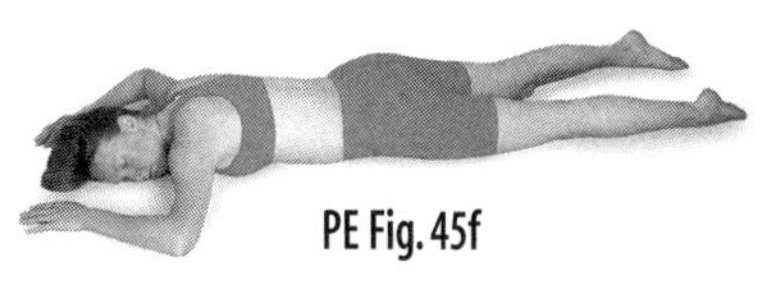

PE Fig. 45f

and apologize when their organs start to rumble, as though their organs were behaving improperly.

Many of the organs are made up of smooth muscles, and it is possible to learn how to relax them. In the same way skeletal muscles hold stress in chronic contractures, so can smooth muscles in the organs, especially in the GI tract, which can become spastic in people prone to internalizing stress there. To alleviate the symptoms, people with irritable bowel syndrome can learn how to relax a spastic colon with touch, awareness, and organic movement.

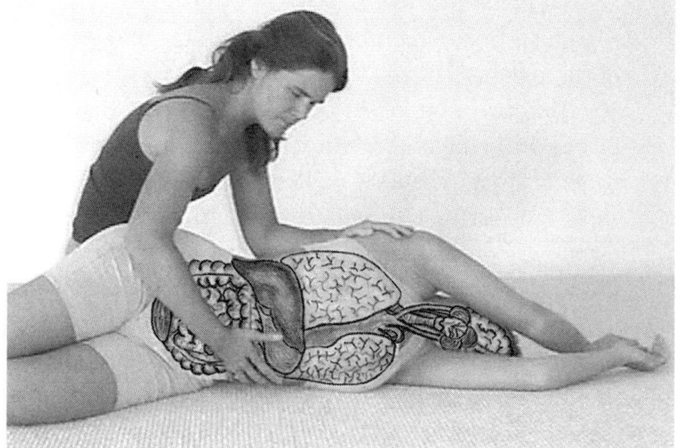

Figure 6.3 A visualization of the inner processes occurring during the Body-Mind Centering exercise of the "organ roll" (see Patterning Exercise #46).

Another condition that stresses the organs is tight fascia around them, which can torque, pull, or place unhealthy pressure on the organs. Fascial adhesions in the organs can be released with gentle massage or with specific techniques such as visceral manipulation.[91] It should be noted that tight fascia around organs or muscular tension in them can account for chronic pain and movement restrictions for which no muscular imbalance can be found.

Fascial adhesions and restrictions in the organs can also be addressed with somatic patterning exercises done with a focus on the organs. For example, a person can learn to target an organ as an axis for motion to stimulate it with new positions and pulls, to breathe into a specific organ to energize it, or to sense weight passing through an organ to relax it. Rolling on the floor in a slow, weighted manner will stimulate sensations in the organs as their weight is

Links to Practical Applications

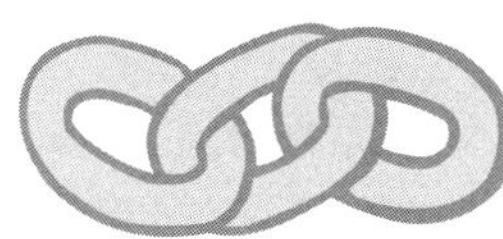

Releasing Tension in Organs

When the organs release tension, they often create short-lived sensations that could be misinterpreted as painful but are, in reality, just unfamiliar. For instance, a dull, passing ache in your chest may be fascia around your heart stretching. Annoying twitches in your muscles, such as those lightning twitches that jerk your body as you are falling off to sleep, may just be neuromuscular releases. And the temporary pains that shoot through your trunk as you move in a new way may just be myofascial adhesions between your organs stretching. Once you start sensing your organs more, the range of sensations you feel in them will expand; therefore, it is crucial that you be able to differentiate between healthy and unhealthy organ sensations to avoid misinterpreting them.

displaced, as well as put them under a broader range of compressive or tensile stresses which can be useful to improve tone in flaccid organs and relax tight organs (Figure 6.3).

Actively sensing the organs is a new concept to most people. Somatic patterning takes organ awareness one step further, using an awareness of movement in and around the organs to relax them, to tone them, to increase motility and body awareness, and to process pain (both physical and emotional). Organic movement is not only helpful in releasing deep holding patterns in the skeletal muscles; it can also be helpful in reversing the maladaptive changes in organs that develop as a result of being under prolonged mechanical stress. For example, slouching compresses the heart, lungs, and viscera. Conversely, good posture plus relaxing and stretching the organs during slow, fluid movements can help to restore organ tone, improve autonomic flexibility, and ground a person in a sensation of inner weight.

Many people, especially women, have been conditioned to misinterpret the sensations of dimensional fullness in the organs as being fat. People obsessed with being overweight often squeeze their organs with chronic muscular tension in an effort to become thinner. This type of holding creates internal stress and puts chronic pressure on the organs. This is particularly true in the abdominal organs, which tend to expand easily because they are not enclosed within a bony container. A person might even have a subconscious disdain for any organ sensations, which could be thought of as a mild self-image disorder. (In an extreme image disorder, anorexia, any body sensations are interpreted as being overweight.) These types of misperceptions constitute a

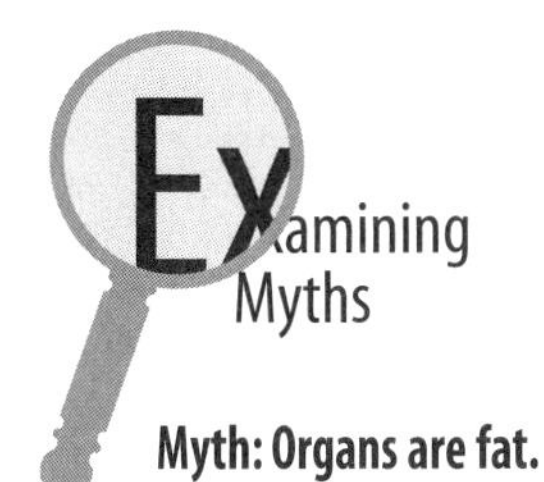

Myth: Organs are fat.

Some people, especially women, consider any volume or fullness in their trunk to be excess fat and think they need to diet. The trunk is filled with organs that have dimension and take up space. Granted, a person may have weak abdominal muscles that allow the organs to sag, but don't misinterpret the natural fullness of healthy viscera for fat.

Patterning Exercise #46: The Organ Roll

(Created by Bonnie Cohen.) This exercise will help you sense and relax your organs with slow, weighted rolling movements. If sensing your organs is a new experience, you may feel new sensations, so don't be alarmed by strange sounds and sensations that commonly arise from the belly as the organs relax.

1. Lie on the floor on your back. Slowly roll from side to side, sensing the weight of your organs sinking toward the ground as you roll (PE Fig. 46a). Make sure to roll slowly enough to sense the weight of each organ shifting and sinking toward the ground. Feel weight pouring into the underside of your body (PE Fig. 46b). The sensations created by your organs will be subtle. You might want to visualize each individual organ as you sense that area move. As you roll over to your belly, make sure to put your arm above your head, sensing the weight of your lungs sink into your ribs. Roll from one side to another, from front to back, stopping and resting in any places where you feel tension or holding.

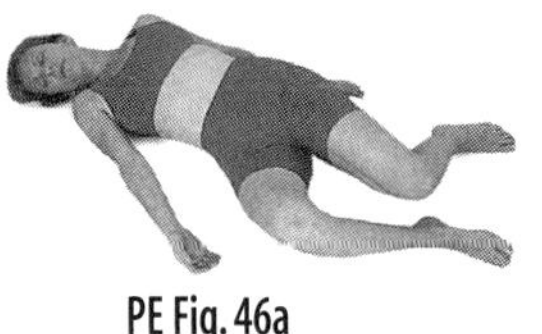

PE Fig. 46a

PE Fig. 46b

2. *With a partner:* Again, lie on your back. Have your partner slowly roll you over to one side, then the other, helping you feel the weight of your organs sinking and yielding toward the ground. Your partner can touch the areas where you need to yield (PE Fig.46c-f).
3. Sit up slowly, sensing your organ weight shifting into the base of your pelvis as you come up.
4. Then switch roles. Slowly roll your partner, encouraging her to feel the weight of her organs sink down toward the floor.

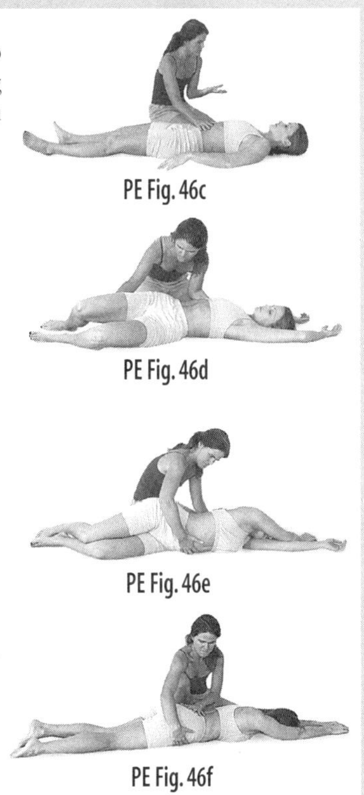

PE Fig. 46c

PE Fig. 46d

PE Fig. 46e

PE Fig. 46f

EMSPress.com

rejection of an essential part of a person, the gut. The word "gut" derives from medieval times when anatomists, who considered organs unimportant parts of the anatomy, gutted their cadavers. It's ironic that these days we say a person has a "gut" when we're referring to fat, yet has "guts" when we're referring to courage.

The Gastrointestinal (GI) Tract

The GI tract is a series of convoluted muscular tubes, pouches, and valves that begins at the mouth and ends at the anus (Figure 6.4). This long tract processes the food we take in and eliminates solid waste. Smooth muscles line the digestive tract organs in alternate layers arranged in circular rings and longitudinal fibers. These muscular tubes milk their contents in the rhythmic motions of *peristalsis,* squeezing and pumping food along the digestive tract in a movement similar to how a snake swallows an egg. If a person eats something too dry to slide down the throat, the sensations of peristalsis become obvious as the esophageal muscles work to milk the lump toward the stomach. When empty, the stomach is about the size of a large sausage; when filled, it digests food with the churning, rippling, mixing waves of peristalsis. Muscular valves open and close to allow materials to pass in and out of the stomach, and, when faulty, may leak stomach acids into the esophagus resulting in a sensation known as "heartburn."

The stomach passes its contents into an S-shaped tube called the *duodenum,* which passes it to the small intestine, made up of about 10 to

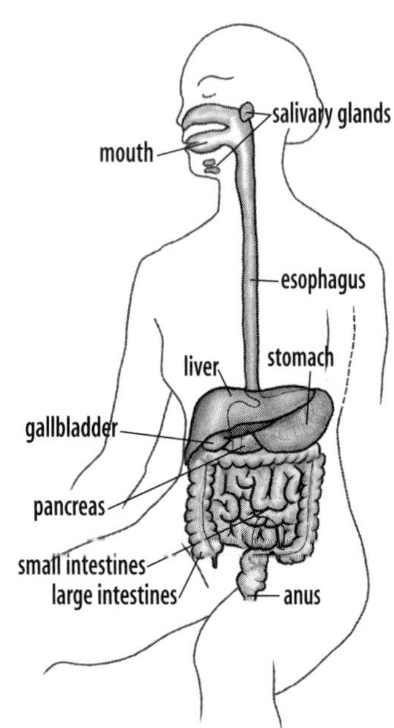

Figure 6.4 Gastrointestinal tract

Patterning Exercise #47: Toning and Stretching Your Organs with Motion

(Adapted from Body-Mind Centering.) ***As we move, the compression and stretching of organs within their cavities tone them. In this exploration, pick an organ you want to relax, tone, or become more aware of.***

1. Place your hands over your liver and use it as a fulcrum for the lateral flexion and extension. Slowly sidebend your spine and sense the movement compress your liver (PE Fig. 47a). Then reverse the movement and sense your liver being stretched (PE Fig. 47b).

PE Fig. 47a

PE Fig. 47b

2. Do the same with any organ, moving in any direction, sensing flexion toward that organ compressing it, then sensing the opposite motion stretching that organ. For example, sidebending will compress the lung on one side while stretching the other lung.

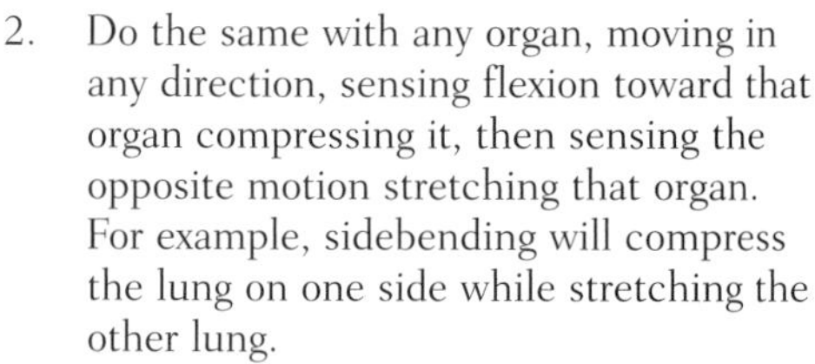

PE Fig. 47c

3. *Counter-rotating organs:* Put one hand on your forehead and the other over your heart. Slowly turn your head side to side and sense or imagine your heart counter-rotating with your brain (PE Fig. 47c).
4. Put your hands over your neck and slowly rotate your head. Sense or imagine your windpipe and esophagus gently twisting inside your neck (PE Fig. 47d).
5. Put both feet flat, knees bent. Then tilt your pelvis under, and feel or sense your abdominal viscera sinking into your lower back (PE Fig. 47e).

PE Fig. 47d

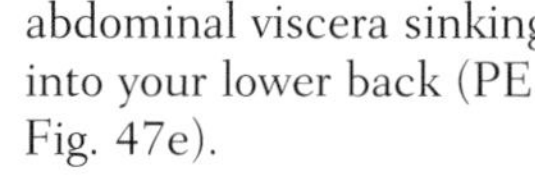

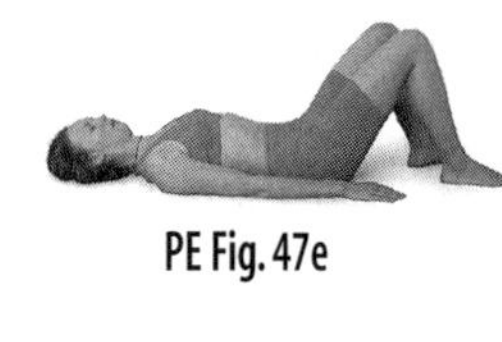

PE Fig. 47e

6. Lift your lower back off the floor and feel or sense weight sinking into your kidneys (PE Fig. 47f).

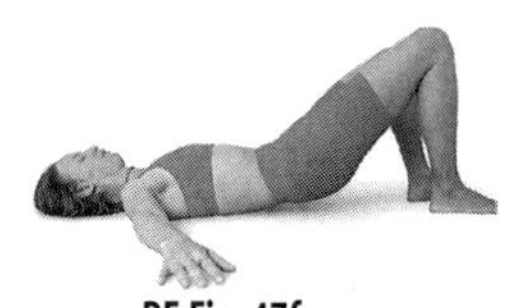

PE Fig. 47f

7. Now lift your lower ribs off the floor and feel or sense weight sinking into the back of your lungs and heart (PE Fig. 47g).

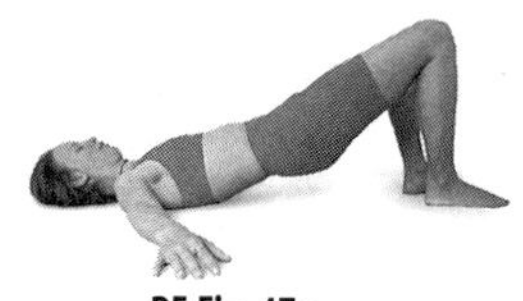

PE Fig. 47g

8. Gradually reverse the motion, rolling your spine back onto the floor one area at a time. As you lower your ribs to the floor, sense the weight of your viscera sequentially sinking through the back of your body into the floor.
9. *Sensing organs fold around adjacent organs:* Lie on your back with your arms out to the sides. Slowly bring your hands together above you and sense or imagine your lungs slightly folding around your heart (PE Fig. 47h).

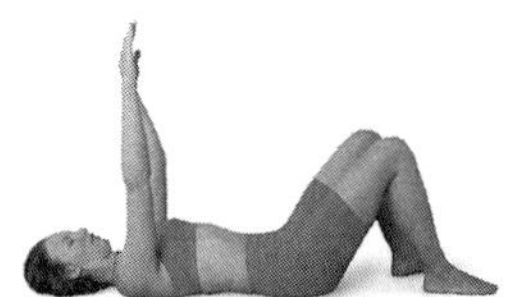

PE Fig. 47h

10. Move your arms in any direction while sensing weight shifting along your back through different areas of your lungs (PE Fig. 47i).

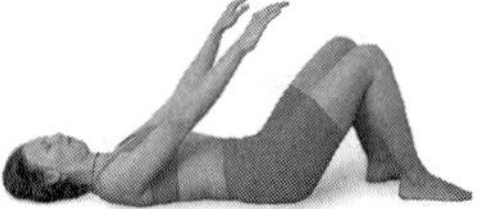

PE Fig. 47i

EMSPress.com

15 feet of muscular tubing lined with convoluted, circular folds that increase the surface area for the absorption of nutrients. The small intestine mixes *chyme* (partially digested food) with digestive juices through a motion called *segmentation*, which pumps and squeezes a localized segment. Intestinal muscle constricts chyme in small sections, and then in progressively larger sections to milk the contents along, while its lining membrane gradually absorbs a combination of nutrients and about 8.3 liters of fluid per day.[92]

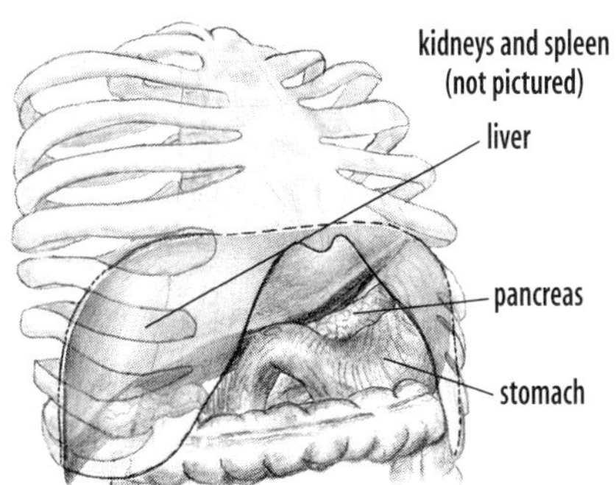

Figure 6.5 Organs under the diaphragm

Then a peristaltic motion (which is much weaker than peristalsis in the *esophagus* and *stomach*) propels the digested food through the *ileocecal valve* into the large intestine. This large muscular tube is about 5 feet long and is divided into an ascending, transverse, and descending *colon*. It cradles the periphery of the *small intestine*, whose bulk is found in the center of the abdomen (Figure 6.4). The colon ends at the large muscular pouch of the rectum and anal canal, which descend along the inside of the sacrum. The anus closes by both an internal sphincter made up of smooth muscle and a protective external sphincter made up of skeletal muscle. Defecation occurs through a combination of voluntary contractions in the respiratory diaphragm, the abdominal muscles, and the external sphincter, which distends the rectal wall. This distension stimulates a *defecation reflex*, which initiates a contraction in the longitudinal muscles that shorten the rectum and increase the pressure inside it in order to expel feces.

Cohen describes an **anal rooting reflex,** which is similar to oral rooting in that an infant will move his tail toward tactile stimulation around the anus.[93] A parent can observe this reflex while changing soiled diapers. The anus responds in a movement pattern similar to how the mouth reaches during oral rooting, moving toward touch; both rooting reflexes underlie spinal movements initiated with either push or reach patterns in the head or the tail.

With aging, the digestive system undergoes a number of changes: both its secretions and motility decline, its muscles and valves lose strength and tone, and it undergoes other physiological changes. Neurochemical changes can lead to inflammation in any part of the long, intricate digestive tubing, or an ulcer, which occurs when acidic gastric juices burn a crater-like hole in a digestive organ membrane. Such changes can also culminate in serious diseases of the *pancreas*, *liver*, or *gallbladder*. Symptoms of dysfunction in the lower GI tract are reduced motility and decreased sensation in any part of the digestive tubing; symptoms of dysfunction in the upper GI tract are a diminished sense of taste, tooth decay, and periodontal disease.

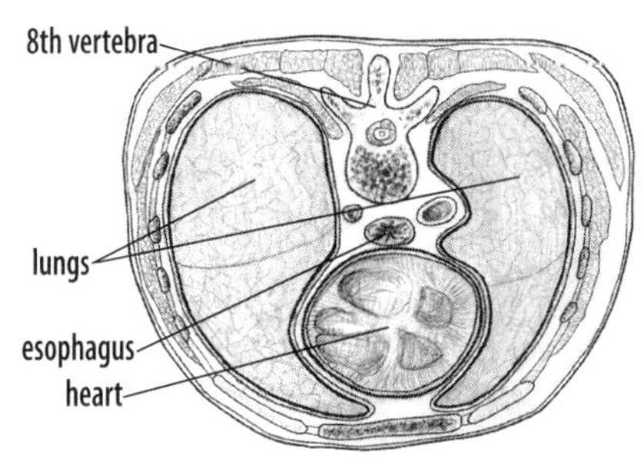

Figure 6.6 Cross-section of the heart and lungs

People can increase their GI health through the combined efforts of diet (unprocessed foods with plenty of nutritional value, fiber, and fluid), learning to relax the intestines, and getting exercise. Anything that increases the motility of the digestive organs and stimulates the intestines, such as stretching, patterning exercises with the organs, and even brisk walking, can improve digestive health. Also, a person can learn to relax yet tone the smooth muscles in the digestive tract, using awareness, biofeedback, or even an organic movement practice.

Breathing exercises also help to tone the digestive organs that lie directly under the diaphragm, which include the liver, stomach, spleen, pancreas, and kidneys. The liver, a vascular bed rich in blood and the second largest organ (the skin is the largest), fills the area under the right side and center of the diaphragm; the stomach, pancreas, and spleen are tucked up under the left side of the diaphragm; and the kidneys sit under the floating ribs (Figure 6.5). All these organs receive a massage from the movement of the respiratory diaphragmatic during breathing.

The Heart and Lungs

The heart is a strong, muscular pump cupped by the lungs and attached to them through large circulatory vessels. Strong ligaments suspend the back of the heart from the front of the upper thoracic spine, and a fascial pouch called the *pericardium* wraps the heart. Both the heart and lungs sit on top of the *respiratory diaphragm* and receive a mechanical massage from its rise and fall. The lungs cushion the heart with their buoyant air spaces and spongy vascular beds, and also massage the heart as they fill and empty (Figure 6.6). The heart and lungs ensure the adequate oxygenation of tissue for normal metabolic processes. The lungs pull in oxygen from the environment, and the heart circulates oxygen within the blood throughout the body.

Cardiac muscles in the heart follow a spiral-shaped pathway. The cardiac fibers are tethered together by strong, interlacing connective tissue fibers that are called the *skeleton of the heart* (Figure 6.7). This ropy skeleton provides a dense, fibrous network that not only wraps the heart but also permeates it, reinforcing the heart's internal fibers and providing additional support around heart valves and vessels. It is interesting to note that since all movements

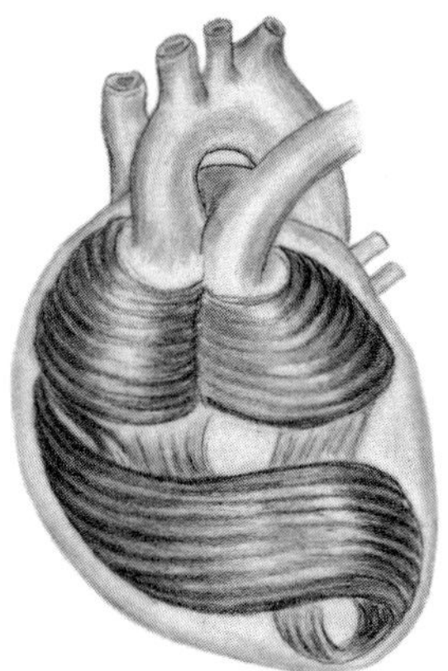
Figure 6.7 The fibrous skeleton of the heart

are some combination of flexion, extension, and rotation, all movements take a spiral-shaped pathway. The spiral shape repeats itself in the skeleton of the heart, in the curved and twisted collagen fibers, in muscle striations, and in trabecular rows of bone cells (see Figure 8.12).

Chapter 5 has a section on lung anatomy and physiology; sections later in this chapter discuss the heart and circulatory patterns, as well as patterning exercises for these three vital organs.

> **Fluidity and Nervous System Balance**
>
> *The following body story told by a skier illustrates the importance of a balance between thinking and being fluid in action.*
>
> I was backcountry skiing when I got caught in an avalanche. First I heard a loud crack, like thunder. Then the ground broke away under me and I began to free-fall in a soft, white cloud of snow. You would think I would have freaked out knowing I was going to die; but it was actually the most exciting experience of my entire life! I completely surrendered into the euphoric sensation of floating. My body was totally relaxed; I felt so fluid and free. Suddenly, a tree appeared and I grabbed it. The snow settled around me, and I survived. The whole thing was a miracle because had I not been in such a euphoric, fluid state, I would have missed that tree.

The Urinary and Reproductive Systems

The kidneys are bean-shaped organs about the size of small fists, which are tucked up under the back of the diaphragm in front of the twelfth rib (Figure 6.8). The rise and fall of the diaphragm massages the kidneys, moving them up and down as much as two inches. Although our kidneys only make up less than 1 percent of our body's total weight, they use about 10 percent of all our oxygen supply while at rest for their enormous job. The kidneys filter about 48 gallons (192 liters) of blood each day, filtering our entire blood supply about 60 times a day.[94] They also produce and drain 1 to 2 quarts of urine a day through two long, thin tubes called *ureters,* into the urinary bladder, a pear-shaped hollow sac located directly above yet slightly behind the pubic bone.[95]

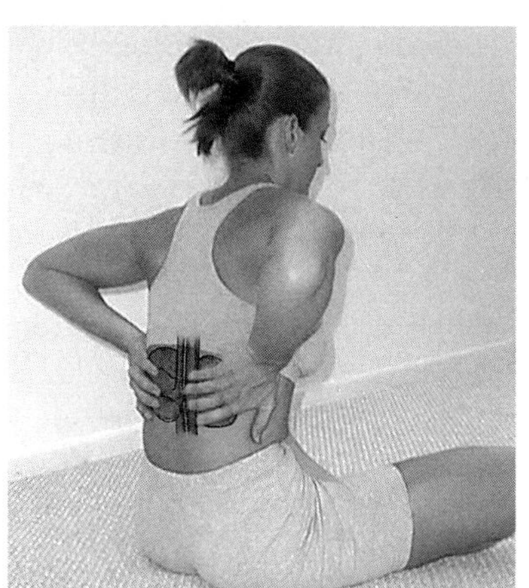
Figure 6.8 Sensing the kidneys

The uterus, which is sandwiched between the bladder and rectum, is a strong muscular sac in women that sloughs off its lining once a month during the menstrual flow. This slightly mobile reproductive sac can tip forward or backward, and seems to have stronger cramping if tipped or if the lower spine is compressed or misaligned. Gynecologists manually manipulate the uterus to reposition it. A woman can do this herself by situating her body in a hips-up position to reposition the womb, then gently massaging the lower abdomen while in this position (Figure 6.9).

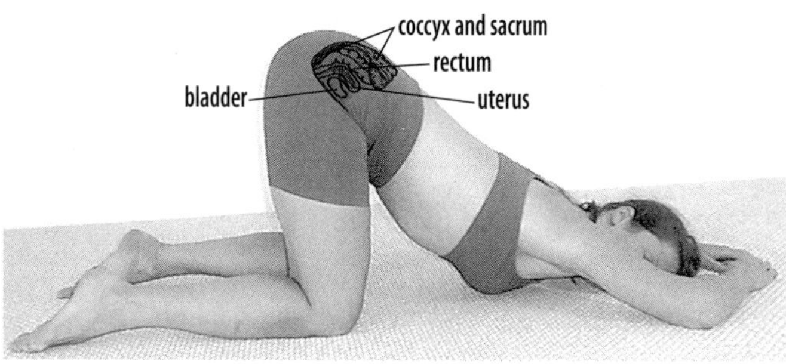

Figure 6.9 Repositioning the uterus

The hips-up position displaces the abdominal organs toward the diaphragm, which helps a person feel a hollow shape in the lower abdomen. In the next chapter, we will discuss how important it is to be able to feel a hollowing of the lower abdomen, which provides feedback that the *transversus abdominis muscle,* an important postural stabilizer, is contracting.

FLUID SYSTEMS

Many schools of patterning address the importance of cultivating fluidity in the body, and do so in a variety of ways, through dance, martial arts, contact improvisation, organic movement practices, and even movement meditations. One of the most direct routes to developing fluidity is by matching the quality of movement in the body with the physiological rhythms of the fluids. This can influence the circulation of any fluid, which will ultimately increase the overall fluidity of a person. In various bodywork methods, such as lymphatic drainage techniques and cranialsacral therapy, the quality of touch that the practitioner uses matches the rhythm and physiological movement of that fluid system.

To match the physiological rhythm of a fluid, a person needs to understand circulation in that system as well as be able to recognize the rhythm through kinesthetic channels of awareness. This perceptual process could be compared to how a musician recognizes a note in music, only he does so through auditory channels. Another difference is that it is possible to isolate a musical note but not a fluid rhythm since all the physiological rhythms are occurring simultaneously. Although we can narrow our focus to access the rhythm of a specific fluid or body system, the rhythms of other systems will be present either in the background or as a more dominant rhythm than the one we are attempting to feel. The following information on the bodily fluids is presented to deepen an understanding of their rhythms and to provide direction for movement and touch explorations focused on fluids.

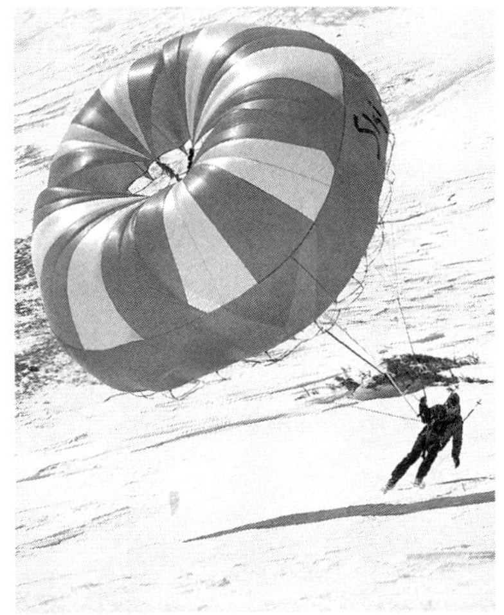

Figure 6.11 Lift

Fluid Forces

A fish moves in the milieu of water, which creates an external fluid pressure around its body, whereas we carry our fluid pressures within our bodies. Our bodies have evolved a rigid bony system to move in the field of gravity against its downward pull, yet our bodies still carry an inner ocean along with a symphony of dynamic internal forces at work. Several fluid forces—**buoyancy**, **lift**, and **drag**—affect our bodies, both internally and externally.

- *Buoyancy,* the upward force of water, counters the downward force of gravity on a body floating in water and keeps it afloat. Considering that the human body is between 60 and 80 percent fluid (depending on the level of tissue hydration), the buoyancy of bodily fluids provides a lot of intrinsic support. Internal fluids keep us "afloat," so to speak, as if we were each carrying our own personal little ocean to float in, one contained by the skin (Figure 6.10). A posture can collapse only so far before hitting the barrier of tissue turgidity created by fluids.

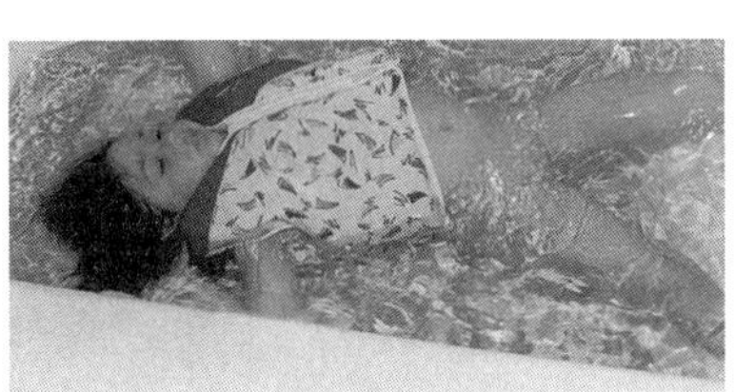

Figure 6.10 Buoyancy (photo courtesy of K. Wasson).

- *Lift* is produced by the flow of a current, either of air or water, on one side of the body moving faster than the flow of the current on the other side (Figure 6.11). When we stick a hand out a car window to surf the air currents, we are riding the forces of lift. When we walk in the same direction a strong wind is blowing, we lean backward into the lift to avoid falling forward.
- *Drag* occurs when a flow meets direct pressure (Figure 6.12). Drag creates a turbulence and resistance that slows the movement down. When we walk or ride a bike into strong wind, we bend down and lower the body to reduce the amount of drag.

The fluid forces are easily felt when generated by external forces. They are also generated by internal forces in our bodies to which we become so accustomed we tend not to feel them. For instance, intra-abdominal pressure created by tone in the muscular sleeve around the abdominal organs creates a turgidity that gives the trunk a supportive lift and counters the radial expansion of the abdominal viscera pressing out.

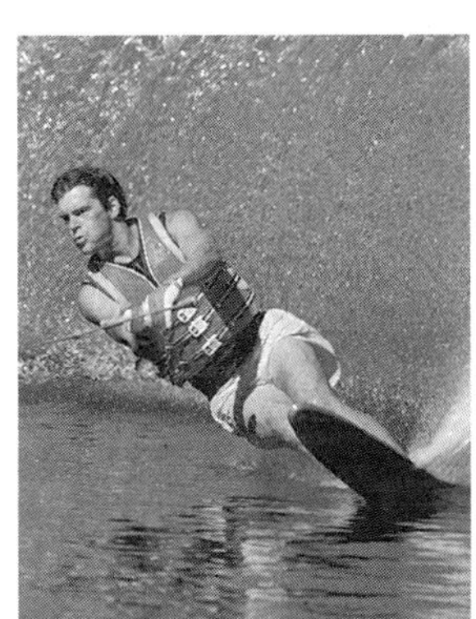

Figure 6.12 Drag

Patterning Exercise #48: Cultivating Spinal Fluidity

1. Begin in a quadruped position, either resting on your hands and knees, or on your forearms, forelegs, and forehead. Undulate your spine in a fluid, carefree manner (PE Fig. 48a-c). Imagine or sense a wave of motion passing from one end of your spine to the other, gently rippling up and down your spine. Make sure the ripple moves through each spinal segment.
2. Explore beginning the undulation at your head, then at your tail. Which is easier?
3. Continue to undulate your spine, sensing the snake-like motion of each intervertebral joint until you feel your entire back loosen up.
4. Explore spinal undulations while sitting (PE Fig. 48d-e).
5. Explore spinal undulations while lying on the floor on your back with your knees bent, feet flat.

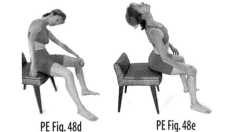

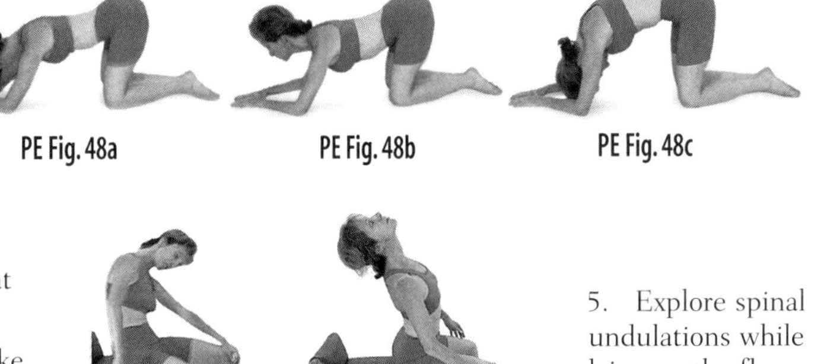

PE Fig. 48a PE Fig. 48b PE Fig. 48c

PE Fig. 48d PE Fig. 48e

EMSPress.com

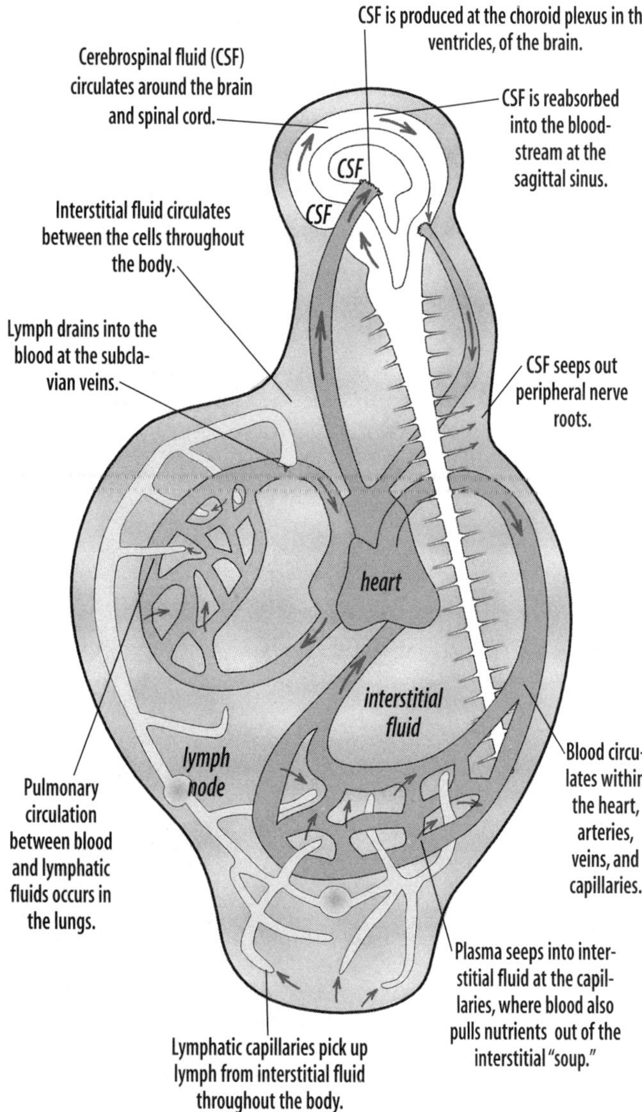
CSF is produced at the choroid plexus in the ventricles, of the brain.
Cerebrospinal fluid (CSF) circulates around the brain and spinal cord.
CSF is reabsorbed into the blood-stream at the sagittal sinus.
CSF
CSF
Interstitial fluid circulates between the cells throughout the body.
Lymph drains into the blood at the subcla-vian veins.
CSF seeps out peripheral nerve roots.
heart
interstitial fluid
lymph node
Pulmonary circulation between blood and lymphatic fluids occurs in the lungs.
Blood circu-lates within the heart, arteries, veins, and capillaries.
Plasma seeps into inter-stitial fluid at the capil-laries, where blood also pulls nutrients out of the interstitial "soup."
Lymphatic capillaries pick up lymph from interstitial fluid throughout the body.

Figure 6.13 Schematic of the circulation patterns between the fluids

In the same manner that water transforms a wilting plant into an upright, turgid structure, the bodily fluids fill the tubes, pouches, and internal spaces within which they circulate. To get an image of this, imagine a water balloon: the more water in the balloon, the more turgid the outer membrane becomes; the less water in the balloon, the more flaccid it becomes.

Air also circulates in and out of the body in cycles that pump the chest and sinuses like a bellows. Although air is a gas and not a fluid, its movement in and out of the body creates a fluid motion that alternates between filling and floating the lungs with air, and then draining out and sinking the lungs. During an inhalation, air fills millions of microscopic air sacs in the lungs, floating the lungs and ribcage; air also circulates in the sinuses, creating a buoyant lift in the skull. Also, the rhythmic up-and-down pumping of the respiratory diaphragm assists the circulation of lymph fluid in the body.

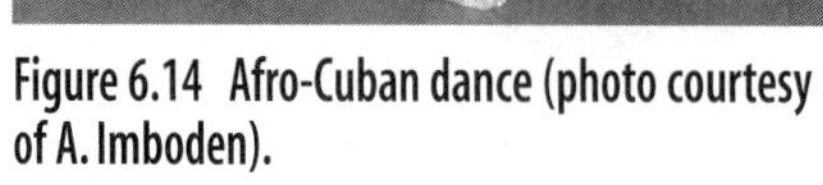

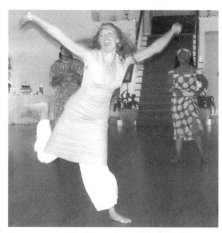

Figure 6.14 Afro-Cuban dance (photo courtesy of A. Imboden).

A person can increase the circulation of the fluids in a number of ways: by dancing or doing rhythmic exercise, exploring fluid or non-structured improvisations, using rocking motions, playing on physioballs or balance boards, or practicing the organic movement exploration described later in this chapter. Also, a fluid-based, organic approach to patterning can loosen up the body during structured patterning exercises. By following fluid responses during patterning, a person develops the ability to let the body release tension in a manner that follows both the grain of the tissues and the tides of fluids.

Several somatic methods use organic movement practices to develop fluidity, among them Automatic Movement, Continuum, Contact Improvisation, and Authentic Movement (see Chapters 11 and 15). The term "practice" is used rather than method or modality here because it better describes the free-form activity of each of these systems. Each practice involves some kind of improvisational movement exploration initiated from a meditative posture that quiets the body and the mind. The participant then focuses attention on the sea of sensations occurring within the body, allowing the organic impulses underlying each sensation to initiate a free-form movement exploration that opens up a stream of evolving, continually changing rhythms, flows, and shapes. (Think of "flows" as the currents of changing shapes sculpted by a movement sequence, similar to the currents underlying ripples on a lake or swirls within an eddy.)

Circulation and Physiological Rhythms

The body systems function in an interactive network of circulatory loops that circulate blood, interstitial fluid, lymph, and cerebrospinal fluid (Figure 6.13). Several pumps power the circulation of fluids—the heart; the rhythmic movements of both skeletal muscle activity and breathing, respectively called the *tissue pump* and the *diaphragmatic pump*; and the pump that circulates cerebrospinal fluid (CSF). Fluids also circulate through absorption and diffusion across membranes, through seepage out of vessels and membranes, and through the skin via sweat and evaporation.

All fluids are, basically, one collective fluid, differentiated by the compartment each occupies at any given time. We may study a bodily fluid as distinct and separate, yet all

Links to Practical Applications

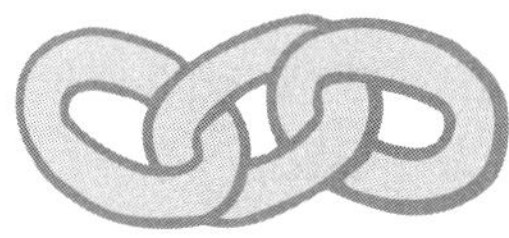

Checking In to Feel Fluidity

During the course of your day, check your internal rhythms to sense the intrinsic movement of your fluids. Sway a little to let go of tension and reconnect with the many fluid rhythms that are constantly going on inside you, or use an awareness of the rise and fall of your breath to pump your fluids and feel inner flow.

the bodily fluids circulate within the same tissue bed contained by the skin. The fluids change compositions and hence, classification, as they pass through permeable membranes that filter specific elements and leave others intact. For example, blood seeps out of capillary vessels and becomes interstitial fluid, interstitial fluid is picked up by lymphatic capillaries and becomes lymph fluid, then lymph fluid drains into the bloodstream and becomes blood plasma, completing a journey through three different fluid beds. Also, blood filters through a barrier in the brain to become the thinner and lighter cerebrospinal fluid that cushions the brain and spinal cord, which eventually is reabsorbed back into specialized blood capillaries and then recirculated back to the interstitial fluid.

Each bodily fluid circulates in a specific rhythm or flow pattern. Each fluid that is moved by a physiological pump has an associated **physiological rhythm** that can surface and become apparent during various activities, just as moods do. For example, the slow tide of the *cranial sacral (CS) rhythm* may dominate while a person is meditating, the lymph rhythm is evident during focused activities such as painting or knitting, and the arterial rhythm underlies the powerful, pulsing beat of many dance forms, particularly African dance (Figure 6.14). Unless a person is adept at feeling a broad range of rhythms or can naturally tune into the circulatory rhythms and the flow qualities of the various fluids, he or she may need to work with a practitioner schooled in fluid rhythms and flow qualities to feel the circulation of bodily fluids. The rhythms of the various fluids will be described throughout the rest of this chapter.

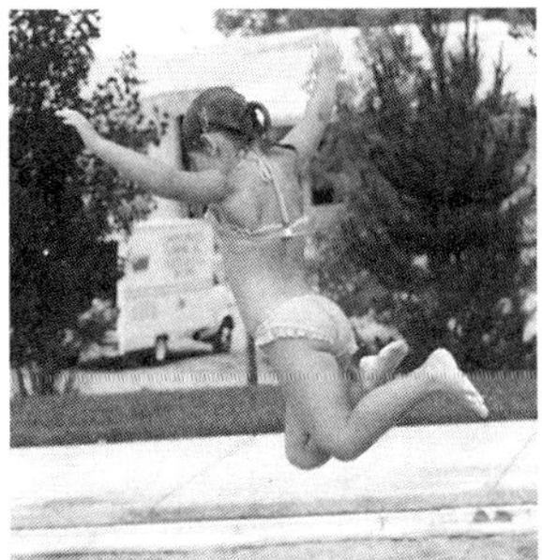

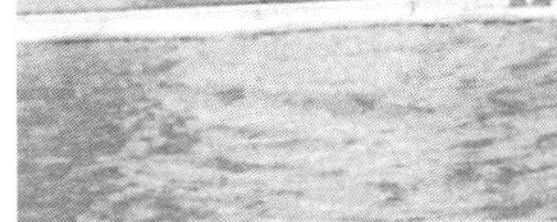

Figure 6.15a A moment of suspension (photo courtesy of K. Wasson).

Flow

The qualities of flow in a movement sequence range on a continuum from **free flow** to **bound flow**. A free flow movement is fluid, ongoing, and open-ended. It is marked by qualities of abandon, spontaneity, freedom, and the seeming absence of control. Free flow movements also tend to have momentum and suspension, and even swing (Figure 6.15a-b). This easygoing quality of free flow conveys a carefree personality, like that of a person who can "go with the flow." It gives people a certain level of flexibility, which allows them to make easy changes in direction and timing. For example, a boxer jumps around to stay loose and lithe in order to be able to shoot out a punch in any direction at any time.

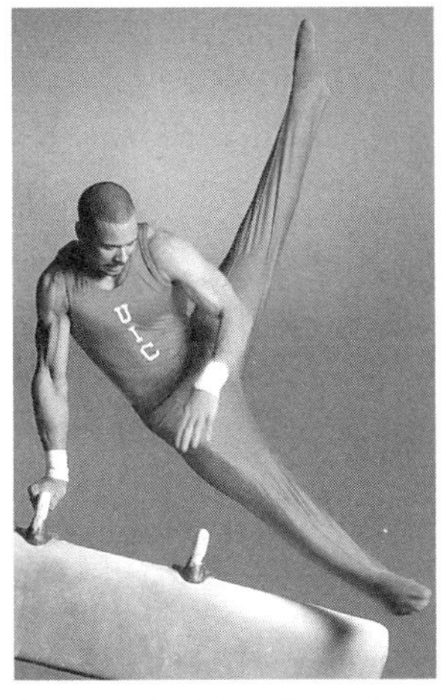

Figure 6.15b A free flow swing of the legs

Fluctuations in flow can be observed in the stream of changing tensions in any sport. A bowler has to bind the flow to aim the ball, then releases the flow to throw the ball; a quarterback binds his flow to aim a football while a running back releases his flow to quickly roll to recover from a fall. Although free flow is usually associated with relaxed, spontaneous movement, too free a flow can be problematic. On a physical level, a person might be too loose and lack joint stability. On a psychological level, a person might be unable to direct choices and feel out of control, without direction, like the proverbial bull in the china shop.

Likewise, bound flow in the body can show up either as areas that are tight, tense, and not relaxed, or as areas that are strong and stable. Bound flow controls a movement during its entire range (Figure 6.16). Slow movements like Tai Chi are usually practiced with bound flow. The more control needed in a movement, the more bound its flow. A person binds the flow to perform precise movements such as drawing, performing surgery, or even walking across a narrow, unsteady plank.

Like any meeting of opposites, a contrast in flow patterns can create conflicts. On a physical level, if one area of the body is too tight and another area too loose, the body will lack continuity of tone. Contrasts in flow even show up in relationships between people. Take for example the contrast between children and adults. Children tend to have more free-flow movement and behavior than adults, who tend to be more directed and controlled, a quality some call maturity. An overtaxed parent might become impatient trying to get an exuberant child to sit still. Since children, especially young ones, lack the ability to bind flow upon command, they need time to make smooth transitions from one activity to another.

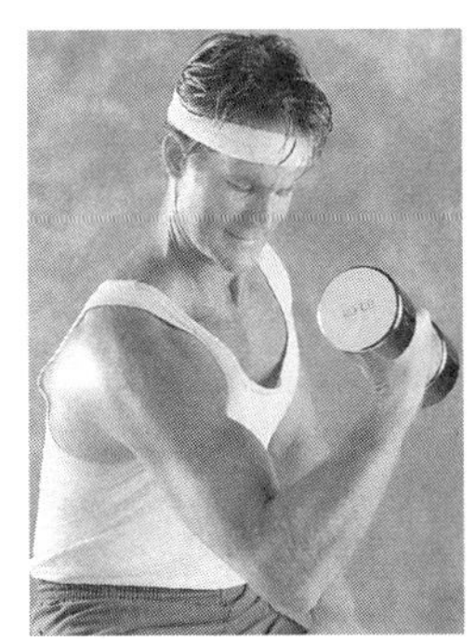

Figure 6.16 Bound flow controls the action

On just a physical level, a child or anyone involved in rigorous activity needs to allow time for the body to settle to avoid jolting it by transitioning too quickly from one activity into a totally different activity. By allowing and even cultivating a full range of fluid rhythms in the body, we can learn to be comfortable with the many fluctuating patterns of flow that show up in balanced body-use patterns, activities, and behaviors.

Accessing the Fluids' Rhythms

Patterning associated with fluid rhythms involves both sensory and motor components. To increase the circulation of any fluid, a person needs to be able to "sense" or feel that fluid's rhythm, and also to "motor" or move in sync with that rhythm. The fluids are a very playful group to explore with movement. Because fluid circulates within all body systems, any work with one or more body system addresses the balance of fluids in some manner. A description of the various fluid rhythms follows:

- Arterial blood surges out of the heart and rushes to the periphery in pulsating surfs.
- Venous blood returns to the heart in waves that have a smooth, waltz-like flow and rhythm.
- Cerebrospinal fluid (CSF) circulates in slow, sustained waves around the brain and spinal cord. Its light tide is so subtle that it produces a floating quality, a quiet swaying that a person might feel during meditation.
- Synovial fluid lines synovial joints and is spread over the articulating joint surfaces during movement. Its slippery lubricant allows joints to move with the loose, rubbery quality that we see in the legs of a tap dancer.
- Lymph fluid moves in a slow, direct, pulsating flow as it is milked through lymph vessels and nodes, a quality that can be clearly felt while receiving lymphatic drainage massage. Deep breathing and rigorous exercise increase the circulation of lymph.
- Interstitial fluid resides in the tight intercellular spaces and presses through them with a quality of surging tension during rigorous motion.
- Cellular fluid quietly sinks and settles as the body comes to rest.

What types of dance, music, sports, or martial arts elicit which fluid rhythms?

Each fluid rhythm can be accessed through touch, movement, and awareness. Some people are naturally adept at feeling a broad range of fluid or dance rhythms. Unless a person has this ability, he or she may need to work with a practitioner schooled in fluid rhythms and flow qualities to feel the circulation and flow qualities of the various bodily fluids.

The qualities of flow in a movement or touch can be varied to access specific fluids and physiological rhythms. For example, lymph and interstitial fluids have more of a bound flow, whereas synovial fluid and blood have more of a free-flow quality. Ideally, a person has access to all fluid rhythms. If one rhythm is weak or absent in a person's movement repertoire, it is possible that the particular fluid circulation may be suppressed. This is especially true when the control of movement is overly cortical and fluidity is sacrificed. When a person is fluid, she can literally "ride the waves" between physical experience and thought, being flexible enough to let the mind relax when the strong sensations of body experience drown out mental activity.

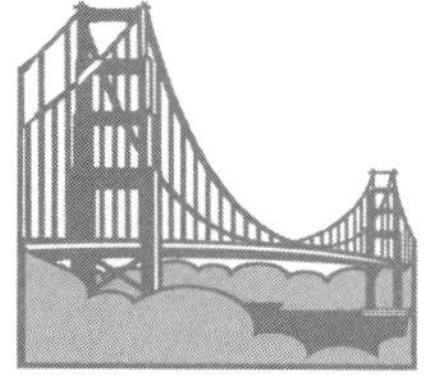

Bridge to Practice

Working with the Body Fluids as an Integrated System

One benefit of receiving bodywork is that it increases a client's awareness of local circulation. The same is true of movement. Movement can be used not only to increase circulation, but also to balance the circulation among different fluids. Generally, a bodyworker uses touch to move fluids, whereas a patterner uses touch coupled with the client's awareness and volitional movements to help the client move bodily fluids.

The fluid that is accessed will vary depending upon the quality of touch of a practitioner, the movement qualities of a client, and on which fluid system the attention is focused. For instance, a cranialsacral practitioner may become so adept at accessing the cranialsacral (CS) rhythm that she remains unaware of the blood-pulse rhythm and works with the CSF in isolation rather than working holistically with all the fluids.

Once you have experienced the physiological rhythm and flow pattern of each fluid, you can access all the fluids with a full-bodied touch that can oscillate among rhythms. You can then vary the quality of your touch to access the weaker rhythms in your client to help your client gain awareness of different fluids.

The most direct way to teach your clients the various fluid rhythms is either to touch or move your client with that rhythm. You can also teach your clients how to access their diverse fluid rhythms. To do this, move your client with a specific fluid quality. Then, while you are still moving him, have your client actively take over the movement. Also, have your client sense or visualize each fluid system as you describe the anatomy of that circulation to him. You might even show him anatomical pictures of the various systems so that he can more clearly visualize them.

Water

Fluids move by flowing, seeping, pouring, surging, or pumping throughout the body. They circulate within the tissues that contain them through the inner sea of cellular and extracellular fluids bound by our skin. All the bodily fluids are water-based, as are all the tissues. Water is the most abundant substance in the body. In fact, an average body is composed, at any time, of mostly fluid. The muscles are 70 to 80 percent water, the brain 85 percent water, the blood 80 percent water, and the bones are 25 percent water.[96] Thus, all our cells live in a water-based

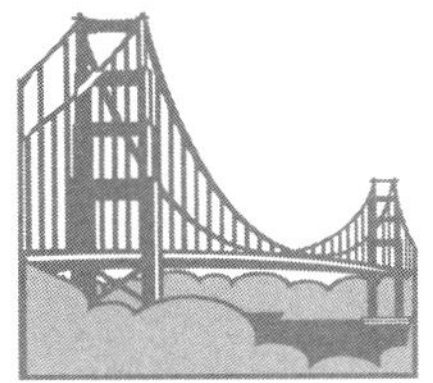

Establishing Rapport with Clients Using Fluid Rhythms

When you touch another person, you are touching a number of different tissues and physiological rhythms. In the same way that you can establish rapport with your client by matching her posture, breath rate, and style of language, you can also establish rapport through touch, a vital skill for practicing successful bodywork. Many bodyworkers have experienced how one client likes a certain quality of touch, such as rocking or friction, that another client finds distasteful. When you match the rhythm and quality of your touch to the dominant physiological rhythms of your client's tissue, you establish rapport through touch.

Once rapport is established, help your client become aware of and move through the fluid rhythms that he does not normally move through, thereby helping him to broaden his range of body awareness and movement possibilities. For instance, suppose a client postures and moves with the slow, sustained qualities of the cerebrospinal fluid, and this person comes to you because he feels too reserved and rigid. First match this fluid rhythm to establish rapport; then transition into a dynamic, pumping, blood-pulse rhythm to help him experience this repressed aspect in his body.

environment and require circulation in order to function. Like the breath, water is always moving in and out of the body, serving three primary functions. Water is a universal solvent, a medium of transport, and the optimal environment in which metabolic processes occur.

Our body's water supply comes both from outside of us, in the fluids we drink and the food we eat, and inside of us: about one-tenth of the water in our bodies is produced each day as a by product of cellular respiration. Water is eliminated through sweat, urine, feces, mucus, tears, and reproductive secretions. To replenish what we lose, an average adult needs to drink six to eight large glasses, about eight ounces each, of water every day. Keep in mind that liquids such as *coffee* and teas and sodas with caffeine are diuretics and cannot be counted as water consumption.

Intercellular and Extracellular Fluids

All the bodily fluids fall under one of two classifications: *intercellular fluid* (located within the cells), and *extracellular fluid* (located outside of the cells). Extracellular fluid includes lymphatic fluid found in the lymph vessels and nodes; interstitial fluid located between cells; cerebrospinal fluid (CSF) found around the brain and spinal cord; synovial fluid within the joints; fluids within the gastrointestinal system, eyes, and kidneys; and serous fluids lining membranes such as those around the heart and lungs.

The bulk of extracellular fluid is either interstitial (any fluid located between the cells) or blood plasma, which is about 90 percent water and 10 percent dissolved substances (solutes such as hormones, enzymes, nutrients, metabolic wastes, gases, and ions). The primary function of extracellular fluid is to provide a liquid medium for dissolving, mixing, and transporting solutes, as well as carrying out chemical reactions. It also provides the cells with a nutrient-rich "soup" from which to draw substances needed for metabolic processes. Extracellular fluid can be observed in the clear liquid that oozes out of a cut or blister.

The properties of intercellular or cellular fluid will be expanded on in the discussion of cellular processes in the next chapter; therefore, it will be mentioned only briefly here. Cellular fluid, or *cytoplasm,* inhabits all cells in all the body systems. Cohen describes the sensate quality of cellular fluid as one of being in a state of quiet presence, a resting state in which the fluid settles within the cells. An awareness of this ubiquitous fluid seems to evoke a state of present-moment awareness, or, as Cohen puts it, "nowhere to go, nothing to do."[97] She teaches her students a skill called "cellular holding" to help sense cellular fluid through awareness and touch (see "Body-Mind Centering" in Chapter 11). By using cellular holding, a somatic practitioner can sense cellular fluid with touch and use it as a ground from which to access diverse physiological rhythms or tissue qualities.

Figure 6.17 The circulatory system

The Heart

A tissue is made up of a group of cells that serve a specialized function. Blood is the only fluid tissue in the body because it is the only fluid with its own specialized cells. The circulatory system for blood functions as a high-speed transport system for the body's trillions of cells. The heart contracts an average of 75 times per minute to pump blood, the thickest and heaviest fluid in the body,

Patterning Exercise #49: Exploring Fluid Rhythms

1. Sit, stand, or lie in a comfortable position. Close your eyes and tune into your body. Sense any subtle rhythms in your body. Once you find a rhythm, give it a quiet sound to make it more obvious and audible. It might be a humming, clicking, or rhythmic sound. It might be a vowel or even a short phrase that you can keep repeating. For example, soldiers use military chants to support marching, mothers use lullabies to support rocking movements, and martial artists use breathing to support thrusts. Use your sound or song to support your intrinsic fluid rhythms. (If you have difficulty making a sound, move silently, or put on some music you like to support your movement.)
2. Begin moving with your sound. You might begin swaying, or pulsing, or even swinging your hips. Keep the movement subtle at first to feel it in the core of your body. Starting with micromovements will give you time to sense internal rhythms and beats in as many parts and layers of your body as you can.
3. Let your rhythm, pulse, or flow permeate your body and increase your circulation. Let it spread into as many nooks and crannies of your body as you can. Let it wash through every nerve, muscle, bone, organ, gland, and even cell. Sense your body as a fluid-filled container, and use your movement to stir and create waves in every part of the container. You could even sense each of your trillions of cells as fluid-filled sacs being swayed, jiggled, and rocked with your movement.
4. Move for at least 10 minutes, up to 20 or 30 minutes. If you are actually moving in sync with the fluid rhythms, your body will loosen up and become freer as you move. The quality and beat of your movement may even change as you transition between with different fluid rhythms.
5. Afterwards, rest for a minute or two and let your fluids settle. Sense the fluids coming to rest.

EMSPress.com

through tens of thousands of miles of *arteries*, *veins*, and capillaries (Figure 6.17). This ubiquitous network of vessels carries a continual supply of oxygen, nutrients, and hormones to all the cells in the body and carries away their metabolic wastes.

The heart pumps blood through a network of *systemic circulation* that transports oxygen to all the organs in the body, including the brain, bones, and muscles, and through a system of *pulmonary circulation* that picks up oxygen from the lungs. The right side of the heart pumps deoxygenated blood from the veins (since it lacks oxygen, blood in the venous return is somewhat blue) and sends it to the lungs for more oxygen.

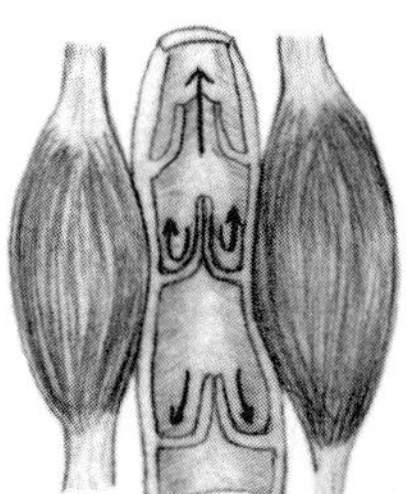

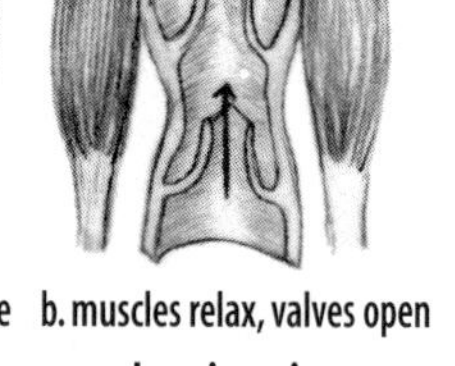

a. muscles contract, valves close b. muscles relax, valves open

Figure 6.18a-b The one-way valves in veins are toned by muscular contractions.

Although arteries generally carry blood away from the heart, the heart has its own circulatory system and vessels. Oxygenated blood is supplied to the heart by the coronary arteries. The left side of the heart receives oxygen-rich blood from the lungs and feeds itself first by pumping this blood through a system of cardiac circulation, then sends the freshly oxygenated blood through the arteries to the cells.

The blood leaves the heart through the *aorta*, a large, muscular tube about the diameter of a garden hose, which progressively subdivides into smaller and smaller tubes, from arteries to *arterioles* to microscopic capillaries. Each arterial vessel has a layer of smooth muscle that contracts to close the vessel (vasoconstriction) and relaxes to open it (vasodilation), regulating the rate of blood flow into the delicate capillaries. Groups of capillaries combine to form small veins called *venules,* which continue to merge into larger and larger vessels, culminating in *veins* that carry blood back to the heart.

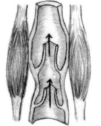

Circulatory capillaries are concentrated in tissues that have an abundance of living cells and high metabolic demands, such as muscles, organs, bones, and particularly the brain (which makes up 2 percent of our total body weight yet uses 20 percent of the oxygen supply). The vital exchange of nutrients occurs through the single-celled walls of the capillaries, where about 20 liters of plasma diffuse out and 17 liters of interstitial fluid are reabsorbed daily. Blood also passes through a network of capillaries across the blood-brain barrier where it is filtered and transformed into cerebrospinal fluid.

Blood pressure is stronger in arterial circulation and weaker in the venous return. The arteries have strong, thick, muscular walls, whereas the veins have thinner, less muscular walls. Because the pressure is lower in the veins, they are lined with one-way valves that prevent the backflow of blood. Also, they rely on the tissue pump—the milking action of working skeletal muscles—and the diaphragmatic pump for assistance in the return of blood to the heart (Figure 6.18a-b). If the valves weaken, blood will pool in the veins, causing their thin vessels to overstretch and become varicose veins.

Blood Distribution

An average adult male has about 1.5 gallons of blood circulating within the body, and an average adult female has about 1 gallon. Distribution of blood varies with levels of activity and changes in autonomic tone. In a resting state, blood is distributed approximately as follows:

- 8 to 10 percent circulates under the skin;
- 25 percent passes through muscles;
- 20 to 25 percent passes through the kidneys;
- 15 percent moves through the intestines;
- the rest moves in the lungs, brain, liver, and elsewhere.[98]

The distribution changes dramatically during a fight-or-flight response, when blood is pulled from the organs, particularly from the intestines, and sent out to the muscles to prepare the body for action, shifting the body from parasympathetic to sympathetic tone. It is extremely important for a person to be able to relax after a sympathetic response in order to allow blood to return in proper amounts to the organs so they can carry out their normal functions.

The bloodstream also carries heat to the body, which is why we warm up when we start moving faster and why people with poor circulation are easily chilled. It is possible to learn how to control circulation using mental directives and sensory awareness (see Chapter 13). Autogenic training is used in treatment for people with Raynaud's disease, marked by chronically cold hands and feet. To practice autogenics, a person learns how to actively warm the limbs by sitting or lying in a relaxed position and systematically focusing on one part of the body while repeating phrases such as, "My hands are heavy and warm; warmth is flowing into my hands." Note the focus on weight to elicit relaxation and the focus on warmth to elicit vasodilation.

Cardiac Health and Heart Rate

Healthy circulation depends on the strength of the heart, the muscles, and the respiratory pump, all of which can improve with cardiovascular conditioning. Cardiovascular exercise and relaxation are essential to cardiac and circulatory health. During intense exercise, the respiratory and circulatory systems are pushed to a higher and more efficient level of performance. This is vital for circulatory health. When a person warms up in a workout, the heart pumps at a faster speed, the lungs work harder and faster as respiration increases in rate and volume, fluid circulation increases, and endorphins may even release in a "runner's high."

The resting rate of the heart for the average person is about 75 beats per minute. It can rise to about 100 beats per minute during mild exercise, and about 150 during strenuous exercise. The heart is a muscle that is also conditioned with training. Efficiency principles apply in conditioning the heart: a person needs to pace herself to warm up effectively. This involves a steady increase in the speed of movement during an exercise routine to increase the level of output without fatiguing the lungs and heart. Then the heart rate can be maintained at a moderately fast yet steady pace, probably between 110 and 140 beats per minute, to challenge the heart without overly stressing and fatiguing it. The rate can be maintained by monitoring the heart with a heart monitor or by setting a pace. Once people recognize their optimal pace, they can regulate it with sensory awareness. Exercising to music or exercise videos also helps with pacing.

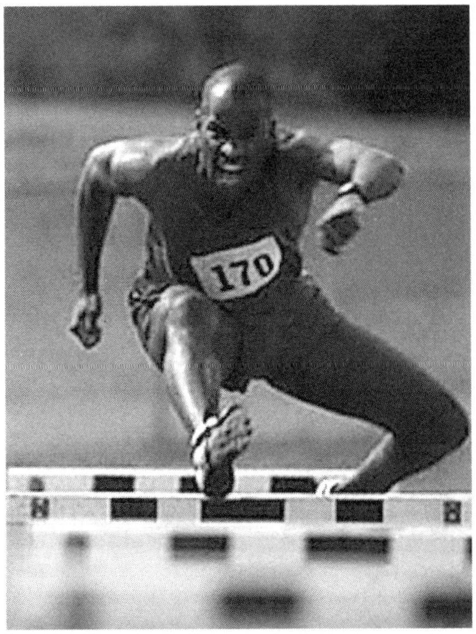

If the rate of exercise is more rigorous than the vital organs can work at, both the heart and lungs will eventually fatigue. Fatigue also sets in when the muscles are not firing in the right order, a problem that becomes obvious when a person uses excessive effort and has poor form. Conversely, exercise done too slowly will fail to develop either muscular or cardiovascular strength.

When form, timing, and efficiency come together, people can achieve a level of metabolic efficiency in a workout or sport that many call a "second wind." It is a state in which the muscles are working so efficiently that they require minimal effort for maximum output, and a person can exercise faster with less effort (Figure 6.19). Runners describe it as a feeling of being able to go forever, of "hitting one's stride." A swimmer described it as a feeling of having "warm water rolling through the veins." In short, it is a state of balance between parasympathetic and sympathetic tone in which the body relaxes yet works harder because it is running more efficiently.

Despite all the emphasis in our culture on improving cardiovascular health, many people still suffer from cardiovascular disease and hypertension, also known as high blood pressure (HBP). Cardiovascular disease is the primary cause of 40 percent of all deaths in the United States, with HBP implicated in about half these deaths.[99] Although the causes of HBP are generally unknown, several conditions are associated with HBP in people without congenital defects. The heart pumps harder when under prolonged stress; the kidneys malfunction and increase fluid in the body; or, the most common condition—one that occurs with aging—plaque builds up in artery walls. Plaque hardens the vessels, reducing their flexibility and constricting them. The heart has to work harder to pump blood through a narrower space, which causes extra

Figure 6.19 A runner at peak performance

wear and tear in the system. As the circulatory vessels harden and weaken, they become more susceptible to blockages and ruptures, making a person more susceptible to strokes, aneurysms, heart failure, and even kidney damage. Narrowing and restriction of the coronary arteries can lead to *angina,* a common condition causing sharp, temporary stabbing pains in the left side of the heart and the left shoulder.

On a more positive note, many of the conditions associated with hypertension and heart disease, such as obesity, stress, sedentary lifestyles, and too much alcohol or salt in the diet, can be controlled. Numerous biofeedback and visualization techniques promote general cardiac and circulatory health. They provide skills to actively control heart rate and circulatory patterning by helping a person learn to slow the heart down at will, relax cardiac muscle tissue, process emotional issues through a felt sense of the heart, and practice nourishing the heart with the right kind of attention.

Researchers at the Heartmath Institute, an organization dedicated to investigating the connections between the heart's physiological rhythms and a person's somatic patterns, have found that the heart has "a mind of its own," so to speak. According to Heartmath, the heart has at least 40,000 neurons that communicate with the brain, and the heart has been known to override unhealthy commands from the brain and produce hormones that regulate blood pressure, kidney and adrenal function, and even certain regions of the brain.[100]

Heartmath founders describe the heart as having a profound information-processing capacity that can be accessed by learning to listen to its natural intelligence in order to activate its harmonious rhythms. These rhythms include beat-to-beat variations (which become random and disordered during negative emotions and become balanced and coherent during positive emotions); energetic patterns (the heart has a strong electromagnetic field, a thousand times that of the brain, which affects every cell in the body); and blood pressure waves (which vary in the arteries, capillaries, and veins). The Heartmath researchers have found that awareness of and attention to the heart can be used to alter its rhythms and access its intelligence, resulting in a peaceful, secure, and solid feeling that is accompanied by clear perceptions.[101] They make an ongoing study of the many people who come for retreats at their California institute to learn healing meditations for the heart.

Circulatory Rhythms

Circulation is affected by breathing. Most people think of breathing as a wind process, an exchange of air passing in and out of the nose, but respiration also occurs through the circulation of fluids, particularly in the bloodstream. Since the blood carries oxygen to each cell, the respiratory and circulatory systems are integrally connected to each other in function. As discussed in the last chapter, respiration occurs *externally* via gaseous ventilation powered by the lungs and *internally* via fluid circulation powered by the heart.

The heart and lungs are not only linked on a physiological level, but also by their physical proximity. The heart sits between the lungs, which are like a pair of hands cupped around a small ball. Their pumping action actually massages the heart on each breath cycle (see Figure 6.6). Heart rate increases during inhalation and decreases during exhalation. The average rate of respiration is 12 to 15 cycles per minute, 30 to 40 cycles per minute in newborns and infants. When breathing speeds up, the heart rate also speeds up. Conversely, calm, even breathing can slow the heart rate, an important skill for a person with heart disease or high blood pressure to foster.

Another surprising physiological state of the heart was described by Dr. Valerie Hunt, a psychologist and physiologist who has done pioneering research on the human energy field. Hunt studied Emilie Conrad, a shamanic healer and founder of Continuum (see Chapter 11), by taking physiological readings of Conrad while she performed a healing and fluid dance-movement ritual. Although Hunt describes Conrad's improvisation as strenuous, she was surprised to find that during it both Conrad's heart rate and blood pressure had dropped. The findings suggest, according to Hunt, that there "are other ways to move that are beyond the classical neuromuscular contraction that we physiologists accept."[102] Perhaps there are also ways to move that can extend circulatory capacities beyond classically accepted parameters so that a person can improve cardiovascular health by influencing its various rhythms. To this end, a person can practice any kind of organic movement improvisations or dance forms to enhance the various circulatory rhythms.

The rhythm of circulation varies with changes in pressure in the arteries, capillaries, and veins. The *arterial rhythm* has a strong, rhythmic pulse found in numerous dance forms, especially African dance. Touch can also match the arterial rhythm; for example, in Swedish massage techniques, the pounding, tapping movement of *tapotement* and the circular kneading of *petrissage* both move in the rhythm of the arterial pulse.

The *venous return* of blood to the heart has a

Links to Practical Applications

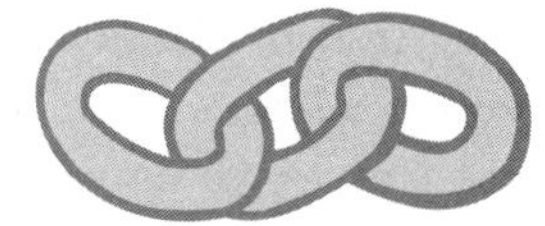

Applying Patterning to Workouts

To apply patterning principles to a cardiovascular workout, begin the workout with a focus on *form* ("What is the shape of my movement?"), *efficiency* ("Am I using the right muscles in the right order?"), and *timing* ("At what rate am I moving?"). Gradually increase your heart rate until you reach your optimal level, then hold it steady there during the entire workout. At regular intervals, check your form, efficiency, and timing, and make adjustments as needed to improve your overall performance.

swing, or waltz rhythm marked by an oscillation between rising and falling, suspending and sinking motions. The long, sweeping Swedish massage stroke called *effleurage* moves toward the heart and matches the venous rhythm, thereby enhancing an awareness of the return of venous blood to the heart.

The *capillary rhythm* has a quality of suspension found in the slow movement of blood at the capillaries where blood pressure is the lowest. Being able to relax and warm the periphery of the body at will improves capillary circulation. Regular cardiovascular exercise increases the number of capillaries in the body to increase oxygen supply to larger, more toned muscles. Also, sustained but still touch will induce vasodilation in the tissues being touched.

Interstitial Fluid and Fascia

Our view of circulatory health can be inclusive of all the fluid rhythms, including the rhythms produced by muscular action. Movement is vital to the circulation of interstitial fluid because the pumping action of working muscles literally squeezes fluid between tightly packed cells. Interstitial fluid floods into the intercellular spaces when the body stops moving after a strong, rigorous activity, such as pumping weights or sprinting. Prolonged inactivity can cause interstitial fluid to stagnate and pool between the cells, resulting in excessive fluid in the tissues and subsequent swelling known as **edema**.

Interstitial fluid moves with a quality of wringing and resistance, pressure, and tension that is similar to pulling taffy, pressing through thick liquid, or kneading clay. To feel this, quickly squeeze and release a fist about ten times in a row, then relax the hand. The unmistakable sensation of interstitial fluid rushing through the hand can be easily felt after this rigorous motion.

Interstitial fluid is also **ground substance,** the fluid in fascia. Ground substance is similar in composition to gelatin; it sets when cold and thins when heated. This unusual property, called **thixotropy**, gives fascia the ability to change from a gel to a fluid and back again. Fascias hydrate and stretch during rigorous exercise both from mechanical forces and from the heat generated by the muscles' metabolic activity. Unfortunately, the thixotropic effect goes both ways. In the absence of an adequate level of activity, fascia can dehydrate and shrink, reducing the space within a facial sheath that a muscle has to move, thereby limiting motion.

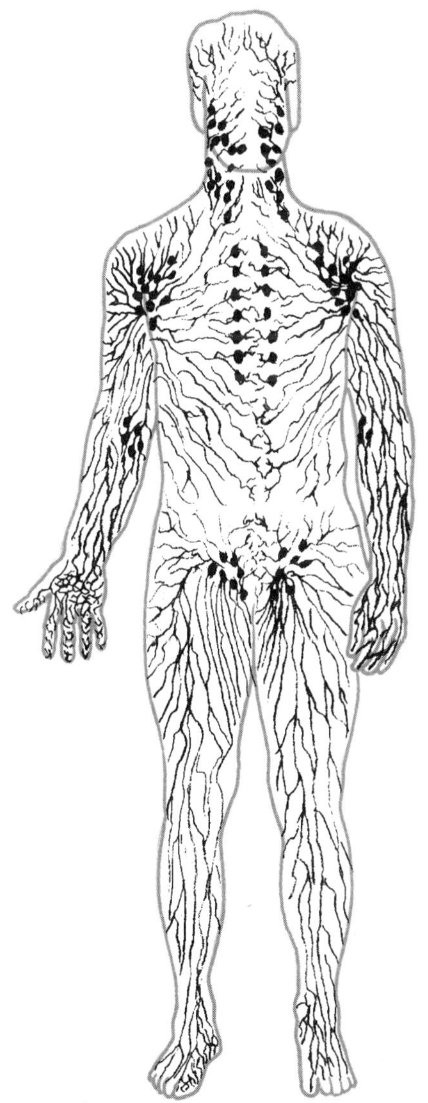

Figure 6.20 The superficial lymph vessels and nodes

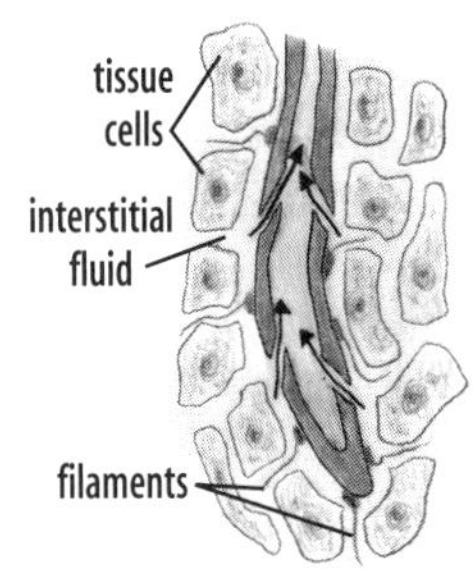

Figure 6.21 A subcutaneous lymphatic capillary

Lymph

The lymphatic system is an important part of our immune defenses because it cleans the interstitial fluid of pathogens and debris. The lymphatics filter interstitial fluid through an intricate and ubiquitous network of vessels that transport lymph to the nodes, where it is cleaned of foreign invaders such as bacteria and viruses (Figure 6.20). The lymphatic vessels draw in about 3 liters (1 to 1.5 quarts) of interstitial fluid and blood plasma each day.

A handful of *lymphoid organs*—the *red bone marrow*, the *thymus gland*, the *lymph nodes*, and the *spleen*—are also part of the lymphatic system. In addition, wandering *lymphocytes* called "scavenger cells" are located throughout the body with concentrations in the blood and small intestines. *Lymphatic capillaries* are found everywhere that blood capillaries are found and are absent in the central nervous system, the bone marrow, and tissues lacking a blood supply. These closed-ended vessels are four to six times larger than blood capillaries and have finger-like projections with slits along each side (Figure 6.21). The subcutaneous vessels are suspended by a network of collagen filaments. Light stretching of the skin stretches the filaments and pulls the slits open, allowing interstitial fluid to drain into lymph capillaries where it begins its journey back to the bloodstream.

All lymph flows in one direction, toward local nodes in specific pathways of drainage called watersheds (Figure 6.22). Everything above, below, or beside a watershed drains in one direction, and one-way valves in the lymphatic capillaries prevent backflow. From the nodes, lymph moves toward the thoracic ducts under the clavicles, where it drains

Patterning Exercise #50: Milking Lymph

1. *With touch:* Begin by placing the fingertips of both hands over the thoracic ducts in the hollow behind your clavicles (PE Fig. 50a). Using minimal pressure, move your fingertips slowly to stretch your skin over the underlying layer of superficial fascia. *Make sure your fingertips remain in the same place and do not glide across your skin.* Stretch your skin in rhythmic, slow and light circular motions until you feel the ducts open (you will feel a distinct warm or cool flush as the lymph begins draining). Use this quality of touch to open and drain all the superficial lymph capillaries.
2. Now place the fingertips of both your hands symmetrically and lightly on your neck or face (PE Fig. 50b). Lightly massage the skin under your fingertips in a series of five slow, circular motions.
3. After each series of five strokes in the same place, lift your fingertips and move to an adjacent area.
4. Proceed with the same technique along a pathway from your face, down your neck, toward your lymphatic ducts.
5. *With movement:* Once you feel confident sensing the physiological rhythm of lymph, find this same quality in your body movement. Begin by sitting or standing quietly and sensing the lymph flow and rhythm. Then slowly move your hands and arms with the rhythm. Use the movement, rather than touch, to milk lymph within your own body. Let the movement slowly spread to your trunk and your legs. You might find yourself rhythmically swaying with a quality similar to a hula dancer.
6. Keep exploring the lymph rhythm until you can feel it throughout your whole body, then rest.

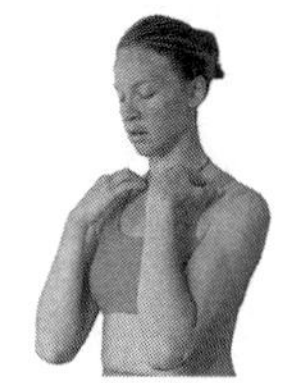

PE Fig. 50a

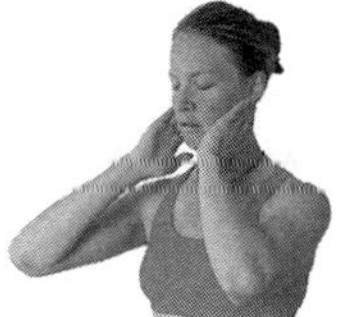

PE Fig. 50b

through the *thoracic ducts* into the *subclavian veins* back into the bloodstream (Figure 6.23). On its way to the ducts, lymph passes through a chain of nodes that are strung like beads along lymph vessels, moving from the superficial nodes lining a subcutaneous layer under the skin toward a deeper chain of vessels, called lymph trunks, along the front of the spine. Each person has from 600 to 1,000 lymph nodes, each about the size of a large raisin. Lymph nodes are made up of fat, connective tissue, and lymph cells, and are scattered in groups throughout the body, with concentrations of superficial nodes in the groin, armpits, breasts, and neck. About 50 percent of the nodes are located in the abdominal viscera, and about one-third are in the neck.

Lymph moves slowly in a resting body, being pumped primarily by the movement of the diaphragm, and moves more quickly in a moving body, being pumped by the squeezing action of working muscles. It is thicker than cerebrospinal fluid yet thinner than blood. Lymph also moves by the force of smooth muscle contraction; each lymph vessel is wrapped in a spiraled row of smooth muscle cells that contract in a wave-like sequence to milk lymph toward the nodes. These alternating contractions not only push lymph forward, they create a vacuum in the vessels that pushes lymph from behind.

We need to keep lymph fluid circulating to continually cleanse our bodies of foreign elements and maintain optimal immune function. The best way to move lymph fluid is through rigorous exercise. It can also be moved mechanically with massage: manual lymph drainage (MLD). MLD practitioners use a subtle, milking touch to slowly knead lymph fluid through the lymph vessels toward the nodes and ducts. Manual lymph drainage requires extremely light pressure, from 1 to 4 ounces, that stretches the skin and pulls on the delicate filaments attached to subcutaneous lymph capillaries to open

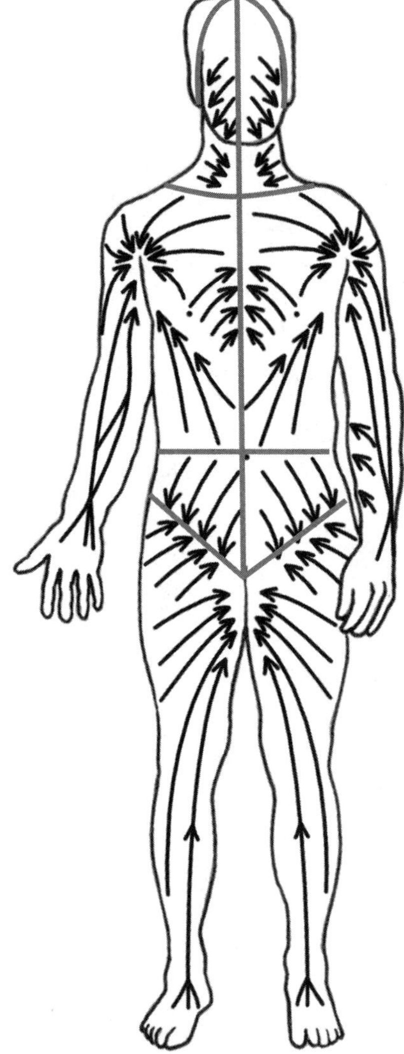

Figure 6.22 Watershed lines (in gray) and the direction of drainage (arrows)

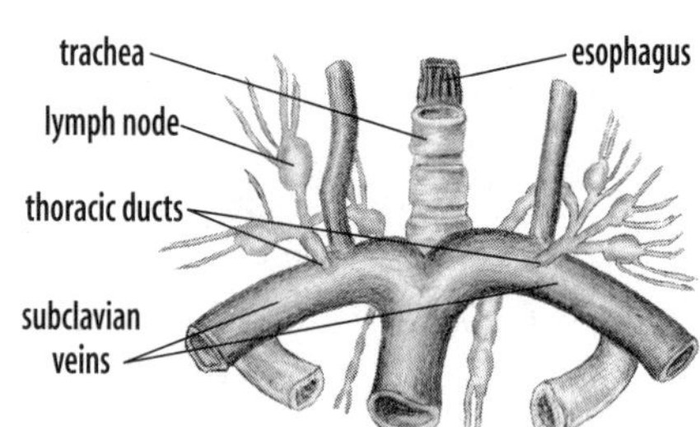

Figure 6.23 Lymph drains into the circulatory system at the thoracic ducts.

them. Light massage around the clavicle, or even light holding with directed intention, can open the ducts in the subclavian veins to allow the lymph to drain into the bloodstream. People describe the experience created by lymph drainage as a sensation of a warm or cool, relaxing wash on the inside of the body, centered in the head and torso.

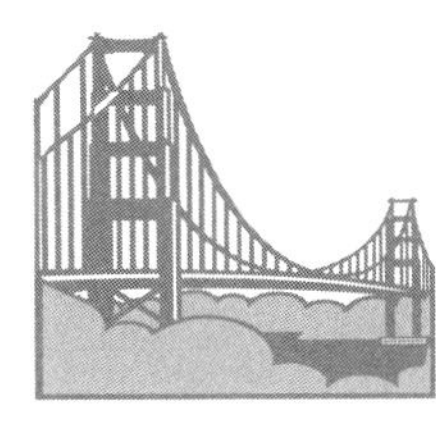

Mobilizing CSF Flow along the Spine

To assess and mobilize the flow of CSF along your client's spine, have your client lie comfortably on her side. Place one hand on her head and the other hand on her sacrum. Use your touch to follow the CS rhythm between these two places.

Cerebrospinal Fluid (CSF)

The cerebrospinal fluid (CSF) is the thinnest and clearest fluid in the body. It fills the caverns and cisterns around the brain and spinal cord to protect and nourish them, serving both mechanical and chemical functions (Figure 6.24). About 3 to 5 ounces of CSF form a fluid shock absorber for the brain, buffering it from blows. Without this protective cushion, minor bumps to the head would easily bruise the brain. The CSF also provides an optimal fluid environment for critical chemical processes to occur in the neurons (nerve cells). In addition, it has circulatory and immune functions, bathing the brain in vital nutrients while picking up and carrying away debris and waste products.

CSF is produced at the *choroid plexus*, a group of clustered capillaries that line the ventricles in the brain and selectively filter blood to transform it into cerebrospinal fluid. CSF circulates around the brain and spinal cord. Ninety percent of this clear light fluid is reabsorbed by specialized blood capillaries in the *sagittal sinus* called *arachnoid granulations*, and the other 10 percent leaks out along the peripheral nerve roots of the spinal cord directly into the interstitial fluid.

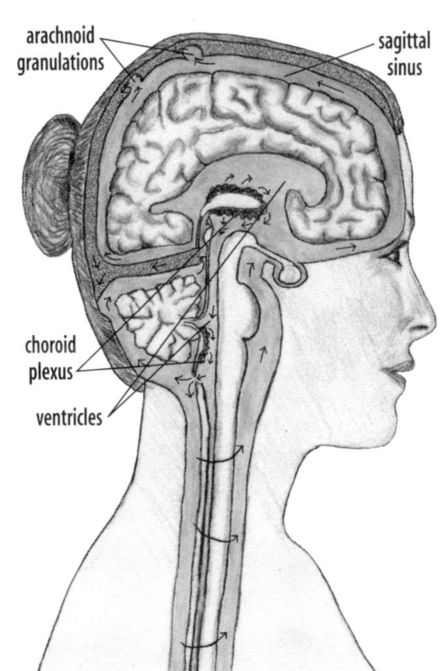

Figure 6.24 Circulation of cerebrospinal fluid

The cranialsacral system is thought to function like a semi-closed hydraulic pump that circulates the CSF around the brain and spinal cord. What powers this pump remains a subject of debate. The *ventricles*—hollow spaces in the brain where the fluid is produced—rhythmically fill with fluid. As the ventricles fill, the cranium widens, stretching the cranial sutures and increasing fluid pressure. Nerves within the sutures are thought to register the stretch and turn the pump off. Changes in pressure may also regulate the pump.

Regardless of how the CSF pump works, CSF moves with a slow rhythm, at about 6 to 12 seconds per cycle, creating a barely perceptible widening and narrowing of the

Patterning Exercise #51: Feeling the Cranialsacral (CS) Rhythm

1. To feel your CS rhythm, sit in a comfortable position. Tune in to your body and notice any subtle movement impulses that you might feel in your head and trunk, such as gentle floating or swaying motions. You might also sense a slight twisting in the head and spine, first in one direction, then the other (PE Fig. 51a-b). If you notice these motions, begin to follow them with your awareness.
2. If you cannot feel any subtle movement, sit as still as possible for at least five minutes. Within this stillness, the CS rhythm tends to arise as a subtle and quiet swaying motion. You may notice that your body is subtly swaying or feels like it is floating. If you feel these sensations, you are probably feeling the CS rhythm. Exaggerate the rhythm a little to feel it more clearly.
3. As you sense the CS rhythm, begin to move with it. Move in a slow, sustained manner, as though you were floating in water. Continue moving and allow the rhythm to spread through your entire body. It may feel a lot like a gentle, organic unwinding or a light, unstructured floating movement that relaxes the entire body.
4. If you cannot feel the CS rhythm, find a CS therapist and have him or her palpate it for you.

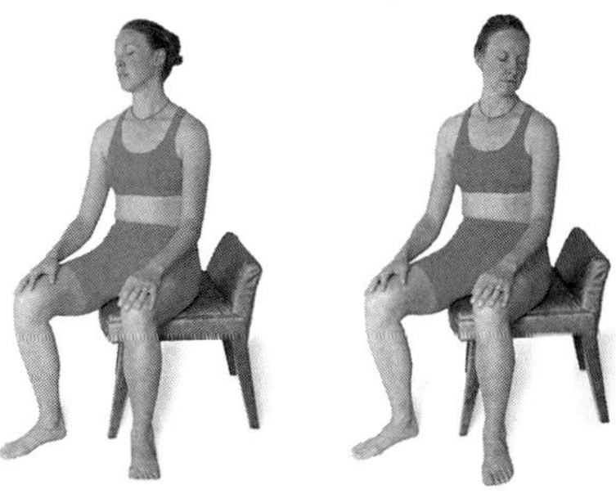

PE Fig. 51a PE Fig. 51b

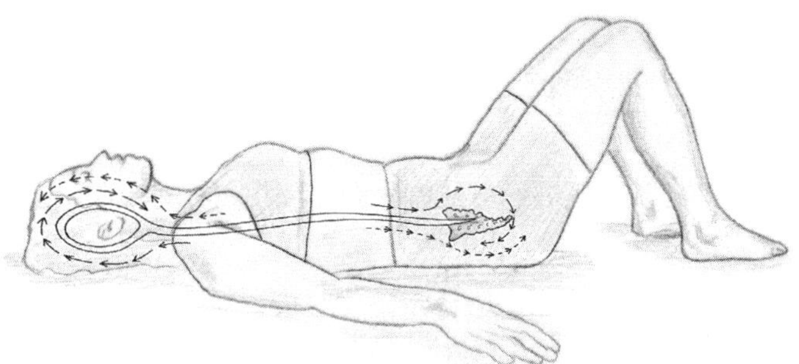

Figure 6.25 Flexion and extension cycles of the spine from the cerebrospinal fluid pump

cranium, and flexion and extension of the spine. This rhythm is also thought to broadcast through the entire myofascial network, also causing a slight flexion and extension in the entire trunk and limbs.

The slow CS rhythm is somewhat hypnotic and very relaxing. It is often compared to a quiet tide that washes through the body in subtle yet powerful slow-motion waves, creating a light, floating sensation. When a person is sitting quietly meditating, the subtle movement of CSF circulation surfaces in a gentle rocking motion. This wave-like motion washes first in one direction, then in the other, creating a slight rotation along the trunk coupled with flexion and extension (Figure 6.25). CSF moves with a quality similar to the slow-motion movements of Tai Chi, a movement quality that can be practiced to release autonomic stress and elicit deep states of relaxation.

Cranialsacral practitioners use the rhythm of the CSF fluid to assess restrictions in fascial membranes around the brain, spinal cord, and myofascial system, and manipulate the rhythm to release membrane restrictions, to improve CSF circulation, and to release tension in the autonomic

Patterning Exercise #52: Loosening and Lubricating the Synovial Joints

1. *Hips:* Lie on your back with both legs out straight on the ground. Begin rolling your legs, turning your feet like windshield wipers and rolling your legs in and out like rolling pins (PE Fig. 52a-b). Keep your toes, feet, and knees relaxed. Use as little effort as possible, isolating the movement in your hips. The movement will spread synovial joint fluid around the sockets, "greasing" your hip joints. You might even imagine the action "unscrewing your hip sockets" and your legs and spine becoming longer. Sense the back of your pelvis becoming wider as you roll your legs in.

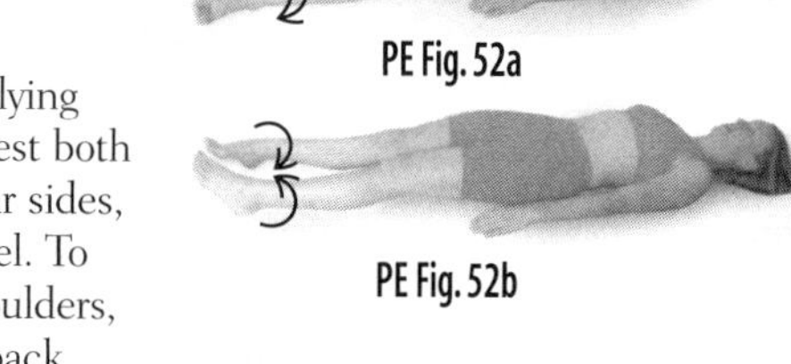

PE Fig. 52a

PE Fig. 52b

2. *Shoulders:* Still lying on your back, rest both arms out to your sides, about chest level. To loosen your shoulders, roll your arms back and forth like rolling pins (PE Fig. 52c-d). As you roll them, relax the muscles around your shoulders. Slightly reach through your fingertips to lengthen your arms. You will probably feel a stretch along your arms as you move.
3. *The entire limb:* Hold your arms or legs above you (PE Fig. 52e-f). Slowly and easily jiggle each pair of limbs. Move as though your bones were rubber and your joints were filled with slippery grease. Progressively jiggle and rotate your hips or shoulders, elbows or knees, wrists or ankles, fingers or toes through their full range of motion. Use the movement to spread synovial fluid as though you were greasing the joints. If moving many joints at once is difficult, just focus on one joint at a time.

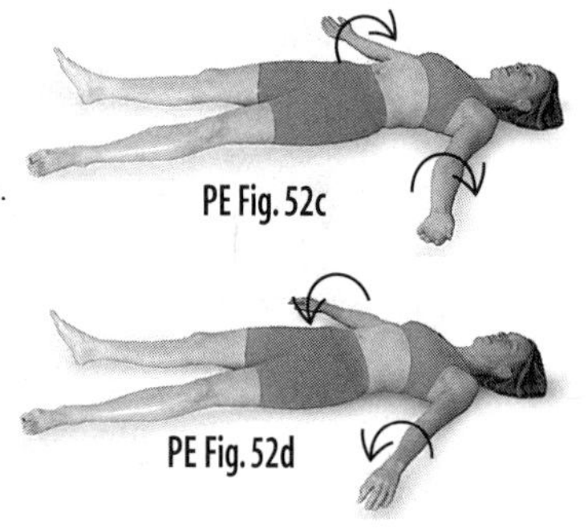

PE Fig. 52c

PE Fig. 52d

4. *The spine:* Either in a sitting or quadruped position, slowly undulate your spine with a focus on mobilizing synovial fluid in the facet joints along the spine.

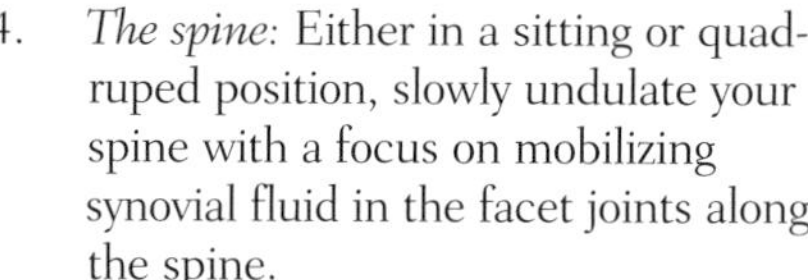

PE Fig. 52e

5. Now stand in a comfortable position and slowly jiggle your wrists and elbows. Move them with loose, circular movements that spread synovial fluid throughout the joints. Let your limbs be weighted while you move. Let the movement progressively spread into your shoulders, and, if possible, into your spine.

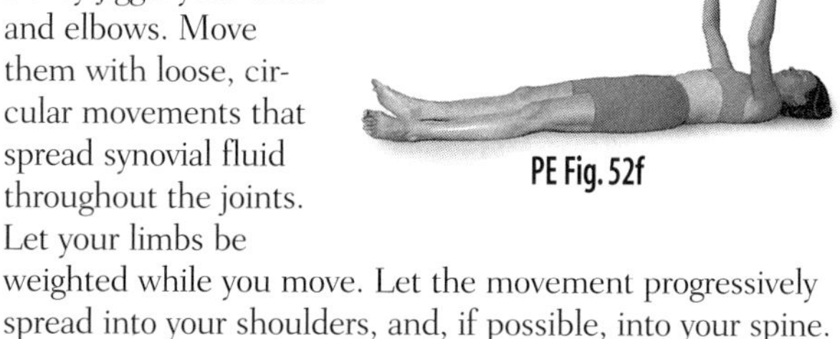

PE Fig. 52f

6. Then jiggle one ankle, knee, and hip, using loose, rubbery circular movement. Repeat on the other leg.
7. *With a partner:* Pick a synovial joint in one of your partner's limbs and hold both bones on either side of the joint. Slowly compress that joint by pressing the two bones together. The compression will be limited be synovial fluid. Once you have reached the limit of compression, gently jiggle the joint to stimulate proprioception in its synovial lining. Then slowly release the compression, allowing the joint to rebound and open. You can practice this in any synovial joint, in the elbows, knees, fingers, toes, wrists, ankles, shoulders, or hips.
8. To move the spinal facet joints, have your partner lie prone. Place your thumbs or fingertips directly over a facet joint (see Figure 10.14 for location of the facet joints), then gently pulse into that joint until it loosens.

EMSPress.com

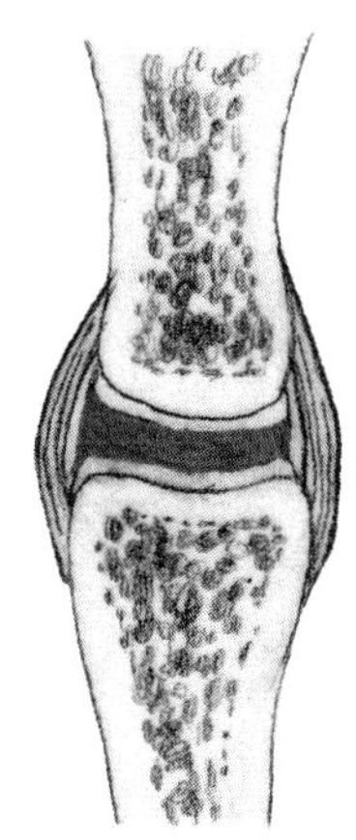
Figure 6.26 A typical synovial joint

nervous system (see Chapter 12). Movement therapists also teach people how to access the CSF rhythm using organic movement meditations for numerous reasons: to become more centered and relaxed, to release tension and trauma, and to process psychological and physiological stress.

Lubricating Joints

The *synovial joints*, the most prevalent type of joints in the body, are found mostly in the limbs and along the back of the spine. A synovial joint is defined as any joint that has space in it, which makes it freely movable (Figure 6.26). Each synovial joint has a capsule filled with thick, viscous *synovial fluid* (about the consistency of egg whites or petroleum jelly), a serous fluid secreted by the synovial lining of this type of joint. Generally, serous fluids are produced by serous membranes and contained within specific structures to lubricate them, such as synovial fluids and the fluids lining double membranes around the heart and lungs. Synovial fluid is also found inside of *bursae,* small sacs located under tendons that reduce the friction from movement and help tendons slide with ease (Figure 6.27).

Synovial fluid lubricates a joint to reduce wear and tear from friction and keeps the joint surfaces from touching each other, thereby cushioning the joint. Like fascia's ground substance, synovial fluid is also thixotropic; when warmed it thins, and when cold or inert it thickens. Synovial fluid also nourishes adjacent cartilage and ligaments, and even has an immune system function. Immune cells within synovial fluid remove bacteria and debris to maintain healthy joints.

Movement spreads a film of synovial fluid over the articulating surfaces of the two bones that meet at a joint. The exact process of synovial lubrication is a matter of speculation and probably occurs in several different ways to accommodate the diversity of synovial joint structures. Compression squeezes synovial fluid out of adjacent cartilage, the counter-rotation of articulating bones presses it out of the area of contact between articulating surfaces, and synovial fluid moves in filmy layers.[103] Adhesive molecules in synovial fluid adhere to each articulating surface within a joint while middle layers slide one over another (Figure 6.28).[104]

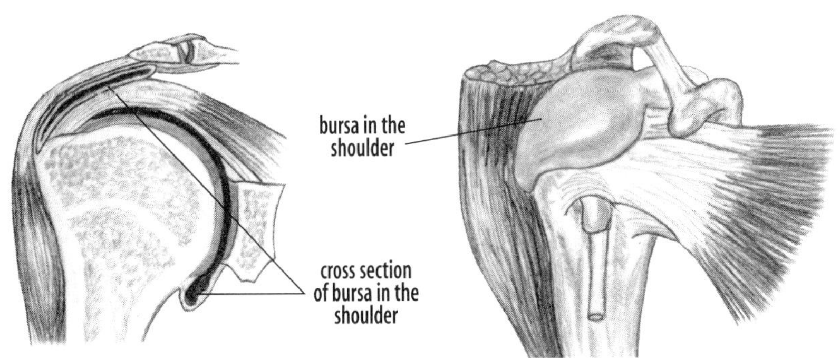

Figure 6.27 A bursa in the glenohumeral joint

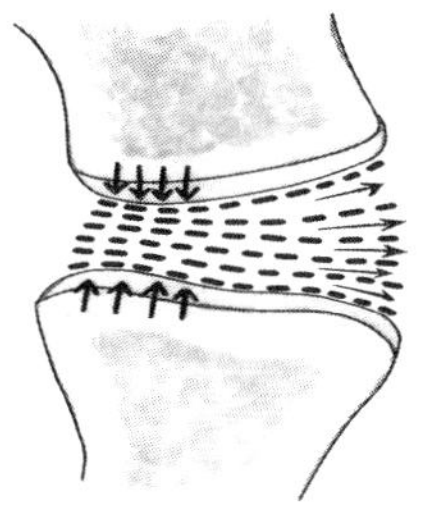
Figure 6.28 The movement of synovial fluid in layers

Synovial joints must go through their full range of motion in order for the fluid to bathe all the articulating surfaces. In the absence of joint motion that distributes this lubricating fluid over the joint surfaces, synovial joints may stiffen and become painful. This pain may be mistaken for arthritic joint pain when in fact movement could alleviate it.

RESPONSIVENESS AND ORGANIC MOVEMENT

The forces of movement translate through soft tissues via myofascial pulls that pass movement from one joint to another in an easily observable manner. The forces of movement also pass through the fluid ground of the tissues in a much subtler and more organic manner, one marked by the level of responsiveness in the body (a concept introduced in Chapter 5). In the same way that throwing a rock in water creates a reverberation apparent in concentric ripples, movement reverberates through the bodily fluids, passing through the fluid beds in sync with the levels of responsiveness in that person. Responsiveness is both a physical and a psychological attribute; it depends on the state of the fluids and on a person's ability to let go of mental constructs long enough to allow the body to move in a fluid manner.

Responsiveness has an inverse relationship to the degree of chronic muscular holding in a person because muscular bracing blocks responsiveness. For example, drunks often sustain fewer injuries from car accidents and falls because they are too relaxed to brace their bodies against the impact. They more or less "go with the flow." Also, people who see a car about to hit them often sustain more severe injuries from car accidents because they had the time to defensively lock their bodies against the impending crash.

Responsiveness is a quality to strive for in somatic patterning because it cultivates effortlessness and fluidity. Organic impulses can make a full sequence through a responsive body. A person might feel the quality of responsive rippling through the tissues while rocking in a rocking chair, or observe it in another person rocking. If the body is respon-

Patterning Exercise #53: Developing an Awareness of Simultaneous Rhythms

The goal of this exploration is to be able to feel several physiological rhythms at once. Since the breath is the easiest to feel, begin with it. You may only be able to sense two rhythms at first and need to work up to three.

1. *Breathing:* Get in a comfortable position. Begin to notice your breathing, feeling the expansion and deflation of your lungs and ribs.
2. Let your body breathe itself. Do not try to control your breathing. Feel your breath like a natural wave that washes up and down your body without your having to do anything to make it happen.
3. Relax as you breathe. If this is difficult to do, pause at the end of your exhalation and wait for the inhalation to come naturally.
4. Rest and let go of your focus on breathing.
5. *Blood:* Focus again on your breathing. Let your focus be light.
6. Then add another awareness: begin to sense your blood. Blood warms the body. Where do you feel warmth in your body?
7. Next, sense the arterial rhythm. Either place your hands over your heart to sense its pump, or put your hand on an artery in your wrist or neck. Check your breathing occasionally as you hold your pulse.
8. Once you are able to sense the rhythm, begin to gently pulse with it, moving your fingers or toes, lightly tapping your hands or feet, or rocking your pelvis. You might even want to sing out the beat, for example, "pump, pump, pump, pump, . . ." or "one, two, three, four, one, two, three, four, . . ." Marching while counting is also a great way to feel the arterial rhythm. Again, become aware of your breathing as you simultaneously feel your blood-pulse rhythm.
9. Continue alternating your awareness between your breath and blood-pulse. Continue pulsing to the arterial beat until you feel the pumping sensation spread throughout your body.
10. Then relax completely. The pulsing moved other fluids in addition to blood, so you may feel other subtle rhythms as you rest
11. *Cerebrospinal fluid:* Sit still, then begin to move very slowly, as though you were floating. This is the quality of cerebrospinal fluid. Make your movement so slow that it is almost imperceptible. The direction of motion is not as important as the quality. Move with a light, easy quality. Let this quality of movement spread through your whole body.
12. As you are moving in the CS rhythm, become aware of the rhythm of both your breath and your heartbeat. Continue moving with an awareness of all three rhythms. If this is difficult, then become aware of only two rhythms at once. With practice it should become easier to sense all three rhythms at the same time.

EMSPress.com

sive throughout, the tissues will rock from head to toes. A fluid rocking motion passes like a wave through responsive tissues, including the muscles and bones, affecting the fluids within them.

The bodily fluids circulating within specific structures (organs and tubes and vascular beds) move by the impetus of organic processes that have a wide range of flow affected by differences in viscosity, hydration, and the type of movement force. Consider the difference between dropping a pebble in water and into thick, viscous dish soap. On a structural level alone, a 150-pound person is made up of about 4 to 5 gallons of bodily fluids. The degree to which the bodily fluids reverberate with each body movement depends upon what degree of responsiveness or holding that person has.

As the qualities of movement vary along a continuum of changing dynamics (strong to weak, heavy to light, free flow to bound flow, large to small, and rhythmic to sustained), so the qualities of responsiveness vary. All actions, particularly rhythmic or repetitive movements, oscillate the body fluids on some level. Responsiveness can be cultivated with rocking, repetitive, or organic movements practiced with awareness and intention. For example, when a practitioner rocks the feet of a relaxed client with the line of force directed toward the client's head, the rocking motion will reverberate through his whole body. Conversely, when a practitioner rocks the feet of a client with a lot of chronic muscular holding, the rocking motion will bypass areas of the client's body that are stiff and held.

Movement explorations of organs and fluids can be used to increase both fluidity and organic movement qualities in the body. Organic movement explorations can be used to release patterns of chronic muscular holding and increase the quality of responsiveness. Organic movement can also be practiced to develop healthy patterns of circulation and motility in the fluids and the organs.

The practice of organic movement was introduced in Chapter 4 as a method to balance the ANS with the SNS by toning the organs while relaxing excessive muscular tension. Organic movement reintegrates the physical and emotional

Links to Practical Applications

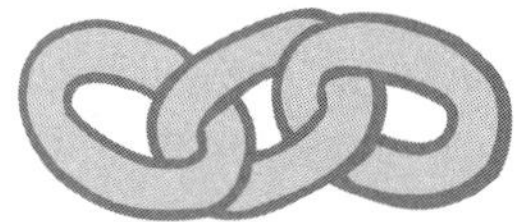

Organic Movement Is Not for Everyone

Since organic movement dissolves the ego boundaries defined by muscular armor, its practice is not for everybody. Many people, particularly those with mental health problems, derive their sense of self from their physical solidity. Boundary dissolution can trigger deep feelings of panic in some people. Therefore, if you feel psychologically unstable, organic movement is contraindicated.

Patterning Exercise #54: Organic Movement Practice

The premise of organic movement is that the body knows the best pathway through which to release tension. Organic movement is a moving meditation that teaches us how to release tension and relax during movement, as well as restore motion to tight areas. Read through the entire exploration before beginning.

1. Find a comfortable place for sitting, standing, or lying down. Make sure that you will not be interrupted and that you have plenty of room so that you do not bump into anything as you move. Practice this exploration for at least 10 minutes, 20 minutes or more is even better.
2. Close your eyes and remain fairly still at first, sensing your entire body, feeling any sensations that arise. When you feel a subtle impulse to move, follow it. Follow any tiny sensation or micromovement that arises. The movements may be subtle and occur in a small one area, or they may be large and sequence through more of your body.
3. *Breathing.* Check your breath periodically, allowing breathing to spread the flow of organic movement throughout your body.
4. Give your body permission to move in any manner that comes up (PE Fig. 45a-c). Let your mind be a passive observer. When you find your mind taking control of your movement, pause for a moment, then focus on tracking any subtle movements you may feel in your body.
5. Make a mental commitment to let your body lead the improvisation and to include your entire body in the process, if not through movement, then through awareness. Oscillate your attention between specific areas and your entire body. If your attention is drawn to tight areas, volley your awareness between what is moving and what is not.
6. If you find that your body stops moving, simply wait and observe the stillness. This is probably a stillpoint (see Chapter 12), which is common during organic movement. Wait for an impulse to move again, then begin moving.
7. Hold the intention to let the organic movement spread through your entire body but not to force it. If it is only in a small area, that is fine. Sense or imagine the circulation of your bodily fluids increasing and washing the motion through your entire body.
8. If you do not feel any organic movement, explore slow, subtle micromovements to get an organic flow started. Or explore slowly swaying or rolling, imagining or sensing your body filled with thick, viscous fluid that slowly pours from one area to the next like lava.
8. Use the organic movement to release tension and unwind. If you feel tension, simply sense it without trying to change it. Breathe into it or around it. Slowly explore subtle micromovements in the tense area. Your myofascial system will slowly start to unwind and unravel tension, so *keep the movement slow and relaxed.* Fast movement will increase sympathetic tone and may wind you into a deeper tension pattern.
9. Look for a natural ending or pause to your improvisation, and stop there. Rest for a few moments. Then slowly open your eyes and gradually stand up, giving yourself time to reorient. Notice any changes you feel within your body and awareness. As you go through the day, check your body for any subtle, organic movements that are occurring.

Note: If organic movement disorients you, balance the formlessness of this exercise by following it with patterning exercises that have mechanical form, such as the pelvic tilt or push patterns.

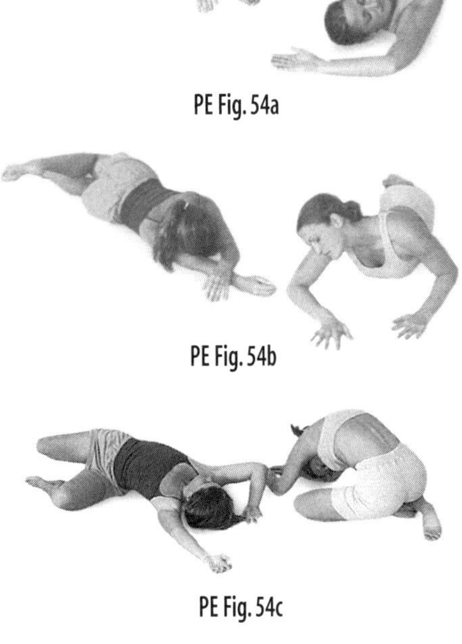

PE Fig. 54a

PE Fig. 54b

PE Fig. 54c

bodies by allowing charge from autonomic tension to be discharged through neuromuscular channels. And it naturally integrates the body and mind by loosening the mind's often-tyrannical control over the body's instinctual processes. This last benefit needs to be underscored because a controlling personality, such as the type A, who becomes habituated to initiating action through thought, may find it difficult to release mental control and let the body lead. Upon being introduced to organic movement, a client in a fast-paced, detail-oriented career described this difficulty as a feeling of losing her sharp edge.

Unlike other animals, whose emotional and physical needs are generally merged, human beings are adept at differentiating physical and emotional needs and thereby suppressing organic impulses for movement. The practice of organic movement can release a backlog of stifled movement impulses. With a diligent practice of organic movement (at least three times a week), the body can catch up on needed rest and eventually dissipate a buildup of chronic fatigue. Such a practice allows the sensorimotor system to become more balanced and movement to become current, freed from the backlog of unfinished, suppressed impulses, allowing an open channel for organic impulses to arise and sequence through the body's fluid matrix.

Organic movement improvisations are especially helpful for releasing stress, both physical and psychological. By sequencing repressed movement impulses, a person can release chronic muscular tensions rooted in psychological armor. For this reason, an organic movement improvisation dissolves ego boundaries defined by muscular armor, which can have a deep effect on a person's psychology. Its ongoing process tends to break down ego-based notions of the body as solid, dissolving the constructs of personality that tend to solidify into muscular armor. Because organic movement practices tend to loosen up ego rigidity, psychological issues may arise. If issues do come up, a person can practice this form to process these issues on a body level, and use cognitive therapy to process the thoughts, emotions, and beliefs that limit the flow of organic movement.

A person who becomes adept at an organic movement practice is often able to move with remarkable fluidity and spontaneity. With experience, a participant in this unique somatic practice learns, at a deep and experiential level, that *the body is not something to be moved, but is actually a moving process,* like a work in progress. Whenever we embody a fluid state, we tap into our natural capacity to undergo deep and profound healing transformations.

Lastly, a point to emphasize: traditional relaxation exercises are usually practiced in a stationary position. The practice of organic movement makes a departure from traditional relaxation exercises because it uses movement to induce relaxation. Although learning how to relax in a stationary position is extremely beneficial, we also need to learn how to relax while we are moving in order to be able to integrate relaxation skills into daily-living activities. Organic movement does just this.

SUMMARY

Fluidity as a quality of motion is not just figurative; it reflects the actual physiological rhythms of the organs and bodily fluids, the intrinsic motion of visceral motility. A physiological pump drives each system of circulation within the body. The heart circulates blood; the tissue pump, which is powered by the rhythmic contractions of both the respiratory diaphragm and working muscles, circulates interstitial and lymph fluids. And the cranialsacral pump circulates cerebrospinal fluid around the brain and spinal cord.

During somatic patterning, each physiological rhythm can be evoked with either a practitioner's touch quality or a person's quality of movement to improve circulatory health and organ tone. Patterning exercises can also be done with a focus on specific organs to improve intrinsic motility and health in that organ. Ultimately, the motility of the organs and fluids creates a sensitivity and fluidity in the body that can underlie and fill out every movement we make. This helps us move in a more relaxed manner and provides a ground from which to practice neuromuscular patterning.

A major drawback of working with organic movement as a singular approach is that following organic pathways in nonstructured, process-oriented patterning does not necessarily assure that musculoskeletal mechanics will improve. Muscle and joint actions are clear and precise patterns that require a degree of mechanical patterning. This can be done in the paradigms presented in the next four chapters on developmental movement patterning, neuromuscular patterning, postural stabilization, and fundamental movement patterns. Developmental patterning (the topic of the next chapter) encompasses both organic and structured patterns of movement; therefore, it can be an excellent way to integrate organic with mechanical approaches.

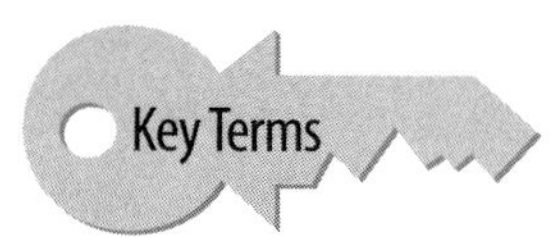

anal rooting reflex
bound flow
buoyancy
drag
edema
free flow
ground substance
lift
physiological rhythm
thixotropy

OVERVIEW OF CHAPTER 7

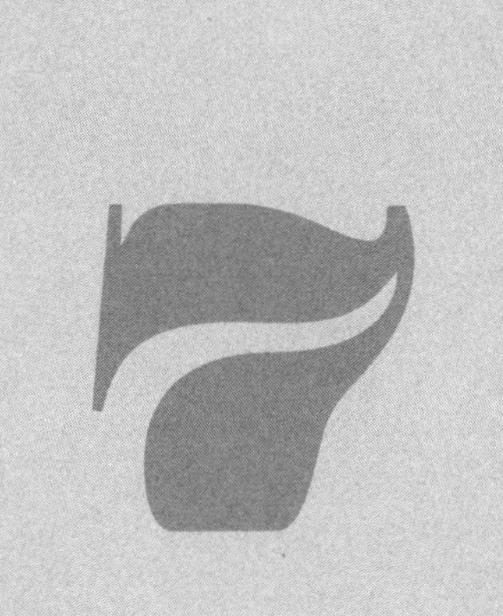

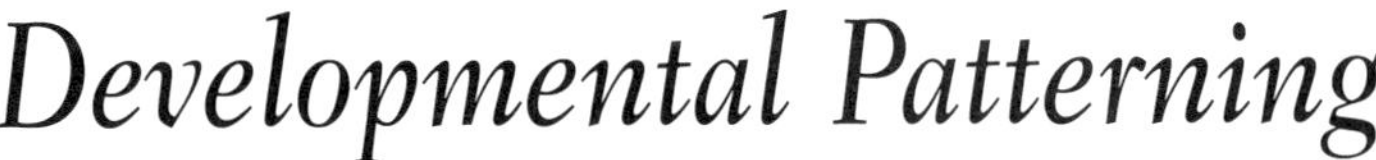

Developmental Patterning

> **Although an infant doesn't [always] establish the most efficient pathway of development, that pathway isn't closed—its potential remains for future development.**
>
> ***—Bonnie Bainbridge Cohen***

As mentioned in Chapter 1, we all move through roughly the same stages of early motor development from conception to walking. This process of *neuromotor* development is complex, yet the stages are predictable. Traditionally, the therapeutic application of developmental patterning has been to treat children and adults with movement pathologies. Developmental movement specialist Bonnie Bainbridge Cohen changed that when she developed an experiential learning process for developmental movement patterns and began teaching her approach to healthy adults. Most of the information in this chapter is based on her work.

Serious problems in neuromotor development can result in severe developmental disabilities and retarded growth, although minor gaps are common.[105] Although we all pass through roughly the same movement stages, each person's journey is unique. Every person has some developmental stages that are strong and others that are weak. But humans are extremely adaptable and can overcome developmental movement gaps with clever compensations. Weaknesses in some stages are balanced by strengths in others. A healthy baby will find her own unique pathway to standing and walking, despite many obstacles. The unique compensations that people learn during neuromotor development underlie the exclusive style of each person's somatic traits.

A study of early motor patterns can be the most direct route to the source of body problems rooted in developmental processes. It leads us on a journey back through the discoveries, moods, and frustrations we experienced in infancy and early childhood. Since this approach is a systematic review of the series of developmental patterns, it illuminates weaknesses and gaps in sensorimotor learning, which can be provocative. This study can take a person directly into the developmental basement of the psyche and stir up deep psychomotor issues. Because early motor development predates verbal and cognitive development, students of developmental patterning often experience gaps as vague and frustrating movement problems that are hard to describe, difficult to comprehend, and overwhelming to feel. The psychological effects of developmental patterning are beyond the scope of this text, yet they are mentioned here to prepare anyone practicing the developmental exercises for these possible ramifications.

Still, the journey through developmental patterning has great value. Developmental patterning can uncover movement gaps, which in turn can point a person to the most effective corrective pattern for a specific movement problem. Developmental patterning addresses the root of most somatic patterns, thus giving us a chance to redo a learning process originally left to chance.

Although this chapter is about patterns of early motor development, adult movement patterns are also discussed to link the two and to provide assistance in identifying the developmental roots of an adult pattern. The developmental patterns are presented in two basic categories: the four neurological actions (yield, push, reach, and pull) and the eight developmental pathways (four correlate with patterns of the prevertebrate species, and four with the patterns of vertebrate species). While the prevertebral patterns and the vertebral patterns are presented here in a linear fashion, motor development consists of a series of revolving spurts, plateaus, and regressions in which the simpler patterns manifest then disappear as they are integrated into more complex patterns, and then reappear in more sophisticated coordinations. Thus, a person could approach developmental patterning in a linear mode or begin anywhere along the continuum by exploring a weak or undeveloped pattern.

THE NEUROLOGICAL ACTIONS

All movements are some combination of four basic **neurological actions**: yield, push, reach, and pull. Each action has a unique tone quality that spans a continuum from passive to active, compression to elongation, and inner to outer focus. One action underlies the next, and the tone of each action builds on the foundation of the previous action. Yield underlies push, which underlies reach, which underlies pull. Most movements involve compositions of all four actions, yet a single action will crystallize and become evident during different stages of a movement sequence.

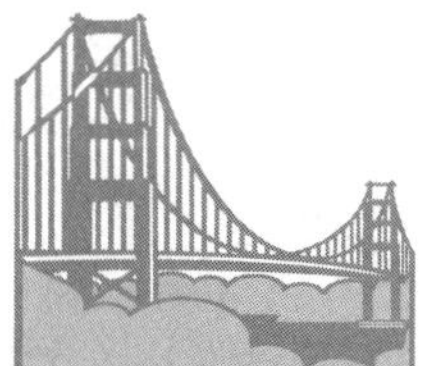

Bridge to Practice

Observing Developmental Patterns

To observe developmental patterns, look at two things in your clients: the *shape* of their movement and the *pathway* it takes.

To look at the shape of the movement, superimpose a stick figure on your client, with imaginary lines through each limb and the spine. What shape stays relatively constant as your client moves? For example, a square shape usually indicates strong homologous pathways. A spine the shape of a question mark usually reflects weak spinal push patterns.

To observe the pathway or sequence a push or reach pattern takes, imagine the spine and limbs like rivers. Movement flows like water in pathways along the riverbeds. The flow can become blocked by rocks and fallen trees (akin to chronic contractions), or have turbulence (akin to instability and spasticity), or be dragged down by sediment (akin to passive or slumped parts). Which pathways does your client move through and which pathways does he move around? Which parts of your client's body does he push or reach through? Which parts does he hold and skip over? In which parts of his body is he tight, unstable, or collapsed? How does this affect the shape and pathway of his movement?

Push and reach patterns organize lines of force in the body, particularly through the skeletal framework. Push patterns take the body into compression and direct force inwards, organizing a compressed relationship between joints that work together in a chain. Conversely, reach patterns move the body out into the environment, stretching out any slack in the myofascias or compression in joints, and lengthening the body. A reach usually culminates in grasp and pull, the most complex of the patterns that draws an object toward the body or the body toward the object. When yield, push, reach, or pull patterns sequence through the entire body, they create a continuity of tone along the pathways of movement. If the force of a push, reach, or pull becomes blocked in a localized area, failing to make a complete sequence from one endpoint (hand or foot, head or tail) to another, the action is incomplete and usually inefficient.

Each person has affinities toward varying combinations of the yield, push, reach, or pull actions. Each action has a tone or personality that shapes the quality of movement in a person's tissues and posture. For example, a power lifter probably has strong push patterns, a ballerina probably has strong reach patterns, and an easy-going relaxed person probably has strong yield patterns. Also, one part of the body can have an affinity toward one action while another part has an affinity toward another, which will be evident in the resting tone of that part. Consider a person with a long, lanky upper body and compact, short legs, who probably has an affinity for push in the lower body and reach in the upper body.

Our upright human posture has a natural affinity toward pushing down with the feet and tail and reaching up with the head. During standing, a supportive push from the legs sends a counterforce up through the spine and head, but only if the force of the push sequences all the way through the spine. Push creates integrity in the intervertebral joints in the spine, particularly if the force of the push is traveling as close to the center of the joints as possible. This integrity provides a stable base for a reach, or extension, with the head.

Ideally, each action sequences through the whole body with continuity. For example, when a person pushes something heavy, the force of the push can travel from his hands through his trunk and all the way into his feet. If he only pushes with his arms and shoulders, the push will not be as efficient.

Each of these actions can also be used as an antidote for body problems: the yield to relax tense areas, the push to stabilize and strengthen loose or disconnected areas, the reach to lengthen compressed areas, and the pull to enhance overall coordination.

Yield

To **yield** is to let down, to surrender on a deep, physiological level, and to generally relax. Some people mistake yielding for collapsing and going limp, but there is a difference.

Patterning Exercise #55: Yielding

1. *Yielding while resting:* Find a warm and quiet environment in which you can deeply relax. Explore yielding in different resting positions—on your belly, your back (called the "corpse pose" in yoga), your side, or curled into a fetal position (PE Fig. 55a-b). Lie in whatever position is comfortable for you, then spend about 20–30 minutes yielding your body's weight into the supporting surface underneath you.

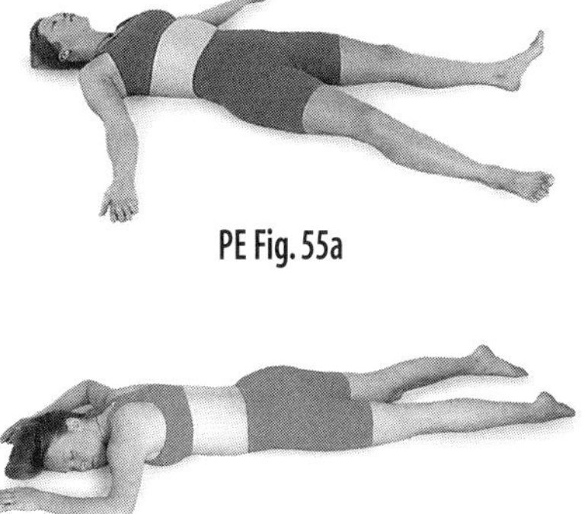
PE Fig. 55a

2. On each exhalation, feel and/or visualize your body sinking down through the floor. Sense and/or imagine your body melting into and merging with the earth. How heavy can you get? How deeply can you let go into the supporting surface under you?

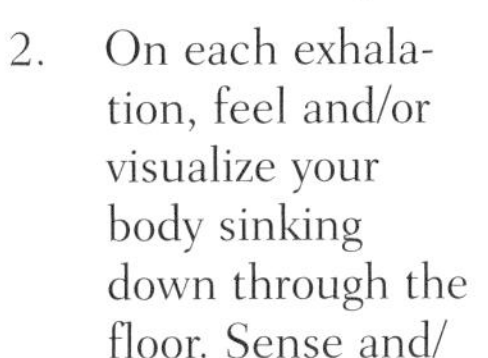
PE Fig. 55b

3. Again, while still focused on yielding and resting, mentally scan your body—head, neck, ribcage, pelvis, right arm, left arm, right leg, left leg—allowing weight to sink through each part. Then mentally scan your organs—brain, throat, heart, lungs, stomach, liver, kidneys, intestines, and bladder—allowing each area to sink and become heavier.
4. *Yielding your upper body while moving your arms:* Lie on your back (PE Fig. 55c). Raise your arms toward the ceiling. Sense your shoulders and upper body sinking and relaxing as you move your arms in different ways, such as moving them in small circles, or slowly folding your arms across your body and then slowly unfolding them.

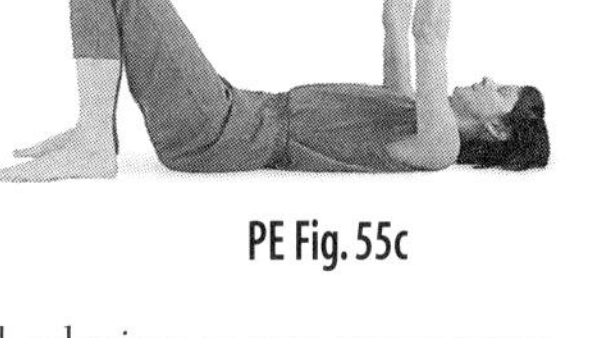
PE Fig. 55c

5. *Yielding your back while moving your legs*: Pull your knees to your chest and let your back relax, sink, and widen (PE Fig. 55d). Slowly lower your legs, one at a time, while continuing to yield in your back. Explore flexing and extending your legs while keeping your lower back relaxed and heavy.

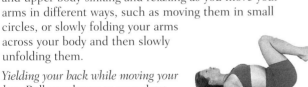

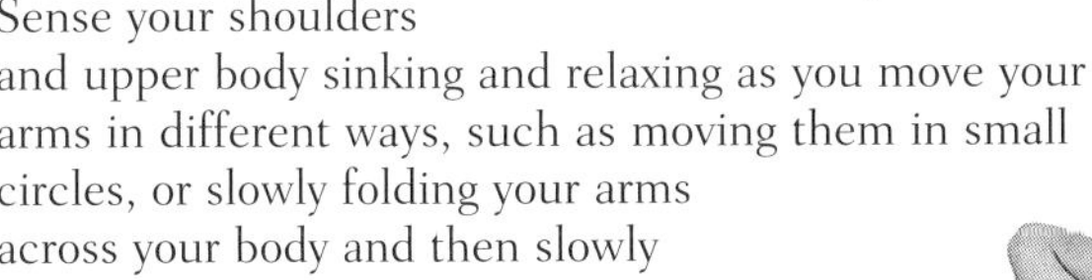
PE Fig. 55d

6. *Yielding organs while moving limbs:* Explore yielding your organs as you move your arms or legs. For instance, imagine your kidneys or lungs as sandbag counterweights on your legs or arms; as you raise a limb, yield and sink through these organs (PE Fig. 55e).

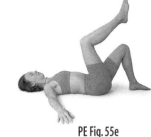

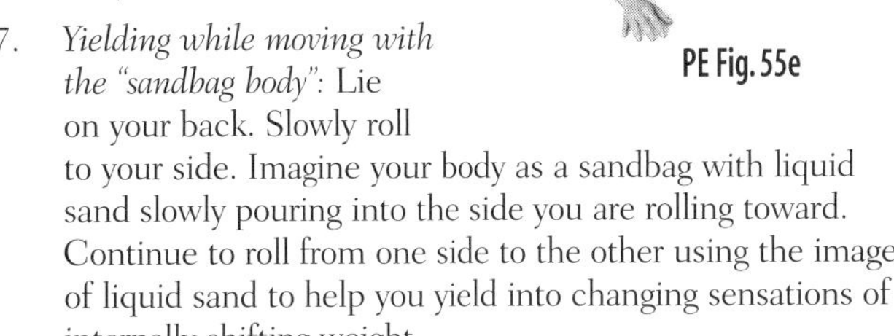
PE Fig. 55e

7. *Yielding while moving with the "sandbag body":* Lie on your back. Slowly roll to your side. Imagine your body as a sandbag with liquid sand slowly pouring into the side you are rolling toward. Continue to roll from one side to the other using the image of liquid sand to help you yield into changing sensations of internally shifting weight.
8. *With a partner:* Have a partner lie comfortably in a prone or supine position. Scan your partner's body and notice where you sense she is unable to yield. To see if you're both on the same page, ask her where she feels tension and wants to yield and relax. Then place your hands on this area, allowing your hands to be heavy and relaxed to encourage your partner to yield and sink in this area (PE Fig. 55f). Gradually move your hands over her whole body to help her yield throughout.

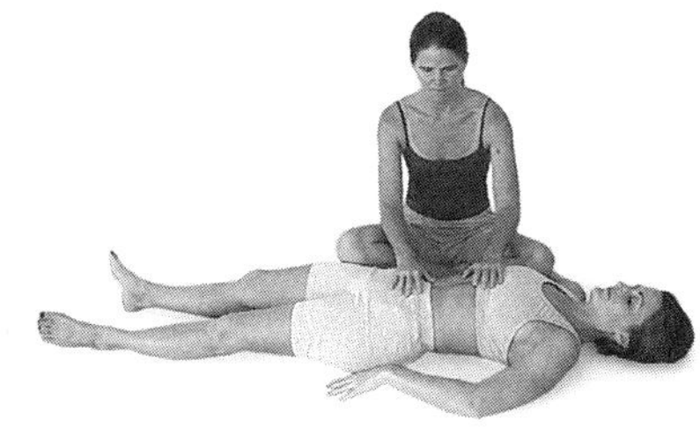
PE Fig. 55f

9. With a partner you trust and are comfortable making physical contact with (a good partner choice for this exercise is a lover because it could bring up intense and perhaps sensual feelings), lie down together in a comfortable position. One of you can hold the other, or cradle each other in a spoon position. Then consciously focus on yielding together, melting and merging into each other as well as into the supporting surface under both of you. Afterwards, discuss how it felt.

The ability to yield reflects the ability of the autonomic nervous system to let down into a deep parasympathetic state of relaxation. Yielding can be learned through practicing relaxation exercises, sensing body weight releasing into the floor, working with nurturing touch, or exploring slow, organic movements. Yielding sets the physiological baseline from which all changes in tone arise, a topic that will be revisited. Since yielding underlies the other three neurological actions, beginning patterning with relaxation training recapitulates the developmental processes.

A primitive reflex that underlies resting tone and is associated with yielding is the **tonic labyrinthine reflex**. It is stimulated by tactile receptors in the skin and the movement of tiny inner ear "stones" called *otoliths*. For example, as a person rolls on the ground, tactile stimulation to the skin and the direction the otoliths fall increase the tone of

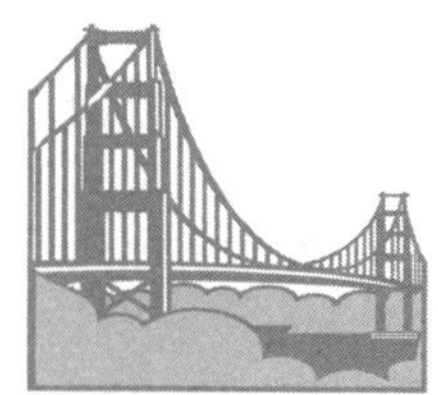

Bridge to Practice

Stimulating Yielding with Touch and Movement

The four steps for eliciting the tonic lab reflex are: 1) slowly and gently move your client's head, 2) wait for the fluid in the inner ear to settle, 3) feel the response and change of tone in your client's body and spine, 4) nudge your client to move with the response.

To stimulate the tonic labyrinthine reflex while your client is lying on a massage table, first help your client sink into the table by using a weighted, mostly passive, fluid and nurturing touch, a quality of touch that encourages her body to trust your hands and to relax and sink under your hands. (See the Patterning Exercise #117 titled "Cellular Holding Exploration with a Partner" in Chapter 11.) Suggest that your client sense or visualize the fluids in her inner ear sinking to the back of her head and toward the ground, like pearls sinking through viscous liquid soap. Also, suggest that she sense the undersurface of her body melting into the support under her, and use your touch to evoke this.

Lastly, teach your client how to practice subtle organic movement while lying or sitting on a massage table or on the floor. (See Patterning Exercise #54.) As she slowly moves, give her a supportive cellular touch that encourages her to yield while moving. Make sure you follow her movement rather than directing her, unless her movement starts to get habitual and produce tension; then give her light nudges to encourage relaxation during motion.

the muscles on the underside of the body. Usually people associate relaxing with a decrease in tone, yet *the tonic "lab" is an unusual reflex because tone rises as the body yields*. This phenomenon is emphasized because it is a state the average person, particularly those with chronic fatigue, rarely reach. Most people function at a rest deficit. Reaching the point where the body relaxes as activity increases seems to be an advanced state of function, one that requires having many traditional elements aligned: nutrition, adequate rest, exercise, mental well-being, and the self-regulation of somatic patterns, including posture and movement.

When a person rolls from back to side to front, the otoliths in the inner ear sink slowly through thick *endolymph fluid* in the direction of gravity and pull on tiny, cilia-like nerve receptors that stimulate the tonic lab reflex. The body yields in the direction that the head is turned, and flexor tone increases on that side. When the otoliths sink toward the face, flexor tone increases along the front of the body. When the otoliths sink to one side and that side yields into gravity, flexor tone balances with extensor tone. When the otoliths sink toward the back of the head, extensor tone increases along the back of the body.[106]

It is very important for the body to be physically supported in order for a person to learn to yield. Newborns need to be held with ample support, especially for the

Patterning Exercise #56: The Tonic Labyrinthine Reflex

This exercise is helpful for grounding, releasing rigidity, and release your body's weight into its supporting surface.

1. Lie on your back with your knees straight or bent. Relax your back. Sense the resting tone of your body (PE Fig. 56a). Slowly roll to your side, then onto your belly. Then reverse the action and roll back to center, then over to the other side. As you roll, focus on the parts of your body making contact with the floor, allowing these areas to sink. *Sensing your contact surface wakes up proprioceptors in the skin.*

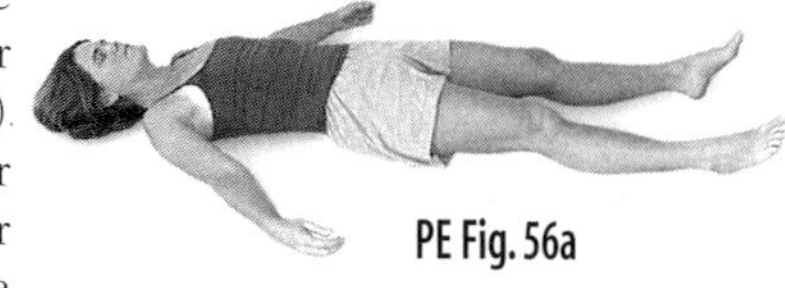

PE Fig. 56a

2. Now slow the sequence down, sensing each step of the exercise. Begin by slowly rolling your head to the right. Sense or imagine the fluid in your inner ear sinking into that side. Wait for and sense any changes in tone that you feel in your body. If the tonic "lab" reflex is active, you will feel your right side become heavy and have an urge to roll that direction. Once you feel this change, roll to the right side and rest (PE Fig. 56b). If you do not feel any change, still roll to the side. It may take awhile to wake up the reflex. *As the otoliths fall to the side, flexor and extensor tone balance each other out.*

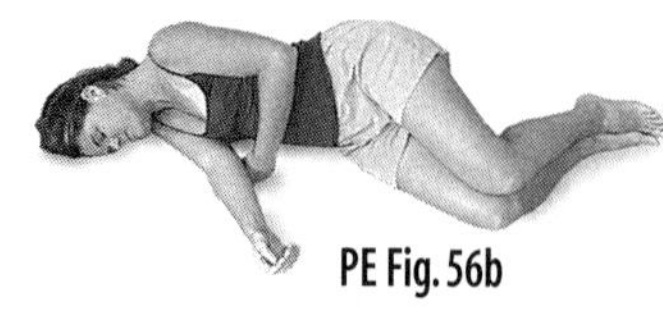

PE Fig. 56b

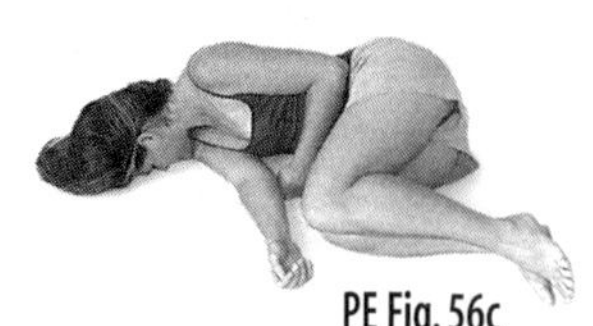

PE Fig. 56c

3. Next, slowly roll your head so that your face faces the floor and rest (PE Fig. 56c). Sense or imagine the fluid of your inner ear sinking toward your face. Wait for any changes in tone. You should feel the tone increase on the front of your body, which will pull your body into deeper flexion. Curl into a fetal curve and rest. *As the otoliths fall toward the face, flexor tone increases.*
4. Reverse the motion by slowly rolling your head back to the side and rest. Sense or imagine your inner ear fluid sinking into your lower ear. Wait for any changes in tone. You will sense your body slowly and spontaneously uncurl from flexion. Roll back to the side-lying posture and rest (PE Fig. 56b).
5. Lastly, slowly roll your head back to the original position, so that your face is facing the ceiling and rest. Sense or imagine your inner ear fluid sinking toward the back of your head. Sense any tone changes in your body, then roll your whole body back to your original position, lying on your back (PE Fig. 56a). *As the otoliths fall toward the back of the head, extensor tone increases.*
6. Repeat steps 2 to 5 on the left side.

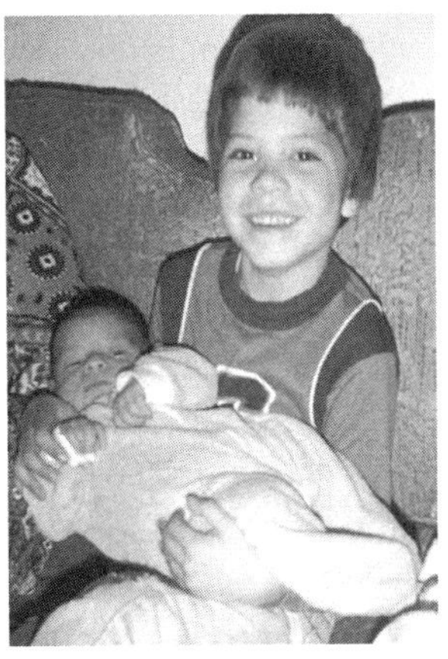

Figure 7.1 A newborn yields into the arms of his brother (photo courtesy of L. Bright).

head, until they develop tonic reflexes and equilibrium mechanisms in the eyes and inner ears to support the head when vertical (Figure 7.2).

The movement of the otoliths within the inner ear along with visual input from the eyes gives a person feedback about where the body is positioned in space. When the information coming from the eyes does not match the information from the inner ear, a person is likely to suffer motion sickness or become nauseous.

Push

Push sends lines of force that either press the body up and away from what is being pushed against, or pushes something away from the body. The push begins when a hand, foot, the head, or tail presses into a supporting surface. During a push, the muscles around the active limb concentrically contract. The compression from the push loads the joints and condenses the tissues (Figure 7.2).

The compression from pushing also provides kinesthetic feedback about where the physical body ends and the outside world begins, increasing internal proprioceptive awareness and establishing a physical sense of containment and the psychological sense of boundaries. calls this sense a "mind of inner attention." In contrast, spinal reach extends the intervertebral joints, increasing the sense of external proprioception, or what Cohen calls the "mind of outer attention."[107] Push is an act of will that requires strength and inner focus. When it is time for the infant to separate from his mother, he literally pushes away from her, and begins to realize his autonomy.

Since our joints can only be compressed to a certain point in the push, once that point is reached, an action naturally sequences into another action. A push can culminate in a reach, or in a recuperative action such as a yield. This sequence is of the utmost importance because a push sustained over a long period will take enormous effort and

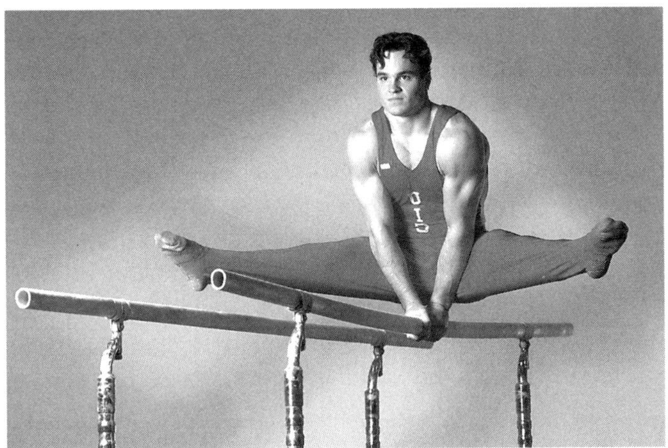

Figure 7.2 Push in the arms and spine, reach in the legs and feet

Patterning Exercise #57: Exploring Push and Yield

Alternate yielding, then pushing, to get a clear feeling of the difference between the two actions. This is an excellent exercise to do while traveling or sitting for long periods.

1. Sit in a chair. To yield, scan your body and relax any parts that you feel tension in, allowing these parts to become heavier. Imagine or sense the area you are focusing on either sinking or melting. Continue to yield. Let your bottom merge into the chair you are sitting on and your feet sink into the floor.
2. Sense the soles of your feet on the floor. Slowly push them against the floor (PE Fig. 57a). Make sure the entire surface of each foot pushes evenly. Push until you feel the counterforce of the push travel up your legs into your trunk, which will create a feeling of lift as it moves up your spine.

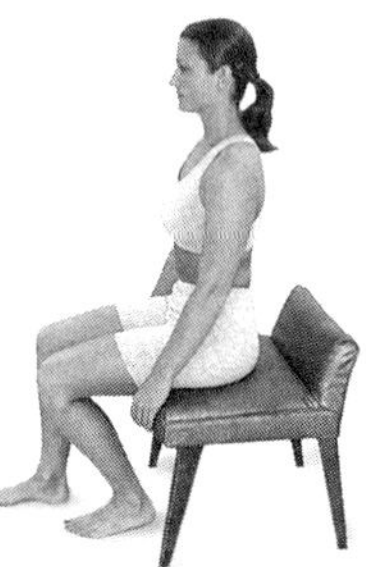

PE Fig. 57a

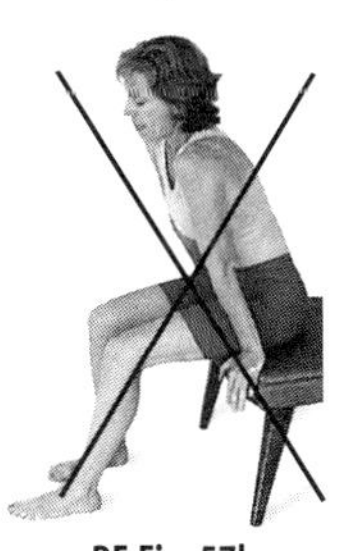

PE Fig. 57b

3. Let the push go, and yield your legs and feet into the floor. Once they are completely relaxed, push again, then yield again. Alternate yielding then pushing both feet at the same time.
4. Put both hands on the sides of your chair next to your hips. Yield the weight of your arms and hands into the chair without collapsing your thorax. Slowly push down through both hands, sensing how the force of the push travels up your arms into your shoulders and down your spine. Yield again, and sense how the yield sequences down your arms. Alternate yielding and pushing several times. Avoid hiking your shoulders (PE Fig. 57b).
5. To stand, push your feet down to stand up (PE Fig. 57c).
6. Sit back down by aiming your sit bones toward the chair.
7. Explore alternating yielding with pushing in any limb (hands, feet, head or tail) from any position.

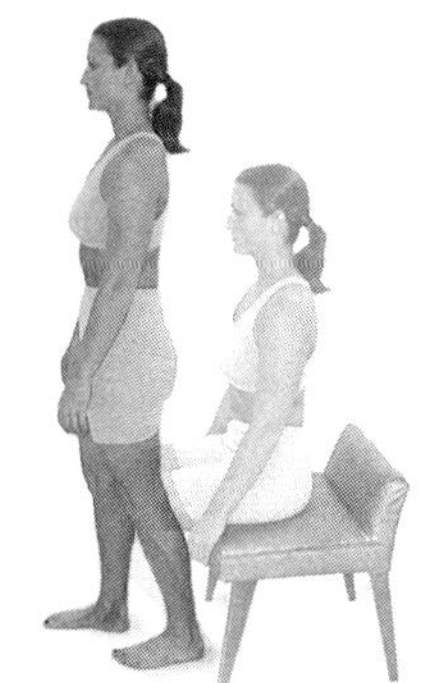

PE Fig. 57c

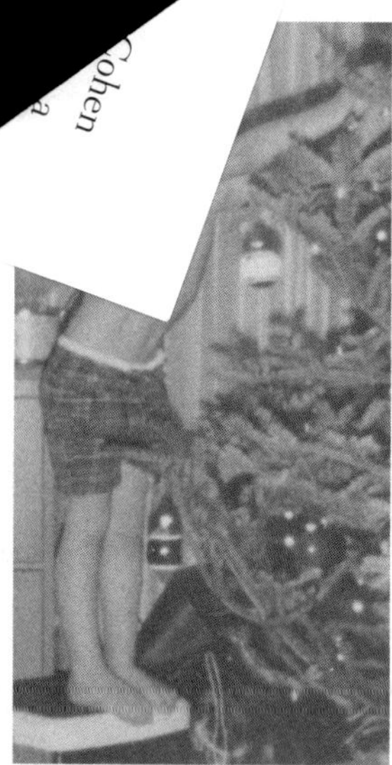

Figure 7.3a Push with the feet sequences into a reach with the arms (photo courtesy of L. Bright).

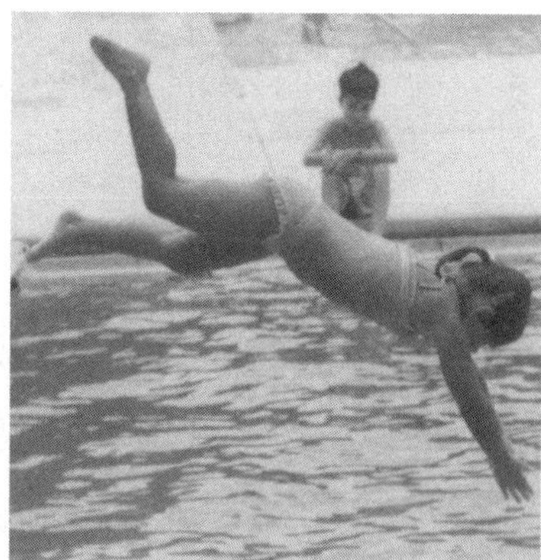

Figure 7.3b A reach and thrust (photo courtesy of K. Wasson).

cause chronic joint compression. A stubborn person who constantly "digs in her heels" may develop tension and pain from the damaging effects of bearing down. Reach elongates the joints, modulating the compression of the push. Yield relaxes the body, modulating the exertion of a push.

A push naturally follows the relaxed and weighted tone of a yield. The usual rhythm of a developing push in an infant alternates between cycles of pushing and yielding, similar to the rhythm of birthing contractions. In birthing, each push-yield cycle of the contractions increases with strength until the final push moves the newborn out of the mother's body. After birth, the baby's motor process progresses in a similar rhythm, only now the baby generates one push after another until he builds enough strength to push up to sitting and standing. Each push recruits more muscle fibers in a contraction, slowly building the tone a baby needs to shift levels. Each yield allows the body to recuperate from the exertion of the push, establishing a natural rhythm between cycles of action and rest. It is important that the push and yield modulate each other because a push without an underlying yield can be stiff, spastic, and tense.

How many endpoints (that is, your head, tail, hands, and feet) can you reach through at the same time?

Reach

Motor development involves simultaneous cycles of yield-and-push, push-and-reach. Whereas the push orients the body toward *weight* and *gravity*, **reach** orients it toward *space* and *levity*. Push compresses the joints and limbs, developing a stable, grounded connection in the body and base from which to reach out. Reach elongates the joints and limbs, extending a person into space and into relationship.

The head has a natural affinity for reach patterns initiated by its refined sensory apparatus—vision, speech, hearing, smell, and equilibrium. Of these five, people are probably the least educated about equilibrium mechanisms, although they are the most crucial for balanced posture and movement. The semicircular canals in the inner ear provide feedback about when the head is upright and when it is not. The head rights on the body in a refined balancing reflex that requires a freedom of motion in the joints between the skull and first vertebra. All too often this freedom is blocked by chronic neck tension, which also restricts blood circulation and nerve supply between the brain and body. Anyone who suffers tension headaches would benefit from learning how to reach with the head and exploring head righting reactions (see Chapter 11).

Push provides a base of support for the reach (Figure 7.3a-b). The transition from a push to a reach involves going from an internal focus to an external focus. Each time a baby pushes, she adds to the inner strength and stability in her body to be able to reach out without tipping over. A baby reaches toward her mother by extending her arms and head, which lengthens the muscles around the reaching limb. In an infant, reach initiates from intrinsic desires such as hunger or thirst, and as the baby grows, from a desire to explore the environment. The reach has an attitude of curiosity, a desire to extend into the unknown and interact with other people, to be connected with something outside of oneself, to be interested and motivated to learn, and to grasp new information and pull it in (Figure 7.4).

Reach extends the body beyond its sphere, pulling the joints open and elongating the limbs. A reach without an underlying push can be unstable and can hyperextend the joints. Although the reach stretches the body, a reach differs from a stretch by the intention of its functional action and its ongoing rate. However, we can reach our way into a position of stretch and increase a stretch by reaching beyond it.

Whereas the push gathers a fixed strength to press away from something, the reach extends toward something with a single momentum and thrust. It is difficult to suspend a reach toward something without hanging in space mid-motion, although we do this when we reach through a stretch. Although reaching out increases the stretch, the motivation to stretch is intrinsic; it comes from a desire to lengthen tight tissues. In contrast, the motivation to reach is extrinsic; it comes from a desire to make contact with something outside of us.

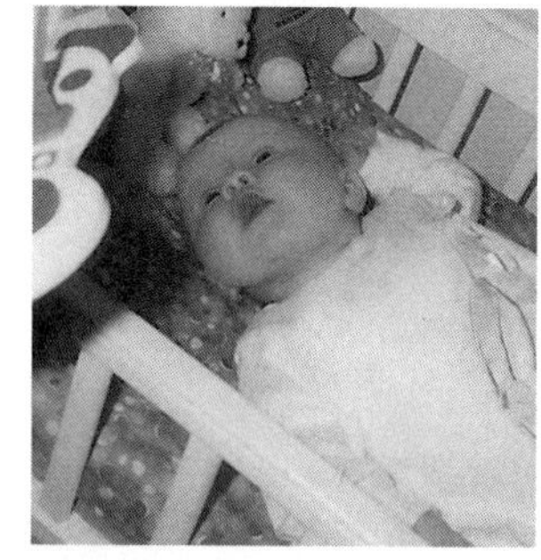

Figure 7.4 Curiosity evokes a reach with the eyes and head (photo courtesy of D. Kolway).

Pull

A reach usually culminates in a grasp and **pull**. A pull occurs when we take hold of

Patterning Exercise #58: Differentiating Push and Reach

1. While sitting on the floor, lean forward and push one hand into the floor as you reach with the other (PE Fig. 58a). Sense how reach elongates one arm while the push compresses the other arm.

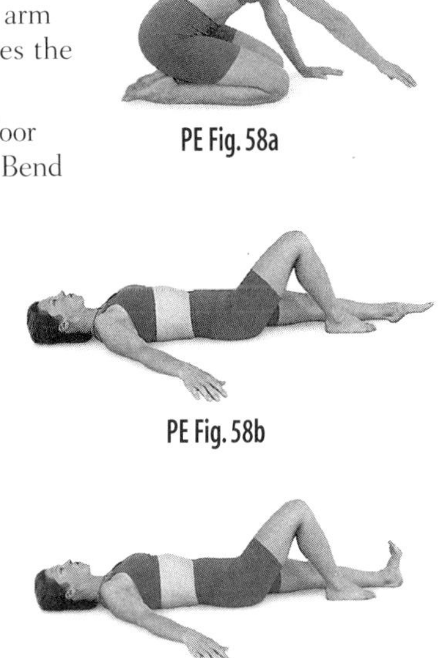

PE Fig. 58a

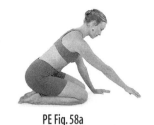

PE Fig. 58b

PE Fig. 58c

2. Lie on your back on the floor in a comfortable position. Bend one leg, placing the foot flat on the floor. Straighten the other leg by reaching through the toes on that foot (PE Fig. 58b). Let the extension of the reach travel into the pelvis, lengthening your hip and back on that side. As you reach through your toes, keep your leg weighted and the back of your knee relaxed. Then push through the heel of the extended leg (PE Fig. 58c). Alternate reaching and pushing with your foot, and feel the difference between the two actions. Switch legs and repeat.
3. Now contrast a reach in the extended foot and leg with a push in the bent leg. Continue to reach through the toes of one foot while you push down through the sole of the other. Sense the contrast in tone between the two actions. How does it affect your hips? Switch legs and repeat.
4. Next, push both feet up toward the ceiling (PE Fig. 58d). Then contrast this with reaching through both feet (PE Fig. 58e). Sense how reach elongates the joints in your legs.
5. Finish by coming back to a spinal action. Do this by bending both legs and placing both feet flat on the floor, then simultaneously push down through both feet (PE Fig. 58f). Sense how the push in a closed chain (with the feet connected to the floor) compresses your joints all the way up through your spine. Compare this with a push of your feet through an open chain (PE Fig. 58d).
6. Explore reaching with one foot while pushing with the other as you walk.

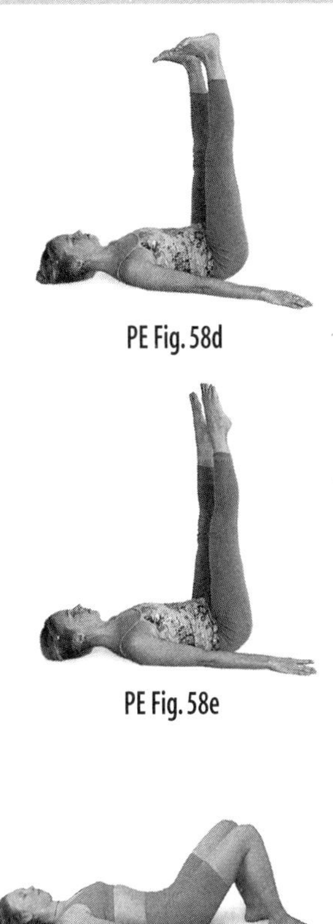

PE Fig. 58d

PE Fig. 58e

PE Fig. 58f

EMSPress.com

something and draw it toward us or draw our body toward it. If the object being pulled on is stationary, our effort will pull the body toward the object (Figure 7.5). If the object is mobile (and light enough), we pull the object toward the body. Pulling leads to a shift in position or the acquisition of something new. Pull is motivated by both biological needs for nourishment and by maturation with its accompanying desires to grasp new experiences, take them in, and learn from them.

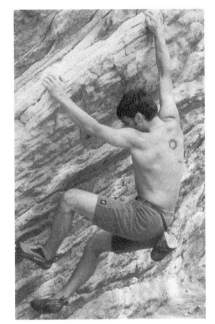

Figure 7.5 Pull with the arms

The action of pulling initiates from a desire to change relationship, either to pull the body from A to B, or to grasp something or somebody we want. The pull establishes lines of tension in the tissues as it sequences through the body. If the pull makes a contiguous sequence, its tensional forces will translate along an entire limb and/or the spine, elongating tissues from one joint to the next along a sequence between endpoints. But the force of the pull can become stuck in one part of the body if a person pulls against herself. For example, when a person stands from a seated position, a strong reach with the head can pull the entire spine up (Figure 7.6a). A simultaneous push with the feet will give the action even more efficiency. In contrast, a person might lift herself out of the chair using her arms, having one part of the body haul another part up in an awkward move made cumbersome by the lack of support from the underlying push and reach patterns (Figure 7.6b).

It is common in patterns of poor posture that one part of the body fixates against the pull of another. There are a lot of variations on this pattern. To name a few, people chronically pull the shoulders up or back, pull the head forward, or pull the elbows back, which distorts the neutral alignment of the spine (Figure 7.7a-b). These postures tend to weaken the integration between the limbs and

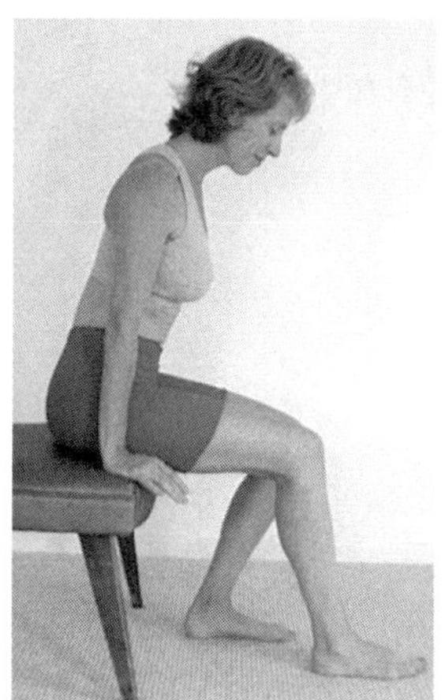

Figure 7.6a Pushing down with the hands and feet is a more efficient way to stand.

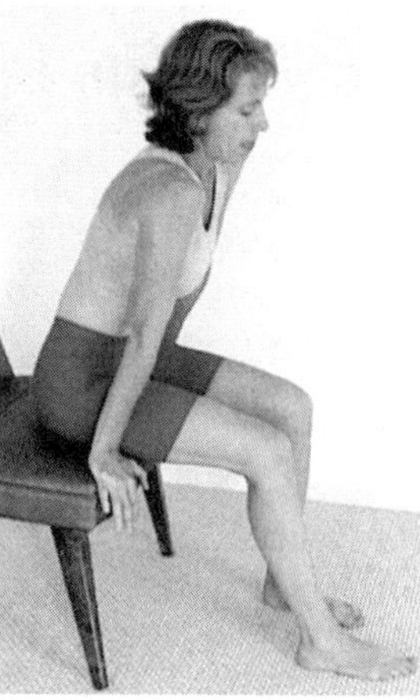

Figure 7.6b Pulling the body up with the shoulders to stand strains the shoulders.

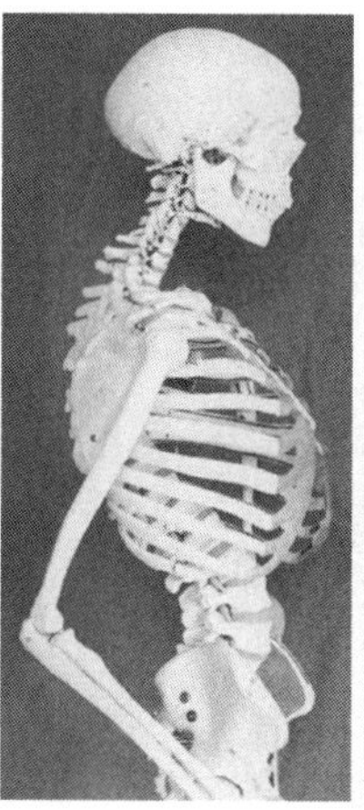

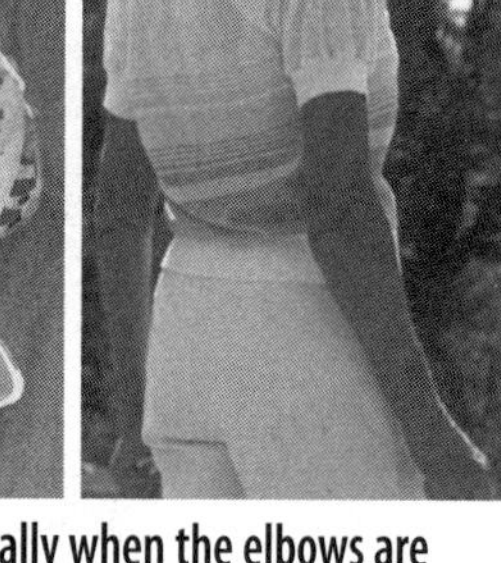

Figure 7.7a-b Usually when the elbows are chronically pulled back, another body part thrusts forward to compensate.

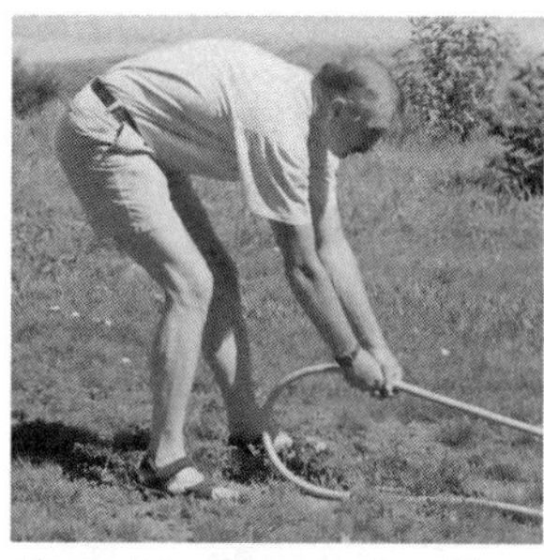

Figure 7.8a This man is pulling his back as much as the hose by bending his spine.

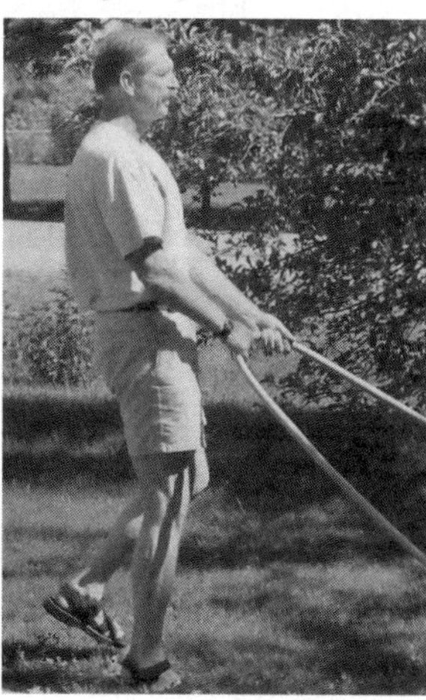

Figure 7.8b Now he protects his back by pulling with a straight back and pushing with his feet.

core, and they block the full sequence of an action, be it push, reach, or pull. Excessive pulls on already weak joints or tendons could predispose a person to injury. Seniors often tear their shoulders when they go to lift something heavy but lack the strength for the exertion. Then the force of the pull, rather than moving the object they intend to lift, pulls and rips the already weak tendons or muscles in their arms or shoulders. Contrast the man in the photo who pulls against himself, and then who pulls the hose (Figure 7.8a-b). A person who habitually holds the shoulders up toward the ears is actually pulling the shoulder girdle up off the rib cage. Older people often do this by pulling their shoulders up to their ears to lift themselves out of a chair. A more efficient way to stand up from sitting would be to push the feet into the ground, allowing the combined push of the lower body and the reach of the head to lift the body out of the seated position (see Figure 7.6a-b).

PREVERTEBRAL PATTERNS

Every person has an innate movement vocabulary that recapitulates the primary patterns of many species that preceded us in evolution. The earliest of these species—such as earthworms, jellyfish, and sharks—lack bony skeletons and hence are classified as prevertebral. The motor responses of the primitive invertebrates are incredibly fluid and amoeboid. For example, the pseudopodia flow of amoebas follows the path of least resistance, achieving locomotion by pushing a tendril out the cell wall, then oozing protoplasm into this newly formed tendril. These early patterns are most apparent in the fluid stream of undulations of newborn babies, yet as adults we can still retain these innate fluid qualities if our bodies remain flexible and intrinsically articulate.

This next section examines the prevertebral patterns of four invertebrates—amoeba, starfish, sea squirt, and lancelet—and their corresponding movements in humans—cellular, navel radiation, mouthing, and prespinal movement.

Cellular Movement

The difference between a response and a reaction is that the former is the result of an impulse to act, whereas the later is a reflexive "knee-jerk" response to a threat. Cellular responses are the building blocks of sensorimotor processes while cellular reactions are the bases of our defense responses. By understanding cellular movement, and even sensing or visualizing it, we can access this deep biological process within us to cultivate a foundation for inner motility in all patterning processes.

In unicellular organisms, such as the amoeba, physiological events occur either inside or outside the cell. The cell wall (*plasma membrane*) separates the organism from its environment. This semi-permeable and selective membrane allows some substances to pass through while keeping other substances out, thus functioning as a primitive nervous system that makes choices to regulate what substances move into or out of the cell. Multicellular organisms such as humans have extensive intercellular spaces (as discussed in Chapter 1). These spaces are filled with interstitial

Links to Practical Applications

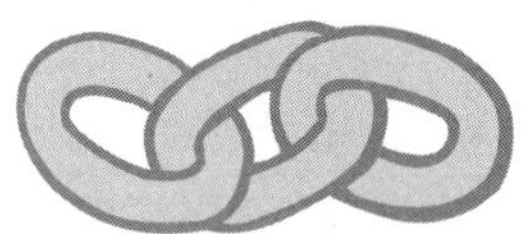

Receiving Touch

When you receive massage or bodywork, although you are passive, explore actively touching the practitioner back with your awareness and notice if it changes the quality of your experience.

Patterning Exercise #59: Exploring Reach, Grasp, and Pull

1. To find energetic support for a reach, imagine something that you really want. It may be figurative, such as joy or good health, or it may be actual. Visualize it being several inches away from your fingertips. Allow your desire or visualization to wake up your fingertips. Feel the sensations this creates in your fingertips, move them a little, then reach from this feeling. Let the reach travel through your arms and into your trunk. How far can you feel the reach sequence into your body?
2. Explore reaching with your head, your mouth, your eyes, your ears, your tail, and your feet, intiating the reach by visualizing something you desire right of reach. How far can your limbs reach before your trunk is pulled along?
3. Now reach and grasp some movable object, then pull it toward you. Notice how your muscles work differently when reaching, grasping, and pulling.
4. Next, grasp onto monkey bars on a playground, or something stable around the house such as a door jam. Explore pulling your body toward it, then pushing away from it (PE Fig. 59b). Feel where you need to yield and push to reach to effectively and pull. Notice how one action cycles into the next. Explore pulling your entire body back and forth. Then contrast pulling while reaching with your tail, then tucking it under and not reaching with it.
5. Reach and grasp a seated friend's hand, then pull her to standing (PE Fig. 59c-d). In what parts of your body do you need to push to get the support to pull her to standing?

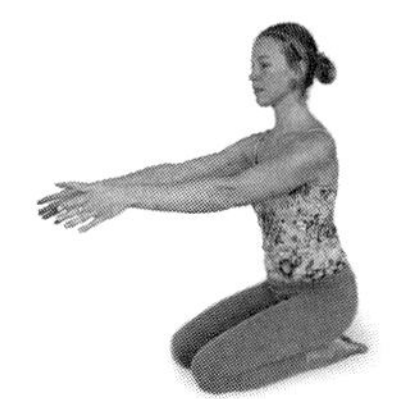
PE Fig. 59a

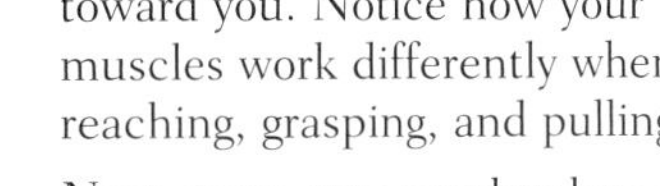

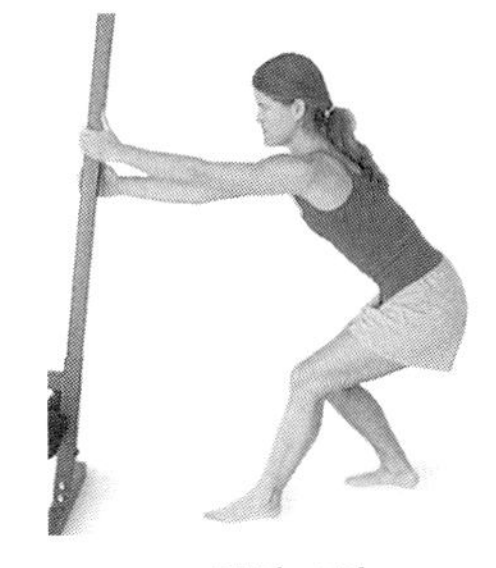
PE Fig. 59b

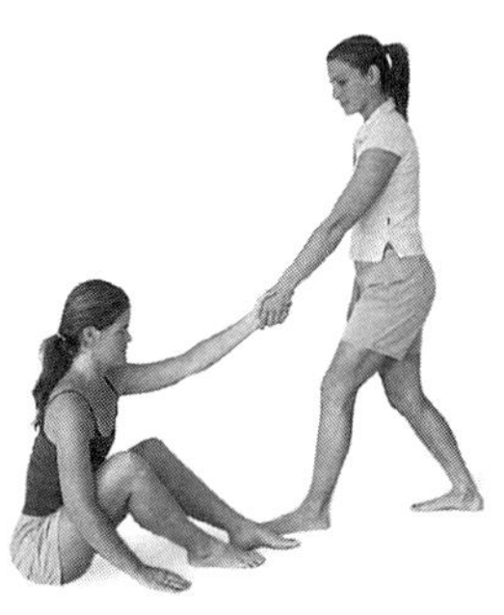
PE Fig. 59c

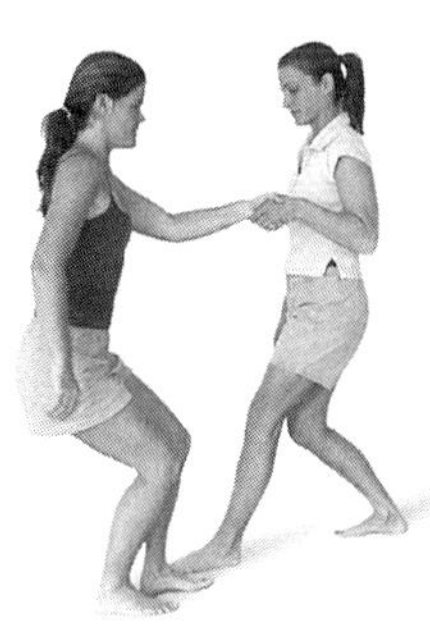
PE Fig. 59d

fluid, which creates an inner "ocean" in an organism. The trillions of cells in the human body communicate with each other within this ocean on a systemic level via a multitude of floating chemical messengers such as hormones.

A point about which scientists have speculated is the idea that a rudimentary level of intelligence exists within cells, and it manifests in their fundamental ability to seemingly "make decisions" about what substances pass through their membranes. Biologist Bruce Lipton refers to this primitive system of cellular information processing as the "organellar equivalent of a brain."[108] Each cell has approximately one million docking sites for hormonal molecules that regulate many metabolic functions. Whether a specific hormone can latch on or not reflects a level of cellular consciousness. Thus each cell within our bodies is a body unto itself, with its organellar equivalent to a respiratory system, a digestive system, a muscular system, and so on. The cells actually breathe, taking in oxygen and expelling waste. Cellular respiration is the basis of cellular metabolism.

When you touch your hand to your face, does your face also touch your hand?

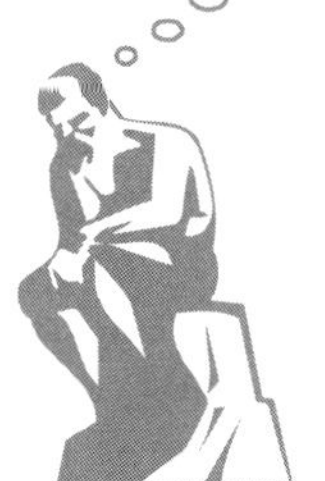

Communication occurs not only across cell walls, but also among many single cells, among large groups of cells within various tissues, and among body systems. Cellular communication even extends between people within a field of somatic, vibrational resonance that people feel as "vibes." Positive vibrations are usually accompanied by an expansive sensation in the body, whereas negative vibrations tend to create a body sensation marked by tightening and contraction. This level of communication occurs most directly during tactile interactions.

As discussed in Chapters 2 and 4, touch elicits deep somatic responses. Tactile experiences are among the earliest stimuli thought to shape patterns of cellular consciousness. Touch elicits one of two basic responses: a movement toward or a retraction away from touch. These two patterns constitute the most primitive movement responses of single-celled creatures, a pattern basic to all systemic responses.

Whether or not a person can actually feel cellular processes is questionable, but we can certainly feel the effects of them. The placebo effect demonstrates the power of the mind to actually change the physiology of cells. Many of the somatic therapies seek to cultivate cellular awareness within movement and touch in order to access the innate intelligence of biological life; to affect it through sensory awareness, intention, and visualization; and to heal and enliven our body tissues. For example, Cohen uses cellular breathing and cellular holding as a basis for feeling cellular responses during somatic patterning (see "Body-Mind Centering" in Chapter 11). Also, people use cellular visualization to boost immune responses and evoke deep healing (see "Psychoneuroimmunology" in Chapter 13).

Navel Radiation

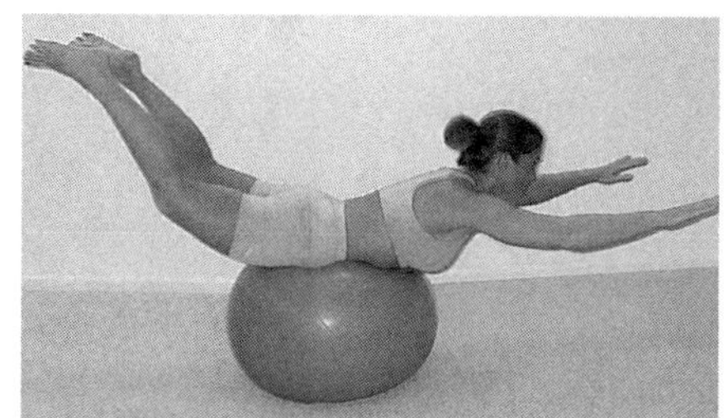
Figure 7.11 The Landau reflex

A cell is generally pictured as spherical with small tendrils extending from the center out. This radial pattern shows up again in the second prevertebral pattern of navel radiation, which is found in the starfish. To visualize the evolution from the single-celled creature to one with limbs, imagine tendrils of the amoeba extending out to form five limbs, and each limb moves in a pattern of radial symmetry to the core. The starfish pattern shows up in some of our earliest motor patterns, when movement begins to differentiate between the core and the limbs.

Newborns and infants often initiate movement at the navel, extending out or drawing in all the limbs in a simultaneous movement that initiates from an impulse in the belly (Figure 7.9). As infants gyrate in a continuous flow of organic, unformed movements, their limbs flex and extend from an impulse that initiates in the center of their bodies. A newborn baby will often throw his head back from movement that actually began in the belly.

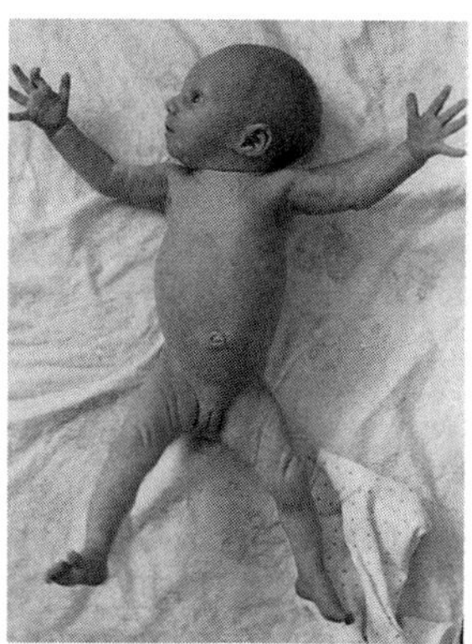
Figure 7.9 The navel radiation pattern (photo courtesy of D. Radandt).

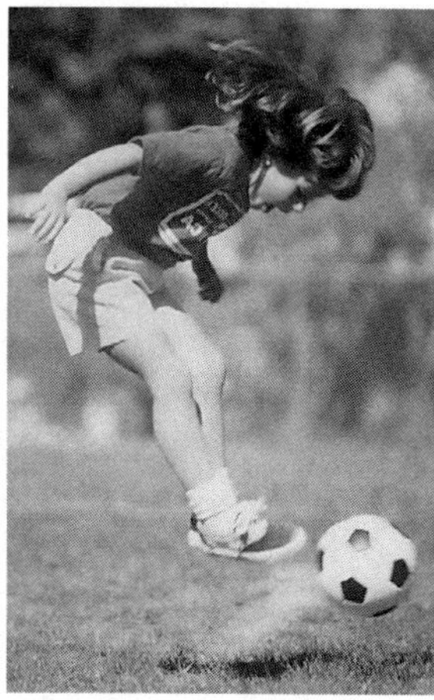
Figure 7.10 A jump centered around the navel (photo courtesy of K. Wasson).

Navel radiation underlies full-body movements that simultaneously extend or condense (draw in) the entire body in one coordinated action (Figure 7.10). Each limb has an equal relationship to the center, a pattern seen in the graceful extension of a sky diver or the tight curl of a gymnast doing an aerial somersault. The pattern is also seen in a jellyfish shooting through the water in an umbrella-like shape.

The photoreceptors on the ends of starfish limbs are reflected in the abundance of sensory nerve endings at the end of each human limb—the fingers, toes, face, and pelvic floor. This configuration enables the arms of a starfish to extend into the environment to gather sensory input. Likewise, our limbs enable us to sequence between our inner impulses and the outer world. Our hands and feet, head and tail, are, metaphorically speaking, the gateways to relationship.

Navel radiation is important for integrating the movement of the extremities with the core of the body. The spatial pathways that emerge in navel radiation encompass all the potential pathways into which the developmental movements eventually differentiate, such as spinal, homologous, homolateral, and contralateral (see Chapter 1 for definitions). If there are any weaknesses in the connection of any limb to the core in the pattern of navel radiation, this will show up in specific weaknesses in a more complex pattern during later stages of development, such as walking or running.

A reflex that underlies the pattern of navel radiation is called the **Landau reflex**. This reflex is obvious when babies lie on their bellies and extend all their limbs at the same time, assuming a "flying position" (Figure 7.11). Holding an infant face down and gently lifting it at the waist stimulates the Landau reflex in which all the limbs simultaneously extend in one action. If the Landau is strong, the core connection of the limbs to the navel will usually be strong, and vice-versa. Also, this early reflex organizes tone in the extensor muscles along the spine; therefore, an imbalance in the spinal muscles can be addressed by practicing the Landau.

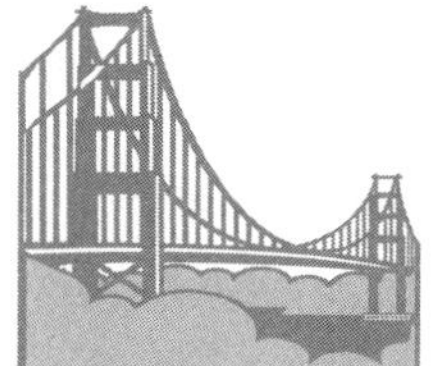

Bridge to Practice

Looking for Full-Body Integration in the Starfish Pattern

You can assess your client's patterns through the starfish template. Watch her as she walks into your office, as you take a history, and during your opening discussion, looking for relationships in the movement between her limbs and navel. Imagine the arms, legs, and spine as "highways" for movement. Along which pathway is the flow of movement strong? Along which is the flow of movement weak? Where are there roadblocks? How do the patterns you observe relate to your client's body problem?

While working with your client, suggest that she tune into a particular pathway. For example, when you give her traction in the neck, suggest that she sense it pulling along her entire spine through her navel down to her hips. Or have her reach through both feet while you traction her neck to make a vertical connection. You can also help her become more aware of the connection between her navel and limbs by slowly brushing each pathway (navel to one hand, the other, to one foot, the other, to the head, and then the tail). Encourage her to relax along each pathway. Be creative in helping your client gain an awareness of the connections along the movement pathways.

Making a full-body connection through all the pathways at once is integrating and helpful to do at the end of a session. To do this, suggest that your client reach through all her endpoints at once while you give each limb (including the head and tail) a gentle pull to take the slack out from her navel to her limbs and spine.

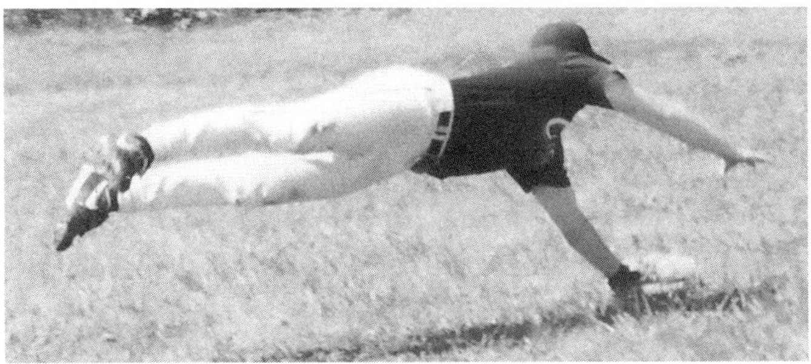

Figure 7.12 The Landau reflex underlies many athletic moves (photo courtesy of E. Foster).

The Landau reflex underlies integrated patterns of full-body extension that we see in many sports that require extension, such as a swan dive or skydiving (Figure 7.12). If a person has strong flexor tone, practicing the Landau could help develop more extensor tone (as in the case of Henry in Chapter 4). The Landau can also help integrate the movement of the limbs with the spine and coordinate full-body extension. The initial phases of the Landau can be practiced to activate and control the deeper stabilizer muscles along the spine, particularly the *multifidi muscles*. (See Chapter 9 for more information on this muscle.)

Mouthing Patterns

As first mentioned in Chapter 1, mouthing patterns recapitulate the patterns of a sea squirt, the primitive invertebrate that lives attached to the bottom of the ocean floor and filters all nutrients and waste products through its tube-like body. The sea squirt even births its offspring out the top. Some sea squirts have small openings on the bottom to secrete waste, which is akin to the bottom of a human's digestive tract—the anus.

The mouthing pattern begins in utero when preborns start to suck their thumbs. A newborn's world revolves around mouthing patterns (Figure 7.13). The smell of his mother's skin stimulates the infant's **oral rooting reflex**, causing him to search for the nipple. Rooting impulses

Patterning Exercise #60: The Landau Reflex

Caution: If you have lower back pain or lower back problems, only practice the initial phases of this exercise (1–3), and consult a physician for an evaluation. Stop immediately if anything causes pain.

1. Lie face down over a large physioball with your eyes closed. (If you do not have a ball, lie on your belly on the floor). Breathe and relax. Allow your limbs and spine to sink and stretch away from your navel on each exhalation (PE Fig. 60a).

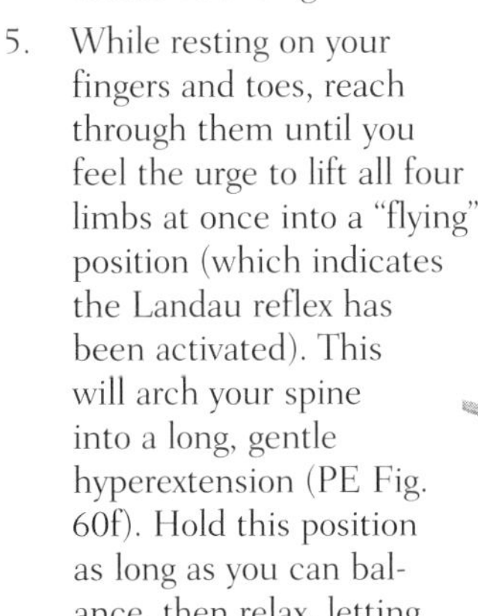

PE Fig. 60a

2. Next, open your eyes and look at the floor (PE Fig. 60b). Feel the length and lift that this optical support gives your spine, especially your neck. (If you do not feel a lift, practice Patterning Exercise #3.)

PE Fig. 60b

3. Now slowly reach all the limbs out simultaneously, including your head and tail, fingers and toes. Keep reaching and rest your fingers and toes on the floor to balance yourself on the ball (PE Fig. 60c). As you reach, sense the connection of your navel to the ball, and balance all your limbs evenly around your navel. Allow the reach to lengthen your spine and limbs. Avoid hyperextension of the spine until you feel intrinsic muscular support in an extended position.

PE Fig. 60c

4. Raise your legs and balance for a moment, then lower them (PE Fig. 60d). Then raise your arms and balance for a moment, then lower them. Then lift your legs with the soles of your feet together and balance a moment, then lower them (PE Fig. 60e). Putting the soles of your feet together provides a midline connection that makes balancing easier.

PE Fig. 60d

5. While resting on your fingers and toes, reach through them until you feel the urge to lift all four limbs at once into a "flying" position (which indicates the Landau reflex has been activated). This will arch your spine into a long, gentle hyperextension (PE Fig. 60f). Hold this position as long as you can balance, then relax, letting your body drape over the ball and elongate. (If the Landau reflex was supporting your hyperextension, your spine will arch effortlessly. If the Landau was not supporting the movement, your back muscles will feel as though they have overworked, most noticeably in the lumbar and cervical regions.)

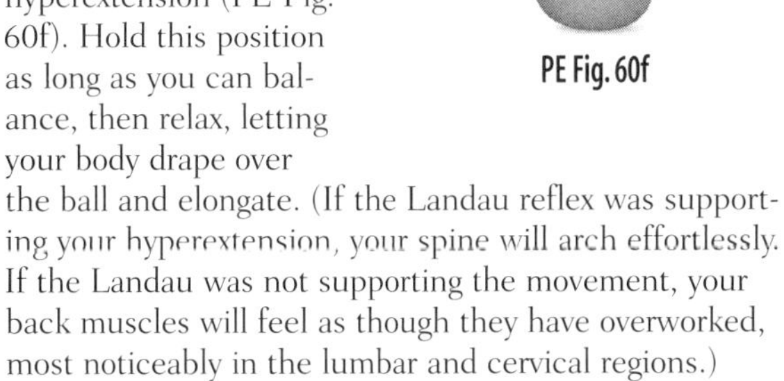

PE Fig. 60e

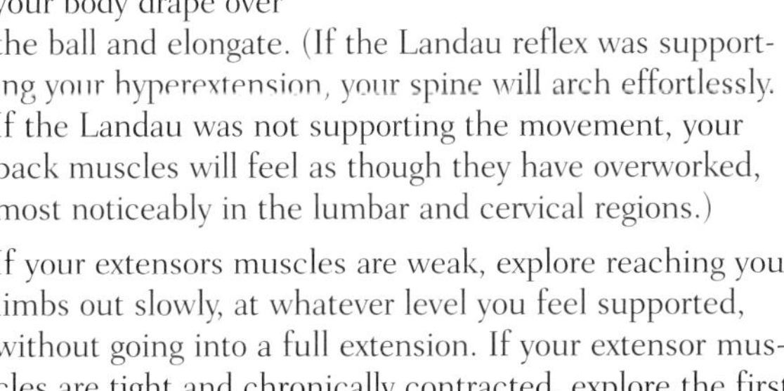

PE Fig. 60f

6. If your extensors muscles are weak, explore reaching your limbs out slowly, at whatever level you feel supported, without going into a full extension. If your extensor muscles are tight and chronically contracted, explore the first 3 steps of this exercise. This develops intrinsic muscles along the spine which helps the larger extensors to relax.

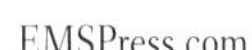

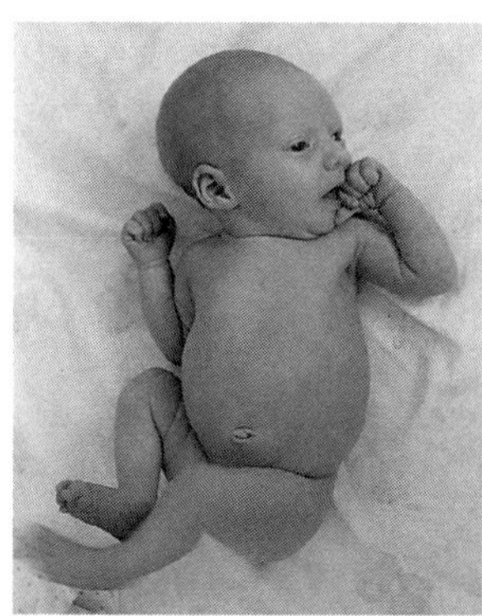

Figure 7.13 Babies spend a lot of time mouthing (photo courtesy of D. Radandt).

initiate a mouthing sequence that works its way through the baby's entire digestive track, milking nourishment along many twisting and bending tubes and pouches in the digestive organs, from head to tail. This process creates incredibly organic spinal movements, obvious as babies quietly wiggle, squirm, and push their inner processes along the digestive tract and spine between the head and tail. It is as though the churning and pushing movements were working paste through a tube. Movement at one end reflects movement at the other end, obvious on a grimacing and squeezing face as an infant pushes a pocket of gas out the bottom.

A starfish grasps its food by extending its primitive gut through a mouth out the end of one limb. Likewise, our mouth is the first limb to reach in the rooting reflex that is active right after birth. It is, in a sense, the end of the digestive tube reaching out. This action not only builds a baseline of tone in the digestive tract; it also has great musculoskeletal implications. Mouthing begins the differentiation of extensor tone along the spine, which is a segmental process, building tone in muscles along one vertebral segment at a time. Babies are born curled into strong fetal flexion; hence flexor tone precedes extensor tone. Extensor tone builds along the back every time the infant lifts her head to reach for the nipple or to look up. When the infant lifts her head to root, the small muscles at the base of the skull contract. The first time the infant lifts and extends her head to root, she rocks the head on the first cervical vertebra, which tones and coordinates muscles at the base of the head. The next time she lifts her head to root, the action strengthens another segment. Each successive movement engages more of the extensor muscles along the spine, and extensor tone progressively builds from the head to the tail. To visualize this process, imagine picking up the end pearl on a string of pearls, then the next time picking up two, then three, and so on. The small muscles along each vertebral segment develop in a similar progression. Thus, mouthing patterns underlie the postural mechanisms involved in head righting, in the development of postural tone along the spine, and in integrated spinal patterns.

How many movement patterns do you do during the day that involve a coordination between your hands and either your eyes or your mouth?

Neuromuscular development follows a set pathway from the center out, the top down, the front to back, and the center or midline to the periphery. Movement initiated by the organs, such as mouthing, underlies neuromuscular coordination. This is apparent when we contrast the strength of the infant's movement initiated by mouthing patterns and associated reflexes with the strength of muscles in a newborn's neck and spine, which are not yet strong enough to hold the newborn's head up. Mouthing movements evoke the **asymmetrical tonic neck reflexes (ATNR)**, which underlie the homolateral patterns that will be discussed shortly. Mouthing movements also pattern **hand-mouth coordination**, which evokes a coupled joint motion of spinal side-bending with flexion. As an infant looks around and simultaneously reaches for the breast to root, this

Patterning Exercise #61: Exploring Mouth and Throat Movement

1. Get in a comfortable position and close your eyes. Become aware of the inside of your mouth, your tongue and teeth, your upper palate, and the inside of your throat. Lightly stroke your lips to wake-up sensation in them (PE Fig. 61).
2. Use your tongue to explore the soft tissue lining of your mouth. Cover the entire surface area: top, bottom, sides, front, and back. Keep your jaw as relaxed as possible as you move your tongue.
3. Next make slow random movements opening and closing your mouth, initiating the movement from the soft tissues on the inside in actions such as yawning, swallowing, gumming, and sticking out your tongue. Use the exploration to loosen and stretch your TMJ, jaw muscles, and tongue.

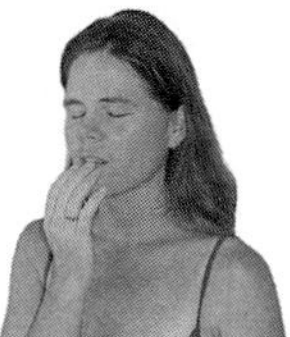

PE Fig. 61

4. Now place your thumb in your mouth (make sure it's clean!) with the pad of your thumb behind your front teeth on your upper palate. Gently massage your upper palate. Then start sucking. Notice how the movement gently rocks your head on your spine and sequences down your throat and neck. Keep your neck as relaxed as possible.
5. Then lie comfortably on your back. Explore turning your head by first reaching to one side with your mouth. (You might need to gently stroke the areas around your lips to wake up rooting reflexes in order to strengthen the initiation of movement with your mouth.)
6. While still lying on your back, explore rolling over. Initiate the movement by reaching with the mouth, then allow your spine to follow. To reverse the movement and roll back, initiate the roll reaching with your mouth. Roll again, yet contrast it from before by leading with the tail.

EMSPress.com

Using Mouthing Patterns to Relieve Neck Pain

A client named Sue came in with chronic neck pain. She had found relief through massage therapy and chiropractic, yet the pain always returned. During a patterning bodywork session, Sue explored both subtle movements of the mouth and tongue, and skeletal movements in the temporomandibular joint (TMJ) while her practitioner held trigger points in the chronically contracted muscles of her neck. The pressure helped Sue relax tight muscles; at the same time, the subtle mouthing movements helped her to engage and organize deeper muscles in her mouth and neck.

Whenever tight muscles release chronic tension, new muscles need to engage to support the area previously held in contraction. In this case, the subtle mouthing movements helped facilitate the intrinsic, stabilizing muscles along the spine, which, in turn, helped facilitate the release of chronically contracted, extrinsic muscles as well as the release of autonomic nervous system tension. Although Sue's neck pain was complicated by numerous factors (facet joint damage, head injuries, car accidents), during this session, Sue became more aware of the tension she held in her mouth. She was then able to use this awareness to begin practicing subtle mouthing movements to relax her neck during the course of her day.

action patterns **hand-eye coordination**, which evokes a coupled motion of spinal side-bending with extension (Figure 7.14). In addition, rooting wakes up tactile receptors around the lips and neck, which in turn strengthen the hand-mouth and hand-eye coordinations that underlie more complex spinal patterns like rolling and turning.

As adults, we follow mouthing impulses every time we eat. The smell or even thought of food can stimulate salivation and gustatory movements in a hungry person. The movement of the mouth is coordinated with the arms and spine so that we can reach out, grasp our food, and take it in.

Prespinal Movements along the Soft Spine

During early fetal development, at about 15 days, the structure of the fetus is similar to a small, eel-like creature called the *lancelet*. This primitive fish has a flexible yet stiff rod called a *notochord* that runs the length of the torso and is, in the fetus, the precursor of the bony spine (Figure 7.15a-b). As the fetus develops, the notochord is gradually absorbed into the spine and becomes the *nucleus* of the *intervertebral discs*.

The early fetus, like the lancelet, has two parallel tubes that run the length of its body on either side of the notochord—a spinal cord and a primitive gut. Since the eel-like lancelet lacks a bony skeleton, it relies on the notochord to serve as a stiffening rod for its soft spine. In the human embryo, the notochord provides a central rod from which the *somites*

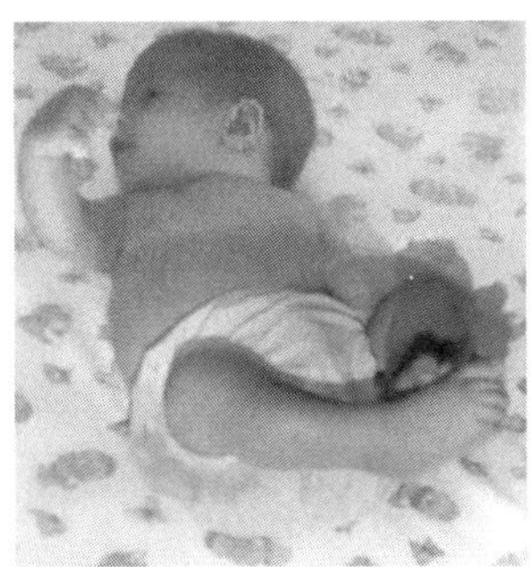

Figure 7.14 Hand-mouth and hand-eye coordinations evoke right-left differentiation (photo courtesy of L. Bright).

Patterning Exercise #62: Hand-Mouth and Hand-Eye Coordination

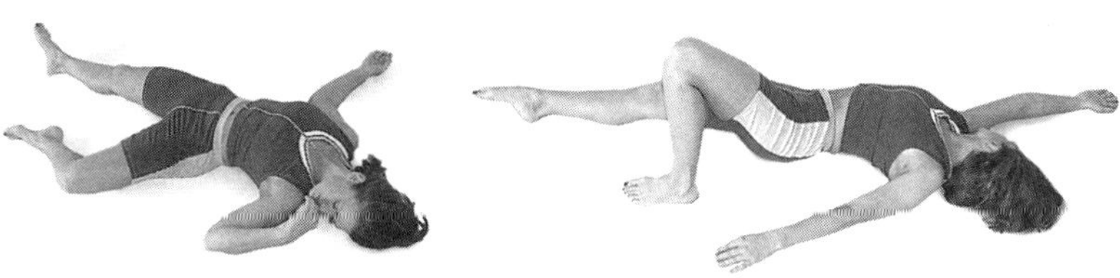

PE Fig. 62a **PE Fig. 62b**

1. Lie on your back. Take a few deep breaths. As you exhale, allow your body weight to sink into the floor. Relax the areas along your back that feel tight.
2. *Hand-mouth coordination:* Bring your thumb to your mouth while turning your head toward your thumb (PE Fig. 62a). Notice how your spine flexes and rotates toward the thumb side.
3. Repeat the same movement on the other side. Turn your head as you bring your thumb to your mouth. The lateral flexion and rotation of your spine should sequence into your hip and leg on that same side. Your tail should point to the foot on the flexed side.
4. Alternate sides until the transitions from side to side are smooth.
5. *Hand-eye coordination:* Still lying on your back, extend one arm along the floor, first out to your side and then above your head. Watch your hand as you move it to establish hand-eye coordination (PE Fig. 62b). Notice how your spine extends and rotates to that side. The extension should sequence into your leg on that side as well.
6. Repeat on the other side.
7. Alternate sides until the transitions from side to side are smooth.
8. Lie on your belly. Take a moment to relax the weight of your organs into the floor. Bring your hand to your mouth, feeling flexion with rotation on that side of your body. Repeat on the other side. Then alternate sides until the transitions from side to side are smooth.
9. While prone, extend one hand along the floor, out to the side and above your head. Watch your hand as you move. The extension should sequence down that side of your body into your leg. Repeat on the other side. Then alternate sides until transitions from side to side are smooth.

arise that eventually develop into the segmented column of vertebrae, ribs, muscles, and nerves along the spine (Figure 7.16).

Like many aquatic species without vertebrae, such as jellyfish, the lancelet propels its long, tubular body through the water like a tadpole, leading with the head and propelling with the tail. Movement ripples along its soft spine with a flexible, serpentine quality. A similar quality of prespinal movement is observed in the squirming, snakelike undulations of the newborn's spine. In the newborn, prespinal movement initiates either along the front of the body in the mouth, or along the back of the body in the sense organs of the eyes and ears.

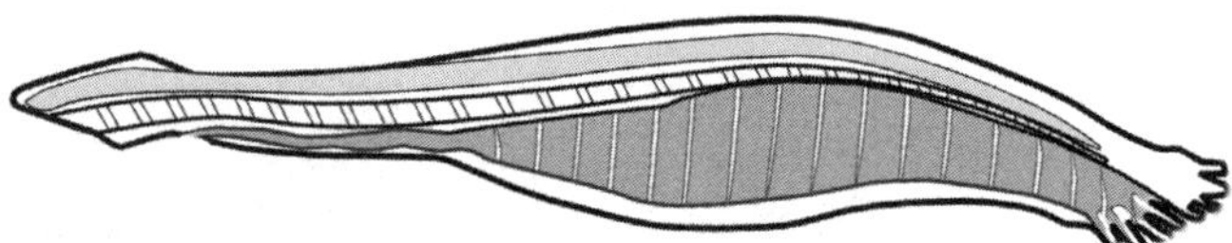

Figure 7.15a The lancelet has an organ tube, a soft spine (lacking bones), and a notochord, which is a primitive skeletal system.

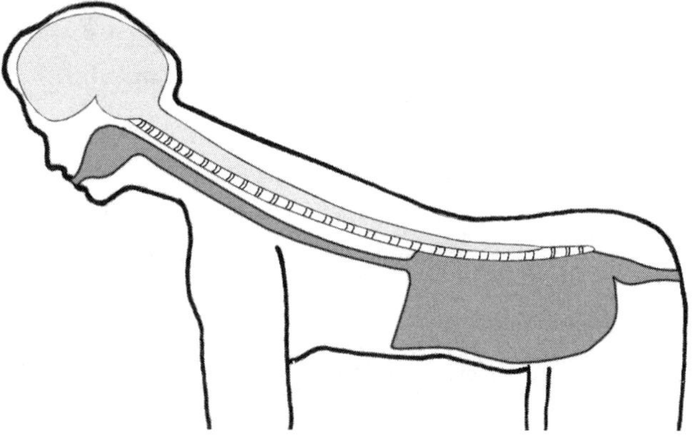

Figure 7.15b The human digestive tube and spine retain the basic configuration of the lancelet.

The prespinal quality of movement is rarely seen in adults. Exceptions are the rippling undulations of a belly dancer or the wavy curves that a hip-hop dancer carves through space with her spine; each gives the illusion that the bony spine is supple and pliable.

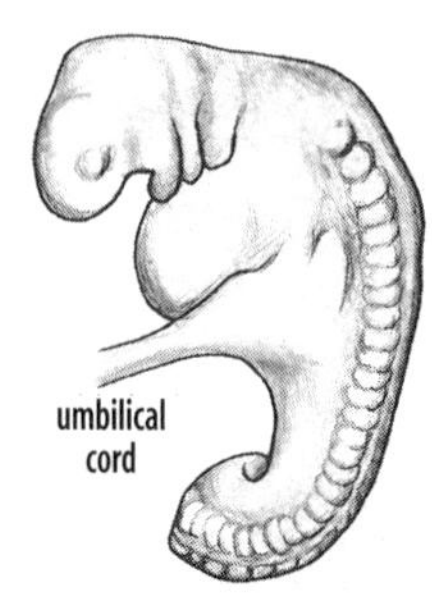

Figure 7.16 Somites on an embryo that is about 28 days old

VERTEBRAL PATTERNS

Recall from Chapter 1 that the vertebral patterns correlate with the primary movements of species that have bony skeletons—the *spinal* patterns of fish, the *homologous* movements of amphibians, the *homolateral* movements of reptiles, and the *contralateral* movements of mammals. The vertebral patterns establish neuromuscular pathways during the exploratory movements of a baby's first few years and gradually build musculoskeletal tone. As a group, the vertebral patterns organize lines of force along skeletal pathways and coordinate neuromuscular pathways for all subsequent and more complex patterns of movement. Spinal patterns sequence through the vertebrae and organize pathways along the core. Homologous patterns of the limbs differentiate movement between the upper and lower body. Homolateral patterns differentiate movement in the right and left side. And contralateral patterns establish diagonal and cross-crawl connections in the body.

Spinal Patterns

As discussed above, the prevertebral spinal patterns begin to develop in the movement through the soft spine while a preborn is in utero, sucking its thumb and squirming in its limited space. The vertebral patterns crystallize at birth when the newborn's head pushes out through the

Patterning Exercise #63: Prespinal Movement

1. Sit or stand in a comfortable position. Imagine a spotlight from the top of your head shining up on the ceiling.
2. Shine the light above you, then begin moving your head in such a way as to slowly draw imaginary shapes on the ceiling with your headlight (PE Fig. 63a-b). Draw whatever shapes are easiest for you—lines, circles, arcs, or figure eights—then reverse the motion.
3. Let the movement of your head pull your entire spine into a wave-like, undulating motion all the way down to your tail in a manner akin to how a kite pulls its tail.

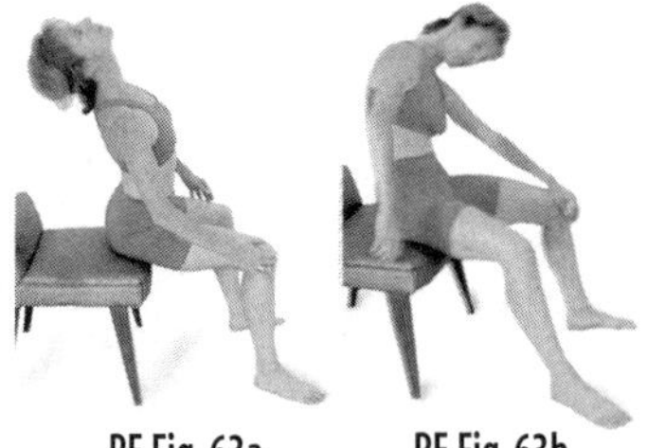

PE Fig. 63a PE Fig. 63b

4. Get into the quadruped position, on your hands and knees. Explore the same quality of wave-like motion in your spine, leading with the top of your head (PE Fig. 63c-d).
5. Then switch and explore leading with your tail. Imagine a spotlight shining from your tail and shine it behind you along various pathways (PE Fig. 63e).

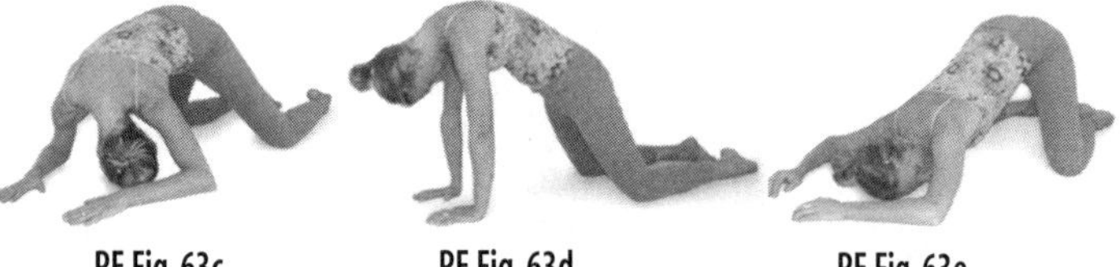

PE Fig. 63c PE Fig. 63d PE Fig. 63e

mother's pelvis and the infant begins looking about with a spinal reach. Over time, the infant moves through many different combinations of spinal flexion, extension, and rotation, pushing, reaching, and rolling over with movements that initiate in the head or tail. Although spinal pushes and reaches are patterns that we all go through, some of us develop either a push or reach with either the head or tail more strongly than others.

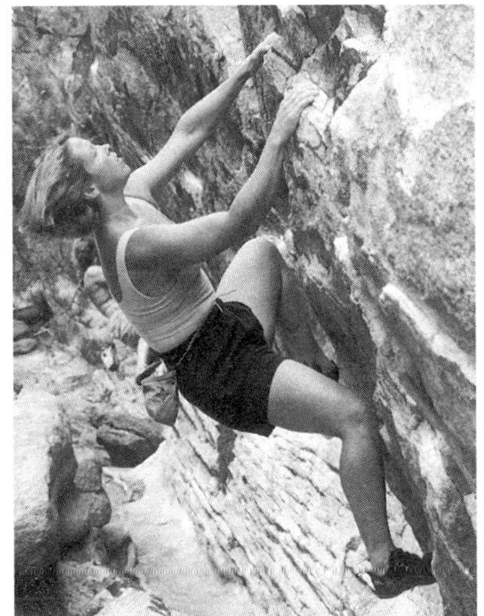

Figure 7.18 A spinal push with the tail gives the climber the thrust she needs to pull herself up.

Spinal patterns echo the movement of a fish, which is guided in its propulsion through water by its specialized sensory receptors along its lateral line that sense water currents. Humans also have an imaginary **lateral line** along the sides of the body, established by spinal movements that differentiate the front of the body from the back (Figure 7.17). A person that is structurally balanced between the front and back has a defined lateral line that bisects the body from the ears to the toes. We clarify the lateral line by making clear movements transitions between spinal flexion and extension.

Perception of a lateral line is subtle and probably most well developed in athletes and dancers who have a clear spatial awareness of their bodies. The clarity or murkiness of the lateral line reflects the strength or weakness of all the patterns, particularly the spinal patterns. If parts of the spinal pushes or reaches become frozen in a held posture anywhere along the spine, creating compression in one area and/or wobbliness in another, this imaginary line becomes blurred as tight fascias and disorganized muscles migrate to either the front or the back of it. Since spinal pushes differentiate the front and back of the body, they can be practiced to develop continuity of tone along the spine and establish a clear lateral line.

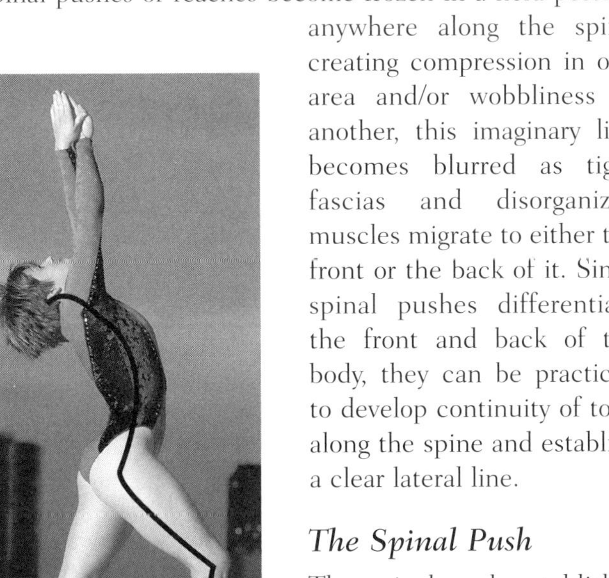

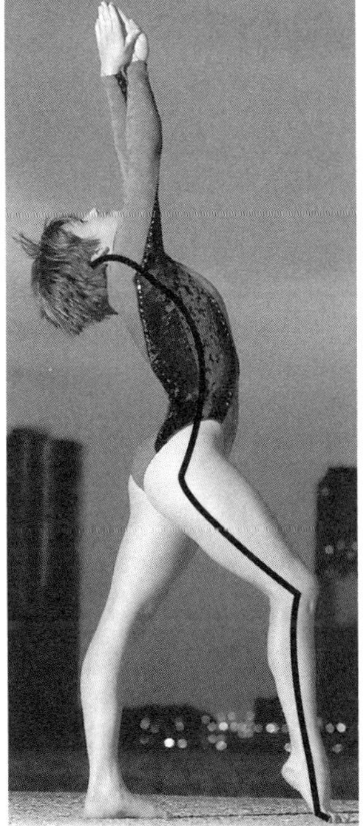

Figure 7.17 The lateral line

The Spinal Push

The spinal push establishes a core strength and stability along the body's spine. Push has been associated with tonic contraction; therefore, push patterns may play an important role in the early organization of postural muscles along the spine.[109] As the push condenses the spine into itself, it compresses the intervertebral joints and engages deep spinal muscles.

A spinal push with the tail initiates with flexion in the coccyx, taking the pelvis into flexion (Figure 7.18). The push then sequences up the front of the spine through the vertebral bodies and disks, ending at the head. As the compressive force of the push travels from one end to the other without breaking anywhere in the middle section, the spinal column flexes and bows as a unified whole.

When the body is supported on the head, as in a head stand, a spinal push with the head takes the spine into extension (Figure 7.19). It initiates at the top of the head, extending the skull on the spine at the uppermost cervical joints, then progressively extends the entire spine, taking the spine into a compressed extension. When an external weight is supported on the head, the spinal push with the head creates an upright, stable posture, such as that which we observe in some elegant tribal women who easily balance loads in baskets on their heads.

The human posture has a natural affinity for reach with the head and push with the tail. A person can energetically push through the head by bearing down through the head, and might feel this action while ducking through a low doorway. Most people feel a push with the tail while defecating; it may sequence all the way to the head, in which case it would flex and curl the entire spine. Women feel a strong spinal push while giving birth. A stubborn child might push through his spine and his feet during a tantrum much like a stubborn mule digs in to avoid being pulled forward. Sumo wrestlers, defensive linebackers, and power lifters usually have an innate and/or well-developed spinal push pattern, which predisposes them to excel at these sports.

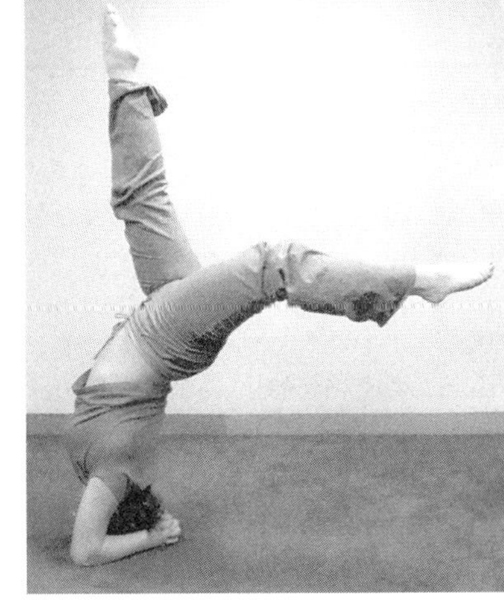

Figure 7.19 A spinal push with the head takes the spine into extension.

A person with a strong spinal push usually has a sturdy trunk and a solid kinesthetic sense of the spine, both physically and psychologically. The spinal push brings one's attention back in, centering a person in

Patterning Exercise #64: Spinal Push

Caution: Do not do this exercise if you have a herniated disc or spinal compression that causes pain. If you have neck problems, be very careful bearing weight on your head, and use gentle pressure to push through your spine. Stop if you feel any sharp or shooting pain. For an easier version of the spinal push, see Patterning Exercise #4.

1. Get into a position in which your weight is supported by your shins, forearms, and forehead (PE Fig. 64a). Without moving, push down through your shins and forearms to sense how the homologous connection through the limbs creates a platform of support for the spinal patterns. Keep this connection during the entire exercise.

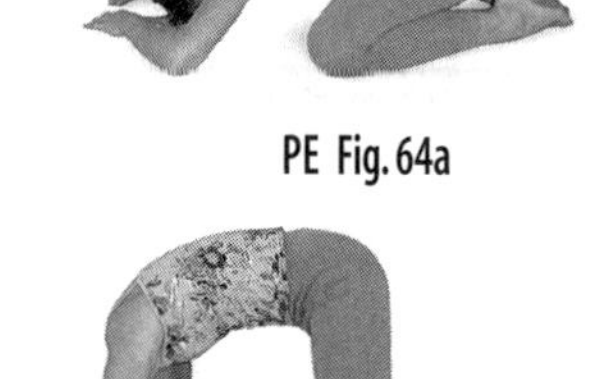

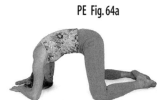

PE Fig. 64a

PE Fig. 64b

2. *Push with the tail:* To begin, take your coccyx into flexion by gently bearing down in the pelvic floor, pushing your tail toward your pubic bone. Continue pushing, pressing each vertebral segment into flexion, one segment at a time, compressing your spine until you are pushing the top of your head into the floor *(be careful not to push too hard)*.
3. If imagery helps you, imagine your spine as a tube of paste with your tail scooping under like a shovel to push the paste through your trunk toward your head.
4. *Push with the head:* Now reverse the action by pushing with your head against the floor. It should rock your skull on your first cervical vertebra, extending it. Then sequentially extend the spine one vertebra at a time until you return to your original position.
5. Alternate between pushing up with the tail, then pushing back with the head. Move slowly at first, sensing the push sequence through each vertebral segment of the spine. Focus on any vertebra that you feel you have skipped over.
6. Once you are comfortable with the action, repeat it in a faster, more fluid manner. Rock between a push with the tail and with the head. This will help you coordinate the action as a more reflexive, organic motion.
7. *Variations on push with the head:* Get a large book and balance it on the top of your head. Or push your head into your hands, sensing the push through your entire spine (PE Fig. 64c). Notice the alignment of your spine. Is it different from your normal alignment? Walk around with the book on your head. Does your walk change? Remove the book, yet still imagine balancing it on your head.

PE Fig. 64c

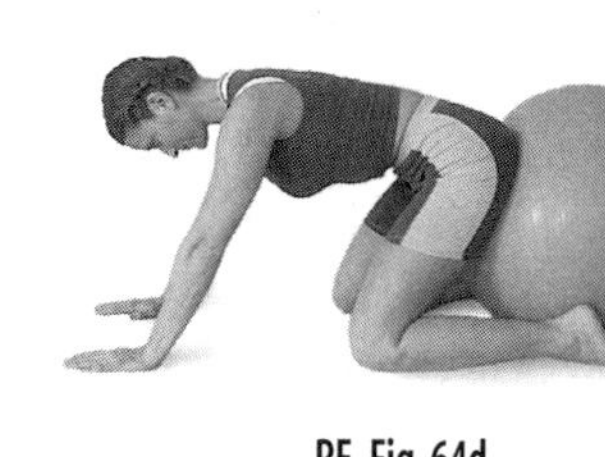

PE Fig. 64d

8. *Variations on push with the tail:* Get in a quadruped position and back your tail up to a surface such as a soft couch or a physioball (PE Fig. 64d). Push, then release. Repeat several times. How far up your spine and how far down your arms does the force of the push travel?

EMSPress.com

the body and mind. A weakness in this pattern can underlie a collapsed spine that lacks structural integrity. The forward head posture, now sometimes called "computer neck," is a classic sign of a weak spinal push with the head.

The Spinal Reach

Like the spinal push, the spinal reach with the head also crystallizes during a normal vaginal birth. Once the head clears the canal, the newborn is free to look around. When a reach with head or tail sequences through the entire column, it elongates and pulls slack out of the spine, taking each intervertebral joint into an open-packed position, and organizing lines of pull along the backbone.

Spinal reaches can be stationary or they can pull the spine through space. As mentioned earlier, we have a natural propensity for reach with the head, which aligns the head over the body and is supported by the head righting reflex. Also, we continually reach out through the perceptual organs of the head to take in the environment around us, a myriad of sights, sounds, and smells. A baby playing peek-a-boo or sound games spontaneously lifts the eyes or ears, elongating the entire spine (Figure 7.20). A person usually reaches through the head during level changes, from lying to sitting and sitting to standing. We also reach with the head to get out of a car, or to stick our head out a door to look out. On a psychological level, a reach with the head expresses alertness and curiosity. It is difficult to be attentive or energized when the head hangs, a posture usually associated with depression or lack of initiative.

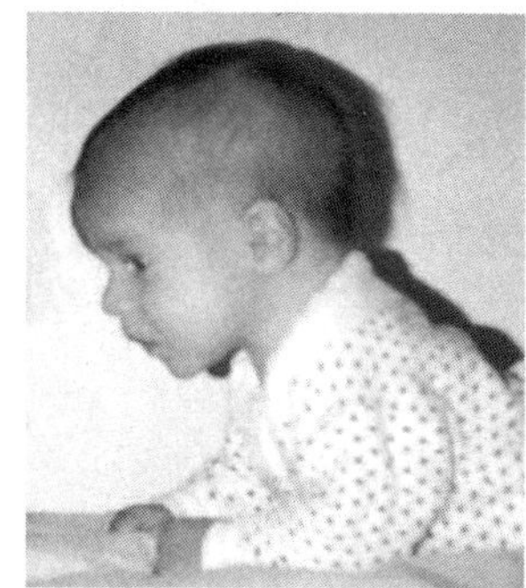

Figure 7.20 A spinal reach with the head (photo courtesy of L. Bright).

On the other end of the spine, a spinal reach with the tail allows us to search the ground under us and adjust our center of gravity accordingly. Adults use a reach with the tail to search for a seat in

Patterning Exercise #65: Spinal Reach

1. Get in a quadruped position. Subtly or energetically reach your tail toward your feet until you feel the reach begin to pull you backward, elongating your spine, so that eventually you will be sitting on your forelegs (PE Fig. 65a).

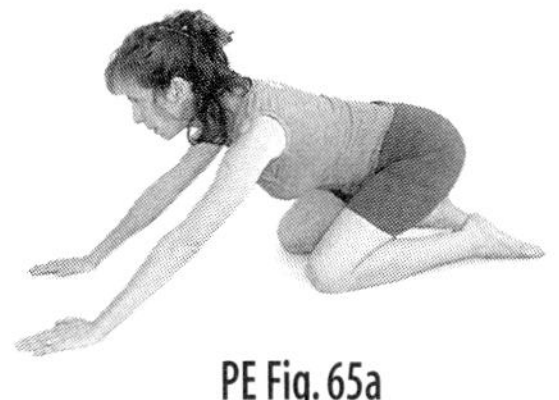

PE Fig. 65a

2. Next, subtly or energetically reach up and forward with the top of your head. Sense the reach with your head elongating your spine, and when it does, return to the quadruped position (PE Fig. 65b).

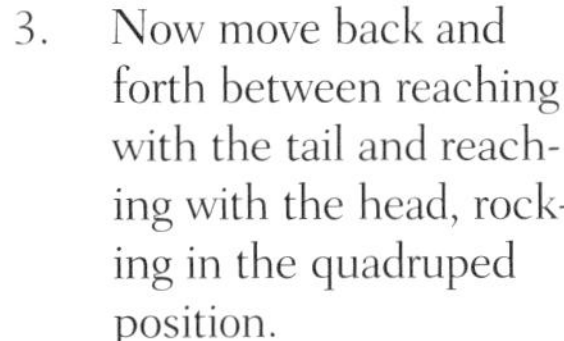

3. Now move back and forth between reaching with the tail and reaching with the head, rocking in the quadruped position.

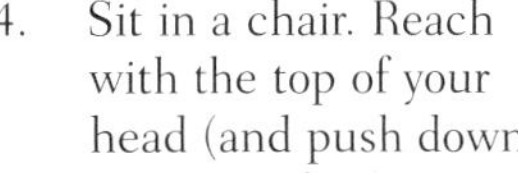

4. Sit in a chair. Reach with the top of your head (and push down with your feet) to stand up. Then reach with your tail to sit back down. Repeat several times, maintaining a simultaneous reach with both your head and tail as you stand up and sit down.

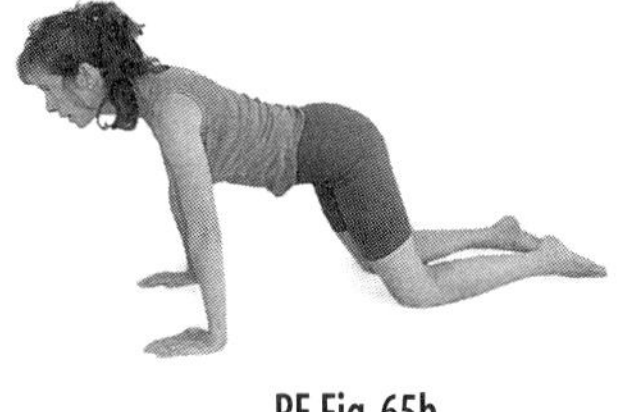

PE Fig. 65b

a dark theater; babies reach with the tail when they sit back into a quadruped position. Reaching with the tail tends to be a vague and difficult pattern for a lot of people to feel. Perhaps humans tend to have a weakness in this pattern because the human coccyx is only a rudimentary tail. If this pattern is weak, sensing a distinct reach with the tail can wake up sensations in the pelvic floor that might be confused with sexual feelings. With practice, reach with the tail can be strengthened, which is helpful because it lengthens the lower spine and helps a person to adjust and balance the lower body to changing positions. It can also bring subtle articulations to the lower pelvis and hips.

An overly strong spinal push coupled with a weak reach can create compression in the spine and limit the range of movement. On a psychological level, this pattern shows up when a person stubbornly tucks the pelvis under and digs in the heels into the ground, refusing to be moved, a pattern also found in the classic masochistic character of Reichian psychology. A weak spinal push, on the other hand, shows up in a backbone that lacks integrity and easily buckles. This pattern is found in the classic oral character type in which a person feels empty and collapsed from a lack of emotional nourishment and support (see the section on "Bioenergetics" in Chapter 15).

The compressive forces of spinal pushes balance the tensional pulls of spinal reaches. Ideally, a person is able to sense the difference between the two actions along the spinal pathway. A balanced combination of spinal push and reach is evident in the flexible grace yet poised strength of certain tribal people who balance heavy loads on their heads and then walk with ease. To cultivate a flexible strength in the spine, a person can explore spinal pushes and reaches, differentiating sensations from the compression of pushing with the tensional pull of reaching.

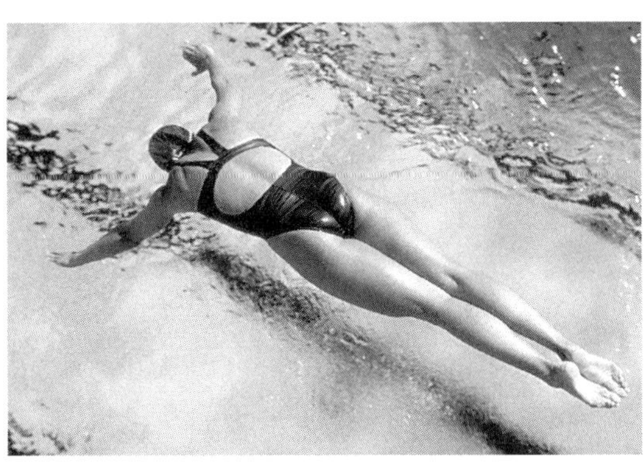

Figure 7.21 Note how the strength and symmetry of the limbs in this homologous pattern keeps the spine centered.

Homologous Patterns

Homologous means the same on both sides. There are four homologous patterns made up of combinations of upper or lower body push and reach patterns. These include a push with both arms, a push with both legs, a reach with both arms, and a reach with both legs. The upper homologous push is one of the first actions a baby takes to make a level change on his own. A baby also scoots backward with a homologous push through both arms, reaches backward with both feet to slide down off a step or stool, or pushes down with both feet to stand up.

The homologous patterns recapitulate the movements of amphibians. Take, for example, the frog, which hops by pushing off its back legs while reaching with its front legs. Children explore homologous movement in the game of "leap-frog." Since homologous patterns are symmetrical, they tend to lack spinal rotation. The frog springs forward, jumping out of the water or into it, without the option of twisting because its pattern lacks a right/left differentiation of movement. In contrast, the next species up the evolutionary ladder, the reptile, can push with one side while reaching with the other, which rotates the spine.

Homologous movements differentiate the upper body from the lower body. Homologous support in the arms and legs provides a platform on which the spine can move along its vertical axis (Figure 7.21). Since homologous patterns lack rotation, they limit spinal movement to flexion and extension.

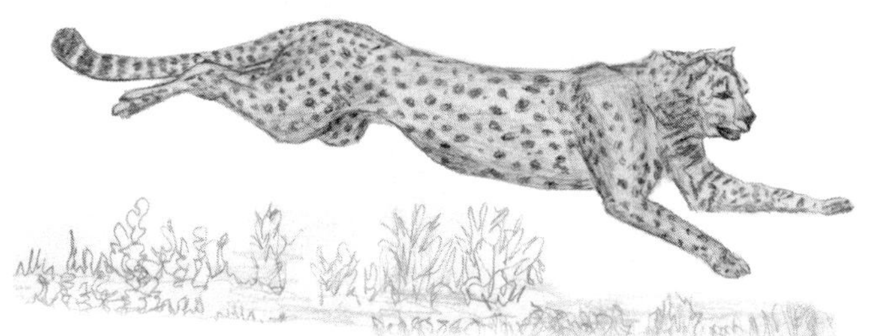

Figure 7.22 At top speeds, the cheetah moves into a homologous stride.

The more parts of the body moving in the same direction, the more direct and strong the movement. Therefore, homologous patterns, particularly patterns of locomotion, tend to be inherently stronger and faster than homolateral or contralateral patterns of locomotion. For example, when a cheetah, one of the fastest runners among mammals, begins chasing his prey, he starts out in a contralateral gait. As he speeds up, his gait shifts to homolateral. When he hits top speed, he begins stretching out his forelegs and hindlegs in a graceful yet incredibly swift homologous gait (Figure 7.22). (The cheetah has been clocked at up to 70 miles per hour.)

What types of exercise are homologous, homolateral, or contralateral?

On a psychological level, the homologous patterns reflect a full commitment to the action. If a baby reaches with both arms, we know that she really wants to be picked up. In our culture, people usually take on a relaxed, one-legged stance, but the homologous person "stands on her own two feet." Two people meeting in mutual homologous stances end up meeting face to face, in direct opposition to each other physically, a position associated with power and confrontation. Most people converse from a comfortable, one-legged stance that actually gives them the flexibility to shift, rotate, and look around.

On a mechanical level, the homologous stance provides maximum musculoskeletal support if the legs are directly under the hips and all the joints are in a neutral position—being neither flexed nor hyperextended—through the knees, hips, and spine. This balanced support is important for a person with an unstable pelvis or sacrum because standing on one leg can twist the pelvis and further destabilize already dysfunctional joints.

In a seated posture, the sit bones replace the feet as our base of support. Sitting with one sit bone higher than the other, which often happens when a person crosses the legs, can twist the pelvis and spine.

In general, homologous postures and movements give the spine a more stable base of support because they lack rotation. Thus anyone having difficulties with unstable spinal joints can benefit greatly from practicing both spinal and homologous movement that stabilize the spine. For example, working out on a rowing machine is homologous because the arms and legs are moving symmetrically. This does not mean that a person should avoid rotational patterns but that practicing spinal and homologous movement will establish a centered core stability for subsequent activities that twist and turn.

Homologous Push Patterns

In adult movement patterns, the spine tends to *support* the body leaving the limbs free to *move*. This supporter/mover relationship is reversed in babies—they tend to support the body through the limbs, freeing the spine for movement. During the upper homologous push, the baby's arms support weight, which frees the head and upper spine for movement (Figure 7.23). Small babies might be found rocking the spine back and forth on the homologous base of the hands and shins. This action resembles a chair or couch sliding back and forth on its gliders.

The upper homologous push establishes lines of force that travel through the arms into the spine, creating a dimensional cross between them, and providing support for extension and hyperextension of the spine. The lower homologous push sends lines of force from the feet through the legs and pelvis into the trunk, extending the lumbar spine. Both upper and lower pushes, when organized and symmetrical, are marked by a widening across the shoulder girdle and/or the pelvic girdle. This widening creates more space for the spine in between the limbs. Take, for example, the cat arch exercise, a basic homologous pattern (Figure 7.24a-b). The posterior muscles along the neck and base of the skull insert along the thoracic spine, thereby rooting the neck between the shoulder blades. Given this, chronic tension between the shoulder blades can restrict head and neck movement, as well as the structural balance of the shoulder girdle.

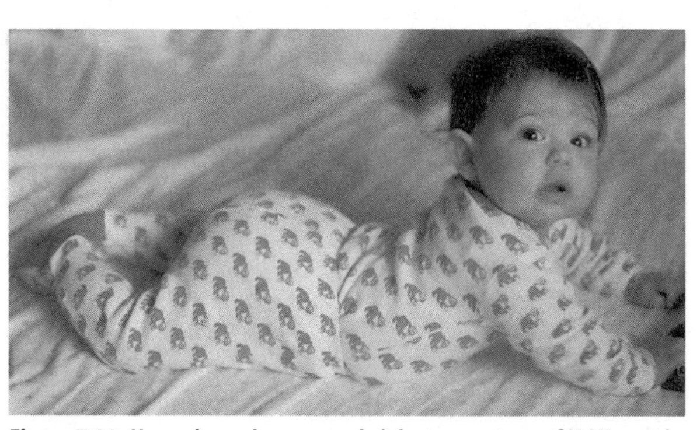

Figure 7.23 Upper homologous push (photo courtesy of K. Wasson).

Links to Practical Applications

Taking a Stance

Notice the position you tend to stand in. Do you rest on one leg or two? Are your knees straight, bent, or locked? How do you stand as you are talking to other people? Explore changing your stance. If you tend to stand on one leg, practice standing on two. Put your feet under your shoulders for optimal support. Try it for several days and see if you begin to feel any different. At the very least, you should feel more supported.

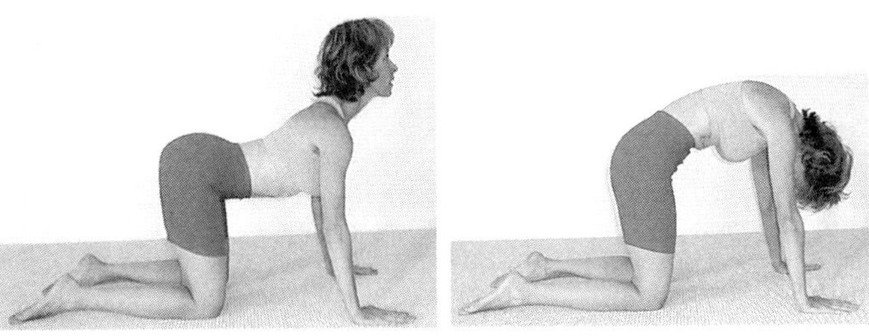

Figure 7.24a-b Homologous support for spinal movement

If a person pinches the shoulders together, the cervical spine will not be free to extend. By reaching through the head and keeping the shoulders wide, a person can lengthen the neck and free the cervical spine during movements that extend and hyperextend the spine.

A strong and balanced homologous push, either lower or upper, helps organize patterns of symmetry in the legs or arms. Our vertical human posture requires a strong lower homologous push to stand on both legs. Look at a room full of people standing around and those with a homologous stance will be obvious: both legs will be planted firmly under the torso. As mentioned earlier, the homologous stance provides a stable foundation, whereas a homolateral stance on one leg provides a more flexible foundation.

The strength of the homologous pathways shows up in the symmetry of the limbs and the relationship the hips and shoulders keep with the spine during movement. For example, when there is a strong underlying homologous support, the shoulders and hips will remain relatively

Patterning Exercise #66: Homologous Push through the Limbs

This exercise will help strengthen lines of force from your limbs into your spine, as well as improve symmetry in your body. If you tend to hike or round your shoulders, the homologous push can also help straighten them out.

Caution: If your shoulders and hips are tight, the prone homologous position will stretch them and you might be sore afterwards; therefore, remain in it only as long as you are comfortable. Also, if you have a lower back pain, this push could aggravate it. To protect your lower back, tuck your toes under and contract your lower abdominal muscles. Skip this exercise if you have a disc problem.

1. Lie on a padded floor on your belly. Turn your head to one side, or rest your forehead on a small pillow or rolled up towel.
2. Put both your arms out to the sides. Bend your elbows so that your forearms are at right angles to the upper arms (PE Fig. 66a). Make sure your palms are flat and all five fingers are touching the floor. Widen and sink across the front of your chest. Reach your elbows out to the sides to widen across your shoulders. Keep your neck long by reaching out the top of your head. Yield into this position by focusing on widening and sinking through your chest, forearms, and hands.
3. *Upper homologous push:* Slowly press your entire hands and forearms into the floor. Sense the force of the push traveling up your arms, into your back, and down your spine. Make sure not to pull your arms up or in, but continue to push them out and down. Gently push, then release. Do this several times.
4. Repeat the push and progress into lifting your head and chest off the floor (PE Fig. 66b-c). Look at the floor to engage optical support for your head. Then rest.
5. Now explore a rhythmic push with the hands and forearms in a motion that rocks the whole body. Then yield in this position a minute before going on.
6. Stay in the same position with one variation: scoot close enough to a wall that you can put your feet flat against the wall with your knees bent (PE Fig. 66d). Keep your knees and thighs relaxed and weighted. Feel the contact your pelvis makes with the floor; widen across the front of your pelvis so that you feel your pubic bone and hip sockets widen and sink into the floor.
7. *Lower homologous push:* Now slowly push against the wall, feeling the push travel up your legs, into your pelvis, and up into your spine. Your heels will come off the wall so that you are only pushing with your toes. Push several times, then release. The push will straighten your knees and inwardly rotate your legs.
8. *Upper and lower together:* Combine the upper and lower push by pushing simultaneously with both your hands and feet, then release. Sense how the forces from the upper and the lower meet along the spine.
9. Then explore rhythmic pushing that rocks the body, alternately pushing with the arms, then the feet.

PE Fig. 66a

PE Fig. 66b

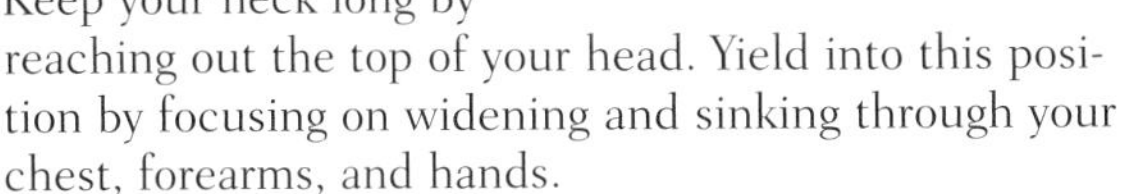

PE Fig. 66c

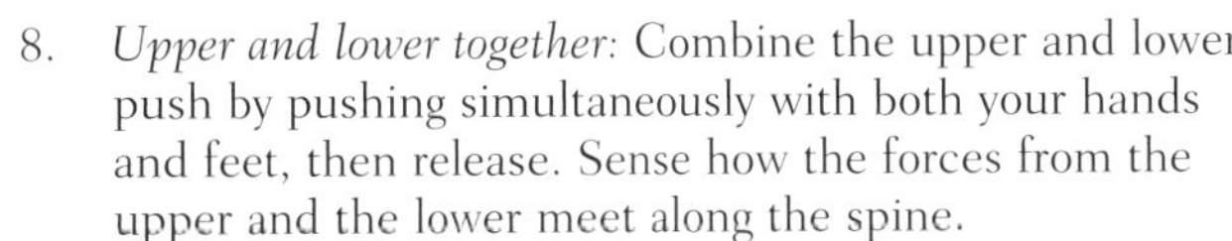

PE Fig. 66d

Feedback: Do your right and left sides push with symmetry? If so, the shoulders and hips will remain square in relation to each other. Get up slowly and stand, then walk around. Do you feel any changes in your posture or movement? (Most people feel that their shoulders and chest seem wider and more open, and their legs more connected to the ground.)

square to the spine, even when a person twists the spine (Figure 7.25). When homologous patterns overpower spinal patterns, the flow of movement between the upper and lower halves of the body along spinal pathways may become disrupted. As a result, a person might habitually hinge in the lower back or neck, resulting in an exaggerated lordotic curve in either place. This hinging pattern is common in forward head posture, where the flow of movement along the spine is lost between the shoulders.

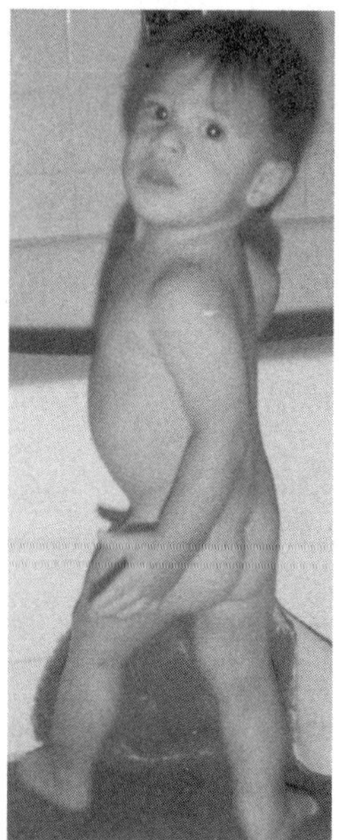

Figure 7.25 With good homologous support, the hips and shoulders stay square to the spine during rotation (photo courtesy of L. Bright).

Homologous Reach Patterns

The homologous push patterns compress the limbs into the trunk, whereas the homologous reach patterns do just the opposite, extending the limbs away from the trunk. Therefore, reach patterns establish lines of tension and pull between the limbs and spine. This relationship can be observed in a baby who reaches in earnest to be picked up and stretches through her whole body. On a psychological level, her action is earnest because reaching with both arms represents a full commitment to being picked up, whereas a baby who only sort of wants to be picked up might just extend one arm in a half-hearted attempt.

When the homologous reach pattern make a full sequence through the core, it pulls the spine along. In adult patterns, the movement of the arms might pull the trunk along during a hug, or extend the spine while reaching for a heavy box on a top shelf (Figure 7.26). Whether or not the homologous reach patterns

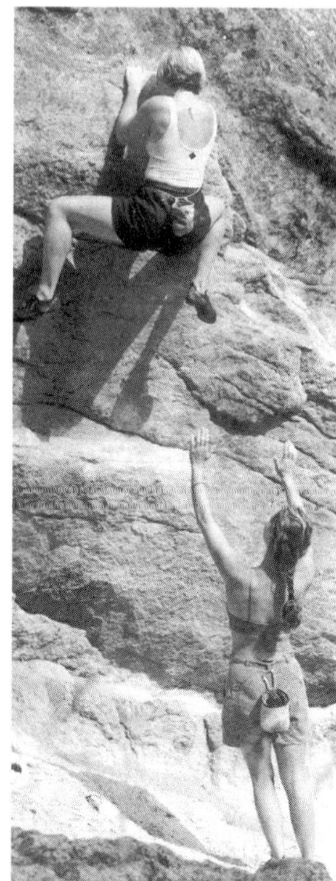

Figure 7.26 Upper homologous reach.

Patterning Exercise #67: Homologous Reach Patterns

To truly reach with your arms and legs, initiate the action in the fingers and toes, then allow the reach to extend the center of your limbs.

1. *Reach with the upper:* Sit either on your forelegs or in a cross-legged position (PE Fig. 67a). Reach with both arms, initiating in the fingertips. Allow the reach to sequence into your spine, pulling you into a quadruped position (PE Fig. 67b).

PE Fig. 67a

2. Return to the original position, then reach again, using more effort so that the reach pulls you up and over your hips, extending your lower limbs so that you land in the upper homologous push position (see PE Fig. 66c).

PE Fig. 67b

3. *Reach with the lower:* Sit on a small physioball or a soft chair. Reach down and out with both feet until the reach extends your body and slides you off the ball or chair onto the floor.
4. Lie on your back with your legs straight. Slowly reach through the toes of both feet, allowing the reach to pull the slack out of your legs, lower back, and spine (PE Fig. 67c).
4. Now reach both hands toward the ceiling. Sense how the reach gradually sequences up your arms and shoulders, pulling the slack out of your tissues. Sense the reach sequencing into your spine and taking out the slack in tissues between your shoulder blades. Explore reaching symmetrically with both arms in many different directions.

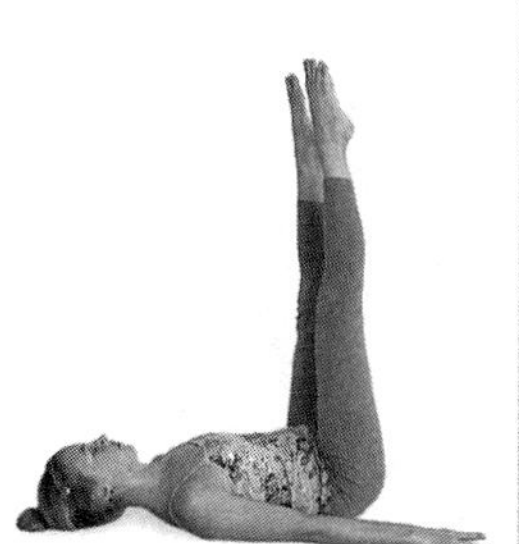

PE Fig. 67c

5. *Alternating upper and lower reach:* Lie over a physioball on your belly, with both legs bent. Slowly reach through both hands until the reach rocks you onto your hands (PE Fig. 67d). Then, with your legs straight, slowly reach back with both feet until the reach rocks you back onto your feet.

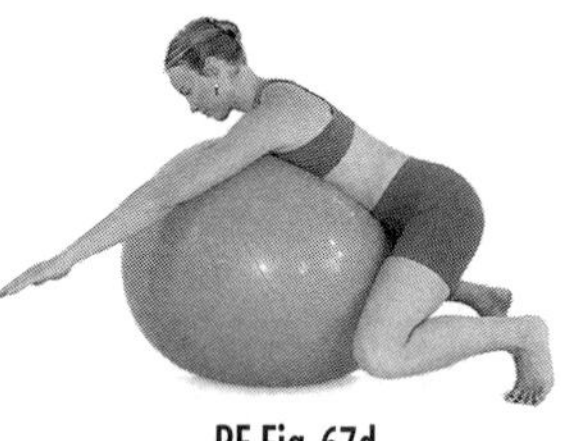

PE Fig. 67d

EMSPress.com

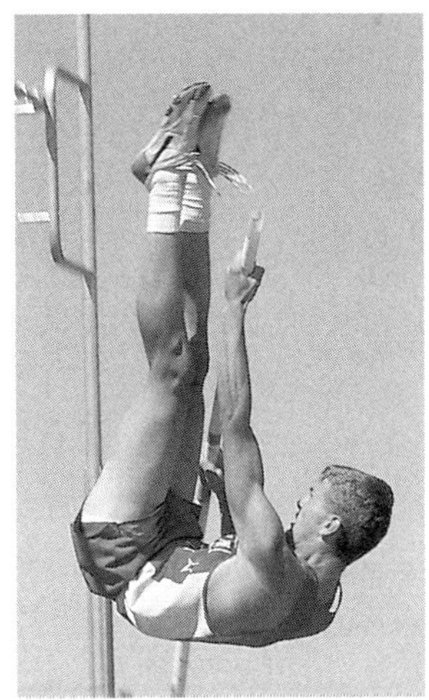

Figure 7.27 A lower homologous reach

of the limbs sequence into the trunk is a matter of personal habit.

The homologous reach with the lower body is probably the least common of the four patterns because our feet are usually planted on the ground. Reach patterns tend to occur in an open chain through the free end of a limb, although it is possible to energetically reach through the feet while still standing on both feet. We reach with one foot while pushing with the other as we walk. A baby might reach with both feet to slide backward off a lap. We also see this pattern in sports. A long jumper reaches with the legs to cover more distance; a pole vaulter builds up momentum, then uses a combination of strong push with the upper, followed by a reach with the lower to thrust the body up and over the bar (Figure 7.27).

Homolateral Pushes

The homologous patterns show up in a square shape between the shoulders and hips, whereas the homolateral patterns show up in side bending (Figure 7.28). As patterns progress to homolateral, they begin to rotate the spine. The homolateral push recapitulates the pattern of a reptile, the first species to adapt to life on land, in its ability to turn right or left via limb initiation. The homolateral pattern initiates from a push with either one hand or foot, which extends one side of the body while flexing the other. There is no homolateral reach because a reach with one hand or foot sequences across the body diagonally, resulting in a contralateral pattern.

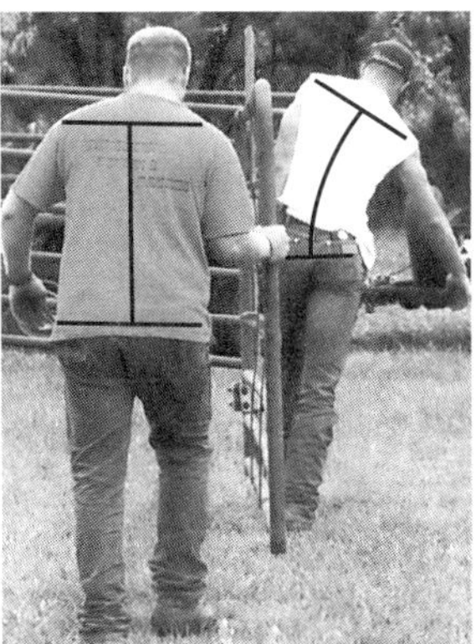

Figure 7.28 Contrast between a homologous pattern (on the left) and a homolateral pattern (on the right)

Homolateral push patterns organize lines of force and movement pathways along the sides of the body. They establish right-left differentiation and lateralization in the body. A push in one limb flexes one side of the body while extending the other, and the spine rotates in between. A shot putter throws a ball with great power harnessed from a homolateral push in the foot. During a homolateral crawl, the right and left halves of the body coordinate a lateral shift by alternating roles of supporter and mover. Hand-mouth and hand-eye coordinations, as well as head turning initiated by visual scanning, underlie homolateral patterns and rotate the spine.

The homolateral push with the arms slides the body backward, while the homolateral push with the legs propels the body forward. Homolateral locomotion appears in a "lizard-like" crawl that is initiated by a homolateral push, with the belly lifted off the ground while the pelvis is still in contact with the ground. During this crawl, the upper and lower girdles move in lateral shifts, causing the tail to swing from side to side pointing to the foot on the flexed side.

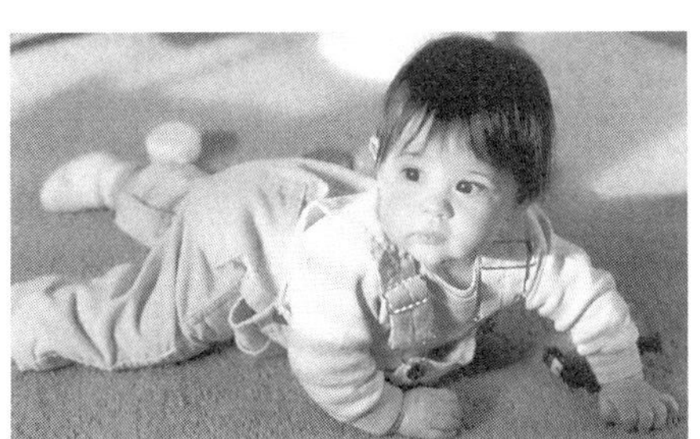

Figure 7.29 The homolateral push (photo courtesy of K. Wasson).

Patterning Exercise #68: Exploring Flexor and Extensor Reflexes

This is an excellent exercise to help you develop flexor and extensor reflexes that can protect you during a fall. Make sure you have a large area to practice in so that you do not bump into anything.

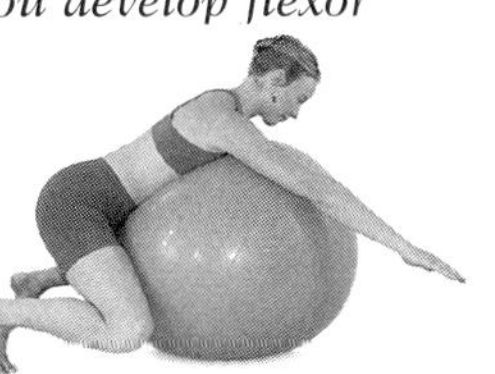

PE Fig. 68a

1. Lie on your belly and chest over a physioball, bend your knees, and tuck your toes under.
2. Push off with both feet and reach out with your hands, landing with your weight on your hands (PE Fig. 68a-b).

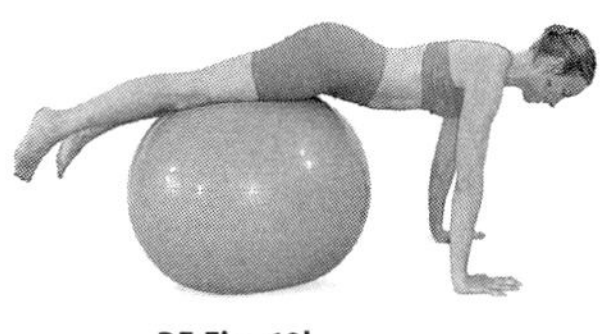

PE Fig. 68b

3. Then push back to your original position.
4. Alternate pushing with feet, then your hands, to roll back and forth on the ball. Remember to reach with your hands while pushing with your feet and vice-versa. Push and roll in a rhythmic, fluid manner.
5. If there are any of the four patterns—upper push, upper reach, lower push, lower reach—that you want to explore, position yourself on the ball to do that movement, then slowly practice the movement.
6. Explore using the momentum of the lower push to lift your hips up over the ball (PE Fig. 68c).

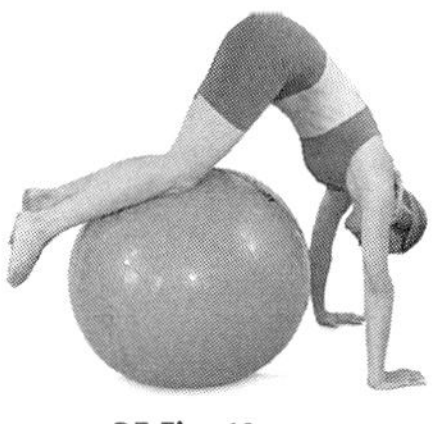

PE Fig. 68c

Patterning Exercise #69: Homolateral Push

This pattern is probably the hardest of the developmental patterns to learn, so do not get discouraged if you find it difficult. With practice, it will become easier.

1. Lie on your belly on a floor upon which you can slide (such as wood or linoleum). (You may need to wear kneepads or thick pants that can pad bony hips and knees.) Begin in upper homologous push position, with both arms out to each side, bending your elbows at right angles. Flatten your hands and palms flat on the floor, making sure each finger is pressing down evenly. Do an upper homologous push to press your thorax and head up off the floor (PE Fig. 69a). Hold this position.

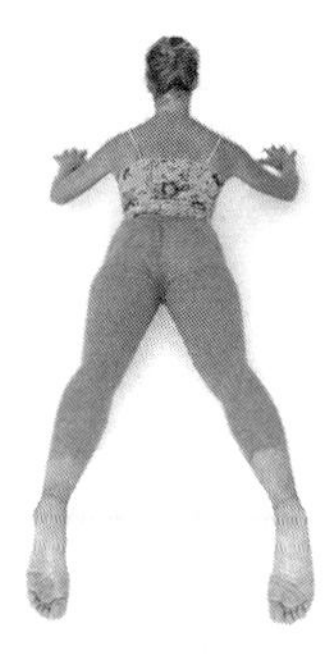

PE Fig. 69a

2. *Upper homolateral push:* Push through one forearm until you feel the force travel into your spine and that side of your body (PE Fig. 69b). Your spine should side-bend away from the side of the push, with your coccyx pointing to the opposite foot.
3. Then push through the other forearm. Your weight should shift to that side of your body as your spine side-bends in the opposite direction.
4. Alternate pushing with one arm, then the other. Let the push slightly roll your pelvis from side to side, but still keep your pubic bone in contact with the floor. Sense when the push sequences through the pelvis and starts to flex the leg on the same side.

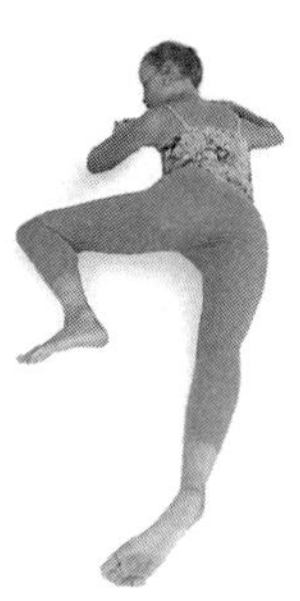

PE Fig. 69b

5. *Lower homolateral push:* Again, begin in upper homologous push position and bring one foot up to the side (PE Fig. 69b). Next, push through the toes on that foot to extend that side of the body. The leg on the other side of your body should naturally flex. Then push through the toes on that side.
6. *This variation is easier:* Lie in the upper homologous push position with both feet against a wall, legs bent. Gently push through one leg, then the other, sensing the force from each foot traveling up that side of your body.
7. *This variation may be even easier:* Lie over a small physioball with both hands on the floor. Gently push with one hand, sensing how that side of your body extends and the opposite knee flexes. Return to center and repeat on the other side. Alternate sides until the transitions are smooth.

Once a baby learns to push up onto his arms, a whole new level of the world becomes available for exploration. An underlying homologous push creates a solid base of support to press the chest off the ground (which keeps lizards from scraping their bellies), while the homolateral push gives the baby support on one arm while freeing the other arm for movement (Figure 7.29). With the ability to move one side of the body independently of the other, the baby expands his range; he is able to turn the upper body in any direction to explore the space all the way around him. To illustrate this point, think of the homologous frog that can't turn very easily; it has to hop in a wide circle in order to face the opposite direction.

During a homolateral crawl, a baby pushes off with one foot that propels that side of the body forward while laterally shifting the weight to the other side. Babies usually crawl in a contralateral pattern but use the lower homolateral push to extend and turn that side of the body toward something they are reaching for. A baby might also initiate the homolateral action by turning her head to look to one side, which shifts weight onto one arm.

The homolateral gait, in which the leg and arm on the same side of the body move in unison, is unnatural in humans and may indicate a neurological disability (take, for example, Frankenstein's monster). When homolateral patterns have an underlying homologous support, although they side-bend and twist the spine, if the rotation is even distributed though each vertebral segment, the spine moves with an even continuity of tone and remains fairly stable throughout the action. Conversely, when the homolateral push lacks homologous support, the spine may collapse and move with chronic asymmetries or excessive rotations in certain segments. Of all the patterns, this one may be the most difficult to learn because it is transitional, halfway between lying down and being up on all fours.

Can you sense in yourself or see in others the underlying tone of a yield, push, reach, or pull? Do certain areas of your body differ in tone from other areas during these actions? Which action do you feel the most affinity for? The least? Which action is easiest for you?

Contralateral Reaches

Four-legged mammals walk with a contralateral pattern in which one paw reaches and pulls the diagonally opposite limb through. Human gait patterns, such as walking or running, are examples of contralateral movement as well. Our gait is initiated by a reach with one foot, which sequences diagonally across the body to the opposite arm. During normal walking or running, the arms swing in opposition to the legs while the thorax rotates with the arm that swings, and the pelvis rotates with the leg that swings.

A movement pattern is only contralateral if it initiates from a reach with one hand or foot and sequences through the waist to the diagonally opposite limb. When a baby crawls in a contralateral pattern (officially called "creeping"), the reach of one hand sequences through the spine along a spiral-shaped pathway, pulling the opposite leg forward. The reach also sequences diagonally, counter-rotating the shoulder girdle with the pelvis.

A good place to observe the intricacy of the sleek counter-rotations of the contralateral movement is in a cat as it slowly stalks its prey. The cat's backbone moves forward in a series of flexible yet controlled and subtly gyrating twists. Each major body mass—head, thorax, and pelvis—moves independently around its central axis, moving the cat's spine through all three planes. In humans, the hips also sequence through all three planes during the bipedal gait.[110] Stability is ensured only by the combined rotational mobility of many joints. In fact, contralateral movement sequences through the combined rotations of more than 130 joints along the spine, as well as numerous joints in the limbs. If each of these linked joints moves in its respective range and contributes its share of motion, the contralateral motion passes in a wave-like progression of rotations and counter-rotations along a series of linked joints from one limb, through the multi-segmented spine, into the opposite limb. Restrictions anywhere along the sequence can cause hypermobility somewhere else, limiting the intricacy and efficiency of the contralateral pattern.

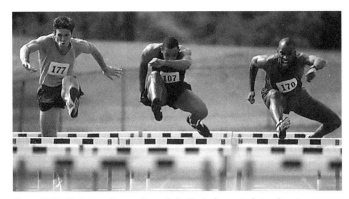

Figure 7.30 Variances in rotations of the limbs in contralateral patterns

Contralateral patterns in humans differ from those in other mammals for several reasons. First of all, the human spine is an upended beam; weight passes from head to tail

Patterning Exercise #70: Quadruped Position and Contralateral Patterning

This exercise will help you check the underlying pathways of support in a neutral quadruped position, then crawl with this support.

1. Get in a quadruped position. Make sure your knees are under your hips and your hands are under your shoulders (PE Fig. 70a). Use a mirror for feedback if you want to check your alignment.
2. Crawl forward and backward, taking note of the movement quality so that you can compare it to crawling after this exercise.
3. In the quadruped position, energetically push through the head and tail and sense a connection along the front of your spine. Then energetically reach through your head and tail to elongate your spine. Rock your spine back and forth, getting a sense of alternately reaching through your head, then through your tail, to elongate your spine.

PE Fig. 70a

4. Relax your lower back. It should hang like a bridge without collapsing. Then lightly pull your lower abdominal wall straight up by lightly contracting it, but keep your upper abdominal wall relaxed so you can breathe fully and easily.
5. Isometrically push down with both hands and feel the support this gives your across your shoulders. This push should lift your shoulders higher than your hips, as well as widen them.
6. Isometrically push down through both forelegs and knees and feel the support this gives your pelvic girdle. Your hips and sacrum. The back of your pelvis should rest easily on your thighs, widening in the horizontal plane.
7. Shift your weight to one side. If you still are energetically reaching with the head and tail and a pushing through your supporting arm and leg, you will be able to balance on one side without sagging or tightening. These underlying pushes will give your body the support you need to make a lateral shift to one side without losing the support of the other side.
8. Slowly reach one hand along the floor in front of you (PE Fig. 70b). Stay supported on your other three limbs. Keep reaching until you feel the opposite leg pull through (PE Fig. 70c).
9. Come back to the quadruped position, then repeat step 8 on the other side.
10. From the quadruped position, slowly crawl, first reaching with one hand, then the other. Make sure to keep your shoulders wide, head up and reaching, and to maintain a strong push through your limbs. Also, make sure to lead each step by reaching with your hands. Let your lower back slightly sway so that the movement can sequence through it.

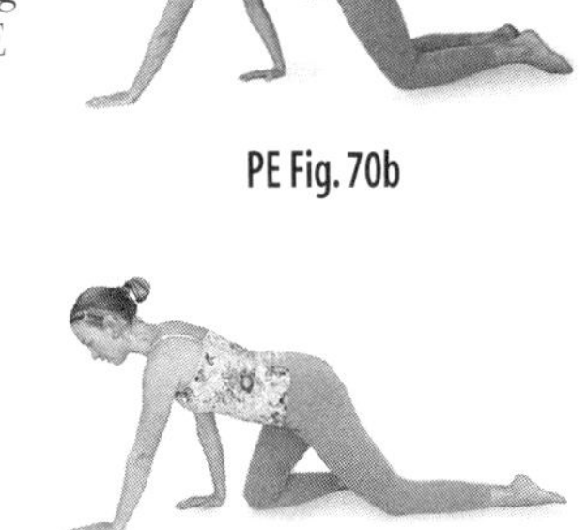

PE Fig. 70b

PE Fig. 70c

Feedback: Compare crawling now with how you crawled at the beginning of the exercise. Is it easier? If so, how?

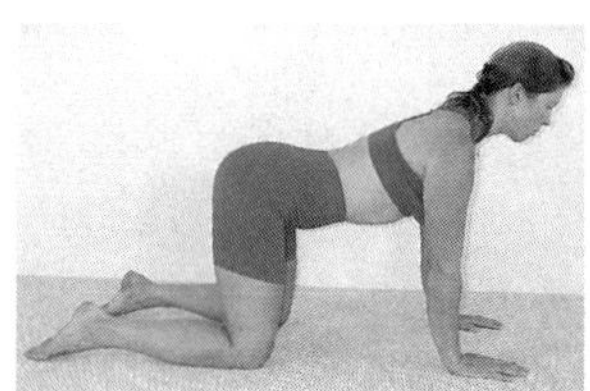

Figure 7.31a The quadruped position with the support of the underlying pushes and reaches balances stability with length.

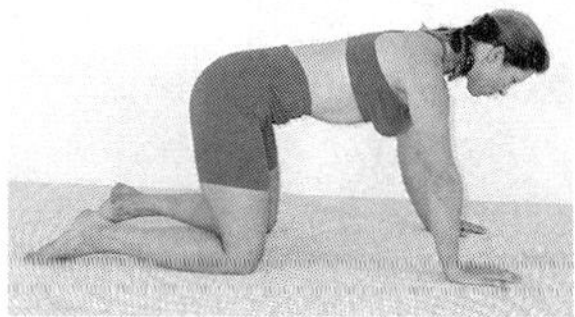

Figure 7.31b The flat back lacks spinal reach and extension, but has strong spinal push.

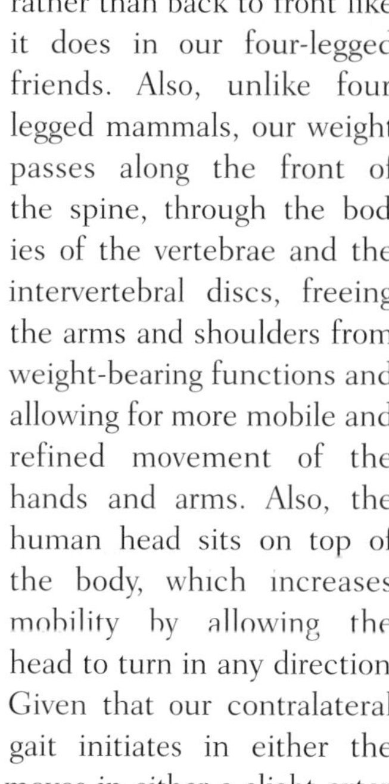

rather than back to front like it does in our four-legged friends. Also, unlike four-legged mammals, our weight passes along the front of the spine, through the bodies of the vertebrae and the intervertebral discs, freeing the arms and shoulders from weight-bearing functions and allowing for more mobile and refined movement of the hands and arms. Also, the human head sits on top of the body, which increases mobility by allowing the head to turn in any direction. Given that our contralateral gait initiates in either the hand or foot, and each limb moves in either a slight external or internal rotation (unlike a quadruped whose limbs lack our rotational capacity), the possibilities for variations in contralateral patterns are broad (Figure 7.30).

A baby can move in any direction from a contralateral crawl. This quadruped pattern is crucial for sequencing between all fours and kneeling or standing. The spine moves forward and up, suspended between horizontal and vertical.

The success of contralateral patterns depends on underlying spinal, homologous, and homolateral support. The strength of the underlying patterns can be seen in the integrity of the spine in a quadruped position, where a person is supported on the hands and knees (Figure 7.31a-b). In this position, a spinal push creates a connection along the front of the spine. A spinal reach extends the head and tail, bringing the head closer to vertical and bringing the hips to a horizontal position. A homologous push through both arms maintains the integrity and width of the shoulder girdle, while a lower homologous push supports the sacrum and pelvic bones. The lumbar spine relaxes without sagging, forming a long bridge between the pelvis and thorax. An underlying homolateral push gives the body the support and flexibility to make a lateral shift to one side without losing the support of or collapsing the other side.

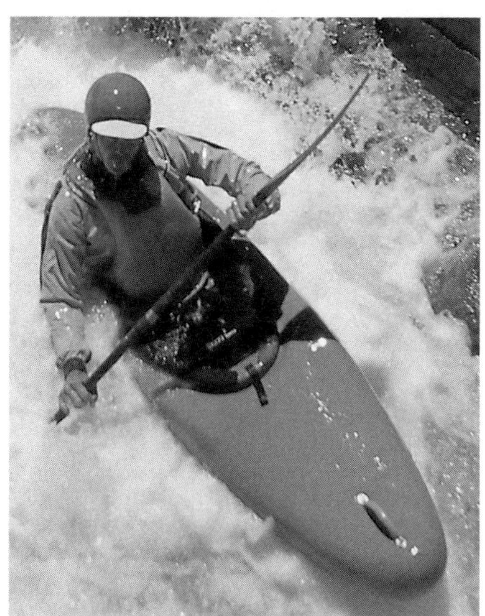

Figure 7.32 A kayaker controls his ride with twisting motions of the waist.

The contralateral pattern is thus the culmination of all the patterns. On a psychological level, it reflects an essential capacity of the uniquely human brain to reach for and take hold of an idea and make something creative (or destructive) out of it. The contralateral ape exhibits a rudimentary mental ability for rational and creative thought, although the contralateral pattern of the ape is more physical than mental. In humans, contralateral patterns are the most developed on both levels. The personality of the contralateral pattern is best seen in the cat, whose insatiable curiosity is always leading it into some kind of trouble. Likewise, on a behavioral level, our contralateral capacities to reach out in any direction drive us to continually explore new territory, to reach out and grasp new information, and to change the world to fit our ideals.

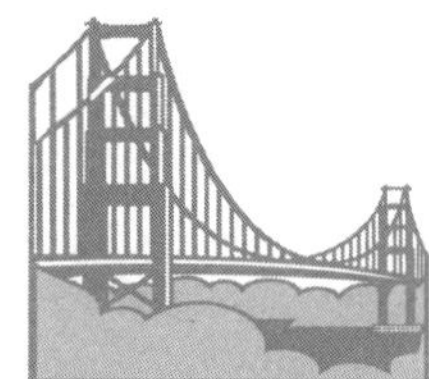

Bridge to Practice

Checking Your Client's Spinal Connection

Have your client lie prone resting his head on his forearms. Is his spine straight or side-bent? Run your hands along the spine to check for rotations from neutral.

Have your client turn his head to one side. Did this change the alignment of the spine? It should have initiated a subtle homolateral side-bend to that side of the spine. Check both sides. If he tends to be off to one side, homologous and spinal reflexes and patterns may strengthen his spinal connection.

Lumbar Reflexes, Rolls, and Gyroscopic Twists

As mentioned earlier, each of the developmental patterns has a number of underlying reflexes. *Lumbar reflexes*, which side-bend and twist the waist, underlie all contralateral patterns. They allow a full sequence to occur between the upper and lower body and between the right and left sides. Although there is no actual reflex called a "lumbar reflex," a number of reflexive responses can be triggered in the sides of the waist. When active, they flex the trunk and rotate it toward the side of the waist in which the response is triggered. Some of these reflexes can be elicited by poking or stroking the front or back sides of the waist, which will cause a reflexive response of side-bending with flexion if stroked on the anterior side, or side-bending with extension if stroked on the posterior side. Other lumbar reflexes are triggered when the chest is rotated against the pelvis or vice-versa. They can be elicited in another person by lifting either her chest or pelvis while she is lying either prone or supine.

In a contralateral crawl or movement, the spine moves through space with a subtle **gyroscopic** turn. Babies

Patterning Exercise #71: Rolls and Gyroscopic Twists

The purposes of this exercise are 1) to establish a vertical connection along the spine while rolling to pattern neck righting on the body (NOB) and body righting on the body (BOB) reactions, 2) to differentiate between simultaneous and sequential movement of the spine, and 3) to differentiate between the initiation of spinal movement at the head and at the tail.

1. Lie comfortably on your back with your knees bent and with enough space to roll over in either direction. Slowly and gently roll your head back and forth from side to side to warm up your neck.

PE Fig. 71a

2. Roll your head and look to one side. Let your spine follow the movement of your neck so that you roll over on your side. Allow your body's weight to yield into your side.

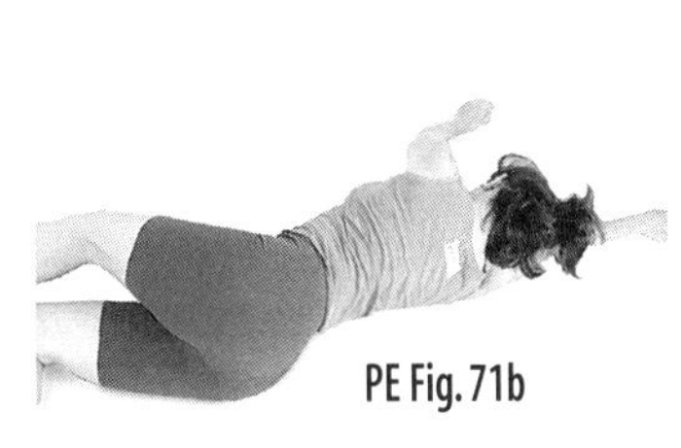

PE Fig. 71b

3. Now reach your hand across and up. Keep reaching until you roll over (PE Fig. 71a).
4. Return to your original position by reaching with your tail to roll onto your back (PE Fig. 71b).
5. Explore the difference between rolling over in one simultaneous action that rolls the spine like a log and in a sequential action that rotates first the head and neck, then the thorax, then the pelvis.
6. Next, lie flat on your back in an X-shaped position. Visualize the surface you are lying on as a square. Then reach your right hand across your body to the upper left corner of the square (PE Fig. 71c). Watch your hand the entire way. Continue to reach until the pull of your hand and the rotation of your neck and thorax roll your body over on to your belly. Reverse the action by reaching backward with your tail and rolling to your back (PE Fig. 71b). Repeat the pattern on the other side.
7. Continue to explore reaching to the corner and rolling over, then rolling back again, until you can move smoothly with ease.

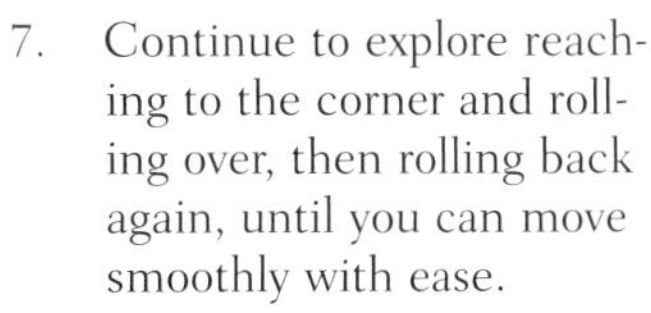

PE Fig. 71c

8. Then bring one knee up to your chest and take it across your body, rotating the pelvis (PE Fig. 71d). Allow this initiation to roll you all the way over to your belly. Reverse and return to your starting position by reaching with your tail (PE Fig. 71b). Repeat the movement on the other side.

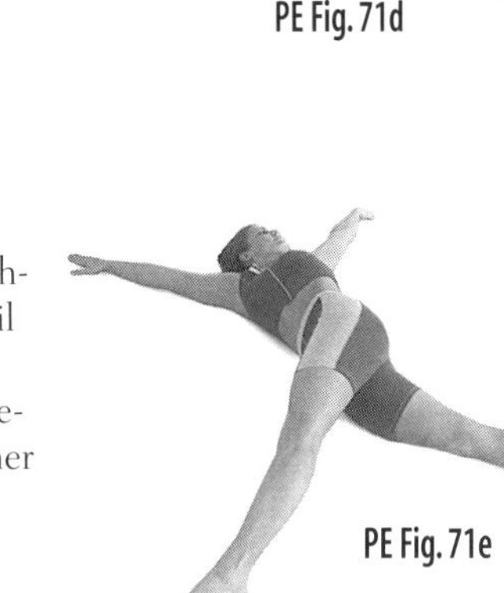

PE Fig. 71d

PE Fig. 71e

9. From a spread-eagle position, reach one foot across and down, and keep reaching until you roll over. To return, reach the arm back and up, and keep reaching until it rolls you back (PE Fig. 71e).

Caution: Explore #10 only if you feel you are very coordinated and in good shape, and have enough room to roll without crashing into something.

10. Lay over a ball and explore rolling over on your waist, extending your limbs for balance. Go both directions.

who accidentally flop over while reaching for something out of their range demonstrate gyroscopic turning. A fish flops around in a gyroscopic twist when out of water.

Gyroscopic rolling and twisting patterns integrate movement between lumbar and cervical areas of the spine. Reflexes that right the neck on the body or right the pelvis and the thorax also coordinate the gyroscopic spiraling of the spine. The **neck righting on the body (NOB) reaction** and the **body righting on the body (BOB) reaction** underlie integrated movement along the central axis of the body and are active during rolling and turning movements (Figure 7.32). For example, suppose someone seated in a chair is looking backward and begins to fall over backward. His torso will twist in the direction he is looking in order to turn his spine to follow his head.

The NOB reaction has two levels—a simultaneous rolling motion or a sequential twisting motion of the spine, which are obvious in the movements of babies as well as adults.[111] The first is a primitive reaction: the baby turns her head and reaches across her body's midline with one arm, which initiates a full-body movement, rolling the baby over like a log, twisting the neck without rotating the spine below the neck. The second level is a mature reaction: the baby turns her head and reaches across the body with one arm, and the spine rolls by twisting in sequential segments,

Patterning Exercise #72: Finding Midline

The purpose of this exercise is to strengthen your connection to midline.

1. Lie on your back. Bring your knees up and hold onto your feet. Gently rock from right to left, shifting your weight from one side to the other without rolling onto your side (PE Fig. 72a). As you go back and forth, sense when you are balanced on midline and when you are in lateral flexion. Ideally, you will feel symmetry in your back while rolling between sides.

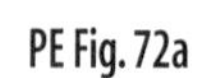

PE Fig. 72a

2. Pull both knees to your chest. Now rock easily along midline from your head to your tail, as though your spine were a bowed leg on a rocking chair.
3. Next, lie on your back with your knees bent. Hold both hands together above your head. Leave one hand in this position and slowly open your other hand out to the side, watching it as you move it. Sense your neck rotating, taking your spine off center (PE Fig.72b). Then bring your hand back to center, watching it and sensing the return to midline. Repeat with the other side.

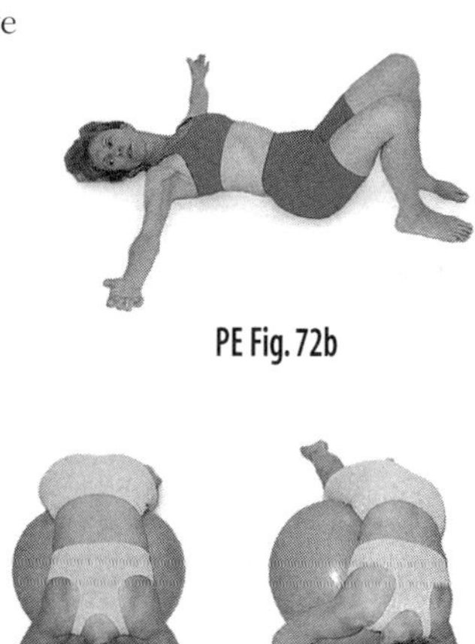

PE Fig. 72b

4. Lie over a physioball on your belly (PE Fig.72c). Roll a little to one side, then the other (PE Fig. 72d). Move slowly so that you do not fall completely. Use your hands to balance. Sense the fall from midline and then the return to midline.

PE Fig. 72c PE Fig. 72d

EMSPress.com

differentiating rotational movement between the head, thorax, and pelvis.

Likewise, the leg and tail initiate the BOB reaction, also in two levels. When the leg crosses midline, it causes the body to roll over either in one simultaneous movement or in a segmented movement sequence in which the rotations of the pelvis, thorax, and head are differentiated. Both the NOB and BOB reactions underlie the ability to roll over and change levels, and both can be practiced at any age to improve the coordination of movement along the central axis of the spine. For example, a person with a stiff spine would benefit from practicing rolling over slowly with sequential rotation along the spine, and from initiating rolling back with the tail to improve coordination in the lower body.

Midline

As mentioned earlier, a movement pattern is only as strong as its underlying neurological pathways. The contralateral pattern, the most complex of all the movement pathways, occurs around a strong central axis of the spine. If the homolateral and contralateral pathways are strong but the underlying pathways are weak, a person may lack a sense of **midline** in the body. Midline is actual, figurative, and neurological; it is the connection between right and left sides, a psychological connection with one's center and core self, and the ability to move off center while retaining a symmetrical connection of the limbs to the center of the body.

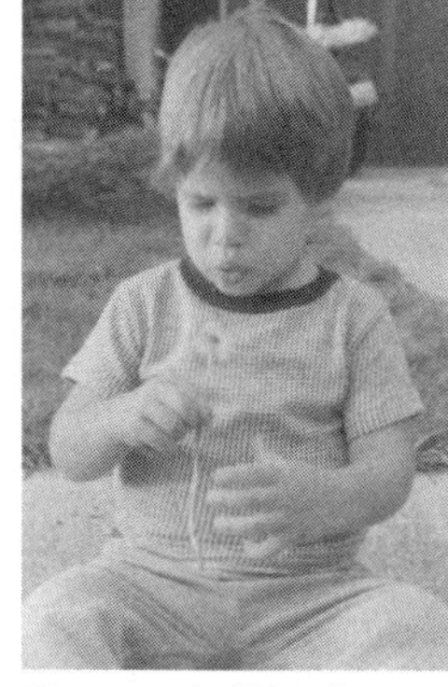

Figure 7.33 Many forms of play bring children to midline.

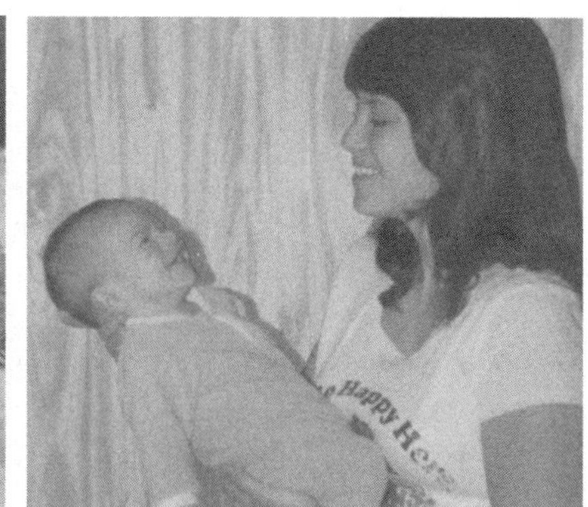

Figure 7.34 Being seen helps a child develop a psychological sense of center (photos courtesy of L. Bright).

The movement of the spine tends to follow the head. Homologous movements usually keep the spine on midline, whereas homolateral patterns twist the spine to one side or the other. When the head and neck are straight (without rotation or side-bending), the spine usually follows and comes to a neutral alignment. When the head turns, the spine usually follows with a subtle homolateral side-bending that is coupled with either flexion or extension.

The midline connection is strengthened through spinal and homologous patterns and through all their underlying reflexes. The homolateral pattern is the first pattern to move off midline. The contralateral rotates around midline. All head/tail reaches and pushes establish movement pathways coordinated along midline. Also, upper and lower homologous pushes and reaches coordinate movement in the limbs above and below the centered symmetry of spinal flexion and extension.

Simple actions bring us to midline: when we eat, we center the body in front of the food and come to midline. Also, when a baby is fed straight on, his spine

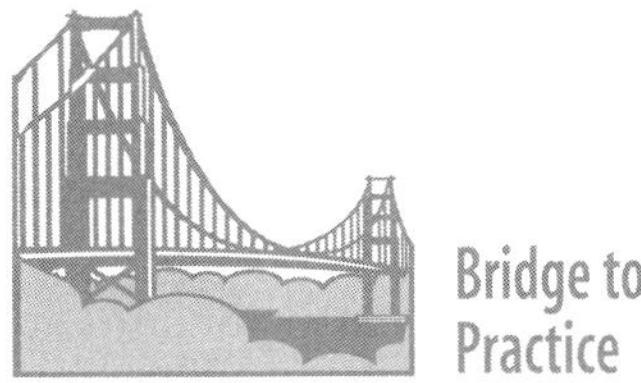

Helping Your Client Find Midline

You can help your client make subtle spinal and homologous connections in his body to help him find midline at the end of a bodywork session. It is usually best to begin with homologous patterns to establish bilateral support for the core before establishing core connections (which can be done by having your client do subtle pelvic tilts while you give him light traction in the neck).

To make the homologous connection when your client is lying prone, put your client in the starting position of an upper homologous push. Have him put both arms out to the sides, elbows at a right angle, with his forearms flat. (His arms may not fit on or may fall off of the massage table. If so, do the best you can with what you have if you can do so safely, or have him lie on a mat on the floor.) Then help him yield into this position by gently pulling his shoulders open to widen them and suggesting that he yield his chest and arms into the supporting surface.

Next, ask him to slowly and subtly push his forearms into the table using minimal muscular effort. Make sure he does not retract his shoulder blades or lift his arms. Put light pressure on the back of his forearms to help give him a sense of pushing from there.

If his chest is tight, the initiation of the push alone will stretch his chest muscles and will suffice to give him a sense of integration between his arms and chest. Or you can guide him to push all the way up, although this type of movement education may be beyond the scope of a bodywork session.

Then have him tuck his toes under and lightly push with his feet to make a connection into his spine from his legs. Suggest he keep his knees on the table while he lightly pushes, and watch his hips to make sure they are symmetrical. If they are not, help him find symmetry in the action.

End with your client on his back. Have him tilt his pelvis and hold it in flexion. Then give him light neck traction, holding the traction while he slowly unrolls and releases the pelvic tilt. Encourage him to gently stretch his lower spine away from your traction to make a connection along the core. If he is moving intrinsically, he may feel the dural tube around his spinal cord stretch.

stays on midline. Conversely, a baby suckling a breast rotates his whole spine around the midline axis to reach the breast.

The eyes converging on a single point in front of the body can bring one to midline (Figure 7.33). For example, when a baby holds a toy with both hands and looks at it, he straightens his spine to face the toy. Midline is also developed by seeing and being seen (Figure 7.34). When the caretaker's and infant's eyes meet, the infant reflexively brings his head to midline.

The **Babkin reflex** is evoked when a caretaker simultaneously presses both of an infant's palms and the baby brings his head to midline while flexing his neck. Similarly, pressure or tactile stimulation on the top of the head or bottom of the tail will evoke a reflexive movement of the spine in either flexion or extension along the midline. A lack of midline coordinations and reflexes can show up in a right/left asymmetry in posture and movement, and also in the lack of a psychological ability to "meet something or someone head on."

DEVELOPMENTAL PATTERNING TO INTEGRATE BODYWORK

The developmental patterns provide an excellent framework for a bodyworker to give a client movement cues while the bodyworker is stretching myofascial tissues. A bodywork client can, while lying on the table, lightly reach or push through any developmental pathway to integrate passive release with active movement and to reorganize the faulty pathways that tightened the client's body in the first place.

The developmental pathways provide a direction for a particular action and can ensure that the client moves through an entire pathway. For example, a bodyworker could have a prone client reach through the hands as he stretches the client's midthoracic area, or have a supine client reach through both feet as he stretches the client's waist. Spinal patterns are also helpful for integrating the core of the body and bringing a client to midline. It is a good idea to always leave a client on midline for integration. This means ending a session with a core connection (via traction) and a core movement (via a pelvic tilt or spinal flexion and extension). To ensure both sensory and motor integration requires both sensing the kinesthetic connection between the head and tail, plus doing a spinal movement (such as a push or reach with the head and/or tail).

At the end of a bodywork session, after a client's muscles have been loosened up and general tensions have been released, it is helpful for the client to move of her own volition to get ready to stand up. This is especially helpful when tight muscles that a client previously used for standing have relaxed; the movement patterns different support muscles. The client's movement organizes new pathways and brings up muscle tone in preparation for standing. The client also learns to move from a passive state to an active state in a conscious way. This avoids the tendency to go back into the old pattern, the one that caused her to be tight enough to come for bodywork in the first place. It also addresses the common problem of clients returning for massage or bodywork session after session with the same problems caused by habitual poor body-use habits.

At the end of a session, the transition point from lying to sitting and standing also presents an opportune time to teach the client a new and more efficient movement to change levels, such as pushing down with the limbs while reaching with the head. Overall, by practicing new ways to move, the client not only learns how to move more efficiently, but she is able to take the stretching and lengthening she received from the bodywork into standing, and hopefully can integrate the new patterns into her daily activities.

SUMMARY

We all go through the same sequence of early motor stages. This series of developmental patterns recapitulates the sequence of evolution that can be traced from single-celled life forms to humans. Each of us had strengths and weaknesses in various stages of motor development, which underlie our body patterns as well as our emotional and cognitive affinities.

Although developmental patterning has traditionally been used to rehabilitate children and adults with neurological damages or disorders, it can be used by anyone to improve the overall coordination of movement. Developmental patterning is helpful for healthy adults who have coordination problems or even postural problems. And it is especially helpful for parents who want to promote healthy motor development in their children.

All movement can be analyzed through the developmental patterns, as will become evident in the study of the fundamental movements presented in Chapter 9. An understanding of the sequence of patterns of early motor development can guide a person during any movement endeavor, be it sports, daily activities, or postural support. A person can practice the basic actions—yielding, pushing, reaching, and pulling—at any time during the day on an energetic level. A person can also direct these actions along specific pathways—spinal, homologous, homolateral, or contralateral—to improve the coordination of movement.

Lastly, each pattern has underlying reflexes that support it. Exploring these reflexes will improve the subcortical coordination of movement and will strengthen neurological tone. More importantly, exploring the reflexes that underlie developmental patterns cultivates the protective and spontaneous reactions we need when our bodies suddenly fall or tip off balance, which can be an invaluable resource for aging gracefully and fearlessly.

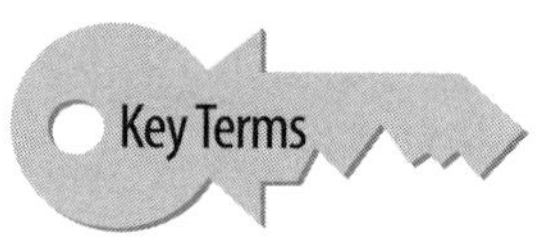

asymmetrical tonic neck reflex (ATNR)
Babkin reflex
body righting on the body (BOB) reaction
gyroscopic
hand-eye coordination
hand-mouth coordination
Landau reflex
lateral line
midline
neck righting on the body (NOB) reaction
neurological actions
oral rooting reflex
pull
push
reach
tonic labyrinthine reflex
yield

OVERVIEW OF CHAPTER 8

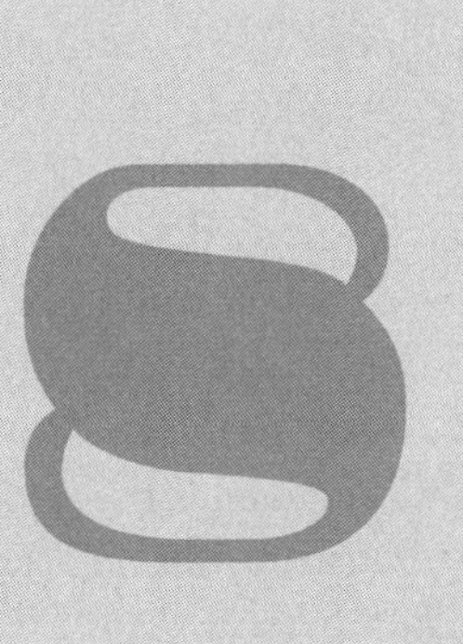

Neuromuscular Patterning

> **The central nervous system deals with man as a whole, never in parts, nor as a sum of parts.**
>
> —*Lulu Sweigard*

The numerous neuromuscular (NM) approaches to patterning all share a single goal: to improve joint and muscle function. Several NM strategies are introduced in this text, such as the developmental movement patterns in the last chapter, the Bartenieff Fundamentals in Chapter 11, and the proprioceptive neuromuscular facilitation (PNF) patterns in Chapter 12.

The complexity of these maps can be obscured by their apparent simplicity. For instance, there are only two PNF patterns of the limbs, called D1 and D2. When considering that they occur in both the arms and the legs, that makes four patterns. Since each pattern has both a flexion and extension cycle, that multiplies the patterns to eight. The patterns can be practice with the elbows and knees flexed or extended, adding more variables. The numerous variables of PNF patterns can be combined in at least a hundred different ways. Multiply these by the various effort qualities and PNF techniques, and the ways to explore PNF patterns extend exponentially. The same is true of developmental patterns and the Bartenieff Fundamentals; they can be patterned in countless combinations.

Given the volume of potential NM patterns, it is only possible to present a fraction of the information that could be discussed on NM patterning in this text. Therefore, this chapter introduces some of the basic elements of NM patterning, such as the use of imagery, joint mechanics, and physiological considerations in muscle patterning and stretching.

TAKING A CORTICAL APPROACH

In a cortical approach to patterning, a person mentally directs the movement while carefully tracking the movement, using sensory input to control motor output. Simply by choosing to do a specific exercise in a specific manner, a person is taking somewhat of a top-down, cortical approach. In an ideal movement sequence, at some point mental control is surrendered to the experience of movement. This is the point at which the mind relaxes and body sensations take over to guide the process.

Muscle and joint function is precise and needs direction to be effective, yet it is important to release mental control at some point during a movement sequence to cultivate a natural and relaxed quality. Patterning done with too much control can easily become stiff and robotic or, at the very least, boring. Cortical and reflexive approaches can be integrated into neuromuscular patterning by oscillating between controlled, directed movement and fluid, organic movement. For example, an exercise can be first practiced slowly with a controlled awareness. Then the same exercise can be practiced with free flow and a certain degree of abandon, perhaps with a rocking or swinging motion.

Cortically controlled patterning is usually directed with an idea or image of how the movement should be. This idea allows the central nervous system to coordinate the best pathway for movement, although the bulk of coordination is subcortical. Using an appropriate image, the nervous system coordinates movement in the whole muscular system toward the accomplishment of a desired goal, not toward the movement of a specific muscle. Although a patterning exercise may be focused on the movement of a specific part, the entire body is affected. Neuromuscular coordination changes the entire system because subcortical activity occurs in muscle groups far from the area of focus. As a result of subcortical changes throughout the body from neuromuscular patterning, the overall integration and coordination of movement improves.

"Awareness Through Movement"

By slowing a movement down, a person can observe and feel each increment of the sequence to identify where along the kinetic chain the movement is faulty, when and where too much effort is being used, and which muscles are dysfunctional—all feedback needed to make subtle patterning adjustments. Moshe Feldenkrais defined and refined a fundamental technique for changing faulty patterns in which a person practices a simple pattern, such as turning the head, slowly with focused awareness in as many different ways as possible. The technique is the same as the name of his style of movement lessons, which he calls "Awareness Through Movement." [112]

In the Feldenkrais Method (see Chapter 11), the same movement is practiced slowly and with awareness while varying the coordination of parts in different sets. For example, a person might explore turning the head, eyes, and arm in the same direction, then turn the head and arm in opposition to the eyes, and then turn the eyes and arm in opposition to the head. By moving through each possible combination, a person eventually uncouples faulty coordinations, differentiating movement between parts and thereby improving the overall coordination of head, eye, and arm movement.

Visualization and Ideokinesis

Visualization can also be used to direct the pathway of a movement. While many different types of images can be used, research has shown that images based on sound anatomical workings are more effective than those based on abstract ideas. This is because the brain is so good at adapting neuromuscular pathways to an idea of how the body "should" be that if an abstract image goes against the grain of sound body mechanics, it may create more problems than it was designed to fix. For example, a student who was also a dancer thought her derriere was too big, so she taught herself how to keep her *gluteal muscles* relaxed, imaging them as "buns melting." Her visualization was so effective that within a month her gluteal muscles became very relaxed, and soon she was suffering from gluteal muscle dysfunction, which created a sciatica-like shooting pain down her hips. The remedy involved learning how to contract and control the gluteal muscles again, both for postural support in a standing posture and to control trunk and hip flexion and extension.

A unique body of abstract images used to improve posture came out of the research that physical educator Lulu Sweigard undertook between 1929 and 1931. In the first part of her research design, Sweigard did a statistical analysis of the X rays of 497 bilateral postural deviations. She also took the same measurements on 200 women before and after they participated in half-hour postural classes for 15 weeks to assess changes in their bony alignment. The women practiced postural exercises using the technique of **ideokinesis**—the process of changing movement using ideation or imagery. The images they used were either anatomical pictures of bones or images of mechanical devices resembling some part of the musculoskeletal system that were anatomically correct, such as the ribcage breathing like a toy accordion, or the pelvis tipping like a bowl of water coming to a level position. They also learned to practice ideokinesis in various positions and during daily activities such as standing or walking.[113]

Sweigard measured the direction and location of their bones in a standing posture and found many changes among the group, but only nine were common. She identified these nine as desired **lines of movement**, which, when used to direct a movement, improve the subcortical patterning of muscular coordination (Figure 8.1). Each woman in the group had undergone:

1. Lengthening down the back of the spine.
2. Lengthening up the front of the spine.
3. Shortening of the distance between the pubic bone and the twelfth vertebra.

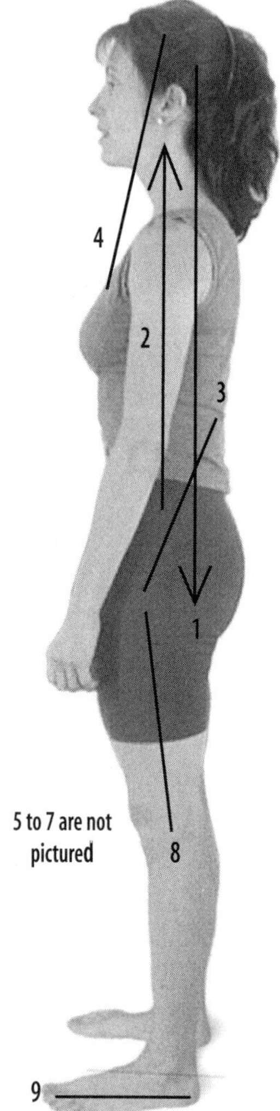

Figure 8.1 Sweigard's lines of movement

4. Either lifting or lowering of the top of the sternum toward or away from the top of the spine. (The direction of this action depended on the relative position of the sternum to the head.)
5. Narrowing of the ribcage.
6. Widening across the back of the pelvis.
7. Narrowing across the front of the pelvis.
8. Repositioning of the center of the knee under the center of the hip socket.
9. Shortening between the big toe and heel, especially during walking.[114]

Afterwards, Sweigard compiled a body of images designed to strengthen these nine lines of movement. What is important to remember about her images is that they are anatomically sound; they won't get a person in trouble as the "melting buns" image described earlier did. The problem with this image is that in a standing posture, the gluteal muscles lightly contract in their role as postural stabilizers. By imagining them melting, the student turned them off. She went against the physiological design of her tissues, which led to a dysfunction. A basic understanding of anatomy and physiology gives a person the ability to discern whether the images are mechanically and physiologically sound. Sweigard made these determinations from her research. Her images are practical and classic, and are still widely used in dance training and somatic education (Figure 8.2a-d).

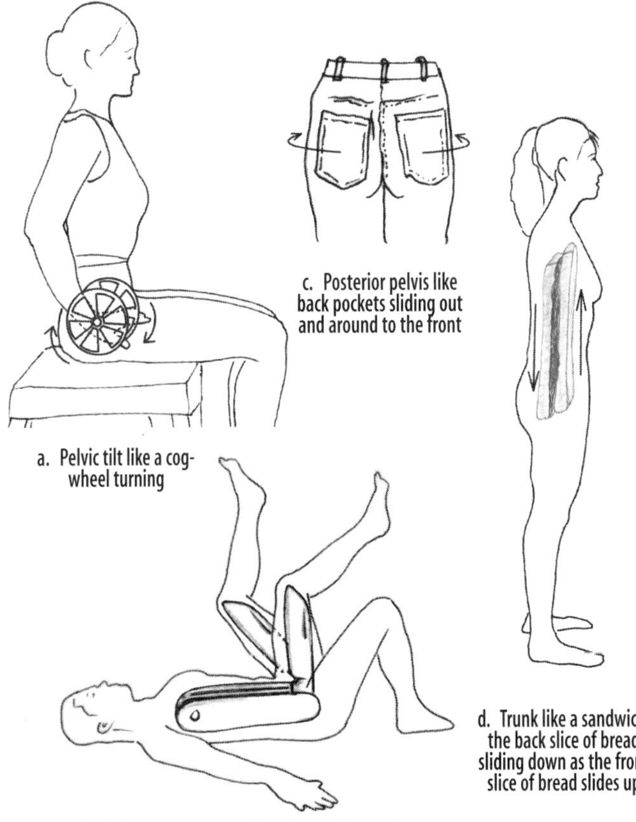

c. Posterior pelvis like back pockets sliding out and around to the front
a. Pelvic tilt like a cog-wheel turning
d. Trunk like a sandwich, the back slice of bread sliding down as the front slice of bread slides up
b. Hip flexion and extension like a jack-knife opening

Figure 8.2a-d Samples of some of Sweigard's popular images that are used to evoke efficient posture and movement

Sweigard emphasized how important it is during patterning exercises *to inhibit any voluntary effort toward the movement until the image initiates the action*. Otherwise, the old pathway will take over and a faulty yet habitual postural correction will dominate the pattern. She also stressed the importance of *beginning each exercise from a position of complete rest* in order to avoid carrying old stress into new actions.

An image creates a gestalt of a total experience. Although anatomically based images are ideal in patterning, not everyone has an understanding of anatomy. Also, the human anatomy is so complex that it may be hard to picture in a simplified version, and focusing on a single part can detract from feeling a full-body pattern. Therefore, Sweigard's images are ideal for patterning because they are both anatomically sound, yet simple enough for a person who lacks an understanding of anatomy to use. Ultimately, the best type of image is the one that works.

Dynamic and moving images, such as wind or water, are helpful in supporting organic or ongoing movements. For example, sensing the body rolling like lava slowly pouring can help a person sense a weighted organic flow, which relaxes a moving body. The image of the legs revolving like pedals on a bicycle can help a walker sustain full flexion and extension cycles. Or the image of the wind blowing under the pelvis can help a hiker climb a hill.

An image that works to change posture and movement one day may not work the next. And because imagery is personal, an image that works for one person may not work for the next. To accommodate changing patterns and needs, each of us needs to keep finding new images. For instance, a man found that by imagining a skyhook lifting the top of his head, his collapsed posture gradually elongated. Yet, after using this image for several weeks, his spine straightened up so much that he reached the end of the postural correction and began to arch over backward. To counter this, he found a new image to correct the hyperextension, one of a buckle anchoring his sternum to his pubic bone.

Memories store experiences in images. A powerful way to use memory while patterning movement is to recall what an efficient and effortless movement felt like. By remembering this, a person can access the neuromuscular circuits needed to coordinate the same movement or recreate that sensation. For example, the memory of feeling relaxed can induce relaxation, the memory of feeling a neutral, balanced spine can induce alignment, and the memory of hitting one's stride in a sport can induce an effortless pace. To improve performance, many athletes and dancers visualize their sport or dance while lying or sitting around thinking about it. Likewise, a visualization of good alignment can be used to guide posture during daily activities.

However, using ideokinesis alone to change movement may not be effective. Imagery needs to be balanced with body awareness and actual movement to be integrated into a well-rounded patterning process. In the effective use of imagery, visualization is followed by a somatic shift, such as a new connection, sensation, or relaxation response. Problems with visualizations occur when the images are static, inappropriate for the action, or when people can become so active in their imaginations that they become mentally too busy to feel sensations in their bodies or to actually move. This last problem is similar to setting goals so high that they are forever out of reach. The further away that the mental image of what a person wants becomes from the actual behavior, the further away the dream gets from reality. Sometimes people use imagery to escape feeling uncomfortable emotions in their bodies. Other times, the mental process of conjuring imagery causes the imagination to become so overactive that a person has trouble getting started, initiating a movement.

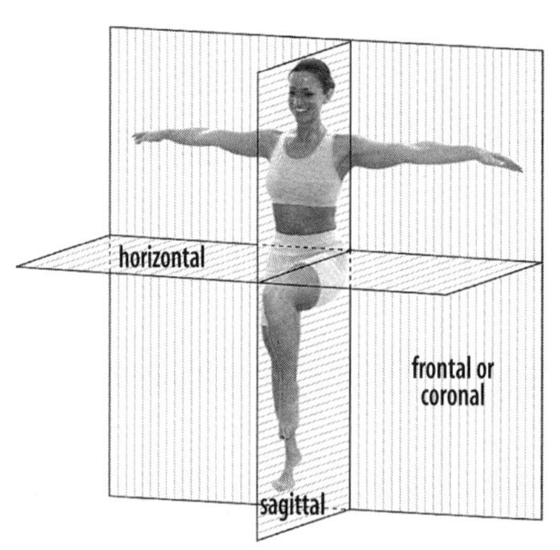

Figure 8.4 The three planes

Keep in mind that imagery is a mental process, while proprioception is a physical process; the use of imagery should be balanced with proprioceptive skills, thus creating a link between mental and physical processes. To integrate ideokinesis with somatic experience, a person needs to also be able to transition between imagining something and actually feeling it by sensing the moving body while simultaneously using imagery to direct the movement. Also, if specific muscles are dysfunctional, imagery or sensory awareness may not be enough to change the pattern. The muscle must be actively contracted or relaxed to change the pattern. To do so, a person needs to develop proprioceptive skills in perceiving changes in muscle tone.

BONES

Since the skeleton is the most clearly defined tissue in the body, patterning can be guided by visualizing the direction in which two bones in a joint move. If the range of motion visualized is accurate, meaning that it is based on the actual mechanics and physiology of a specific joint, then that image will probably call up the most efficient neuromuscular program for that joint. To reiterate, imagery of the bones should be done in conjunction with actually sensing the moving bones.

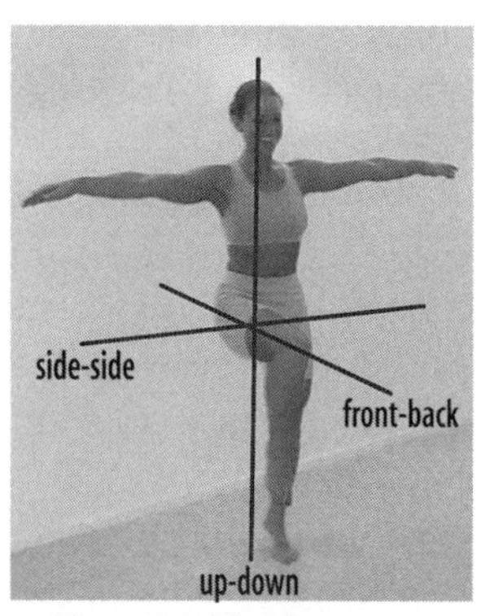

Figure 8.3 The three axes

Sensing the bones during patterning tends to evoke qualities of effortlessness and spatial clarity. Also, since bones are the densest tissue in the body, sensing them can enhance an awareness of the sensation of weight during motion. Recall from Chapter 4 that sensing weight in the body, whether at rest or during movement, elicits a relaxation response, which helps a person release excessive muscular effort and tension in both the skeletal and smooth muscles. A person can also gain feedback about how working muscles are pulling on a joint by tracking the direction that the bones move, and using this feedback to direct and change faulty patterns.

Skeletal Architecture and Physical Forces

Each of the three major body masses (head, thorax, and pelvis) has an affinity for movement in a different plane predisposed by the nature of that mass's well-defined architecture. A plane is a combination of two of the three axes: up-down (vertical), front-back (sagittal), and side-side (horizontal) (Figure 8.3). An easy way to remember the three planes is with Bartenieff's analogy of the "door," "wheel," and "table" planes. She describes the door or **frontal plane** as the plane of presentation, the wheel or **sagittal plane** as the plane of locomotion, and the table or **horizontal plane** as the plane of receptivity (Figure 8.4).

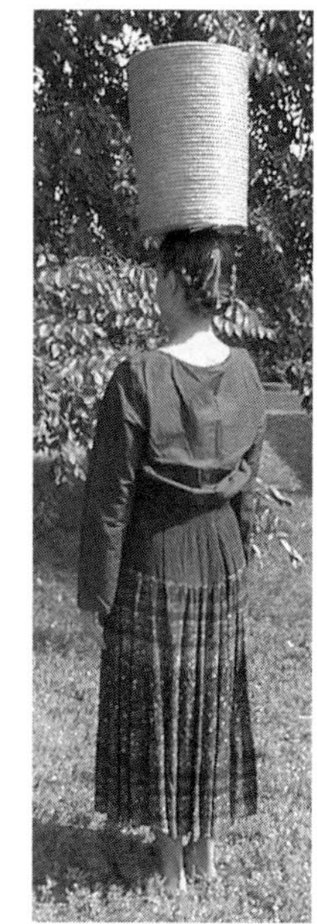
Figure 8.5 A top load

Geometrical balance in the planes is obvious in the dimensional balance of a well-integrated body, which has a proportional fullness from front-to-back, side-to-side, and top-to-bottom. Structural balance is built into the skeletal architecture and is evident in how each of the three body masses supports weight and has an affinity for motion in a specific plane.

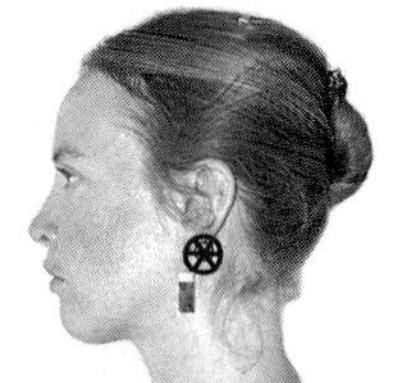
Figure 8.6 The axis for movement between the head and neck

- The **top load** of the head sits atop the spine; its weight transfers directly through the compression structures of the vertebrae and disks (Figure 8.5). The cervical spine easily rotates in the *horizontal* plane,

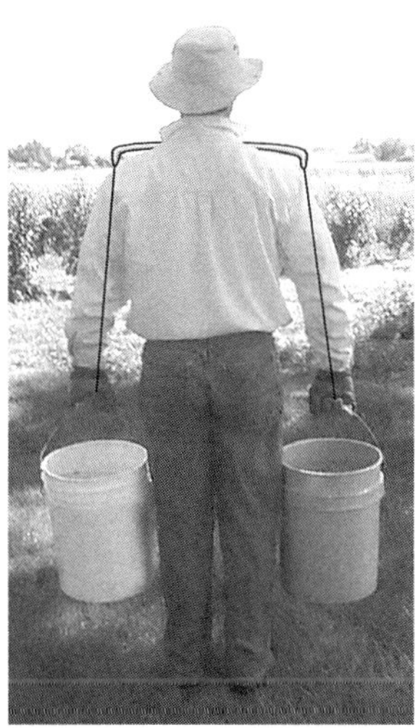

Figure 8.7 Ideally, the shoulder girdle is seated on the thorax along a horizontal axis like a weighted yoke.

pivoting on joints in the upper cervical vertebrae and at the base of the skull (Figure 8.6).

- The **side load** of the arms hangs like a yoke from the tensional pulleys of soft tissues attached to the shoulder girdle (Figure 8.7). Like spokes on a wheel, the muscular pulls on the shoulder socket must have even tension to seat and move the arms in the center of their socket. The shoulder muscles function like straps on a harness, steering the arms through a wide range of movements. Since shoulders are oriented in the *frontal* plane, the arms hang beside the body. Although this seems obvious, consider how the arms migrate to the front or back of the body in slumped or retracted postures.
- The **braced arch** of the pelvis is supported by a keystone arch made up of five bones (Figure 8.8). The sacrum is buttressed between the pelvic bones that are then buttressed between the legs (Figure 8.9). The pelvis is oriented in the *sagittal* plane, and the legs move through cycles of sagittal locomotion similar to a wheel (Figure 8.10).

Dimensional Balance in Movement

Balanced movement is three-dimensional: it sequences in all three planes, through the hanging and swinging structures of the arms and legs, the compressive structures of the

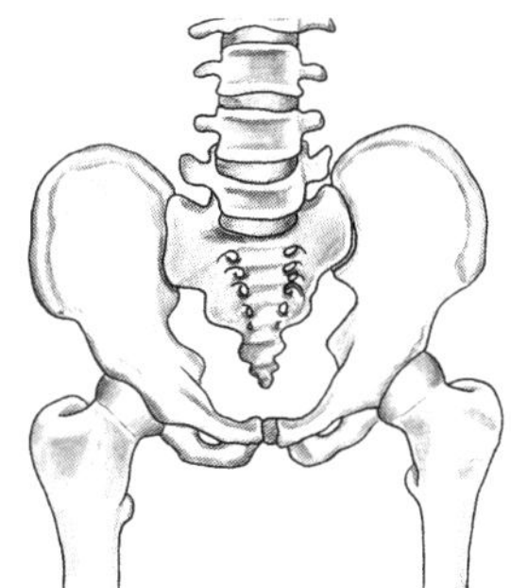

Figure 8.8 The pelvic bones function as a braced arch.

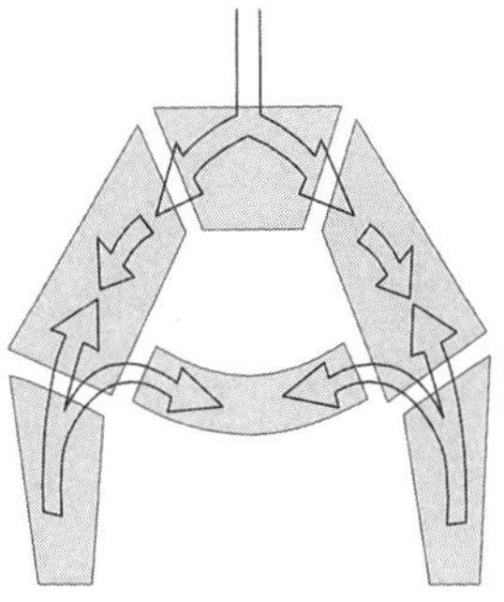

Figure 8.9 Directions of forces buttressing the braced arch

hips and spine, and the tensional webbing of the myofascia (Figure 8.11). The connective tissues of the body make up a three-dimensional grid in which the top needs to be balanced with the bottom, the right with the left, and the front with the back. The complexity of the grid extends into the microscopic level; each cell has a three-dimensional network of collagen fibers that function as a pseudo-cellular skeleton. Friction on a cell wall actually pulls on the grid and somewhat flattens the cell.[115]

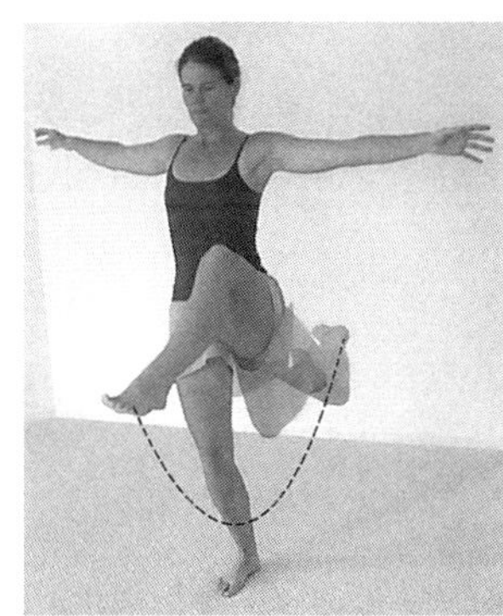

Figure 8.10 The hips flex and extend in the sagittal plane.

Geometrical balance even extends into the bones on a cellular level. The cells within spongy bone are organized along *trabecular rows*, which develop according to the lines of tension that pass through that bone (Figure 8.12). Bones are both elastic

Patterning Exercise #73: Sensing Weight in the Bones

1. *Arms:* Lie on your back. Raise both arms toward the ceiling (PE Fig. 73a). Draw small circles in the air with your hands, sensing weight in your shoulders as you move. Use the sensation of weight to relax any excessive muscular tension you may feel in your neck, back, and shoulders.
2. Slowly open your arms toward your sides, again sensing weight in your shoulders as you move. Once your arms are open, slowly return to the starting position, sensing weight in your scapulae and ribs as you move (PE Fig. 73b-c). Afterwards, relax and breathe for a moment.

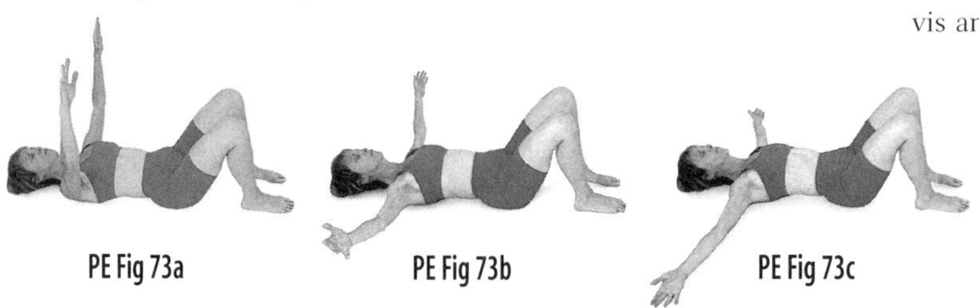

PE Fig 73a PE Fig 73b PE Fig 73c

3. *Legs:* Lift one foot toward the ceiling (PE Fig. 73d). Sense weight sinking into your hips and pelvis as you lift that leg.
4. Next, explore drawing a small circle with your foot in the air, allowing the sensation of weight to sink through your leg. (Imagine your leg filled with sand that is sifting toward your hip.) Allow the sensation of weight to stabilize your pelvis and release excess tension around your hip.
5. Slowly lower your foot back to the ground, again sensing weight in your pelvis as you move (PE Fig. 73e). Repeat with the other leg.

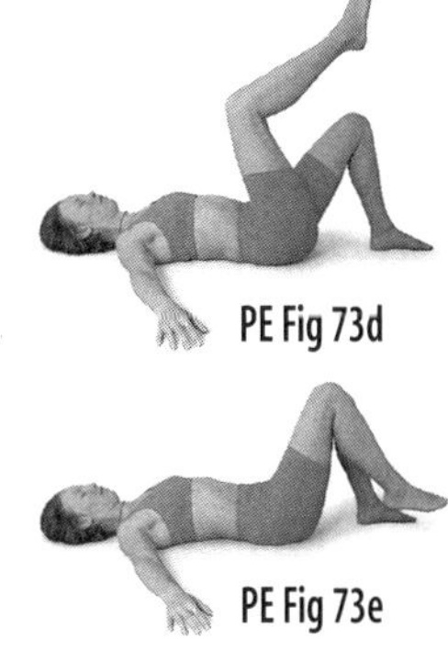

PE Fig 73d

PE Fig 73e

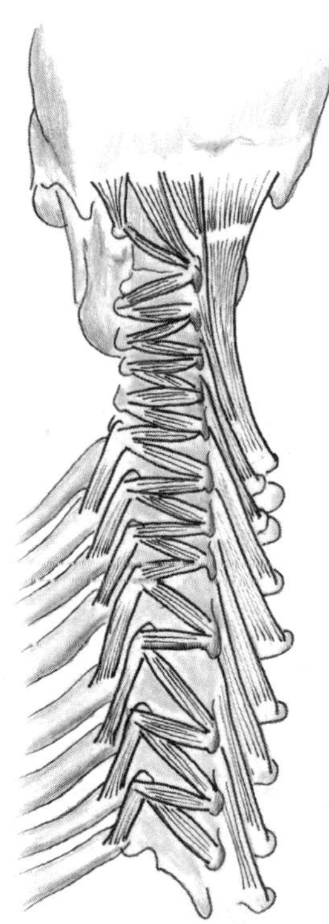

Figure 8.11 The scaffolding of intrinsic muscles along the spine

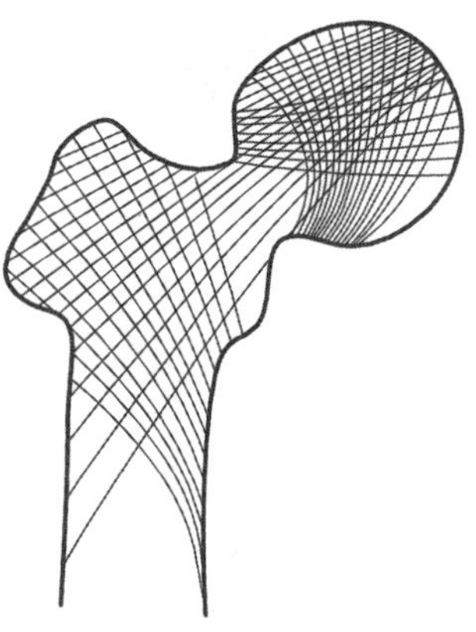

Figure 8.12 The trabecular rows of cells in the femur

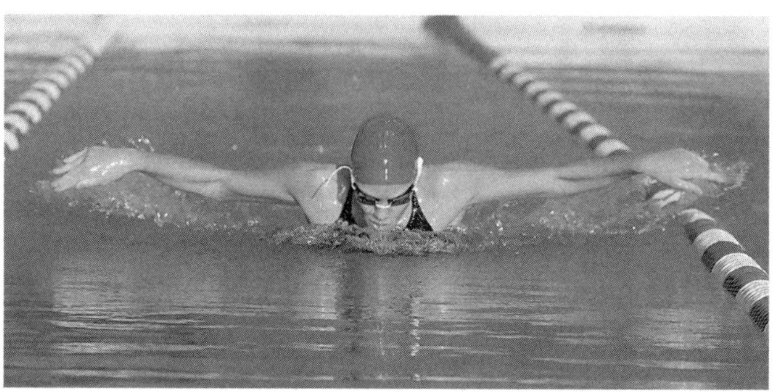

Figure 8.13 Symmetry in action strengthens the dimensional cross made by the horizontal pull of the arms and the vertical thrust of the spine.

and able to resist a certain amount of stress; *trabeculae* reflect the direction in which the forces of muscular contraction pull on a bone and to which it adapts by thickening or bending. Illustrating this point, the trabecular rows in the femurs of amputees, who lack weight-bearing stresses, atrophy and elongate from the stretching forces of the hanging limb.[116]

Spinal movement sequences along the body's central axis, whereas homologous patterns organize lines of force and movement pathways across the shoulder and pelvic girdles, integrating the girdles with the spine. Homologous movements underlie right and left symmetry in the body by creating a unified axis between the two arms across the shoulders and between the two legs across the pelvis (Figure 8.13). The axis of the arms across the torso creates a **dimensional cross** in the body, establishing horizontal support through the arms that intersects the vertical axis of the spine and legs. The lower homologous push in both legs sequences through a vertical thrust through the hips and up the spine. The stronger the integrity of the dimensional cross, the more support for the subsequent lateralization of homolateral movement on either side of the body. (See Chapter 7 for descriptions of homologous and homolateral patterns.) A person with a strong homologous pattern will have relatively square spatial balance between the four corners of the shoulder and hip sockets.

Ideally, the arms and legs make a sturdy homologous connection to the trunk through the hips and shoulders, transferring forces along their respective axes. The movement forces of the legs transfer through the hips into the sacrum along oblique pathways, sending a vertical thrust into the spine. The movement forces of the arms transfer into the body along the horizontal axis of the shoulder girdle.

In the system of movement analysis developed by Rudolph Laban called Labanalysis (see Chapter 11), students participate in movement improvisations to explore the effort qualities and spatial pulls of movement within each dimension and plane, and through three-dimensional curvilinear pathways (Figure 8.14). Irmgaard Bartenieff, a prominent Laban analyst, stressed the importance of clear spatial intention as a motivator of integrated movement. Having a clear perception of the spatial pathway along which a person is moving brings clarity and efficiency to neuromuscular patterns. For example, if a person knows and can feel where up and down are, this person will probably have a posture where the head is on top and pelvis underneath, and will be more likely to move with

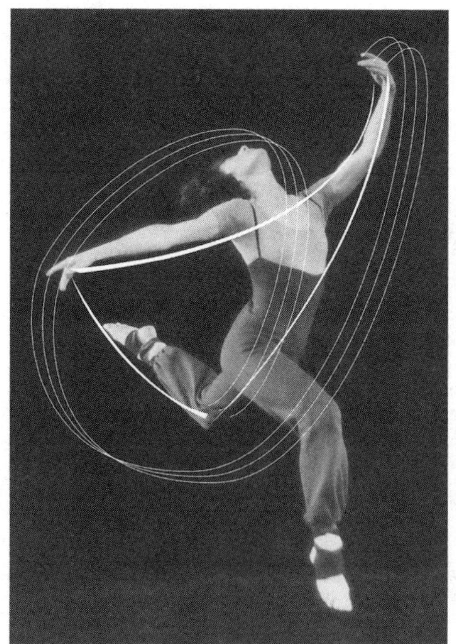

Figure 8.14 Three-dimensional movement traces a three-ring in space, a shape that passes through the corners of all three planes.

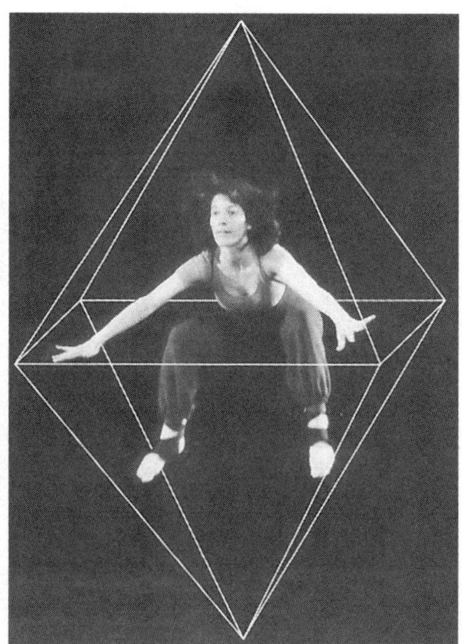

Figure 8.15 The spatial pulls of this dancer's jump make the shape of a tetrahedron (photos courtesy of M. Seereiter).

a balanced relationship between the head and the pelvis. In Laban studies, students learn to feel dimensions and spatial tension in their bodies and to recognize the geometric forms inscribed by their movement pathways (Figure 8.15). By becoming familiar with three-dimensional spatial configurations, we can more readily recognize dimensional balance in form and function as well.

Laws of Motion

The seventeenth-century British physicist and mathematician Sir Isaac Newton observed that an apple falls to earth by the same force that keeps the moon in orbit around the earth. Newton formulated three **laws of motion** that govern the movement of physical bodies and demonstrate how matter relates to force via a gravitational pull between objects. The first *law of reaction* states that for every action there is an equal and opposite reaction. The weight and downward exertions of our body are met by an upward push of **ground reaction force.**[117] With every step we take, the ground provides upward resistance to the downward force of the foot.

A clear illustration of these counterbalancing forces can be found on a beach where evidence of ground reaction force is sculpted in the footprints in sand. Walking requires more effort because sand provides less resistance than cement. To accelerate forward, a person must push back; therefore, the toe imprint is deeper than the heel print. The strength of opposing forces is reflected in the depth of the toe print; someone running would leave a deeper impression in the sand than someone walking.

Even a book resting on a table exerts a downward force by its weight, and the table meets it with an upward ground force. Due to the second law of gravity, the book remains on the table until another force acts upon it. The *law of inertia* states that a body remains in a state of rest or of uniform motion until an unbalanced force acts upon it. We experience inertia when we have been sitting for too long and find it difficult to get up. We also feel the impact of inertia when a driver hits the brakes and we lurch forward unexpectedly.

If an earthquake were to shake the room in which the table with the book is resting, the third law of gravity would cause the book to shimmy or fly off the table. The *law of acceleration* states that the "acceleration of an object is directly proportional to the force causing it."[118] The rate at which the book comes off the table is directly proportional to the strength of the earthquake, and inversely proportional to the mass of the object. A large, thick book needs a stronger tremor to move it off the table than a small paperback.

Mechanical Stresses

Opposing stresses push and pull on the body during all activities. The normal rigidity of joint capsules and tonic contractions of stabilizer muscles prevent the total displacement of joints from the stresses acting on them. Our bodies are always under a number of **mechanical stresses,** which include:

- *Tension.* Two opposite forces parallel to the axis of the joint pull the ends of the joint apart, creating tensile stress. Reach and pull patterns of movement generate tensile stresses from within; external forces such as traction generate tensile stresses from without (Figure 8.16).
- *Compression.* Two opposite forces parallel to the axis of the joint press in on the joint, creating compressive stress. The weight-bearing joints in the spine, hips, and legs are always under compression from the combination of the body's weight and ground forces. Lifting a heavy load creates external compression on the body (Figure 8.17).
- *Shearing.* Two parallel forces perpendicular to the axis of a joint press on the joint in opposite directions, causing it to shear. For example, pressing two stacked blocks sideways in opposite directions will create a shear between them (Figure 8.18). The head forward posture causes a shear in the lower cervical vertebrae.
- *Torsion.* Two parallel forces perpendicular to the axis of the joint pull away from each other in opposite directions, creating a torsion in the joint (Figure 8.19). For example, twisting two ends of a board in opposite directions will torque the board. Chronic asymmetrical contractures can cause torsion in the spine.
- *Bending.* The combination of tensile, compressive, and shearing stresses bends a structure. In all the previous stresses, one weight mass still rests above another. *Bending is the most harmful* of all the stresses on the spine because it displaces one mass off of another. Once bent, the spine can no longer support weight and the muscles have to chronically contract to shore up the collapsing structure. Bending occurs in abnormal curvatures like scoliosis, in which the vertebrae and discs adapt by becoming distorted in shape, which will eventually damage them (Figure 8.20).

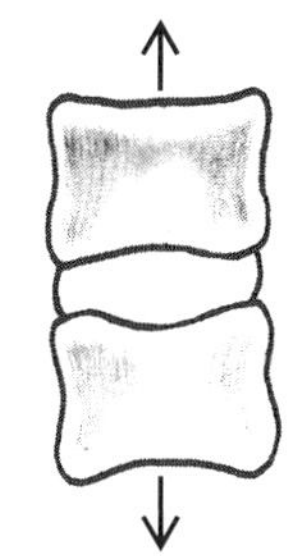

Figure 8.16 Tension

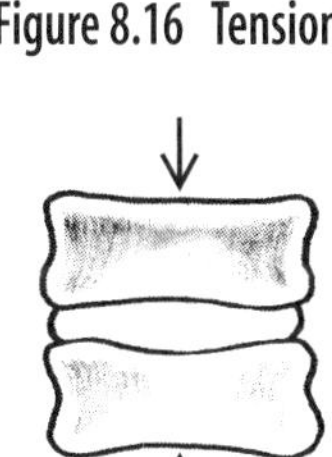

Figure 8.17 Compression

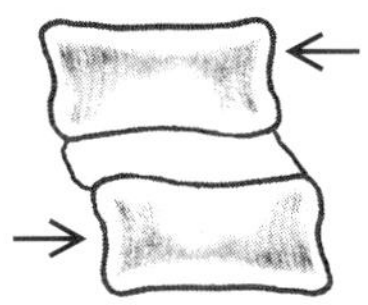

Figure 8.18 Shearing

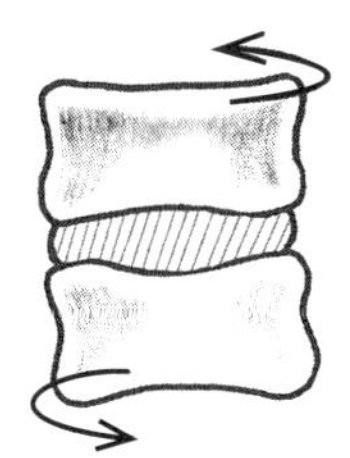

Figure 8.19 Torsion

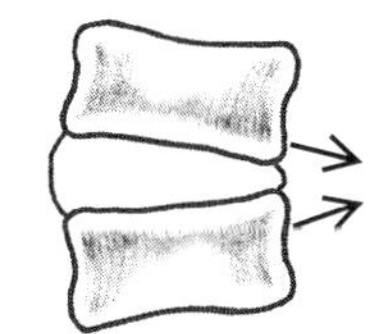

Figure 8.20 Bending

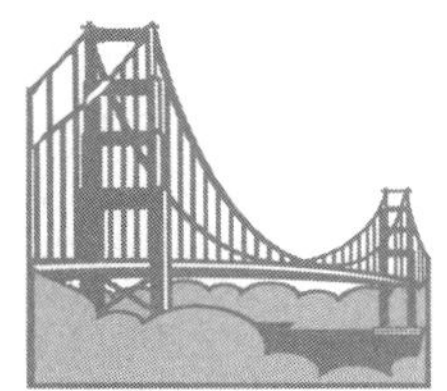

Bridge to Practice

The Relationship between Massage and Movement

It is common for some beginning massage students to question the need for understanding mechanical movement. By understanding the mechanics of movement, you learn not only to use your own body more efficiently, but also to simulate the mechanical stresses of movement in your client's body in numerous ways. You can approximate (compress) and distract (pull apart) joints. You can push, pull, and twist soft tissues. You can use wringing motion to stimulate circulation with shearing forces. You can rotate and bend joints within their appropriate physiological range to improve synovial circulation, stretch tight joint capsules, and stimulate proprioception. And you learn to be sensitive to the end range of motion so that you can effectively stretch your client's tissues.

Therefore, it greatly benefits the massage practitioner to understand the mechanical range of motion in the body. You will be able to improve your own body mechanics while you are working, thereby reducing stress in your body; and you will understand the physiological range and limits within which you can passively move your clients' joints and stretch their muscles.

If our joints are stable, sturdy, and resilient and our muscles and bones strong enough to withstand mechanical stresses, they will be strengthened by them. Our joints are made stable by the chronic contractions of stabilizing muscles (see Chapter 9), and by the integrity of the joint capsules and surrounding ligaments. If our joints and tissues are unable to withstand specific stresses, these stresses can disturb the dimensional balance of the muscles and joints and, over time, cause the structure to buckle.

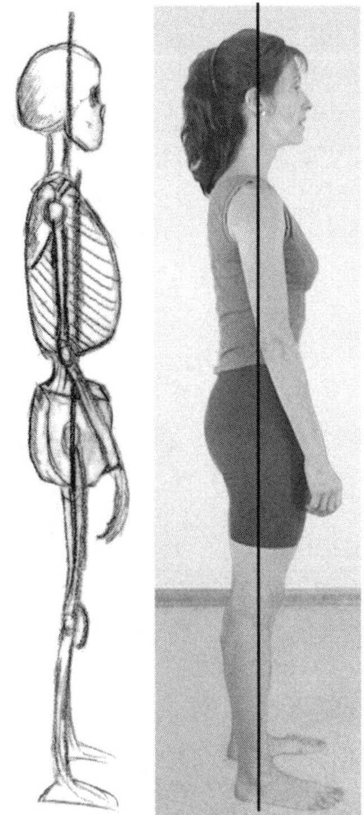

Figure 8.21 The line of gravity

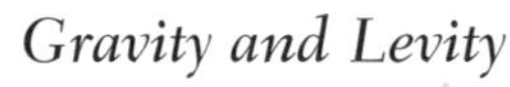

Gravity and Levity

Our bodies are literally anchored to the earth by the pull of gravity. The pull of gravity is so constant we rarely notice it, until the dynamics change. For example, its pull startles us when we lose our grip and drop something heavy or inadvertently step off a short ledge. Without **gravity**, all bodies would be weightless and would float. Bones evolved as rigid struts in soft tissues to withstand the constant gravitational force that draws all bodies toward the center of the earth. In the absence of gravitational pull, the bones de-mineralize and weaken, a problem discovered in astronauts returning from extended stays in outer space.[119]

Efficient movement passes along a **line of gravity**, an imaginary vertical axis that passes through the **center of gravity (COG)**—the point in each body mass around which all parts are exactly balanced (Figure 8.21).[120] The center varies slightly in different people, depending on the displacement of each body mass from the vertical axis while in a neutral posture. In a balanced pelvis, the COG lies behind and below the navel, midway between the front and back. It is usually lower on women because of greater width and weight in the pelvic girdle. In a balanced thorax, the COG lies several inches above the diaphragm, anterior to the 10th thoracic vertebra midway between front and back. In the skull, the COG lies several inches behind the third eye (between and slightly above the eyebrows), approximately in the area of the *pituitary gland*.

Levity counters gravity. Levity is the lift unique to living organisms that evolved rigid skeletons for support to stand and move in the gravitational field. It is associated with spatial and perceptual support. We generate levity from within the body, from the breath filling and expanding the lungs, from the buoyancy of the fluids, and from the lift produced by and head righting reflexes, and by postural muscles. The degree of levity each person has reflects the strength of that person's extension and reach patterns.

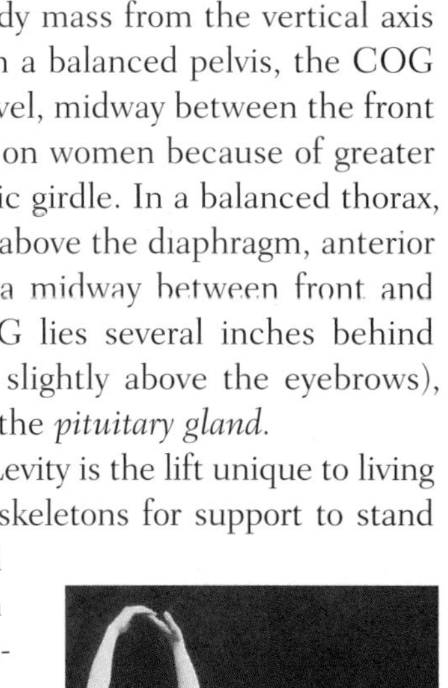

Figure 8.22a Intentional spatial reach for tensional support (photo courtesy of M. Seereiter).

Like gravity, levity is so constant that it may go unnoticed until some uncontrollable force, such as a low ceiling, a heavy weight on the shoulders, or a depressed mood restricts our upright proclivity. In the same way that plants grow toward the sun, the human is also oriented upwards. This innate upwards pull gives us a feeling of lightness on both a physical and psychological level, from the lift of postural support and from the expansion a person feels when experiencing joy, hope, curiosity, happiness,

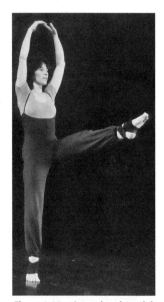

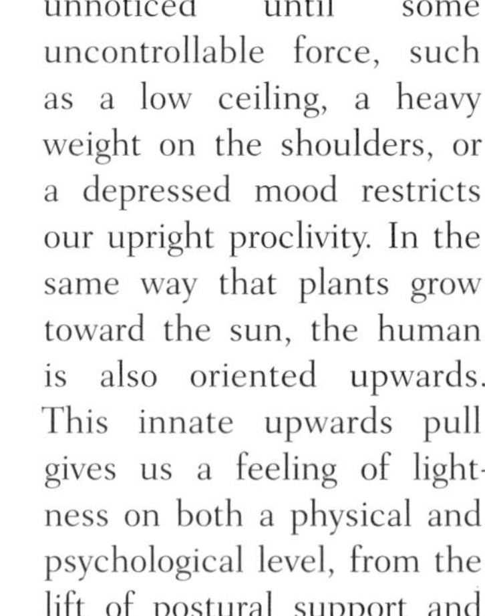

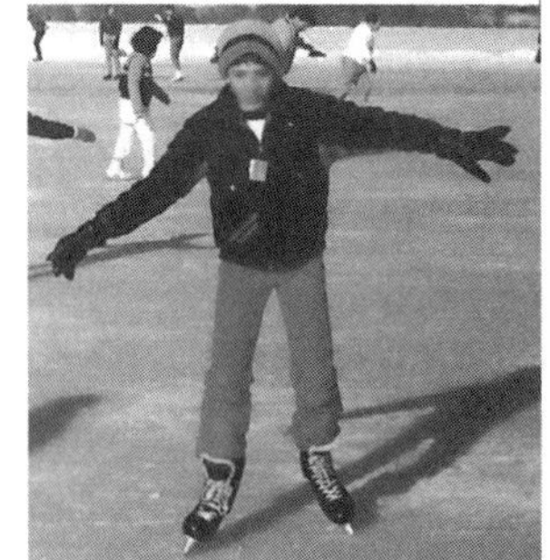

Figure 8.22b Reflexive spatial reach to balance (photo courtesy of L. Bright).

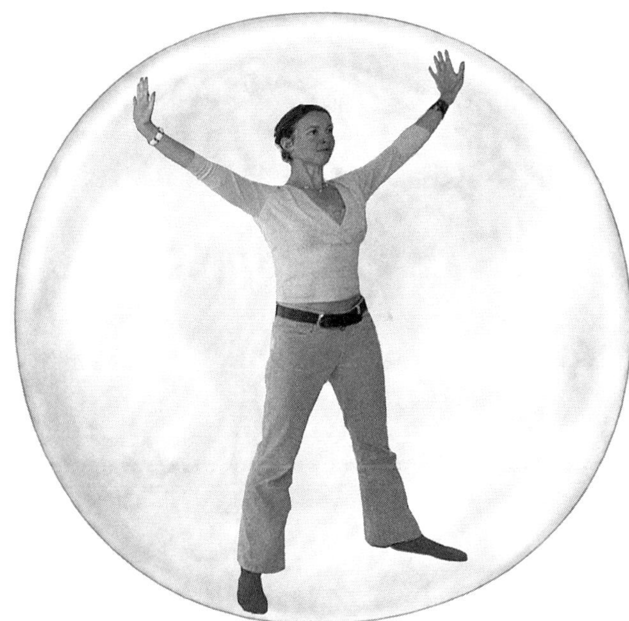

Figure 8.23 An individual's kinesphere is made up of all the points in space around the body that the person can reach from a stable base of support.

and enthusiasm. An upward and outward **spatial tension** from levity provides a tensional support that we employ whenever we reach out, for example, extending a limb to maintain our balance, or reaching the head up to elongate our spine (Figure 8.22a-b).

We can observe spatial tensions in the shape of a person's **kinesphere**, which is all the space an individual habitually moves within while maintaining a fixed base of support (Figure 8.23). The shape of the kinesphere reflects how a person orients to both gravity and levity. Some people occupy their kinesphere fully, others tend to shrink to one corner of it, others hyperextend beyond their reach, and others pull toward the back edge of it. The weighted feeling of gravity gives a person a feeling of being grounded and stable. Without this, a person might relate more to the upper half of the body and kinesphere, in the extreme case being unstable and even psychologically "spacey." Without levity, a person might relate more to sensations of inner compression, in the extreme case being literally dragged down and compressed, or "heavy."

Balance between Tensile and Compressive Stresses

Tensional forces generated by movement or postural habits translate across muscles, tendons, and joints, and along fascial planes, passing through the fabric of the entire body. The fascial system provides a network of tensional support for all our tissues and organs similar to how a web supports a spider. The main difference is that our web is internal, made up of an intricate three-dimensional lattice of connective tissue fibers (collagen and elastin) that permeates every tissue and cell. This fibrous network is so pervasive that if every one of the six trillion cells in the body were removed, a structure made up of collagen fibers would be left that still resembled that person. The scaffolding of connective tissue fibers permeates each cell within us with millions of fibers; if scaled to size, a spider's web would barely fill one corner of one cell.

The geometric balance of myofascial tissues, with its pervasive web of collagen fibers, gives the body a certain amount of tensional support. Chronic contractures shorten fascias and distort the skeletal balance (Figure 8.24a-b). Considering that the tensional pulls and distortions in one structure (cell, tissue, muscle, bone, or any other body element) broadcast through the fabric of the entire body, the possibilities for distortions of dimensional integrity are endless, just as a snag in a sweater can distort the shape of the sweater along the axis of any of its fibers.

Compressive forces pass from one bone to the next through a series of linked joints, such as the stack of intervertebral joints of the spine that load into axial compression (Figure 8.25). In a neutral joint position, compressive forces pass through the relative center of each spinal disc and vertebral body. Recall from Chapter 2 that the neutral zone of a joint is the

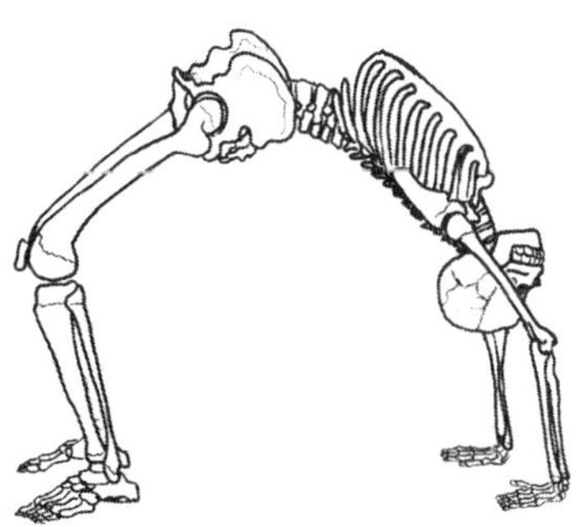

Figure 8.25 Compression passes from the hands to the feet in this closed-chain action.

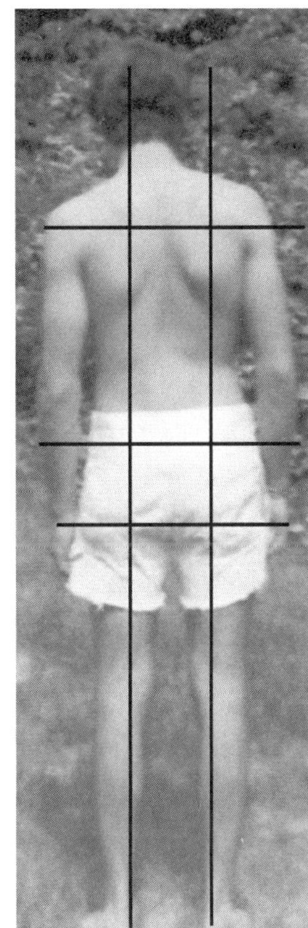

a.

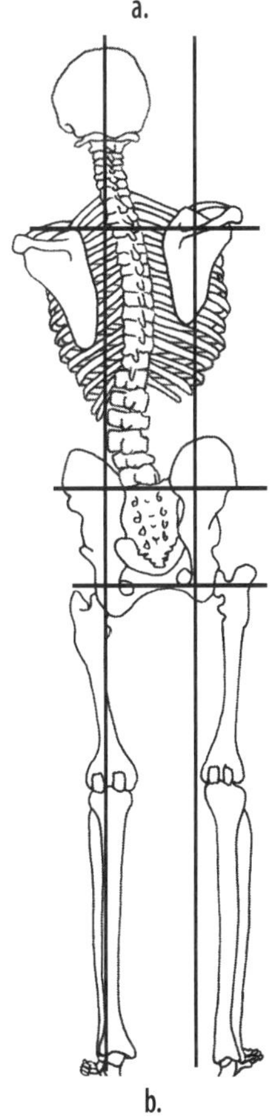

b.

Figure 8.24a-b Asymmetrical myofascial pulls put mechanical stresses on skeletal balance, as evident in this scoliosis.

range in which the joint can move without being restricted by the joint capsule or surrounding ligaments. When a compressed joint has an unstable neutral zone, movement can result in excessive shearing, torsion, or bending that will stress and may eventually damage that joint.

Ideally, opposing forces are balanced with a joint. Each part of the human body relies on balance between compressive and tensile forces for healthy functioning, particularly in the pelvis because it must simultaneously transfer weight from the spine to the legs while having enough flexibility for the legs to swing freely under the trunk during locomotion. Compressive forces in joints are generated by the forces traveling through them, tensional forces by the pulls of muscles. The effect of these two forces on a joint depends on the architectural design of that joint, and also reflects the relative ratio between stability and mobility in that part of the skeleton. For example, the pelvic girdle needs to be extremely stable to transmit forces between the legs and the spine. To this end, the pelvic girdle is stabilized by the tensional pulls of the lower abdominal muscles, which draw the hips together in the front like a corset, and by the compressive forces of the sacrum wedged between the pelvic halves at the *sacroiliac (SI) joints*. In contrast, the shoulder girdle is far more mobile. The shoulder is stabilized primarily by the tensional pulls of its muscles and ligaments and its joint capsule, all tensional forces which allow far more mobility in the shoulders than hips, but with far less stability.

Links to Practical Applications

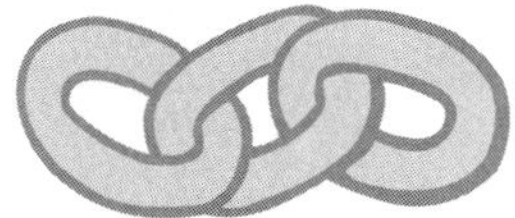

Using Spatial Tension for Postural Support

During the course of your day, whenever you feel yourself slouching, reach the top of your head toward the ceiling, sensing your spine elongate and pulling the slack out of your soft tissues.

Synovial Joints

A bone articulates with another bone at a joint. Strong fibrous joint capsules and ligaments bind the articulating surfaces of two bones together in a joint. The closer the bones fit together, the more immovable the joint. The looser the fit, the more play and mobility in the joint. There are three main types of joints: *immovable* (e.g., cranial sutures), *slightly movable* (pubic symphysis), and *freely movable* (synovial joints). Slightly movable joints, such as the sacroiliac joints around the sacrum, stabilize the body, whereas highly movable joints, such as the hip sockets, provide bony articulations that serve as fulcrums for rotary movement.

As mentioned earlier, synovial joints are the most numerous and freely movable joints in the body. They are found mostly in the *appendicular skeleton* (the limbs and girdles of the pelvis and shoulder), whereas the slightly movable or immovable joints are found in the *axial skeleton* (the spine, the rib cage, and the skull). Some synovial joints, such as the knee and the jaw, have cartilaginous discs within them that reduce friction between bones and absorb shock. The discs and synovial fluid in the knees enable them to withstand up to seven times the weight of the body.

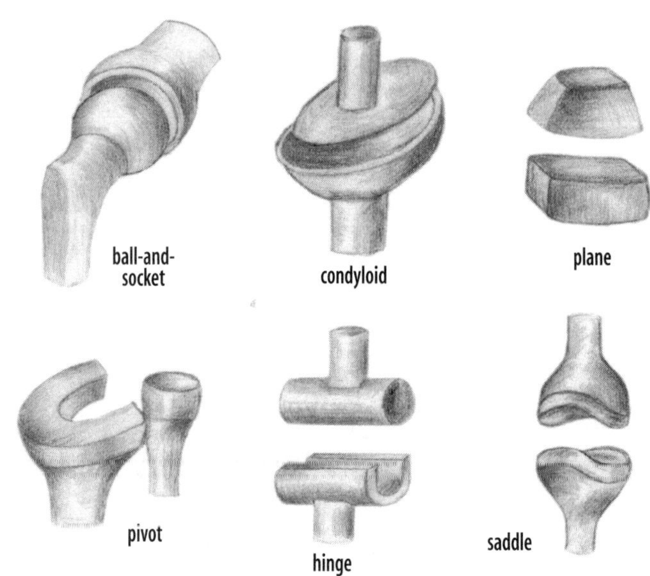

Figure 8.26 Six types of synovial joints

There are six types of synovial joints: *hinge, pivot, saddle, condyloid, plane*, and *ball-and-socket* (Figure 8.26). Synovial joints function as levers for motion. A lever is a rigid straight arm or semi-rigid curved arm that pivots around a fulcrum. Each synovial joint has concave and convex surfaces that connect in male/female pairs.[121] If the two ovoid surfaces of contact were even and consistent, the joint would have congruous joint surfaces, allowing one bone to pivot around a fixed point on the other bone (Figure 8.27).

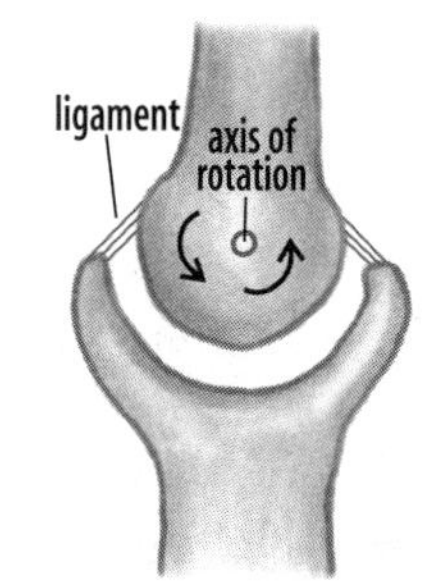

Figure 8.27 A ball-and-socket joint gliding around a relatively fixed axis of rotation

Since all joints have irregular, incongruous surfaces, there are no totally congruous joints in the body, although the hip joint approximates a congruous joint. In all synovial joints, one articulating surface tends to be larger than the other (Figure 8.28). This allows the bones not only to *spin* (like a top), but also to *roll* (like a wheel), and *glide* (like a mortar in a pestle) (Figure 8.29a-c). When a joint spins, it rotates around a fixed spot, an action that a ball-and-socket is well suited for. When

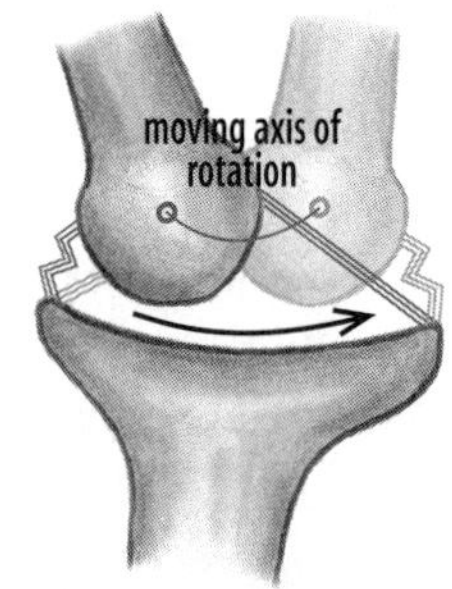

Figure 8.28 An incongruent joint rolling around a moving axis of rotation

Patterning Exercise #74: Differentiating Spinning, Rolling, and Gliding

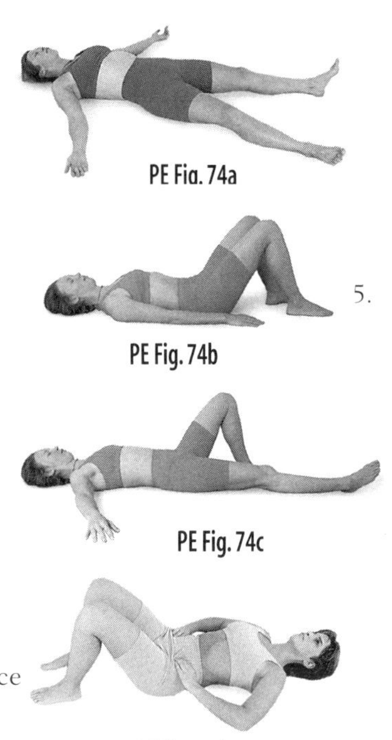

PE Fig. 74a

PE Fig. 74b

PE Fig. 74c

PE Fig. 74d

1. *Hips:* Either lie supine or sit. Then, with both legs straight, begin to roll your legs (PE Fig. 74a). Turn your feet back and forth like windshield wipers, rolling on your heels. Use this oscillating motion to spread synovial fluid in your hip sockets, as though you were greasing the socket. This action will *spin* the femur in the socket around a mostly fixed point.
2. Now, flex then extend one hip several times (PE Fig. 74b-c). As you repeat this action, sense the joint action in your hip socket. The femur will *roll* in its socket. Compare the difference between this movement and the previous spinning action.
3. Start with your knees bent, leg parallel (PE Fig. 74d). Next, open your knees out to the sides (PE Fig. 74e), then bring them back to center. Do this numerous times. Compare how this action *rolls* and *glides* your femurs in a different direction than the previous motion.

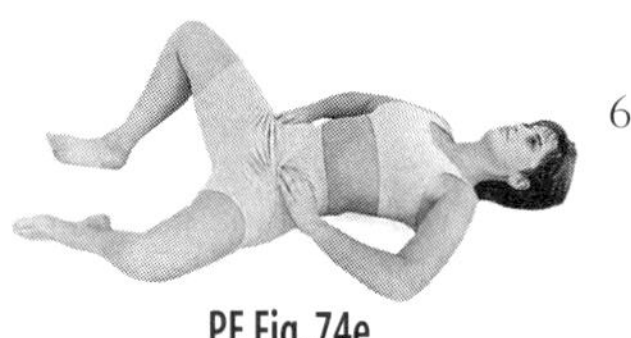

PE Fig. 74e

4. *Arms:* Put your arms out to each side, bend your elbows at a right angle, and externally rotate your arms so that the back of your hands are lying flat (PE Fig. 74f). Next, keeping your elbow at a right angle, turn your arm like a crank, lowing your hands to waist level (PE Fig. 74g. Then raise them and return to the original position. Repeat several times, sensing how this action *spins* the joint, turning the humerus in its socket.

PE Fig. 74f

PE Fig. 74g

5. Now, straighten both arms to your sides, with your elbows straight but not locked. Roll both arms like rolling pins, back and forth around the axis of the middle finger (PE Fig. 74h). Reach through your middle finger as you move to take the slack out of your joints. You will probably feel stretching sensations, maybe even nerve sensations, along your arms at certain points in the movement. This action also *spins* the glenohumeral joint.

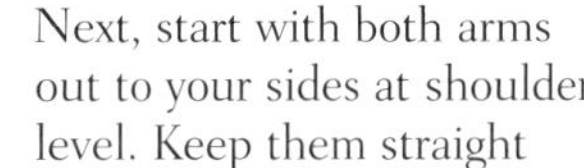

PE Fig. 74h

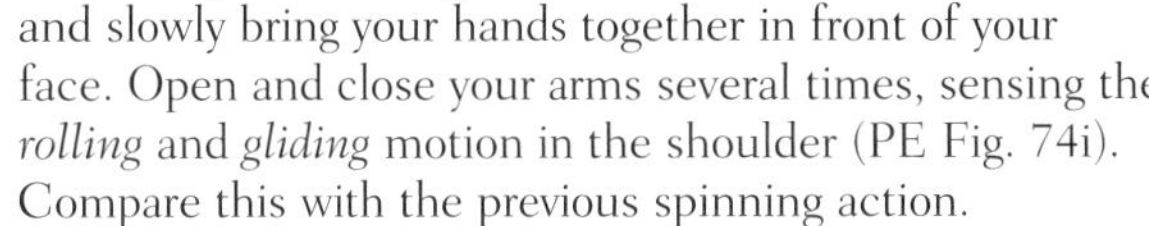

PE Fig. 74i

6. Next, start with both arms out to your sides at shoulder level. Keep them straight and slowly bring your hands together in front of your face. Open and close your arms several times, sensing the *rolling* and *gliding* motion in the shoulder (PE Fig. 74i). Compare this with the previous spinning action.

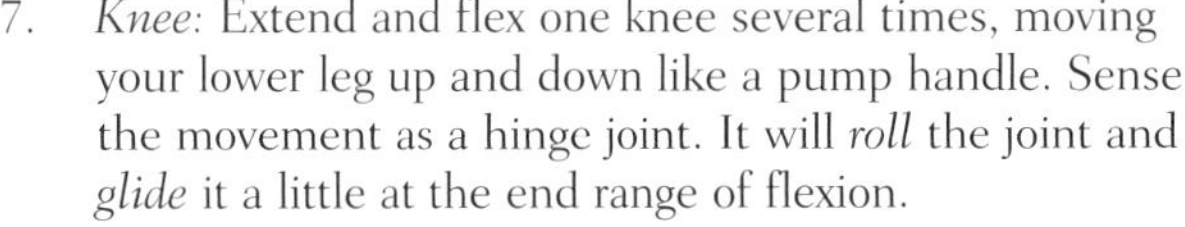

7. *Knee:* Extend and flex one knee several times, moving your lower leg up and down like a pump handle. Sense the movement as a hinge joint. It will *roll* the joint and *glide* it a little at the end range of flexion.

EMSPress.com

a joint rolls, one articulating surfaces rolls over another along the surface area of its circumference. For example, a tire might roll six feet in a single revolution. When a joint glides, the articulating surfaces slide over one another like a tire sliding on ice.

Most joint movements are a combination of all three motions. During knee flexion and extension, the condyles of the femur simultaneously roll and glide over the meniscus on the tibia. They may even rotate a fraction, although too much rotation in the knee will damage it. As joints move, their incongruent surfaces press synovial fluid toward the open area of the joint; therefore, habitual limitations in the range of joint motion will limit the area lubricated by synovial fluid.

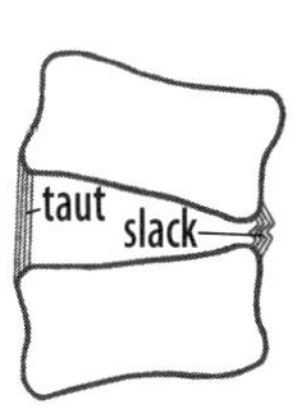

Figure 8.30 Taut and slack ligaments on a flexed joint

Muscles and ligaments surrounding a joint have a dual role: they must provide support while moving one surface on another. The ligaments around a resting joint are slack; movement twists them and pulls them taut (Figure 8.30). Ligaments protect a joint by restricting its range of motion, although they can be overstretched beyond their elastic range, in which case they become lax and damaged (a common problem in a slouched posture). Since ligaments are *avascular* (without a blood supply) and rely on the vascular supply of synovial joints for circulation, once overstretched they are slow to

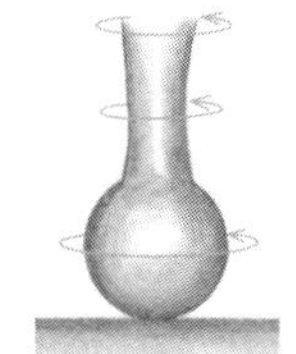

Figure 8.29a Spin

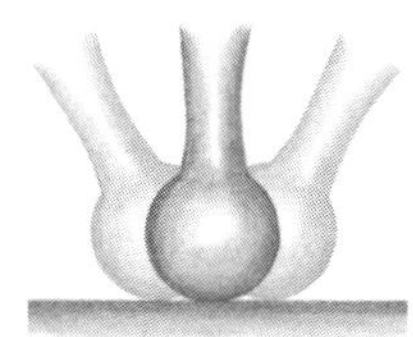

Figure 8.29b Roll

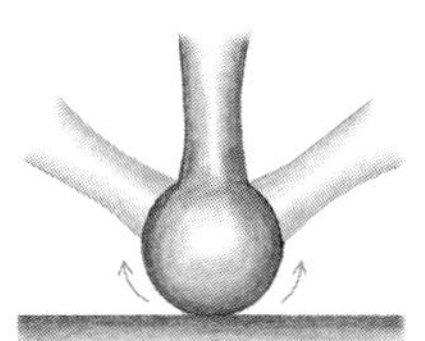

Figure 8.29c Glide

Patterning Exercise #75: Checking Gluteal Muscle Function

This exercise can facilitate and strengthen inhibited or weak gluteal muscles (denoted by a flat derriere).

1. *Lying down:* Lie on your stomach with both legs straight. Place one hand on your right gluteal muscle. To stabilize your lower back before moving, contract your lower abdomen by slightly lifting it off the floor. Then lift that leg about an inch off the floor (PE Fig. 75a). Avoid rotation in your leg or pelvis, hiking in your hips, and any change in your lumbar curve (it should be maximally elongated but not flat). First the hamstrings should contract to initiate the movement, then the gluteal muscle, then the deep muscles along either side of your spine will contract.

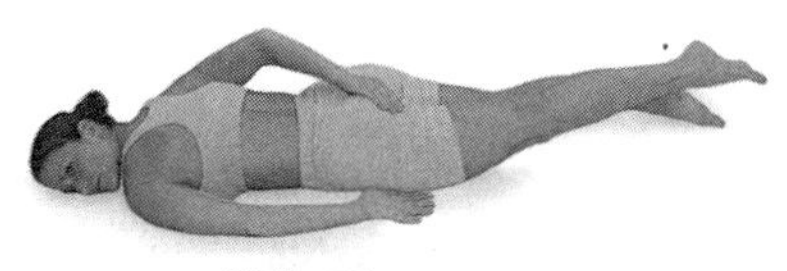

PE Fig. 75a

2. Lower your leg and relax. Repeat on the other side with the other leg.
3. If the gluteal muscle fails to contract, get it to fire by mentally directing it to contract. Keep your hand on it to monitor a change in tone (it will bulge when it contracts). If this does not work, stand up and apply rigorous cross-fiber friction across it with your fingertips for 20 seconds (this may cause temporary discomfort). After doing this, lie back down and again lift your leg. Your gluteal muscle should fire. If it does not, you may need the help of another person to stimulate the muscle with friction, or to simply palpate it and provide you with feedback about its tone as you attempt to contract it.
4. *Standing up:* Stand in a neutral posture. Lightly contract your lower abdomen to protect your back. Then put your hands on your buttocks to monitor your gluteal muscles (PE Fig. 75b). Completely relax them, then slowly and lightly contract them with a light tonic contraction, without externally rotating your hips or squeezing your buttocks together. The contraction needs to be gradual to make sure the tonic fibers are working. If your gluteal muscles contract suddenly, the fast (phasic) fibers are working.

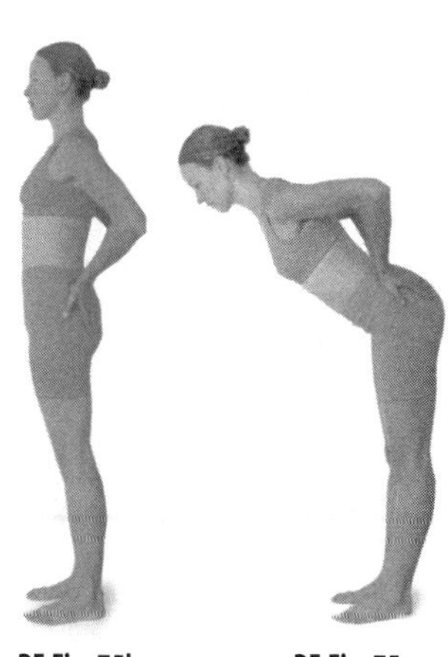

PE Fig. 75b PE Fig. 75c

5. Once you are able to contract the gluteal muscles at will in a neutral standing posture, slowly bend forward at the hips until your spine is level with the ground (PE Fig. 75c). Your gluteal muscles work eccentrically to control the rate at which you lower your body. Return to standing, feeling the gluteals contract concentrically to bring you back up.
6. Practice the standing exercise to engage gluteal support while leaning over, especially during daily activities such as leaning over a sink to brush your teeth or, for bodyworkers, leaning over a massage table.

heal and their protective capacity of preventing a joint from movement past its range declines.

MUSCLES

Muscles move joints, control the range of motion, and stabilize joints. Every physical problem rooted in poor posture or faulty body-use habits involves some kind of muscular imbalance. Most muscle imbalances can be addressed with several basic remedies: controlling postural muscles, strengthening prime movers (the major muscles carrying out an action), coordinating timing between the tonic and phasic contractions, and/or stretching the overly tight myofascia that restricts motion. The effectiveness of any of these approaches is based on a person's ability to feel muscles, that is, *muscle proprioception.* This is the ability to feel and differentiate whether a muscle or group of muscles is contracting, relaxing, or stretching, and how each action is carried out. Since we can only control the action of muscles when we can actually feel their tone or tension change, developing an ability to perceive the various types of muscle action is crucial to building a sensory foundation for effective motor control.

Muscle Fibers and Function

A muscle fiber is classified according to the speed at which it contracts and the way in which it produces *adenosine triphosphate* (ATP), the molecule that provides energy to muscle fibers. Each muscle is made up of varying combinations of the different types of *myofibrils* (muscle fibers). The three most common fibers will be discussed here: *slow oxidative fibers, fast oxidative 2a fibers,* and *fast glycolytic 2b fibers.* Muscle fibers use some type of fuel to produce ATP. Oxidative fibers require oxygen to process ATP in an *aerobic* process. Glycolytic fibers can metabolize ATP without oxygen, using sugar in an *anaerobic* process. Anaerobic processes fuel the first 30 seconds of strenuous muscle activity after that, aerobic processes take over.

Slow fibers are found in high concentrations in muscles adapted to anticipatory, tonic contractions. Muscles classified as postural stabilizers have predominantly slow fibers.

They are resistant to fatigue and are therefore well suited to the sustained holding required for postural stabilization. Fast fibers are found in high concentrations in muscles that generate movement. Muscles classified as mobilizers have predominantly fast fibers. Mobilizers are the prime movers that many people are familiar with from strength training. Their contractions always produce movement, they work harder under moderate to heavy loads, and they fatigue faster than slow fibers. There are two types of fast fibers: the fast 2a works well under moderate loads and fatigues at a moderate rate, while the fast 2b works well under high loads but fatigues more quickly.

The types of fibers that are active within a muscle determine that muscle's physiology and how it is best adapted to work (Figure 8.31). Since certain muscles have greater concentrations of slow or fast fibers, they have been classified as tonic or phasic muscles. Yet these classifications can be misleading because every muscle has a combination of all three types of muscle fibers, so a muscle can have both tonic and phasic functions.

Together, all three types of fibers work on a continuum that ranges from light, isometric contractions to controlled, eccentric contractions to strong, quick, concentric contractions. For example, the large gluteal muscles in buttocks are nicknamed "power packs" because the fast fibers can generate quick, powerful hip extensions. The 2b fibers in the gluteals also work with eccentric contractions that control the rate at which the body is lowered during a forward bending movement. And the slow fibers in the gluteals work in light isometric contractions in a standing posture to stabilize the hips.

Type of fiber	*Speed of contraction*	*Function*	*Properties*
slow oxidative	slow & sustained-tonic	postural support low load activities	resistant to fatigue
fast oxidative 2a	medium-phasic	eccentric control mid-load activities	quicker to fatigue
fast glycolytic 2b	fast, spurt- phasic	concentric work high load movements	quickest to fatigue

Figure 8.31 Major types of muscle fibers and their properties

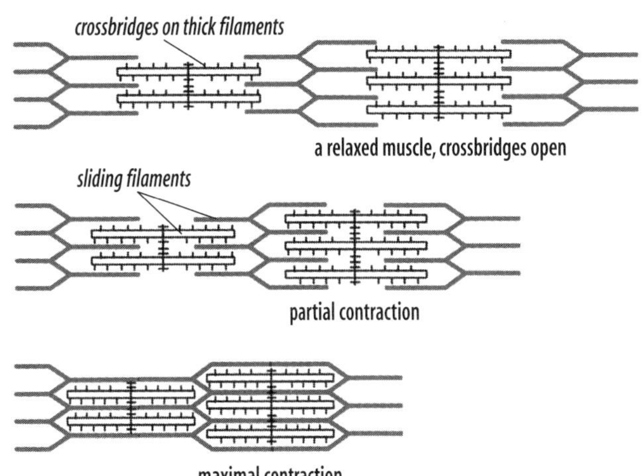

Figure 8.32 Schematic of the sliding filament theory of muscular contractions

Muscle Contraction

A **motor unit** is a motor neuron plus all the muscle fibers it innervates. The combined work of many motor units within a muscle produces a muscle contraction. Despite the complexity of muscle physiology, a skeletal muscle is really only capable of two actions: it can either *contract* or *relax*. A muscle cannot actively stretch, although it can be put on a stretch by an outside force.

Exactly how a muscle contracts is unknown, although the *sliding filament theory* is the generally accepted theory. It states that during a contraction, a nerve impulse to the muscle creates an electrical impulse in it that initiates the release of calcium ions. These ions open receptor sites on the *crossbridges* of the sliding filaments in muscle fibers, which are arranged in parallel rows. Crossbridges have arms with heads on

Patterning Exercise #76: Proprioceptive Skills: Contract, Relax, and Stretch

An effective way to feel a muscle change tone is to contrast contraction with relaxation, then with stretching.

1. *Contrasting contraction and relaxation:* Pick any muscle and contract it as hard as you can. (Imagine your muscle like a sponge and squeeze it as hard as you can.)
2. Now relax the muscle slowly. (Again, imagine your muscle as a sponge returning to its original shape.) Keep focusing on relaxing until you feel the muscle completely relax. If this is difficult, contract it again under a load, perhaps lifting a limb or an external weight to make the muscle work harder. Then relax it again.
3. Continue to contract and relax it until you feel a clear contrast in sensations between the two states.
4. *Feeling stretch:* Put the same muscle on a slow stretch. Sense the difference in sensation between relaxing and stretching the muscle.
5. Progressively contract, relax, and stretch other muscles in your body, refining your proprioception of each muscle by actively contracting, relaxing, then stretching it.

the end that can swivel in either direction. During a contraction, the muscle twitches as the crossbridges on one row chemically bind to the crossbridges on another row to pull the fibers together into a contraction (Figure 8.32). As a muscle contracts, its motor units fire repeatedly, binding, releasing, and binding again in repetitive twitches that ratchet the fibers together or apart. The fibers overlap during a concentric contraction and are pulled farther apart during an eccentric contraction.

Although the phasic contractions typical in bodybuilding are usually fast, muscles do not just turn on and off like flipping a light switch. Contraction is a graded process, a continuum of recruitment of motor units. All movements involve a coordination of all kinds of contractions occurring in sequences with varying timing, strength, and duration.

Anticipatory, tonic contractions occur in preparation for movement. For example, in the moment before a power lifter bends over to lift a barbell, deep, intrinsic muscles along his spine begin firing in preparation for action. Anticipatory contractions are so automatic that we tend not to feel them. Likewise, when a muscle is chronically contracted for a long period, we habituate to the absence of changing tensions in it and tend to lose awareness of it until the chronic contraction starts causing pain. A simple tool for restoring sensory awareness and control to a chronically contracted muscle is to contract it even more, then relax it. Since the muscle is already in a state of partial contraction, the active contraction will probably feel weak, but it can increase proprioceptive feedback of that muscle's tone, plus make the already subconscious contraction conscious and bring the muscle under a person's control. Each time the contract-relax cycle is repeated, a little more control is gained over the muscle and it relaxes a little bit more. With practice, a person can teach a specific muscle to relax more than it is chronically contracting, thereby gaining control over the degree of contraction or relaxation.

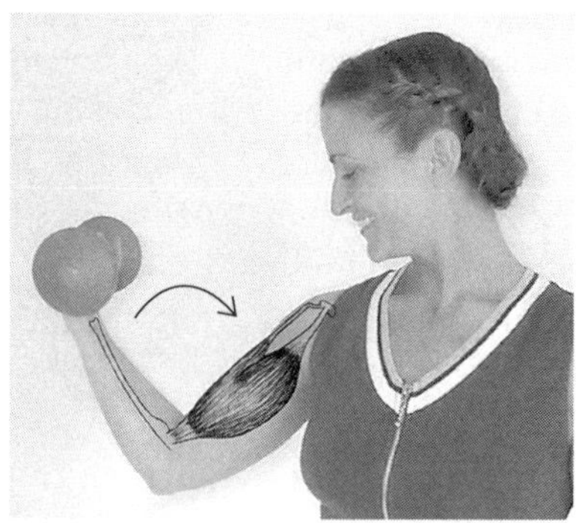

Figure 8.33 A concentric contraction

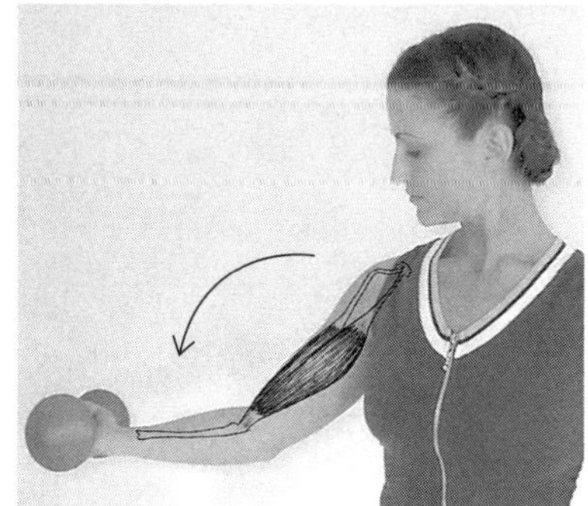

Figure 8.34 An eccentric contraction

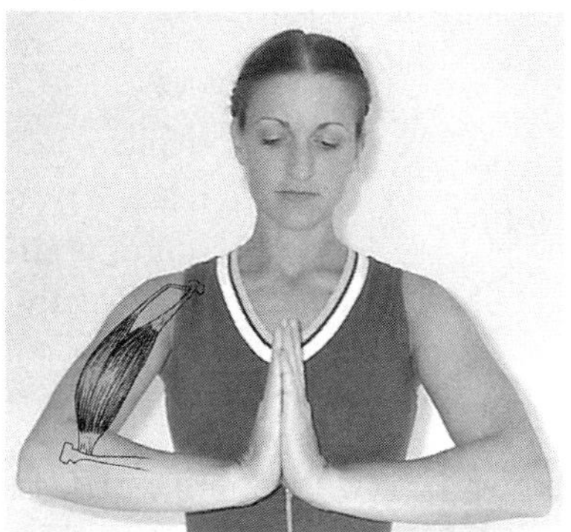

Figure 8.35 An isometric contraction

Types of Contraction

Recall from Chapter 2 that there are three main types of muscle contraction: concentric, eccentric, and isometric.

- In a *concentric contraction,* the two ends of muscle pull closer together because the strength of the contraction is greater than the load or weight in the moving part (Figure 8.33). During a concentric contraction, the muscle shortens as the number of motor units firing increases to recruit more power to lift a load. This type of contraction generates joint movement and accelerates a movement.

Patterning Exercise #77: Developing Isometric Control

1. While sitting or standing, put your hands on your lower abdominal wall (PE Fig. 77a).
2. Using all your strength, pull your lower abdominal muscles back toward your sacrum as fast and hard as you can in a phasic contraction (PE Fig. 77b).
3. Then completely relax them and let your belly hang out (PE Fig. 77c).
4. Now contrast this phasic contraction with a tonic isometric contraction. Start by placing your hands on your lower abdominal muscles to monitor them. Then *slowly, very slowly and lightly,* pull your abdominal wall back toward your sacrum and hold it there (PE Fig. 77a). *Use only one third of the effort you used for the concentric contraction.*
5. Continue to hold this light isometric contraction while you breathe deeply. How many seconds can you hold it?
6. Relax completely. Then repeat step 2 several times to get the feel for slow, tonic isometric contraction.

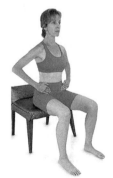

PE Fig. 77a

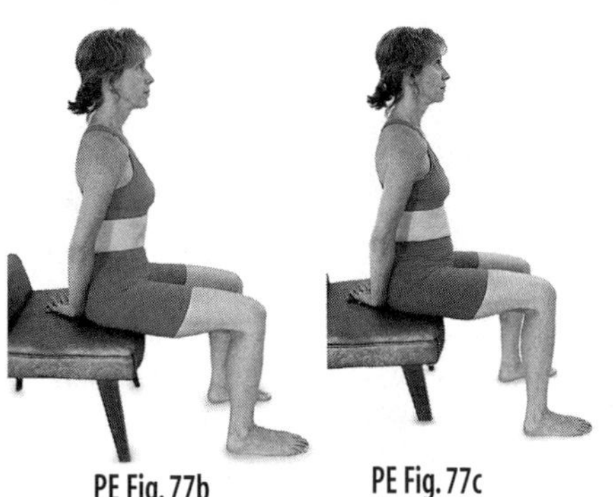

PE Fig. 77b **PE Fig. 77c**

- In an *eccentric contraction*, two ends of a muscle are pulled farther apart when an extrinsic load on the muscle is greater than the intrinsic force of the contraction. (Figure 8.34). The muscle slowly lengthens and the number of motor units firing gradually decreases to control the rate at which the muscle responds to the force acting upon it. This controlled movement prevents joint damage by decelerating movement. Since fewer motor units are firing during an eccentric contraction, the muscle works harder. Eccentric contractions are often referred to as "negative work" because rather than the pull being generated by the muscle, the pull is done to the muscle. Since the pull elongates the muscle, people often mistake eccentric contractions for stretching.
- In an *isometric contraction*, the muscle remains the same length. (Figure 8.35). Because the length of the muscle remains the same, isometric contractions do not generate joint motion. Isometric contractions are ideal for postural control are done slowly and lightly, then held in a sustained, tonic contraction. During this type of contraction, motor units fire round-robin like flickering lights.

Feeling the difference between contraction and relaxation is a relatively simple skill that builds with practice. Differentiating the sensations produced by different types of contractions is a bit more difficult. The reason for this is that the harder and faster muscles work, the more proprioceptive feedback they provide and the easier they are to feel. Phasic, concentric contractions are the easiest to feel because they occur in strong, quick bursts and they produce obvious movements. Light isometric contractions used in postural education are more difficult to feel because they do not generate motion and are slower and weaker.

For example, it is easy to feel the *biceps brachii muscle* working concentrically when we pick up or lower a heavy weight because the weight and arm motion provide obvious visual and kinesthetic feedback. But try contracting the biceps isometrically without moving the arm. This is incredibly difficult to do because there is no movement or resistance to provide proprioceptive feedback that the muscle is actually contracting, plus the biceps brachii has relatively few slow twitch fibers. In the absence of movement, the best way to get feedback that tonic contractions are actually occurring is by palpating the muscle's belly; it will tighten and slightly bulge when contracting isometrically.

The sustained, subtle isometric contractions of stabilizer muscles are particularly hard to isolate and feel when the extrinsic muscles are overdeveloped. A person can become so accustomed to the strong sensations of phasic contractions that they drown out the subtler sensations of tonic contractions. Also, strength training usually leaves control of the postural muscles to chance. A person can lift weights without using the postural stabilizers and may not even have an awareness of them. If the stabilizers

Patterning Exercise #78: Contrasting Different Types of Contraction

Note: Pull your lower abdominal muscles straight back and hold them there during this entire exercise to stabilize and protect your lower back.

1. *Feeling concentric contraction:* From a standing position, slowly arch your back and look up at the ceiling (PE Fig. 78a). Feel how the *erector spinae muscles* along your spine contract concentrically to hyperextend and arch your spine (PE Fig. 78b).

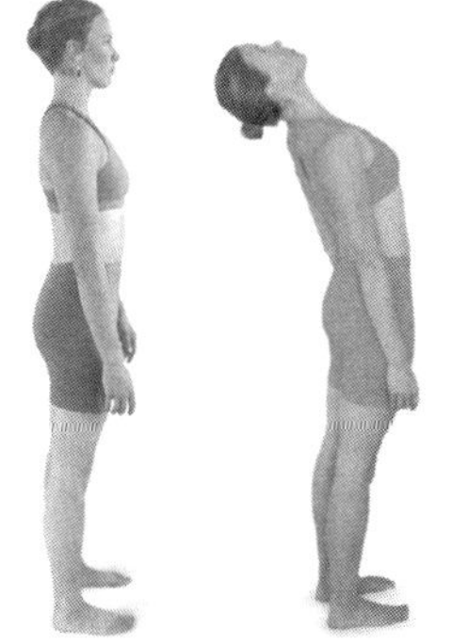

PE Fig. 78a PE Fig. 78b

2. Return to a neutral posture and feel the extrinsic part of the erector muscles relax.
3. *Feeling eccentric contraction:* Next, slowly roll down your spine, one vertebra at a time (PE Fig. 78c-d). Feel the erector muscles along your spine working eccentrically to control the rate at which you lower your body.

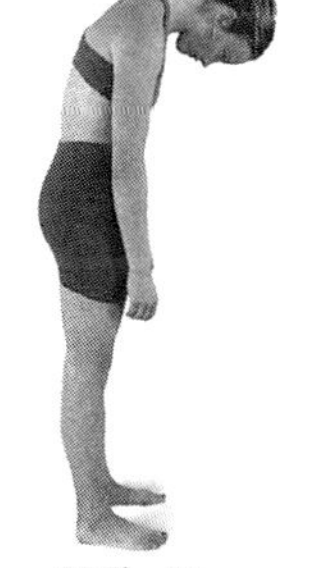

PE Fig. 78c

4. *Feeling relaxation:* Once you have rolled about 90 percent of the way down, your erector muscles will start to relax. Feel this transition point, where the muscles along your spine go from being eccentrically contracted to relaxed (PE Fig. 78e).

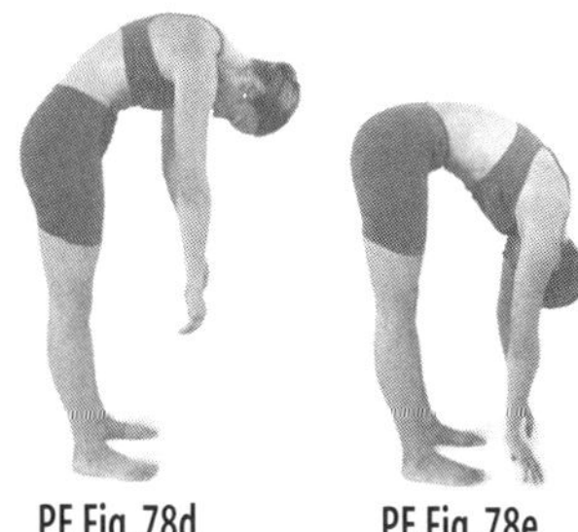

PE Fig. 78d PE Fig. 78e

5. *Feeling stretch:* After the erectors have relaxed in this rolled-over position, the weight of your body will pull on them and stretch them. Feel this transition from relaxed to stretching. If you are unable to feel this transition, roll your spine up several notches and feel these muscles working to pull you up, then roll back down, again feeling your erectors work eccentrically to lower you, then feel them relax, and finally feel them stretch.
6. Reverse the movement and roll back up to your original neutral standing posture.
7. *Feeling isometric contraction:* While standing, contract your erectors isometrically. Monitor them by putting your hands along the sides of your lower back and feeling the erector muscles bulge as you contract, then relax.

are working, the weight lifter will have a sturdy, well-aligned spine, but if they are inhibited, the weight lifter will probably have a compressed core, distended abdomen, and poorly aligned spine.

If a person lacking structural integrity or joint stability takes up strength training to correct these deficits, he might develop a rigid outer sleeve of overactive mobilizers while further displacing unstable joints. A person with scoliosis (s-shaped curvature of the spine), for example, will need to develop the muscles asymmetrically to balance the uneven muscular pulls and displaced joints (Figure 8.36).

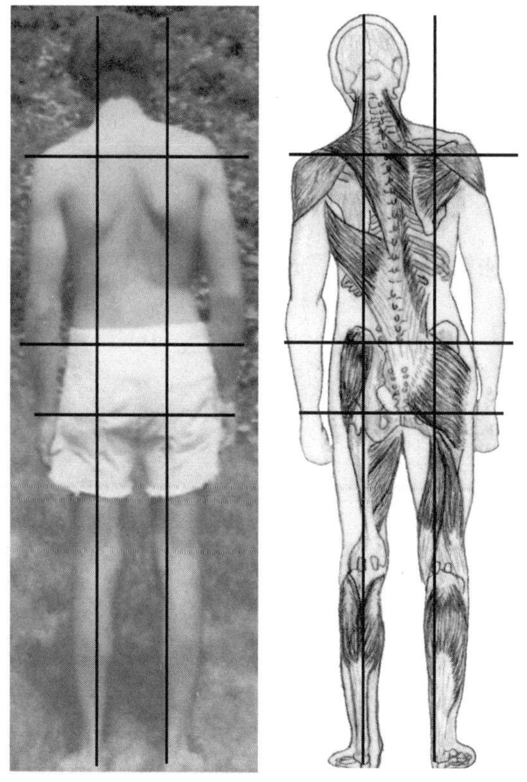

Figure 8.36a-b Muscular asymmetries in scoliosis (see Figure 8.24a-b for the effect of scoliosis on skeletal alignment).

Muscles are *elastic* and *extensible:* they return to their original shape after contracting or extending, and elongate when pulled by an outside force (a heavy weight or the contraction of another muscle). At the end of range of an eccentric contraction, a muscle has extended as far as it will go and has a minimal number of motor units working. The fewer motor units working, the harder each motor unit has to work to carry a load. For example, it is much harder to hold a ten-pound weight stationary at the waist level than at the shoulder level because fewer motor units are working in the arm when it is at waist level. Lifting with extended muscles, particularly in the spine, leaves a person susceptible to soreness and injury. This is why it is recommended to keep the spine straight rather than flexed while lifting something heavy, and why eccentric exercises are recommended for learning control of joint range of motion but not for strengthening.

A muscle can shorten to about one-half its normal resting length and lengthen to about one and a half times its normal resting length. Obviously, a longer muscle will be able to shorten or extend a greater distance than a shorter muscle. Muscle fibers have various shapes: *serrated, fusiform* (*single* or *double belly*), *strap, spiral, pennate* (*bipennate* or *unipennate*), and *circular,* (Figure 8.37). The distance that a muscle's origin (where it attaches to a bone) and insertion (where it inserts on another bone) are from the joint it acts upon determines the angle of its pull and the strength of its lever arm. For example, long strap or pennate muscles, such as the *hamstrings muscle* group on the back of the thigh or the *quadriceps muscle* group on the front of the thigh, generate strong pulls and a greater range of motion. In contrast, tuscles with short fibers that attach close to a joint, such as the *lumbar multifidus muscle,* generate weaker pulls that increase axial compression in the joints they act on without generating joint motion.

Patterning Exercise #79: Eccentric Control versus Concentric Power

1. *Moving the arm:* While sitting or standing, raise one arm in front of you to shoulder height (PE Fig. 79a). Sense your shoulder muscles working concentrically as you lift your arm.
2. Then *slowly* lower your arm. Sense the same muscle groups working eccentrically to control the rate at which you lower your arm. They will decelerate the movement as they elongate.
3. Now quickly lift and lower your arm several times. Sense how the speed of your concentric contractions creates a momentum, accelerating the movement.
4. *Moving the legs:* Either sitting, standing, or lying down, slowly raise one knee toward the ceiling. Sense your hip flexors working concentrically to lift your leg.

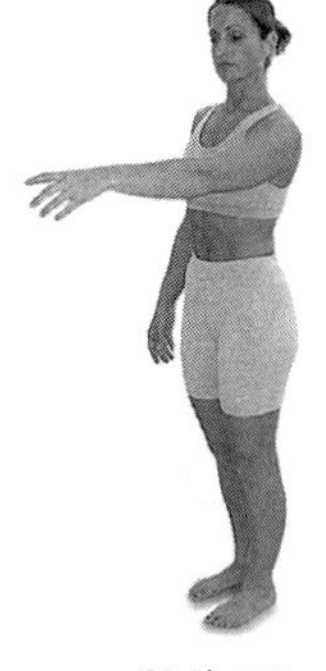

PE Fig. 79a

5. Then slowly lower with control. Now, sense the hip flexors contracting eccentrically to control the rate at which you lower your leg.
6. *Controlling rotation:* Lie on your back with both knees bent, feet flat, and legs parallel. Contract your lower abdominals to protect your lower back. Slowly lower both knees to one side (PE Fig. 79b). Sense how the oblique muscles wrapping your waist control the action, elongating on one side while working eccentrically, and shortening on the other side while working concentrically.
7. Next, slowly reverse the movement and raise your knees, sensing your obliques working concentrically. Repeat on the other side, then alternate sides, controlling the movement through its entire range.

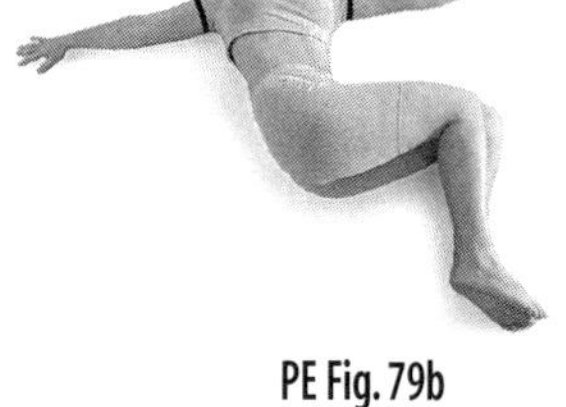

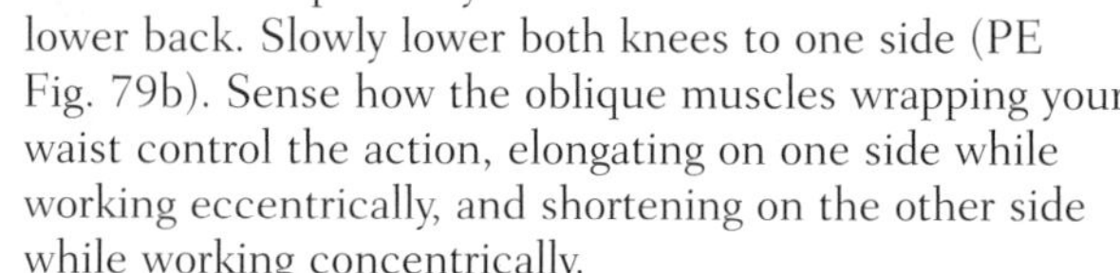

PE Fig. 79b

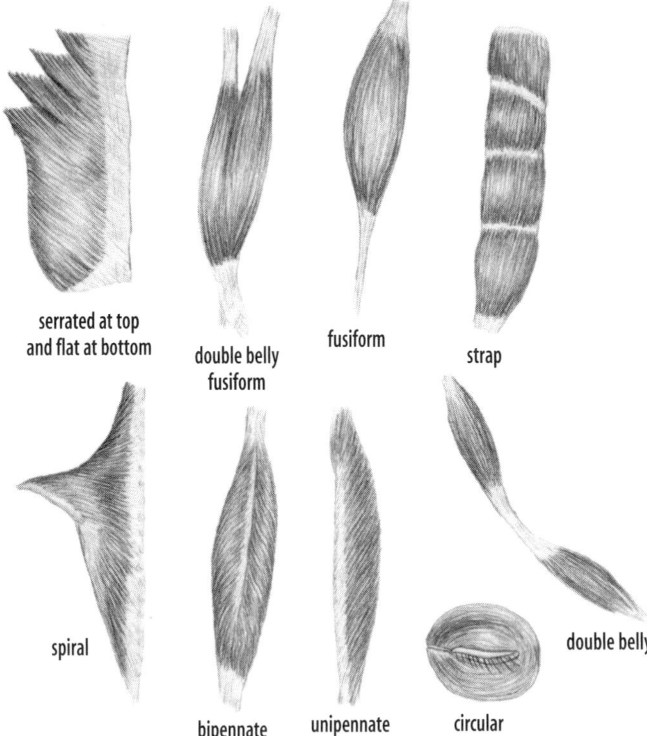

Figure 8.37 The various types of muscle shapes

A muscle is generating its strongest force but is on its greatest slack during the end range of a concentric contraction; a muscle is generating its weakest force on its greatest tension at the end range of an eccentric contraction.[122] When weight lifting, for example, the *triceps brachii muscle* is at its greatest tension at the end range of elbow flexion, when the hand is closest to the shoulder; and the biceps brachii muscle is at its greatest slack at the end range of elbow extension. Without the weight, the biceps brachii would probably relax at the end of its extensor range. Given this dynamic, we can prevent muscle pulls and injury, heavy objects should be lifted or carried close to the central axis, where the force of the contractions will be stronger and the tension on the muscle minimal.

The nervous system can organize various types of contraction in a muscle, some better suited than others to a particular muscle or specific action. Therefore, it is helpful to understand the type of contraction a specific muscle is suited for to work that muscle within its appropriate physiological range. For example, phasic (fast) contractions generate movement while tonic (sustained) contractions stabilize joints. Concentric contractions are best suited to lift weight, eccentric contractions are best suited to control the rate at which a body part or a weight is lowered, and isometric contractions are best suited for postural support. Problems develop when phasic contractions in mobilizer muscles are used for postural support because they fatigue quickly, may spasm, and their strong pulls can displace, buckle, or even damage the joints they pull across. Conversely, if stabilizers are trained to work in quick, phasic contractions, a person may not develop the muscular control necessary for adequate postural support or to control the rate of movement.

A muscle develops according to how we train it. This applies to all neuromuscular education, whether it be muscular relaxation, postural education, or strength

Patterning Exercise #80: Exploring Proprioception while Walking

To change the proprioception of muscle work, some change in dynamic needs to be made during the action, such as slowing it down, altering the routine, or focusing on one aspect of the movement cycle.

1. *While walking:* Focus on how you push off the back foot and toes while you reach with your front foot. Are the push and reach simultaneous? Which is stronger? Are the push and reach symmetrical from right to left?
2. Feel how you roll through each foot. What is the path on the bottom of your feet that you roll across? From the center of your heel through all five toes? Or on the outside or inside of your feet?
3. Now focus on the swing of your legs and arms. Do they swing in opposition? They will do so only if you are walking faster than one cycle—two steps—per second.
4. Now focus on your spine. How stable is it? Are there any places along it that tend to buckle or wobble as you walk? Gently and slowly contract and pull your lower abdominal wall in as you walk. Does that change the stability in your lower body? Gently reach out the top of the head while you simultaneously and lightly pull your shoulder blades down your back and widen them. Does that change your posture or gait pattern?
5. Focus on breathing in for four counts, then out for four counts as you walk. What does counting do to your speed and rhythm? Feel the inhalation lift your chest, then feel the exhalation sink your chest without collapsing it.
6. What shape do your hips carve through space as you walk? Focus on the lateral (side-to-side) shift of the pelvis. Does this change the shape? Now focus on the bilateral swing of the pelvic bones (one going forward while the other goes back). Does this change the shape?
7. Change your focus and lean back a little. How does your gait change? Then lean forward a bit. What happens? At what point do you feel like you are carrying your upper body in a balanced manner over your pelvis? At what point is your whole body over your feet?
8. Lastly, focus on the movement of your sacrum. What pathway in space does it draw as your walk? Now feel the forward and backward shift of the sacrum on each cycle. If you cannot feel this, imagine a hand on the back of your sacrum giving you a little push forward on each step. Does this change your gait?

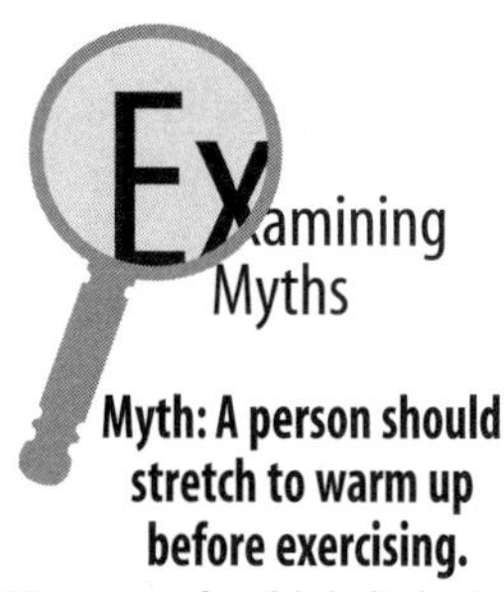

Myth: A person should stretch to warm up before exercising.

Most people think it is best to stretch before exercising to warm up the body, although the opposite may be true. Exercising warms up muscles and their associated fascias, making them more supple and responsive to stretching. Therefore, explore stretching *after* exercise, when the myofascias are warmed-up. Or take a hot bath or apply a hot-pack to tight myofascias, then stretch them.

training. Strength training develops a muscle group in the range of motion in which it is worked. For example, many conditioning programs focus on strengthening the *oblique muscles,* whose fibers are oriented diagonally, with sit-ups (Figure 8.38). Strengthening them in this manner will tone them concentrically, but their primary function is the eccentric control of rotation. When the obliques become too short from phasic contractions, they limit rotation. To develop them appropriately, a person needs to practice slow, controlled twisting movements of the waist that work the obliques within the extended, eccentric range for which their fibers are well-suited.

Although many of the examples of muscle activity presented so far describe the isolated action of agonist and antagonist muscle pairs, it is actually difficult to contract a single muscle. It is also unusual that normal movements during activities of daily living move a single joint in isolation. Rather, muscular effort is distributed along kinematic chains that pass muscular pulls from one joint to another in a coordinated effort. The active muscles work cooperatively in continually changing roles as agonists, antagonists, stabilizers, or synergists. One action cycle leads to another in a revolving chain of activity. Once a muscle group reaches its shortest point in contraction, it cannot shorten any further. This is similar to holding the hand in a tight fist until it can close no further; it can only open. Hence, that action cycle ends.

Muscles work in such an efficient and automatic manner that we become so accustomed to the sensations they produce and barely notice them. We do, however, tend to notice them when the dynamics of our habitual movements change, such as when we take on a new activity, slow a movement down, or lift a heavier load. Thus, consciously changing our habitual patterns is a basic patterning tool to help us become more aware of how the muscles and joints work.

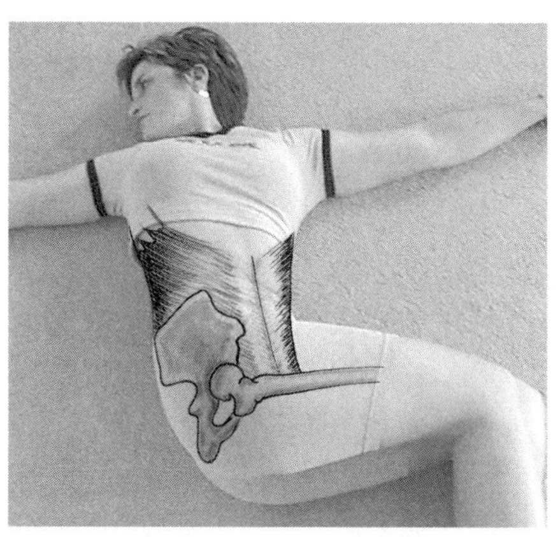

Figure 8.38 Oblique muscles wrapping the waist control rotation of the lumbar spine.

What is the difference between the sensation of a muscle that is working eccentrically, one that is relaxed, and one that is being stretched?

The sensations of changing tensions and pulls generated by the network of extrinsic muscles and their fascias, which wrap the entire body, translate through the fabric of the soft tissues. They could be compared to the sensations a person feels when moving in a closely fitting wet suit or in tight stretch-knit clothes. A pull from a bend in the hip or knee or elbow can stretch fascia in an area remote to the movement, which can be felt along the back or across the shoulders. We can increase our proprioceptive skills by taking the time to notice the sensations that working muscles produce and the changes in sensations that occur when we alter habitual dynamics, such as rate, force, direction, or range of motion.

Stretching Muscles or Fascia

Mechanical movement restrictions usually come from a combination of two sources: from dysfunctional contractile tissues and adhered non-contractile tissues. Recall from Chapter 2 that fascial adhesions form when connective tissue fibers build up in myofascias. A muscle that is chronically contracted over time develops a fibrous build-up both in it and in its associated fascia. When a pocket of fascia enveloping a specific muscle or group of muscles becomes fibrous, it shrinks, reducing the space within which that muscle or group of muscles has to elongate, thereby restricting the range of motion.

An important aspect of assessing how to stretch a movement restriction is determining whether it is caused by fascial restrictions or by chronically contracted muscles. Usually it is a combination of both, but one system predominates in most cases. Mechanical processes of stretching will lengthen inflexible fascias and restore elasticity to them, but no amount of stretching will release a chronically contracted muscle. A chronic contraction has a neurological source; the muscle is over-facilitated, meaning that its motor units are firing too much. Rather, releasing a chronically contracted muscle requires more than passive stretching, it requires active techniques that access the neurological control of a muscle and, basically, turn the muscle off (this process is described in the section on muscle reflexes that follows). Once a chronically contracted muscle is turned off, it relaxes and can then be effectively stretched.

It is of the utmost importance to wait until a muscle completely relaxes before stretching it. Stretching a contracted muscle can damage it because

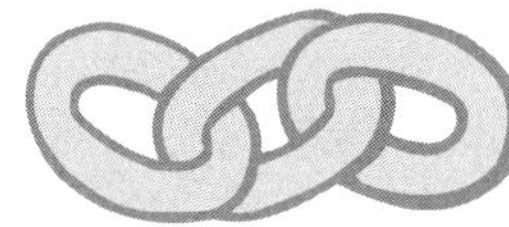

Links to Practical Applications

Assessing Whether a Restriction is Muscular or Fascial

To differentiate between restrictions caused by muscle tension and by fascia, relax a problem area as much as you can. Then stretch that area to its end of range. Next, contract the area you just stretched. Then release the contraction and stretch it again. Does it stretch farther? If so, then muscle tension from chronic contraction was restricting the motion. If not, your restriction is probably due to tight fascia. Restrictions to stretching are usually a combination of both though one is usually predominant.

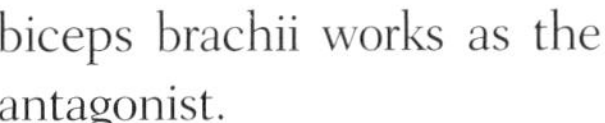

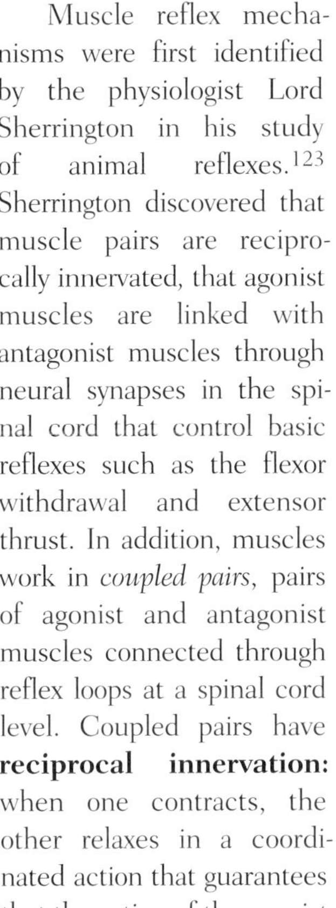

when it is contracted, the crossbridges of the sliding filaments in the myofibrils are held together by chemical bonds. Thus, stretching a contracted muscle can tear its crossbridges. Most people feel this as a "muscle pull," although it is actually microscopic tears in myofibrils. Muscle relaxation occurs as the motor units firing within a contracted muscle turn off, a progression that may take time, patience, and awareness to feel.

Similarly, a muscle can be damaged when the pull on the muscle increases while that muscle is working eccentrically and the strength of its contraction is decreasing. For example, if a person is carefully placing a heavy bucket on the ground and a fifty-pound rock falls into the bucket, it is likely that this person will sustain some kind of soft tissue injury. Unless she drops the bucket, muscles in her arms or back will probably spasm while being yanked hard by the force of the unanticipated weight, and will tear. More commonly, a person will tear soft tissues trying to lift or lower an object without using enough force. To avoid this type of stretching injury, a person should be careful to lower weight slowly and with control. Also, weight should be moved with the joints in flexion rather than at or near the end of extension range, when the muscles are working eccentrically.

Reciprocal Inhibition and Innervation in Coupled Pairs

For clarity of discussion of muscle reflexes, the role a muscle plays relative to a movement needs to be revisited. A muscle is classified as an *agonist* when it initiates a specific action. For example, when lifting a weight, the biceps brachii initiates the action of lifting, so it is the agonist and prime mover in that action. On the other side of the joint, the triceps brachii works to counter the pull of the agonist, so it functions as the *antagonist*. When the movement is reversed, they switch roles: the triceps brachii works as the prime mover or agonist, while the biceps brachii works as the antagonist.

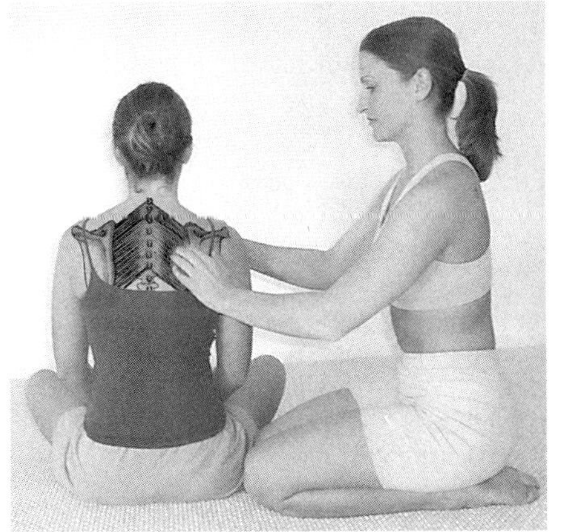

Figure 8.39 Cross-fiber raking of the rhomboids

Muscle reflex mechanisms were first identified by the physiologist Lord Sherrington in his study of animal reflexes.[123] Sherrington discovered that muscle pairs are reciprocally innervated, that agonist muscles are linked with antagonist muscles through neural synapses in the spinal cord that control basic reflexes such as the flexor withdrawal and extensor thrust. In addition, muscles work in *coupled pairs*, pairs of agonist and antagonist muscles connected through reflex loops at a spinal cord level. Coupled pairs have **reciprocal innervation:** when one contracts, the other relaxes in a coordinated action that guarantees that the action of the agonist always affects the antagonist. This feature of the neuromuscular system coordinates involuntary, subcortical movements, which are crucial for our very survival. The spinal cord reflexes trigger instant motor reactions that are protective. For example they jerk our bodies away from such dangers as fire or an attack, and catch our bodies during a fall. If we had to think our way through these life threatening processes, we might not survive.

Another principle that Sherrington discovered is called **reciprocal inhibition.** This means that the contraction of an agonist can inhibit its antagonist by initiating relaxation in the antagonist. To apply this principle to stretching techniques, a muscle will stretch more if its antagonist is actively contracted. For instance, if a person is trying to stretch the hamstrings muscles along the back of the thigh, contracting the quadriceps muscles along the front of the thigh tends to increase the stretch. In this case, the antagonist is contracted to facilitate the relaxation and stretch of its agonist.

Another important protective reflex mentioned briefly in Chapter 1, the *stretch reflex,* prevents a muscle from being overstretched. When a muscle is stretched, the sensory fibers

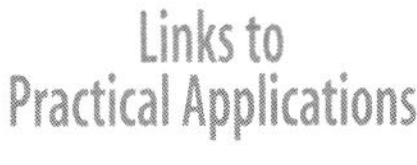

Links to Practical Applications

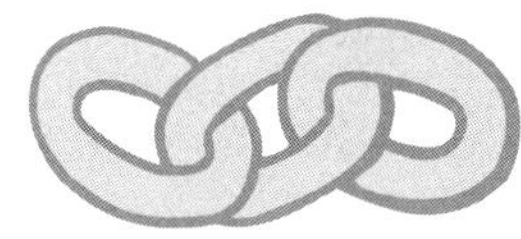

Stretching Fascia

To stretch fascia with bodywork, you need to hold sustained pressure and stretch on the tight fascia for at least 30 seconds, 90 seconds for a ligament.

To effectively stretch muscles, first contract a muscle for at least 8 seconds, then relax it for 8 seconds, then stretch it for 8 seconds. To do this accurately, count out loud, saying, "contract one one-thousand, two one-thousand, three one-thousand, . . . ; relax one one-thousand, two-one-thousand, three one-thousand, . . . ; stretch one one-thousand, two one-thousand, three one-thousand, . . ." This will help you train yourself to wait until a muscle relaxes before stretching it, and to differentiate the sensations of contraction, relaxation, and stretch in a muscle.

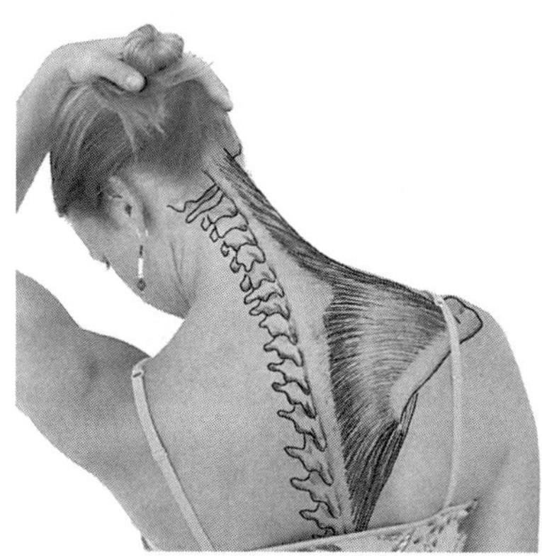

Figure 8.40 Stretching the upper fibers of the trapezius muscle

in that muscle called *spindle fibers* register a change of length and tension. If the muscle begins to stretch beyond its physiological range, the stretch reflex triggers a protective contraction. Understanding the stretch reflex can enhance the effectiveness of stretching by teaching us to hold a stretch steadily and long enough to overcome the reflex. Short, quick stretches, such as bouncing over and touching the toes to stretch the hamstrings, can actually shorten muscles by triggering the stretch reflex in them and causing them to contract.

Stretching Techniques

Stretching is effective in releasing chronic contractions, although recall from Chapter 2 that a muscle can have a stretch weakness from a posture that stretches it to its outer range. For example, the muscles between the shoulder blades can become overstretched in a rounded shoulder posture. In fact, muscles with stretch weaknesses often become taut because the body lays down collagen fibers in the overextended muscle to stiffen and protect it, causing the muscle and its tendon to become ropy and stringy. In an area where a flat muscle is under extreme tension (usually from the pull of an overactive antagonist), a band of fibers may become so built up and thickened that it feels like a cord, a sort of makeshift tendon in the belly of the muscle. For example, a person can usually find a few ropy areas in a flat, oblique muscle called the *rhomboid muscle* by raking the fingers down the area between the spine and shoulder blade (Figure 8.39). The tendon-like ropes in muscles will feel like cords as the fingers pop over them.

When stretching muscles, it helps to jimmy the body through slightly different positions to target the tightest fibers in a muscle. It is also helpful to keep shifting the position of stretch a few degrees in one direction or the other to access all the fibers in a muscle, particularly in large, flat muscles like the *trapezius muscle*, whose fibers span a broad area (Figure 8.40). Bodyworkers use cross-fiber friction to loosen fibrous build-ups in muscles. People can also do cross-fiber friction on their own knotty muscles and tendons using a blunt, rounded object such as a knuckle, elbow, or a Theracane (see Figure 2.21).

Some stretch techniques, such as ballistic or sustained stretches, mechanically pull on fascia while others work with muscle reflexes. Facilitated or inhibitory stretch techniques put Sherrington's principles into action; they access the neurological mechanisms that control nerve impulses to the muscle, turning off nerve stimulation so that a muscle can relax before stretching. A description of each type of stretch follows:

- In a **ballistic stretch**, a person uses short, quick bouncing movements. This type of stretch is controversial because putting a muscle on a quick stretch can trigger the stretch reflex that causes a muscle to contract, thereby shortening the muscle.
- In a **sustained stretch**, the stretch is held from 30 seconds to two minutes, long enough to override the stretch reflex and put mechanical tension on tight fascia.
- In a **facilitory stretch**, a person first contracts the muscle to trigger the secondary response of relaxation, then stretches the muscle. A popular facilitory technique is the **contract-relax technique** in which a muscle is first contracted against resistance, then relaxed, then stretched. Ideally, a muscle is contracted with an isotonic contraction, which involves resistance through a range of motion. If this is not possible, an isometric contraction will suffice.
- In an **inhibitory stretch**, the antagonist of a targeted muscle is contracted in order to elicit a relaxation response in the agonist (the muscle being stretched). A popular inhibitory technique is called the **contract-relax-antagonist-contract (CRAC) technique**, in which first the contract-relax-stretch described above is done (see Figure

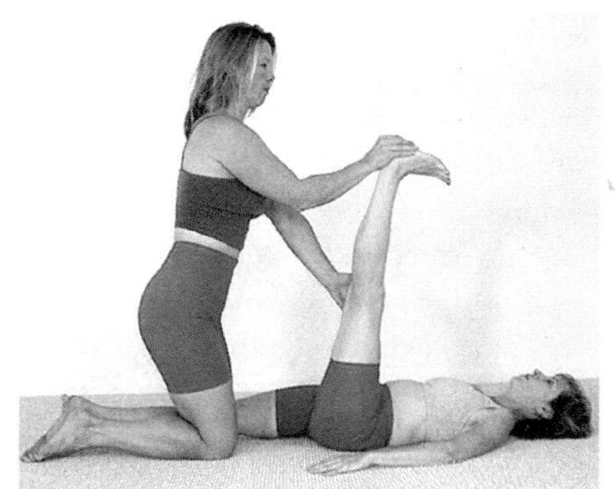

a. Practitioner stretching hamstrings while client is passive

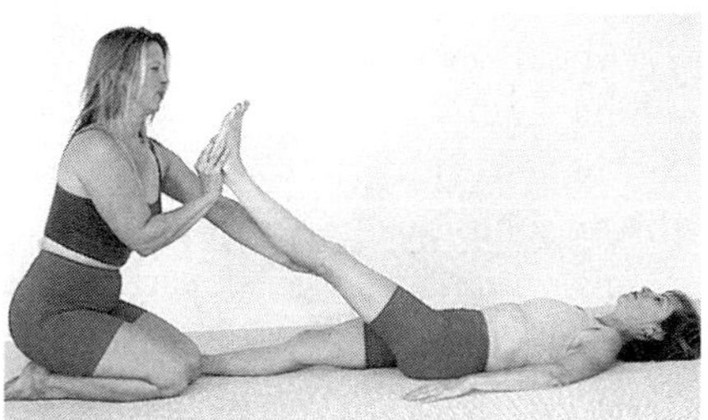

b. Practitioner providing resistance for client to contract against

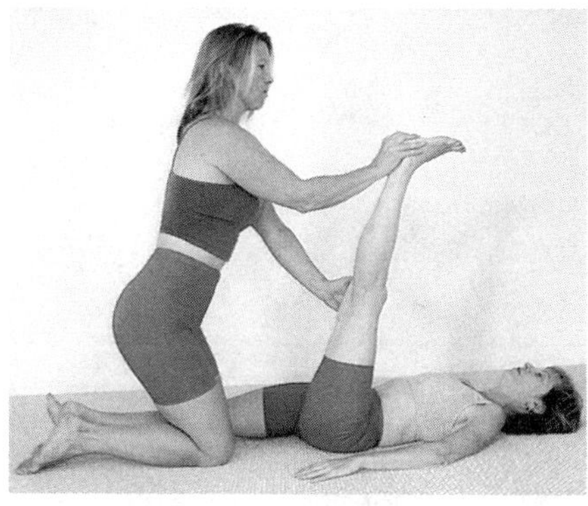

c. Practitioner stretching client's hamstrings as client contracts antagonist, the hip flexors

Figure 8.41 a-c A practitioner using contract-relax-antagonist-contract (CRAC) to stretch the the client's hamstrings muscle

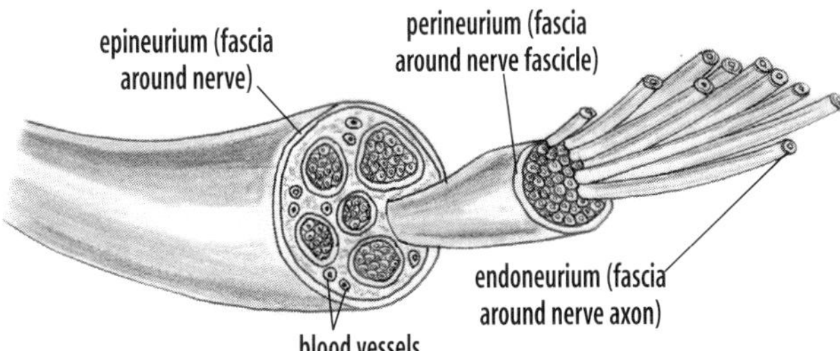

Figure 8.42 Schematic of a peripheral nerve and its fascias

8.41a-c). Then, during the stretch, the antagonist muscle to the muscle being stretched is contracted to increase the stretch. For example, when the hamstrings are being stretched, the hip flexors along the front of the thigh and hip are actively contracted.

PERIPHERAL NERVES AND STRETCHING

As we move, the nerves are subject to various stresses and pulls from their surrounding myofascial tissues. For this reason, peripheral nerves and their protective connective tissue sheaths are somewhat elastic; they elongate to accommodate the changing shape of the body during movement (see Figure 2.19). For example, during hip flexion, the nerve roots slide within their *dural sheaths* out of the *vertebral foramen* up to 12 millimeters.[124] Three layers of connective tissue surround each *nerve axon*, each bundle of axons, and the entire nerve (Figure 8.42). These sheaths protect the nerves with their tensile strength and contribute to the elasticity of nerve tracts. The sheaths and the nerves are arranged in crimped accordion-like bundles that uncurl as the nerve is being stretched. The elasticity of a peripheral nerve enables it to stretch from 6 percent to 20 percent of its resting length.[125]

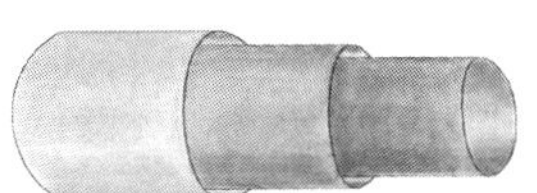

Figure 8.43 Schematic of a peripheral nerve as a tube within a tube

As mentioned in Chapter 2, myofascial adhesions and joint restrictions can impinge or entrap nerves, interfere with their normal function, and cause pain. Stretching can help restore the normal slide to nerves, although several precautions need to be taken. If a stretch exceeds a nerve's elastic capacity, the peripheral nerve fibers and their protective sheaths may sustain microtears. If a stretch causes nerve pain that wasn't previously there, a person needs to see a doctor because this may indicate nerve irritation. Also, stretching should never be done on swollen or inflamed tissues.

To avoid injury to the nerves, a person should stretch slowly and with awareness. Stretching can be done in a way that puts subtle traction on the peripheral nerves. A person may feel pulling and tingling in the nerves as restrictions begin to release. These symptoms will be temporary and should decrease with regular stretching. Also, if myofascial adhesions around the peripheral nerves restrict their freedom, the myofascial stretches described earlier can be applied.

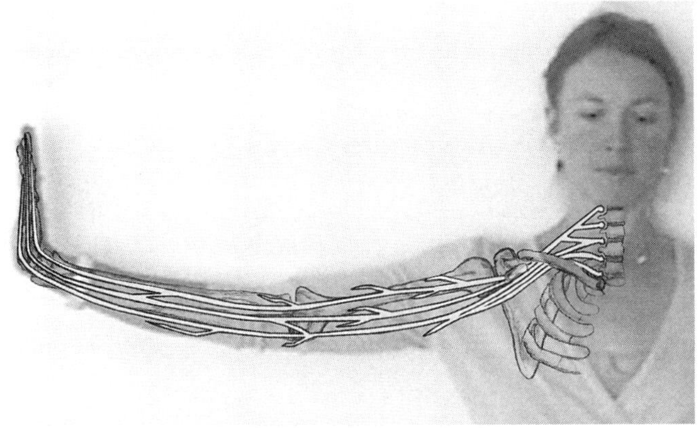

Figure 8.44 Stretching tissues around the brachial plexus

Since stretching pulls on both myofascia and its associated nerves, it could be done with a focus on both. One helpful image for stretching both tissues is to imagine the limb being stretched having a core and sleeve (a concept that comes from Rolfing), like a tube within a larger tube, while sensing the nerve tracts sliding within their myofascial sleeve (Figure 8.43). The foreground and background of the image can also be switched, with a focus on elongating the myofascial sleeve around peripheral nerve tracts, then vice-versa.

An accurate picture of each *nerve plexus*, or network of peripheral nerves, will greatly assist a person in using stretching to release neural tension. The *brachial plexus* leaves the spinal cord from the fifth cervical to the first thoracic vertebral foramina. The brachial plexus passes between the lateral third of the clavicle and the first rib on its way to the arm (Figure 8.44).

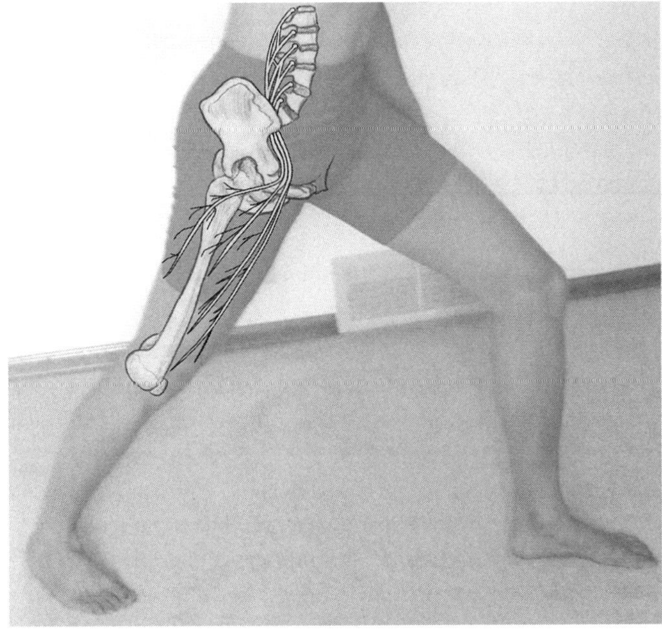

Figure 8.45 Stretching tissues around the lumbar nerve plexus

Patterning Exercise #81: Stretching Restrictions around Peripheral Nerves

Caution: As stretching puts tension on nerves, you might feel tingling, shaking, or shuddering sensations. As you continue to stretch, these sensations should pass, although this could take time if you are tight. Always stretch slowly and carefully. If you feel or have any known nerve irritation or damage, or a stretch creates new pain, then these stretches are not advised.

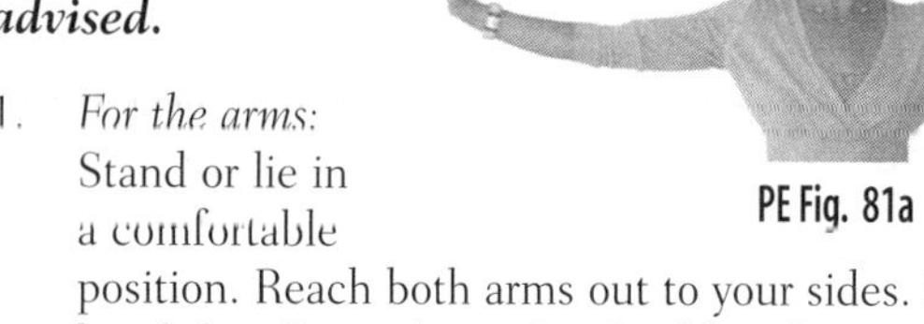
PE Fig. 81a

1. *For the arms:* Stand or lie in a comfortable position. Reach both arms out to your sides. Slightly bend the elbows, keep the shoulders down and relaxed, and keep the arms slightly in front of the body to avoid pinching the shoulder blades together. To stretch, slowly push your palms away from you as you pull your fingertips back (PE Fig. 81a). Hold this stretch for at least 20 seconds, then relax.
2. Explore extending your wrist, then turning your hands and flexing your elbow to find the position where you get the best stretch (PE Fig. 81b).

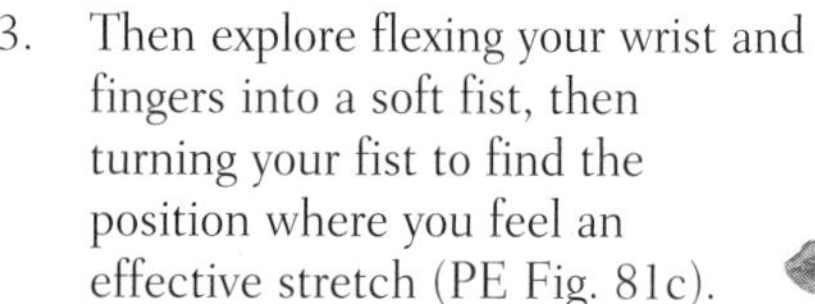
PE Fig. 81b

3. Then explore flexing your wrist and fingers into a soft fist, then turning your fist to find the position where you feel an effective stretch (PE Fig. 81c).

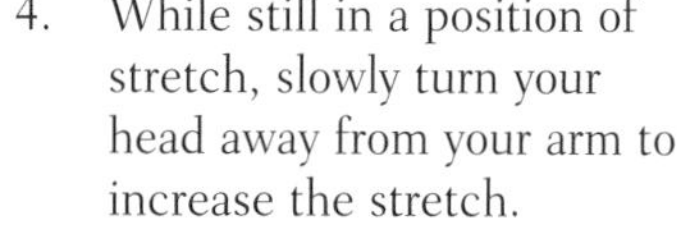
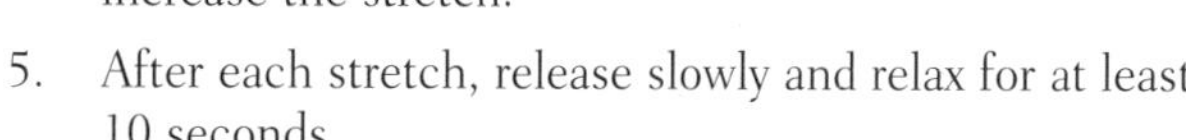
PE Fig. 81c

4. While still in a position of stretch, slowly turn your head away from your arm to increase the stretch.
5. After each stretch, release slowly and relax for at least 10 seconds.

Note: During the next series of exercises, contract the muscles on the front of your thighs to avoid hyperextending and overstretching the back of your knees. Also, contract your lower abdominals to protect your lower back.

6. *For the lower body:* Sit comfortably on the floor, with both legs straight and feet together. (If you cannot straighten your knees while sitting, place a small pillow or rolled up towel under them.) Push your heels away as you pull your toes back toward you (PE Fig. 81d). Breathe into the stretch, holding it for as long as you can comfortably. You may feel tingling in your hips and legs.

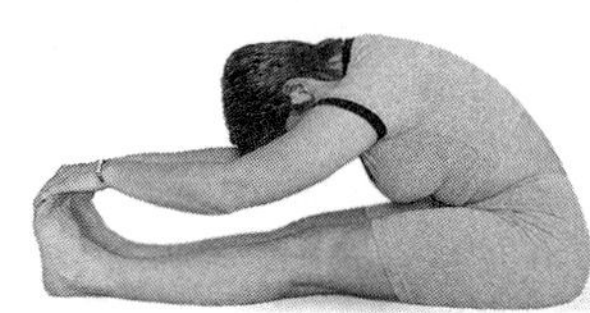
PE Fig. 81d

7. Stretch around the nerves in the lower back by lifting your thorax up away from your pelvis and pulling your spine away from the thighs. Stretch the area around the sacral nerves by contracting your abdominals and feeling the back of your sacrum open. Stretch around the sacral nerves and coccygeal nerves by widening your sit bones and pelvic floor.
8. Standing, roll down through your spine, head first, one vertebra at a time. Make sure to pull your lower abdomen in. As you reach the end of the stretch, reach the top of your head toward your knees or shins to take slack out of your spine. Lean forward to increase the stretch on the back of the legs, hips, and sacrum (PE Fig. 81e).

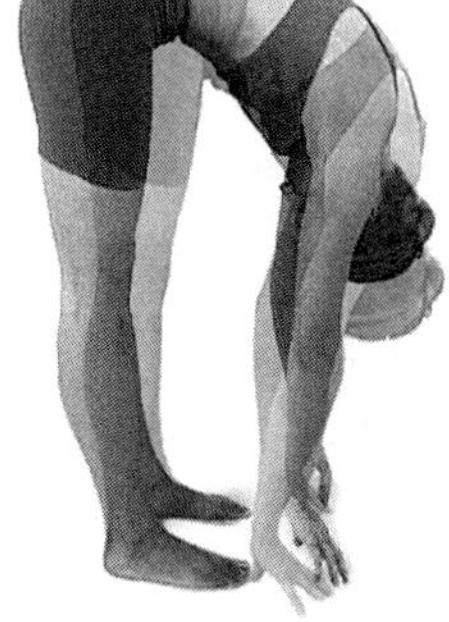
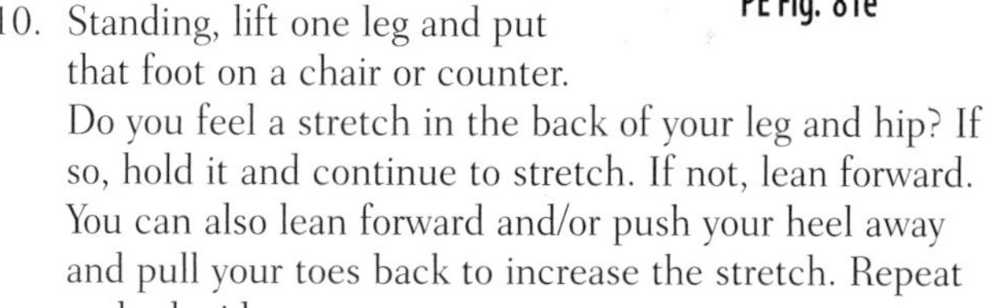
PE Fig. 81e

9. Lying on your back, extend your legs and push your heels toward the ceiling while pulling your feet toward your head. You should feel a stretch along the back of your legs and in your buttocks. Hold the stretch and breathe. Do both legs together or one at a time.
10. Standing, lift one leg and put that foot on a chair or counter. Do you feel a stretch in the back of your leg and hip? If so, hold it and continue to stretch. If not, lean forward. You can also lean forward and/or push your heel away and pull your toes back to increase the stretch. Repeat on both sides.

The spinal cord ends at the twelfth thoracic vertebra, where it diverges into a bundle of nerves resembling a horse's tail, called the *cauda equina,* which gives rise to the lumbar and sacral nerve plexuses. The *lumbar plexus* exits the lumbar spine through the *lumbar vertebral foramen*, passing behind the abdominal organs and through the torso at the inguinal area (close to the front of the hip socket), and continues into the *femoral nerve*. It innervates the muscles of the thigh (Figure 8.45).

The *sacral plexus* passes out the front of the *sacral foramen*, converging in the back of the hip at the *sciatic nerve*, and descending along the back of the thigh and lower leg, ending at the foot (Figure 8.46). The sciatic nerve is large, about the diameter of a person's finger; it passes under the *piriformis muscle*, a strong external rotator of the hip. When overly tight, the piriformis muscle can put pressure on the sciatic nerve resulting in hip and leg pain, which can be alleviated with effective stretching.

The *coccygeal plexus* has small tendrils that arise from the end of the sacrum and coccyx, an area that is difficult to stretch but can be stretched with extreme hyperextension of the tail.

Stretching with a focus on lengthening peripheral nerves is helpful for people who have the symptoms of nerve entrapment, such as tingling or numbness in the fingers or toes. Usually the numbness or tingling will subside when the person puts the limb in a position that takes the pressure off the nerve and effectively stretches on a regular basis. If the symptoms do not subside, a person should consult a physician to determine the degree of the problem. Also, slow, deep tissue bodywork, such as Rolfing, is an effective way to release myofascial restrictions around peripheral nerves. If the restriction is caused by faulty body-use habits, the movement pattern needs to be changed or the restriction will return.

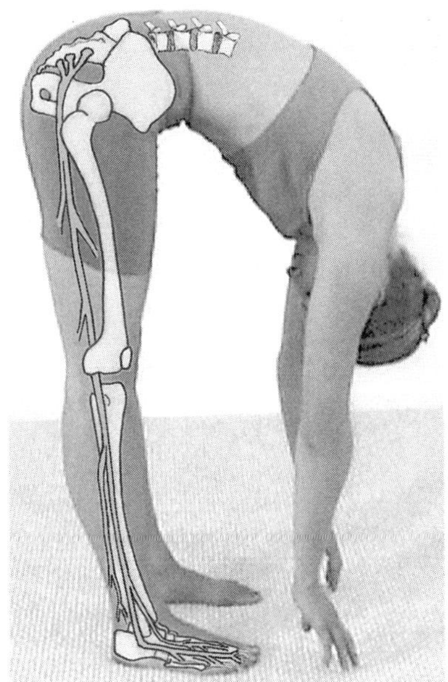

Figure 8.46 Stretching around the sacral plexus

SUMMARY

Neuromuscular patterning skills require not only a basic knowledge of neuromuscular anatomy but also a general understanding of body mechanics. This includes the biomechanical workings of joints and muscular contractions that maintain posture and generate movement. Through a basic understanding of anatomy and mechanics, a person can use anatomically based visualizations to coordinate movement during patterning. Since the bones are probably the most clearly delineated tissue, having a clear picture of the skeleton can enhance patterning.

On top of having a cognitive understanding of neuromuscular mechanisms, a person also needs proprioceptive skills. In short, we need to be able to feel something before we can change it. Therefore, neuromuscular patterning requires an ability to actually feel how muscles are working. Skills in muscle and joint proprioception involve being able to accurately sense if a muscle is contracting, relaxing, or elongating, and whether it is working as a postural stabilizer or as a prime mover. Other skills in neuromuscular patterning include being able to feel and ultimately exert some control over what rate and in what order a muscle in a chain of muscles contracts.

Ultimately, all patterning affects the neuromuscular system on some level. Whereas this chapter has focused predominantly on skeletal anatomy and the methods of neuromuscular patterning, Chapter 9 delves into the function of specific muscles that maintain upright posture, and Chapter 10 covers the fundamental movement patterns that underlie all our actions.

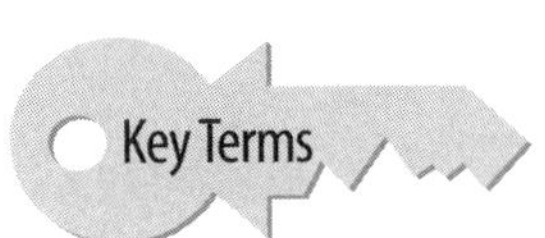

ballistic stretch
braced arch
center of gravity (COG)
compressive forces
contract-relax technique
contract-relax-antagonist-contract (CRAC) technique
dimensional cross
facilitory stretch
frontal plane
gravity
ground reaction force
horizontal plane
ideokinesis
inhibitory stretch
kinesphere
laws of motion
levity
line of gravity
lines of movement
mechanical stresses
motor unit
reciprocal inhibition
reciprocal innervation
sagittal plane
side load
spatial tension
sustained stretch
tensional forces
top load

OVERVIEW OF CHAPTER 9

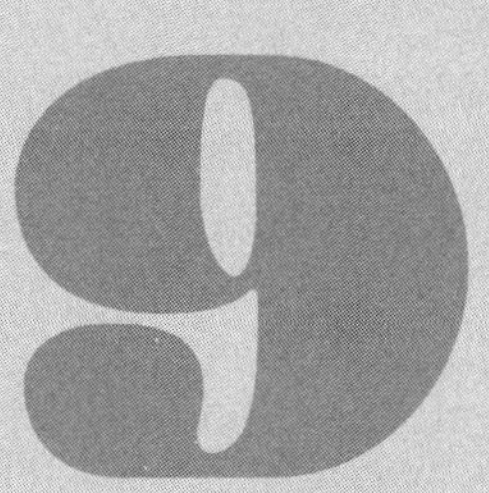

Postural Stabilization

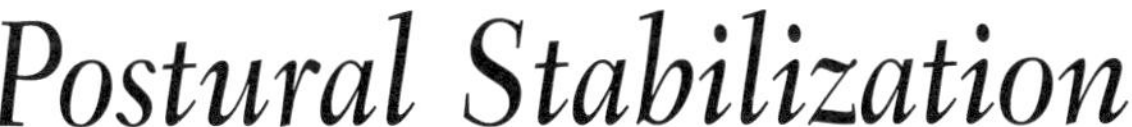

A building is only as strong as its foundation.

—*Anonymous*

Although chronic muscular contractions can lock a person's body into a dysfunctional holding pattern, we need a certain amount of muscular holding to maintain an upright posture. This type of holding comes from the tonic contractions of muscles that function as postural stabilizers. Tonic contractions maintain the body in a stable, upright position against the pull of gravity; therefore, the muscles that function as stabilizers are often called "anti-gravity" muscles.

The uniquely upright human posture has been discussed in numerous sections throughout this text. Although references have been made to the family patterns and developmental processes that shape posture, to the skeletal alignment of healthy posture, and to the detrimental effects of poor posture, few references have been made to the actual muscles that work to maintain good posture. In this chapter, we will begin to look at the postural muscles and how they stabilize the joints upon which they act. An understanding of how the muscles actually work has a tremendous impact on the effectiveness of patterning done to improve postural stability, both for the practitioner and the layperson.

Most of the somatic pioneers recognized the importance of cultivating good posture for overall health and well-being, particularly Alexander, Rolf, and Pilates (see Chapters 11 and 12). They also recognized the primary elements that lead to healthy posture: ease and economy of motion, body-mind integration, coordination, and a balance between stability and mobility (Rolf and Bartenieff emphasized this balance). To date, the somatic methods for postural stabilization have focused primarily on several aspects of patterning: sensorimotor awareness, tonic function, the use of imagery in eliciting alignment changes, the control of core muscles and intrinsic muscles, and the relaxation of extraneous muscular effort. Thus the somatic theorists' ideas and methods concerning posture and stabilization have been a standard in the somatic field upon which subsequent generations of somatic practitioners and teachers have elaborated.

In the last twenty years, however, orthopedists and physical therapists have been refining stabilization theories and methods (see Chapter 12). One of the more sophisticated applications of stability training in rehabilitation was developed by a group of physical therapists in the United Kingdom. In light of their research-based work, called Kinetic Control, it becomes obvious that many of the original somatic theories and methods for stabilization need updating. For example, a central theme of the Bartenieff Fundamentals, Rolfing, and Pilates Conditioning has been that the *psoas major muscle* is a primary hip flexor and postural integrator. But according to the newer research, the psoas major is not only *not* a primary hip flexor, it is also one of a handful of lumbar stabilizers with no more or less importance than the other stabilizers.[126]

What somatic patterning can bring to these traditional medical approaches is both sensory awareness skills and the integration of a focus on the function of parts into full-body patterns. Conversely, what the traditional medical approaches can offer somatic patterning is the benefit of sound research findings on the function of specific muscles.

The growing prevalence of stabilization as a topic in both the somatic world and among those in the medical community points to its central role in maintaining biomechanical health. Two important elements of modern life make it extremely important today. One hundred years ago, the life expectancy of the average person was about 45 years. Now we are not only living longer but are also generally more sedentary than previous generations. Thus, postural stabilization is crucial for our adaptation to the relatively recent demands of longer lives and sedentary lifestyles. People might be able to tolerate prolonged sitting if they are physically fit, but not if they have poor posture or abusive postural habits. Therefore, it is imperative that the postural muscles be working if a person sits a lot because weak intrinsic muscles coupled with weak extrinsic muscles can lead to double trouble.

A person lacking extrinsic muscle tone can still have healthy postural tone, which is the subject of this chapter. Keep in mind while reading it that although the stabilizer muscles are presented here one at a time, it is literally impossible to isolate the action of one muscle. Also, training for postural stabilization muscles is progressive. It begins with stationary isometrics done while maintaining a neutral spine, to which progressively more difficult exercises are added. To this end, the isometric exercises presented in this chapter can be integrated as an underlying support for the fundamental movement patterns presented in Chapter 10.

This chapter introduces a number of fundamental theories and stabilization exercises developed by physical therapists and integrates them with traditional somatic approaches.[127] Keep in mind that the application of stability training to rehabilitation is a specialized field that requires a thorough evaluation of joint and muscle dysfunction, which is beyond the scope of somatic patterning and of this text. This chapter is simply an introduction to stabilization theories and exercises for both the layperson and the somatic practitioner.

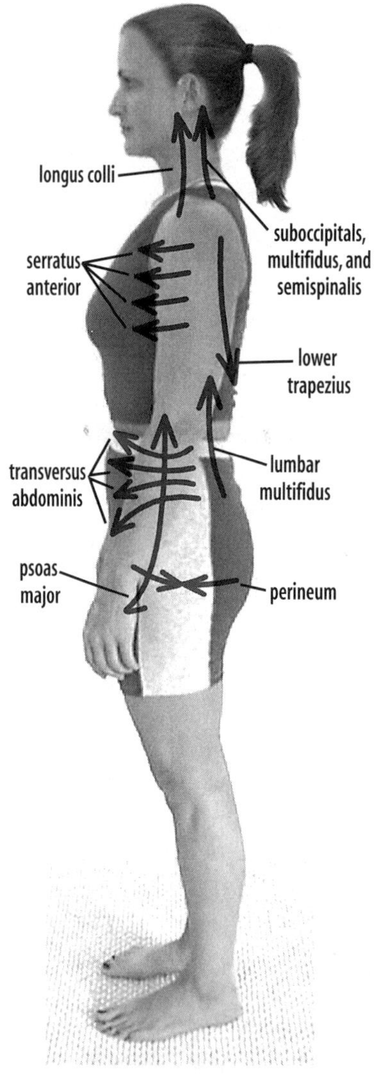

Figure 9.1 Location and pulls of the muscles that function as primary postural stabilizers

PATTERNING FOR POSTURAL STABILITY

Before talking about specific muscles, a few points about patterning postural stabilizers need to be emphasized. Since support precedes movement, it is only logical that neuromuscular patterning begin with learning how to control the stabilizer muscles. Also, the stabilizers work independently of movement or direction and need to fire prior to movement; hence, learning to control them is first practiced in a neutral, nonmoving posture.

Patterning for postural stability occurs in a training progression that builds one level of skill upon another. First, light isometric contractions of the stabilizers are practiced in a nonmoving, extended, neutral posture. Next, this neutral spinal alignment is maintained while doing simple movements such as a pelvic tilt or hip flexion. Once these fundamental skills are mastered, slow, controlled, rotational movements of the spine and limbs are added to the training progression. At advanced stages of training, increasingly more complex exercises are practiced while maintaining core stability in the spine. At all stages of training, a person is encouraged to practice the simple isometric contractions throughout the day during common daily activities. Since the exercises are isometric, they can be done while sitting or standing; therefore, a person can practice a single exercise a dozen or more times during the course of his or her daily activities.

Think of this progression by using the metaphor of three layers of muscles, and imagine the movement from inner to outer layers as the development from simplest to most difficult stabilization exercises. (In reality, there are many layers of muscles. The layer a muscle inhabits does not necessarily determine its function, although some generalities do apply.) The deepest layer is made up of the intrinsic, anticipatory muscles that contract isometrically to establish support and stability for the spine prior to moving (Figure 9.1). The middle layer is made up of the muscles that work eccentrically to control movement and prevent joint damage from habitual movement beyond a normal end range. The outer layer is made up of the large, extrinsic muscles that work phasically, in on-off bursts, to lever bones through space and actually move the body.

Although the postural muscles are usually intrinsic and the prime movers (muscle that generate motion) are usually extrinsic, these layers are still somewhat figurative because most muscles work in various capacities. Every movement we make involves the coordinated combination of muscles in all layers and joint motion in all the planes. For example, postural stabilizers are analogous to a rider standing in a train gripping a pole for stability before the train takes off. As the train hits bumps and rounds curves, the person has to adjust his grip to keep from falling over. Likewise, the muscles change function according to the demands put on them. For example, the same muscles that work eccentrically to lower a heavy weight work concentrically to lift the weight.

Guidelines for Patterning Postural Stabilizers

Like learning any other motor skill, learning to pattern muscles to work effectively as stabilizers is a progressive process that requires a training program. First a person learns to control one postural stabilizer and practices it, then adds another. As the learning curve grows, the person is able to work with many diverse and intricate parts of a body pattern, oscillating between working one isolated area to coordinating a connection of movement between parts.

Control and coordination are key words. In postural stabilization training, a person is learning to control, meaning to turn on and off at will, the tonic contractions that support and stabilize the joints in a neutral position. Coordination is timing. To coordinate an efficient action, a person needs to be able to control the recruitment order of muscular contractions, contracting the stabilizers prior to the mobilizers, then contracting the mobilizers along an organized kinematic chain. For example, when extending the trunk from a flexed position, first the *paravertebral muscles* along the spine contract, then the *gluteal muscles*, next the *hamstrings muscles*, and finally the *soleus muscles* on the back of the calves.[128]

Because the muscles that function as postural stabilizers usually lie close to the joints or the spine, they are often referred to as "core" muscles; hence, training in stabilization is called "core training." It is important to differentiate core training from "core strengthening" or "core conditioning." Core training is used to establish control over the recruitment order of postural muscle contractions, whereas core conditioning is used to strengthen muscles in and around the center of the body. Although muscular strength contributes greatly to postural stability, recall from the last chapter that strengthening exercises train muscles to contract phasically and thus are not as effective as core training for the tonic control of postural muscles.

Although the control of specific muscles may seem difficult at first, progressive training builds control and gradually becomes easier. Success lies in the ability to replace bad habits with good ones, which requires making the correction enough times that the amount of time spent in an aligned and balanced posture exceeds the amount of time spent in a poor posture. It is important to note that stabilization exercises are not just for people who suffer from joint instability or for people who sit a lot; anyone can benefit from learning them. Since any movement is only as efficient as the underlying postural fitness of a person, patterning to improve postural control is bound to improve performance in any activity.

Using Minimal Effort

Although stabilization exercises are easy and require no sweat, several issues commonly arise when people first learn them. A major problem is that isometric exercises take a commitment to repetition, precision, and concentration to be effective, all of which can be mentally taxing. To overcome this difficulty, a person can intermix the isometrics with more dynamic patterning exercises that work the body while relaxing the mind. And, since these exercises are subtle and hard to feel, it may be useful to work with a partner, having one person giving the other person feedback. Also, a person can use subtle rocking or swaying movements while practicing isometrics to keep the body from getting stiff from excessive mental effort.

When first learning to do light isometric contractions, most people tend to use too much muscular effort and mistakenly use phasic contractions. Part of this problem comes from the relative lack of sensory feedback from light tonic contractions. Since tonic contractions are subtle and hard to feel, a person is encouraged to palpate the muscle targeted for training while contracting it to receive tactile feedback as to whether or not it is firing, the speed of its firing, and how much effort is being expended. Although it is difficult to contract a single muscle during a movement, learning control over a muscle that functions as a postural stabilizer involves first isolating a contraction in that muscle while in a *non-moving* posture.

Recall from the last chapter that all skeletal muscles have some combination of both slow and fast motor units, and that a muscle will develop in accordance with how it is trained. Slow isometric contractions generally recruit slow twitch fibers; slow, controlled movements recruit both slow and fast 2a fibers; and strong, fast movements recruit fast 2b fibers. This point needs to be emphasized because *in order to make sure the slow twitch fibers are firing when training postural stabilizers, an isometric contraction must come on slowly, in a sustained manner.*

The ideal amount of time to hold an isometric contraction is about ten to twenty seconds. Each muscle can be trained in sets, with about ten contractions in each set. However, one effective contraction is better than an entire set of ineffective contractions. Although a person is encouraged to keep the tonic contractions of the postural muscles on whenever upright, while training it is important to relax completely after each contraction in order to refine a sensory awareness of the difference between when a muscle is working and when it is relaxing.

Diaphragmatic Breathing

A common issue that people face when first learning to do light, sustained isometric contractions is the tendency to hold their breath. Therefore, a person is encouraged to practice deep yet relaxed breathing during all of the stabilization exercises. Diaphragmatic breathing also helps a person stay relaxed, thereby preventing the use of excessive effort.

Recall from Chapter 5 that the *respiratory diaphragm* functions as a postural stabilizer; it follows, then, that diaphragmatic breathing is crucial for achieving the desired results in training stabilizers. Since the respiratory diaphragm is attached to the lower ribs, a hallmark of diaphragmatic breathing is an expansion of the lower ribs around the entire circumference of the body.

It is important to stress the difference between diaphragmatic breathing and belly breathing. Although the abdomen will expand slightly during diaphragmatic breathing, belly breathing reduces intra-abdominal pressure by overly extending the abdomen. Conversely, intra-abdominal pressure is increased by the tonic contractions of postural muscles wrapping the abdominal wall and pelvic floor during diaphragmatic breathing. This makes the torso more turgid (like filling a balloon with air), thereby lightly stiffening the torso and providing more support to the spine.

Inhibiting Phasic Contractions and Stretching

If, during any of the stabilization exercises, the muscle being contracted isometrically bulges out in a strong, quick contraction, the fast twitch fibers are working, indicating that a person is not training postural muscles. As discussed in Chapter 8, tonic, isometric contractions should be practiced using about one-third of the maximum perceived effort, even less if the strong and quick phasic contractions override tonic contractions. Also, when fast fibers dominate and produce phasic contractions during any of the stabilization exercises, a person will need to inhibit contractions in the over-facilitated muscles.

As first mentioned in Chapter 2, if stabilizers are chronically inhibited, mobilizers take over their job. Since mobilizers are not suited for tonic contractions, they may become stuck in a tight and chronically shortened span that compresses and may even twist or bend the joints they span. Once mobilizers are chronically contracted, it is difficult to facilitate stabilizers until the chronic contractures are turned off, which can be done with inhibitory stretches. Recall from Chapter 8 that it is difficult to stretch a muscle that is firing; therefore, it must be relaxed before it can be put on a stretch and elongated.

Links to Practical Applications

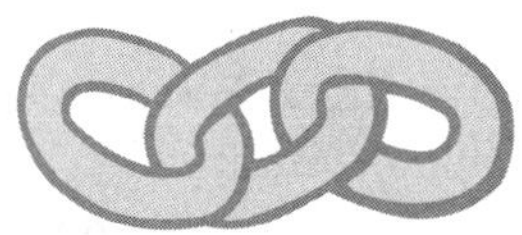

Tracking Isometric Contractions

The tricky part about gaining control over stabilizing muscles is being able to feel their weak and slow isometric contractions. Therefore, it is recommended that, while doing any of the postural stabilization exercises in this section, you use tactile feedback to monitor whether or not the targeted muscle is actually contracting. Put your hands on the targeted muscle: as it contracts, you should feel it slowly tighten and bulge under your hands. Also, make sure it contracts slowly. If it hardens or bulges quickly, you are doing the exercise incorrectly by using fast muscle fibers.

The best results from stretching come from knowing what kind of stretch to use when. Since ballistic stretches are controversial, they are not recommended to stretch myofascias, although they can be used to warm up the body before an activity. The following are guidelines for what type of stretches to use when:

- If fascial restrictions and fibrous build-up in the muscle cause rigidity, use a *slow sustained stretch*. The stretch should be held long enough to override the stretch reflex in the muscle (a reflex that causes a muscle to contract after being put on a quick stretch), from 30 seconds to 2 minutes. Hold the stretch long enough to feel a sensation of the myofascial tissues elongating.
- If myofascial restrictions are caused by muscle weakness from immobility, use a *facilitory stretch*, such as the contract-relax technique. To do this, put the muscle in a position of stretch. Then contract it, relax it, and stretch it even farther.

Patterning Exercise #82 Diaphragmatic Breathing

Note: The hallmark of diaphragmatic breathing is the lateral expansion of the lower ribs.

1. Sit, stand, or lie in a comfortable position. Take in several deep breaths and notice what moves first (your abdominal wall, your lower ribs, your solar plexus, etc.).
2. Place your hands on the sides of your lower ribs (PE Fig. 82a). As you inhale, expand your lower ribs into your hands to engage the diaphragm (PE Fig. 82b). Then exhale and relax.
3. Continue to breathe like this until you feel you can initiate breathing with the lateral expansion of your ribs.

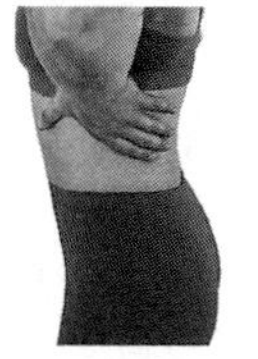

PE Fig. 82a

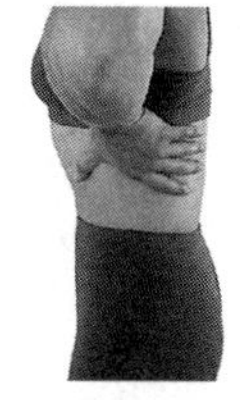

PE Fig. 82b

EMSPress.com

- Lastly, if myofascial restrictions are caused by the over-facilitation of a muscle, use an *inhibitory stretch* such as the CRAC technique (described in Chapter 8). To do this, repeat the contract-relax technique—contract the muscle, then relax it, then stretch it. While it is stretching, actively contract its antagonist.

Spinal Stabilization and Neutral Posture

Recall from Chapter 2 that the spine moves more efficiently from a stable, neutral posture because this is a position of mechanical advantage. There are several considerations for achieving the optimal spinal alignment. First, the body's weight needs to be carried as close to the central axis as possible. Second, the postural muscles need to work in a manner that maintains the spinal curves at their maximum length. And third, they need to co-contract as a unified system. If any one of the postural stabilizers fails to fire, the chain of underlying support will be compromised, reducing the integrity and stability of postural alignment. This will make subsequent movement less efficient because when a postural stabilizer is inhibited, the larger mobilizer muscles take over its job. This forces the mobilizers to support the body as well as move it. Recall from Chapter 8 that the mobilizers have predominantly fast motor units; they will rapidly fatigue when stuck in tonic contractions to stabilize the body. In addition, their chronic contractions will reduce the economy of motion because if they are held in contraction, they are not free to move through normal contraction/relaxation cycles.

Unlike quadrupeds, whose tonic muscles are distributed over a horizontal spine, our postural muscles are distributed along a single column (Figure 9.2a-b). The quadruped's tonic muscles work like straps pulling each functional segment (two adjacent vertebrae and their shared disc) up on its own axis to prevent it from buckling. Our postural muscles are distributed along one vertical axis and co-contract in synchrony toward the unified goal of verticality.

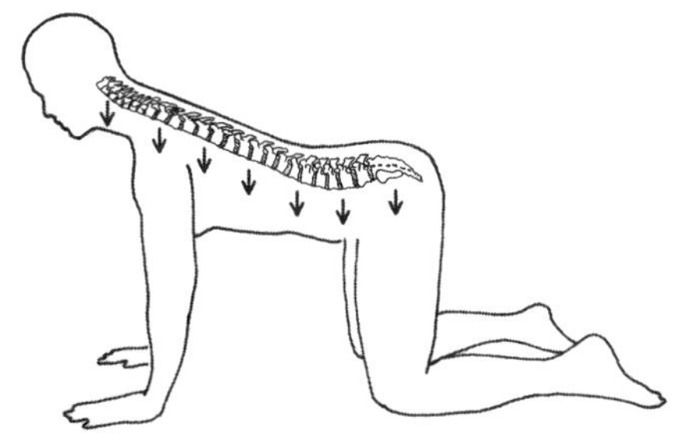

Figure 9.2a The gravitational pull on the quadruped spine travels through each vertebra.

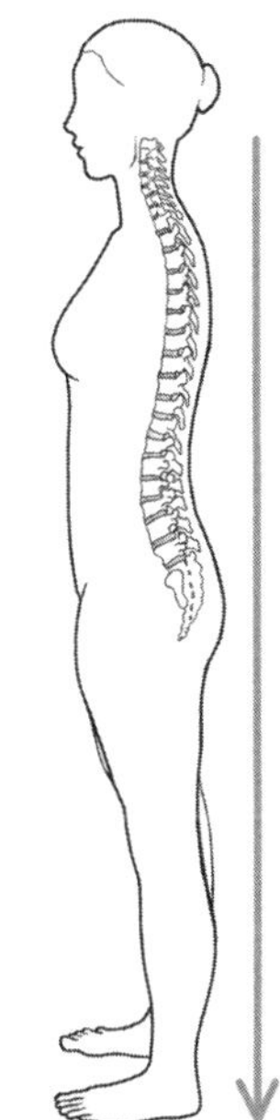

Figure 9.2b The pull on the human spine is unified because it travels through a single vertical axis.

Although the arrangement of human postural muscles is much more efficient than that of quadrupeds because the force of each muscle is distributed along a single column, the downside of this arrangement is that instability in one segment transfers stress along the entire column. Conversely, the stability of a single segment contributes to greater balance in the entire spine.

The push patterns presented in Chapter 7 on developmental movement, particularly the spinal push, facilitate the deep tonic contractions that increase axial compression along the spine and through the limbs. If a person successfully coordinates movement in all the push patterns during early motor development, and the push patterns are strong, chances are good that that person will develop a stable

Patterning Exercise #83: Hip Hinge in Forward Bending

This exercise (adapted from Sahrmann) is helpful for learning to keep your spine stable as you move. It can also be used to assess where the spine is unstable.

1. Stand or sit in a neutral, vertical posture.
2. Stabilize your spine in neutral by lightly pulling your lower abdomen straight back, then lightly contracting the deep muscles along the front and back of your spine. Reach out the top of your head to elongate your neck and engage the cervical stabilizers (PE Fig. 83a).
3. Take several breaths while maintaining this stable position.
4. Keeping your spine long, straight, and stable. Lean forward by bending at the hips (PE Fig. 83b).
5. Come back to neutral, then slowly lean forward again. Explore this action several times while concentrating on maintaining a neutral spine (described in step 2 above).

Feedback: Can you keep your spine neutral as you lean forward? Does your spine break or bend anywhere along the column? Check your posture in a mirror or put a yardstick along your back and keep your spine against it as you lean forward. If you have trouble initiating the movement, explore reaching behind you with your tail, or bending only at your hips, creasing in the front of the hips. To avoid rounding your back, keep your shoulder blades and chest wide, your legs parallel, and reach out the top of your head. Keep your spine as long as possible.

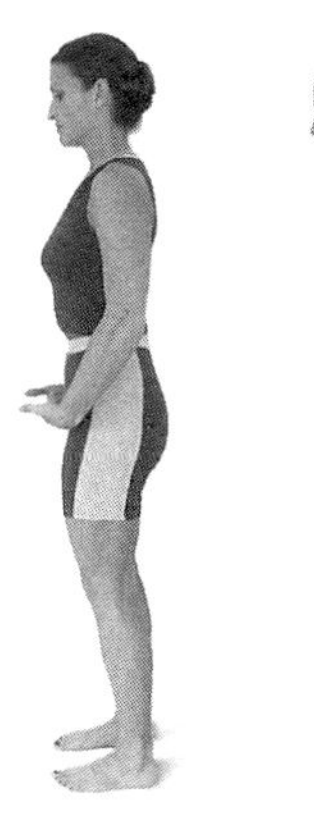

PE Fig. 83a

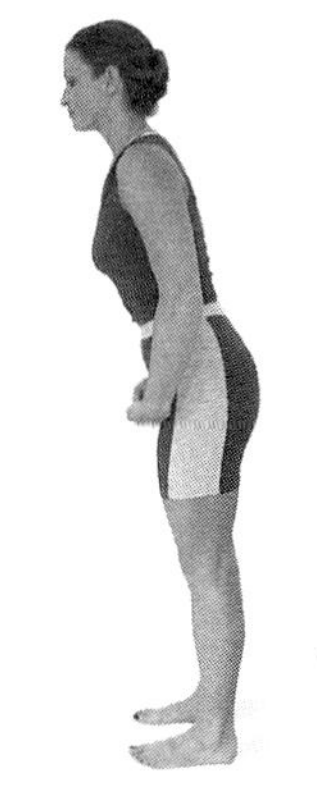

PE Fig. 83b

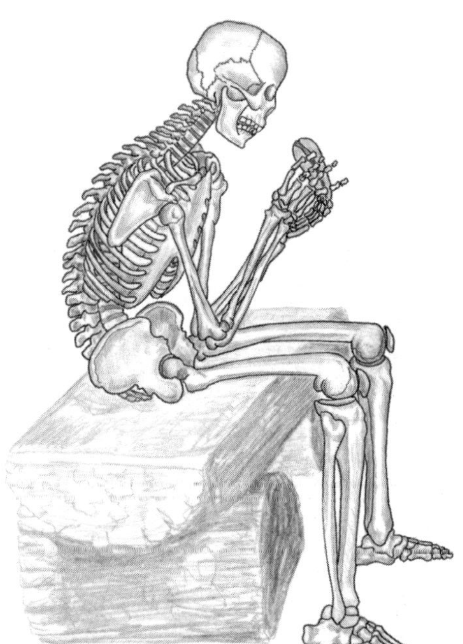

Figure 9.3a A common cause of low back pain comes from the prolonged stress that bending puts on the joints and discs.

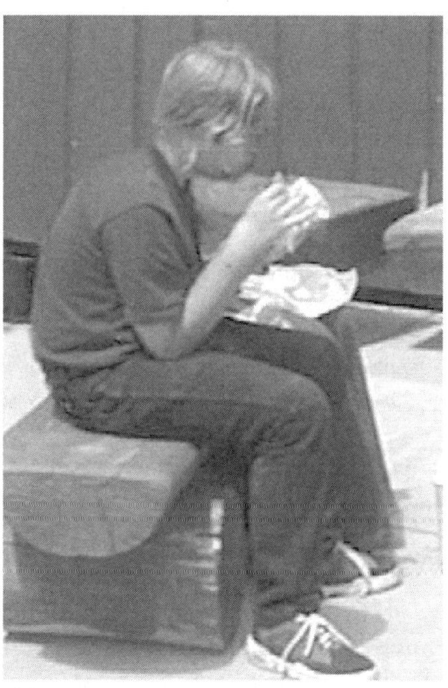

Figure 9.3b Postures that bend the spine often become habitual in childhood.

spine that is well-aligned in a neutral posture. If the push patterns are weak, particularly the spinal pushes, a person may lack stability through the entire column. Stability can be built by practicing spinal pushes, although patterning the stabilizers while in a neutral spinal alignment is probably a more direct route to stabilization.

A balanced, neutral spine and pelvis ride over the legs in a manner similar to how an experienced rider stays balanced on top of a horse. The rider is responsive to the movement of the horse; she is not thrown or jarred by the quick pulls and turns of the horse's legs. Likewise, a stable spine is responsive to the motion of the limbs; it remains balanced and connected during all movements. For example, during a forward bending movement, the hips pivot on the legs and the spine rides on top. If a person habitually bends forward by flexing somewhere along the spine, usually in the upper or lower back, the *intervertebral joints* and *facet joints* at the apex of flexion bend and become stressed by the habitual angle. A common cause of lower back pain is slouching (Figure 9.3a-b). This abusive posture compresses the sacrum and puts the lumbar spine on a prolonged stretch, overstretching and weakening the surrounding ligaments and tissues and gradually displacing the lumbar discs posteriorly.[129] Slouching also puts the upper spine under bending stresses, often causing chronic pain in the thoracic spine and neck.

The Dissociation of Joint Motion

Newborns generally move with full-body patterns. Later, as early motor development progresses and a baby gradually becomes more coordinated, he is able to control the movement in his various parts. This process of differentiation continues throughout motor development and provides us with the ability to isolate the action of a single joint. A moving joint rotates around an axis that can change from moment to moment. Ideally, the axis of rotation is within that joint's physiological range. But rigidity from chronic myofascial tensions can restrict range of joint motion and stiffen a joint, limiting its axis of rotation, resulting in a compensatory instability in an adjacent joint. Like water flowing through rocks, the force of a movement passes along a kinetic chain, bypassing rigid joints and knocking unstable joints off their central axis.

It is important that each joint is stable yet moves within its physiological range so that the forces of movement can sequence evenly through each joint in a kinematic chain (such as the foot, ankle, knee, hip, and spinal joints during walking). If one joint in the chain is restricted, another will become hypermobile and unstable to compensate, and vice-versa. Muscles compensate for instabilities by becoming chronically contracted, thereby limiting the range of motion in the joints they span.

To make certain that the forces of movement are distributed evenly through a series of joints, a person can practice dissociation exercises to gain control over a single joint or groups of joints. The **dissociation of movement** is a basic patterning skill in which a person isolates the movement of one area from another to gain control over that area. The isolation can be done with one bone in a joint, or with a joint adjacent to another joint, or with a section of the spine (lumbar, thoracic, or cervical in relation to the rest of the spine). Dissociation is the opposite of integration (the coordinated movement of all parts in synchrony), although it is a vital skill that contributes to coordinating and integrating movement within full-body patterns.

During any movement, some part of the body functions as a support while another part moves, whether it be two bones in a joint, adjacent joints, or sections of the spine. Dissociation exercises can also be used to create a balance between the supporting and moving parts of a synovial joint. The two articulating bones in a joint move in a cogwheel relationship. Depending on the movement, one cog will be stationary providing the other cog with a stable base to rotate around, or both cogs will counter-rotate in opposite directions. Of course, this analogy does not apply to dynamic, gymnastic movements where the center of support is in motion, such as an aerial somersault, flip, or dive. Yet in most of our daily activities, our feet rarely leave the ground together and our base of support remains stationary.

Patterning Exercise #84: Spinal Dissociation

During this exercise, focus on moving one part of your spine independently from the other parts.

1. *Pelvis:* Start in a neutral seated posture (PE Fig. 84a). Keep your thorax and head stationary in a neutral position as you flex and extend your pelvis under them (PE Fig. 84b-c). To monitor your upper body, hold your hand on your sternum and keep it in the same position as you move your pelvis. Rock your pelvis forward, then backward, then to center, ending in the neutral, middle position. Repeat this movement several times until you can dissociate the movement of your pelvis from your upper body and can sense when your pelvis is in a neutral.
2. *Thorax:* Next, keep your pelvis and head stationary in a neutral position, then lift your sternum forward. Next, pull it back, then move it to neutral (PE Fig. 84d-e). Move your sternum and thorax independently of your pelvis and head. Stop with your thorax in the middle.
3. *Head*: Now, keeping your pelvis and thorax stationary in a neutral position, move your head straight forward, backward, and then to the center (PE Fig. 84f-g). Repeat several times until you can dissociate the movement of your head from your thorax and pelvis, and can sense when it's in the middle, in a neutral position.
4. Finish with a fluid movement of your spine, flexing then extending the whole spine at once to release any tension you might have incurred during the exercise.
5. Repeat steps 1 to 3 standing with your back against a wall. Use the wall for feedback.

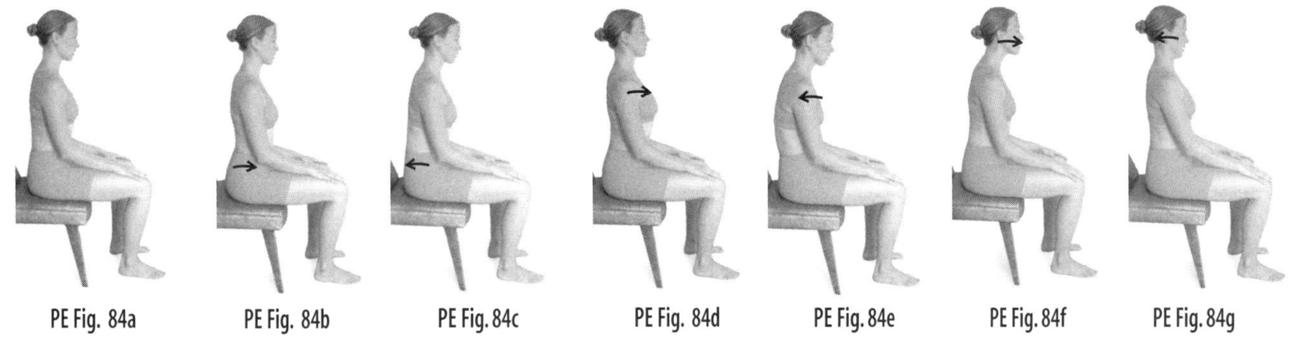

PE Fig. 84a PE Fig. 84b PE Fig. 84c PE Fig. 84d PE Fig. 84e PE Fig. 84f PE Fig. 84g

EMSPress.com

Dissociation exercises can be practiced in a single joint by focusing on the rotation and counter-rotation of the moving bones. This focus enhances the proprioceptive awareness of the supporter/mover balance in a joint when a person senses the nonmoving bone as a base of support for the moving bone. For example, before a person moves her leg, she could focus on the weight in the hip and use this sensation to help anchor and stabilize the pelvis (Figure 9.4). Or she could focus on the mobile ball of the femur turning in a stable hip socket.

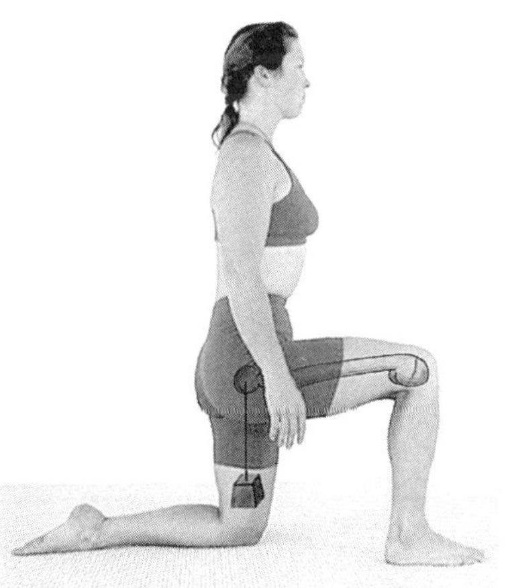

Figure 9.4 To dissociate the movement of the thigh from the hip, imagine a weight on the head of the femur to anchor it.

Dissociation can be used in patterning any synovial joint. It can also be done with an awareness of the organs as a counter-support for a moving bone, which will combine skeletal awareness with organ awareness. For example, a person could sense the weight of the lungs as "sandbags" on the arms, feeling the lungs sink as an arm raises in order to keep the shoulder relaxed. Or a person with an excessive lumbar curve could sense the weight of the abdominal viscera sinking back during hip flexion to release tension in the lower back and elongate the lumbar curve.

Dissociation skills are helpful to learn to control movement in an area, increase skeletal proprioception, bring clarity and ease to joint actions, and release excessive tension around a moving joint. Yet it should be noted that there is a major drawback to patterning based solely on joint motion and skeletal awareness. It can be incomplete by itself because most joint imbalances, excluding those caused by injury or neurological damage, are usually caused by muscular imbalances. A dysfunctional muscle can only be changed by actively controlling that muscle.

Assessing Which Muscles to Train

One way to make a general assessment of which postural muscles need work is to stand in a neutral posture next to a full-length mirror and check the skeletal alignment from the side. If all the postural muscles are doing their job, one body mass will be aligned over another. Body masses (head, thorax, and pelvis) that fall either in front of or behind the line of gravity will indicate areas that need work. The following list offers some general guidelines for determining which muscle groups to train:

1. If the lower abdomen protrudes, train *transversus abdominis* and *perineal muscles*.
2. If the lower back is flat, train the *psoas major muscle*.
3. If the lower back is hyperextended and the pelvis tilted forward, train the *lumbar multifidus muscle*.
4. If the buttocks are flat, train the *gluteal muscles*.
5. If the neck is forward of the body and hyperextended, train the *posterior neck stabilizers*.
6. If the neck is flat, train the *anterior neck stabilizers*.
7. If the scapula wings and the shoulders are rounded, train the *middle* and *lower trapezius* and the *serratus anterior muscles*.

Assessing which areas need stabilization can be complex in cases where a person has multiple instabilities and injuries. This assessment is usually done by orthopedic doctors and physical therapists who specialize in manual therapy that addresses movement and stability dysfunctions. Although these general guidelines can help a healthy person decide which postural muscles to work with, anyone with chronic pain from unstable joints is encouraged to first consult with a physical therapist and/or orthopedic doctor for a medical diagnosis.

Once the problem has been medically assessed and the dysfunctional muscles identified, a person can embark upon a training program that targets specific muscles. The training exercises presented in this chapter help a person locate and isolate each muscle that functions as a local stabilizer. If these muscles are difficult to feel, a somatic patterner can help a person build the refined sensory awareness needed to control tonic contractions and postural alignment. A somatic patterner can also help a person to integrate mechanical neuromuscular exercises with organic processes to keep the body fluid and relaxed while learning to control postural muscles.

Patterning Exercise #85: Dissociating Movement of Hip and Shoulder Joints

These exercises are presented using a supine position so that you can relax your back muscles. They can also be practiced in a side-lying, sitting, or standing position.

1. *Hips:* Lie on your back in a comfortable bent-knee position with your legs parallel and feet flat. Put your hands on your hips, one on each pelvic bone. Gently press your hips together to internally rotate the pelvic bones (PE Fig. 85a). The amount of rotation will be barely perceptible; it is made possible by a slight give in the sacroiliac joints on the back of your pelvis. Hold your hips together using your hands and muscles of your lower abdomen while you slowly and simultaneously lower both knees to each side (PE Fig. 85b). Sense the counter-rotation of your externally rotating femur heads against the internal rotation of your hip sockets.

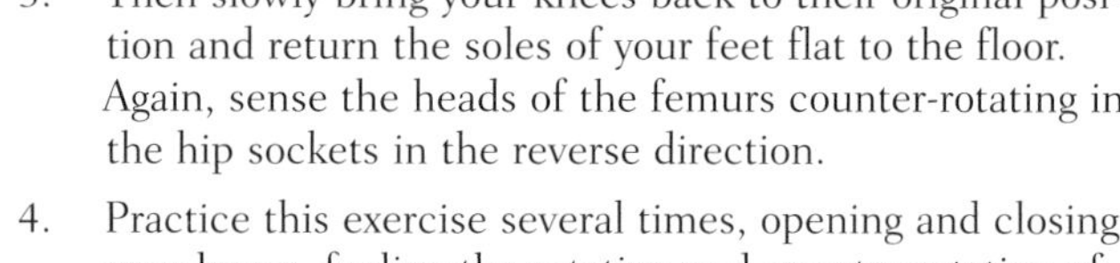

PE Fig. 85a

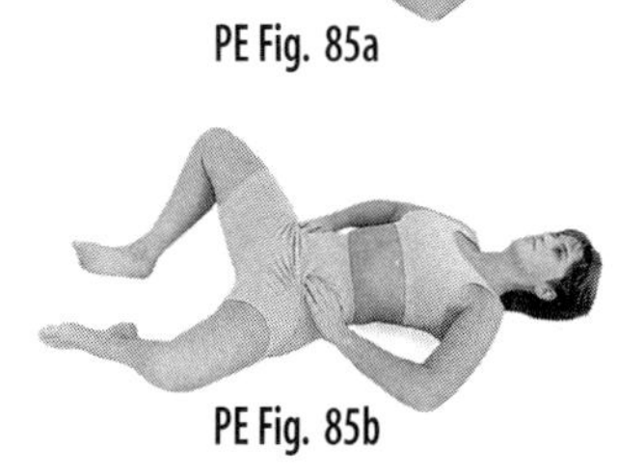

PE Fig. 85b

Caution: Skip the next step if you have problems with sacroiliac pain and/or instability.

2. Once your knees are at the end of range, gently pull your hips apart to externally rotate the pelvic bones and hip sockets.

PE Fig. 85c

3. Then slowly bring your knees back to their original position and return the soles of your feet flat to the floor. Again, sense the heads of the femurs counter-rotating in the hip sockets in the reverse direction.
4. Practice this exercise several times, opening and closing your knees, feeling the rotation and counter-rotation of your femurs in your hip sockets.
5. *Shoulders:* Again lying on your back in a comfortable position, put both arms out to your sides, about mid-chest level. Gently flatten the corners of your shoulders to the floor (PE Fig. 85c). This should externally rotate your scapulae and press them onto the floor.
6. Keeping your scapulae still, slowly raise your arms to the ceiling until your hands meet above your face (PE Fig. 85d-e). Sense the counter-rotation in the ball and socket between your humerus (upper arm) and scapula.
7. With your arms still raised, widen between your shoulder blades, and slightly internally rotate the scapulae. Then slowly open your arms while maintaining the width between your shoulder blades. Make sure to keep the front of your chest open. Repeat the exercise several times, sensing each shoulder like a hinge, unfolding and folding as you open and close your arms.

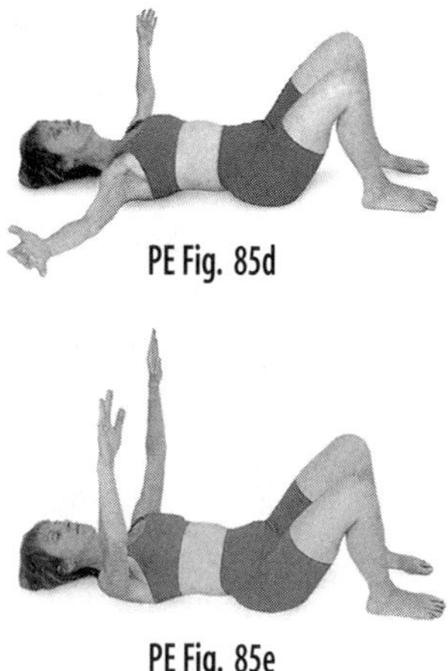

PE Fig. 85d

PE Fig. 85e

THE PELVIS AND LUMBAR STABILIZERS

The local stabilizers of the pelvis and lumbar spine include the transversus abdominis muscle, perineal muscles (often called the "pelvic floor"), psoas major muscles, and the lumbar multifidus muscle.

The transversus abdominis wraps the waist like the control panel of a girdle, and the perineum spans the pelvic floor like the skin of a drum, connecting the pubic bones and sit bones to the coccyx. Together they form a muscular sheath that wraps the front, back, sides, and bottom of the waist and pelvis (Figure 9.5). When contracted, they compress the abdominal viscera to keep it from spilling forward.

The psoas major and lumbar multifidus muscles sandwich the lumbar vertebrae. Together, their simultaneous contractions stiffen the lumbar vertebrae in a neutral position, elongating the lumbar spine to its maximum length, which gives us a lift in the waist while maintaining the natural lordotic curve of the lumbar spine.

The Transversus Abdominis and Perineum

Although research about the human movement capacity is extensive, research on the stabilization function of muscles is sparse. However, a body of information about the function of the transversus abdominis is growing. This thin, flat muscle envelops the entire abdominal wall like a form-fitting sleeve and plays a vital role in the stabilization of both the lumbar spine and the sacroiliac joints, as well as maintaining intra-abdominal pressure (see Chapter 5). A team of Australian researchers specializing in the study of the stabilizing function of muscles found that only 10 percent of people with chronic low back pain could successfully control the transversus abdominis muscle, whereas 82 percent of those without pain could control it. Their numerous studies suggest that learning to control this crucial stabilizer can not only alleviate low back pain, but can reduce its reoccurrence.[130]

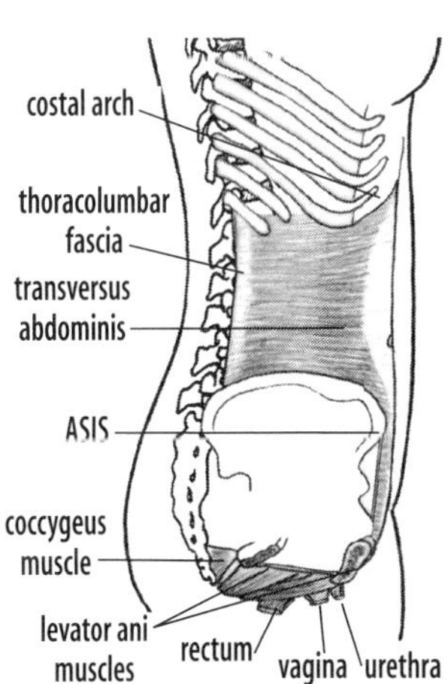

Figure 9.5 The transversus abdominis and perineal muscles create a muscular wrap and sling the contain the viscera.

The posterior fibers of the transversus abdominis arise from the thick *thoracolumbar fascia* of the lower back. Thus, the muscle's contraction increases tension in the fascia that helps to stiffen and maintain a normal lumbar curve (Figure 9.5). The lower anterior fibers attach along the anterior rim of the pelvic bowl and stabilize the *sacroiliac joints* by pulling the *anterior-superior-iliac spines (ASIS)* together, preventing the pelvic bones from flaring out (Figure 9.6a-b). The upper anterior fibers attach along the entire *costal arch* and pass across the midline of the body, criss-crossing from right to left in an arrangement that resembles a corset.[131]

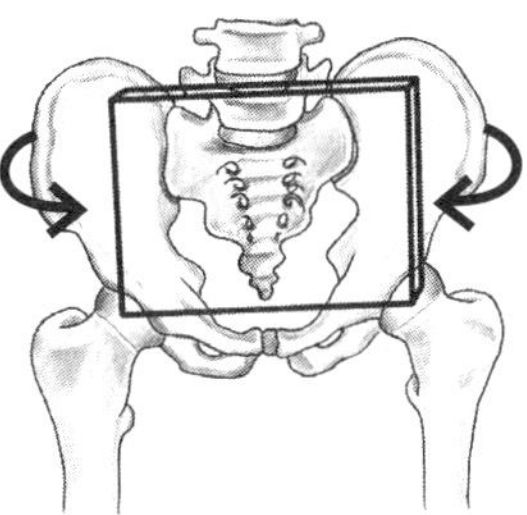

Figure 9.6a The transversus abdominis muscle draws the pelvic halves together.

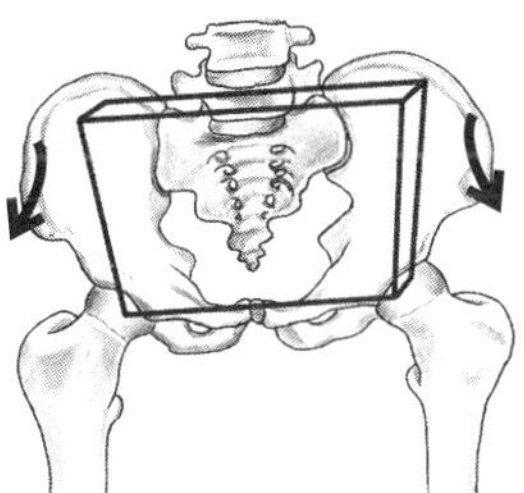

Figure 9.6b Muscle weakness can lead to a flaring out of the pelvic halves.

As the transversus abdominis contracts, it draws the lower abdomen straight back toward the sacrum, hollowing out the lower abdomen (Figure 9.7). Several of the movement modalities reviewed in Chapter 11 emphasize the hollowing action for maintaining control in the core of the body. Laban Movement Analysts stress the importance of initiating each of the Bartenieff Fundamentals with a subtle hollowing of the lower abdomen to connect to the core of the body during integrated patterns. Also, all Pilates exercises are taught with a focus on keeping the navel hollowed by pulling it back toward the front of the spine to build core strength during conditioning exercises. Both Bartenieff and Pilates were ahead of their time in emphasizing the importance of hollowing out the lower abdomen to build core connections in the body, although they initially taught that the psoas muscle initiates this action, which we now know is incorrect.

The psoas major, which will be discussed shortly, has vertically oriented fibers, whereas the transversus abdominis has horizontally oriented fibers that wrap the waist like a cummerbund. When they fire, these fibers pull the navel straight back, securing a horizontal integrity in the pelvis. Along with the horizontal fibers of the perineal muscles of the pelvic floor, the transversus knits a horizontal foundation for the vertical lift provided by stabilizers along the spine. Together, the horizontal and vertical fibers balance each other like two arms on a dimensional cross. Weakness in the control of one group will reflect in the other. In other words, it is impossible to get a postural lift along the spine if the abdominal wall

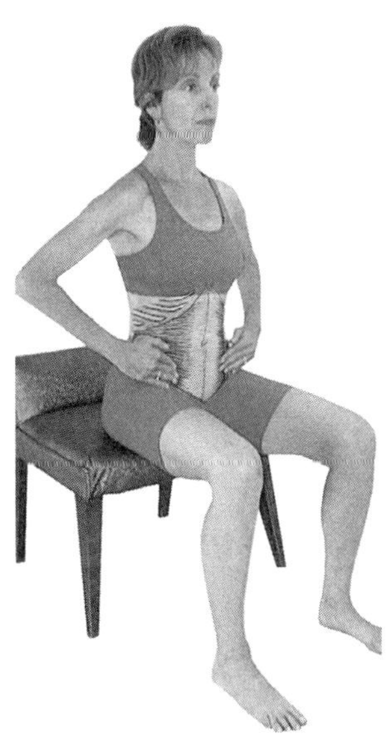

Figure 9.7 Palpating a contraction of the transversus abdominis muscle

sags, and a sagging spine can put undue pressure on and even collapse the integrity of the abdominal wall.

Because of its broad span and attachments, and its crucial role in stabilization, the transversus abdominis is usually the first muscle trained in stability training, preceded only by exercises to establish diaphragmatic breathing. Ideally, the transversus abdominis should be engaged during all exercises and activities.

When the transversus abdominis is inhibited or fires late, phasic muscles in the abdominal wall take over its function in a **substitution pattern**. Common substitution patterns to look for when isolating its contraction include any movement of the abdominal wall up or down, which indicates that the *oblique muscles* are firing; or flexion of the trunk, which indicates the *rectus abdominis muscle* is firing. The rectus abdominis is typically strengthened to stabilize the lower back, although using the rectus abdominis for stabilization creates a threefold problem. It is a phasic muscle, so it will tire easily. It is also a major trunk flexor, so its chronic contraction will flex the trunk and disturb the neutral alignment of the spine. Also, since the rectus abdominis attaches to the sternum, its chronic contraction will depress the ribcage and interfere with normal breathing (Figure 9.8).

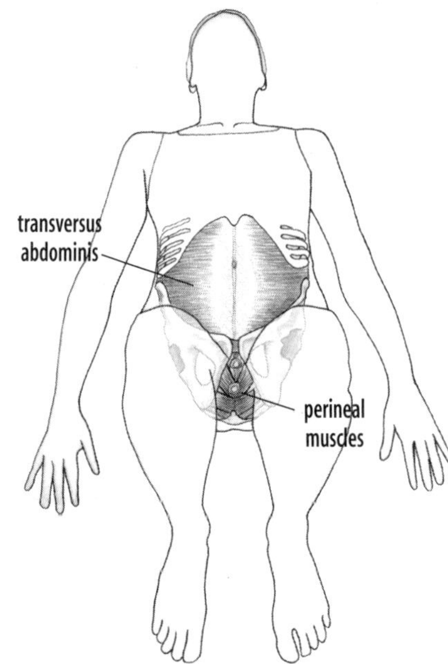

Figure 9.10 The transversus abdominis and perineal muscles co-contract

Likewise, a problem with chronic oblique contraction is that the oblique muscles attach to the lower ribs, and their contractions will restrict the expansion of the diaphragm during normal breathing. This pattern is marked by a cinching of the torso above the waist and by muscular ridges along either side of the rectus abdominis muscle (Figure 9.9). Overworking the oblique muscles can make it difficult to isolate a contraction in the transversus abdominis. To differentiate between work in the transversus abdominis and the oblique muscles, a person can watch the lower abdominal wall in a mirror while it is being contracted to see if it moves straight back, up, or down.

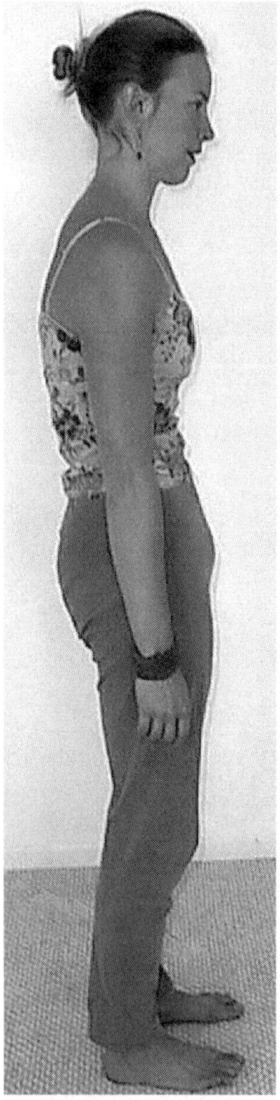

Figure 9.8 Contraction of the rectus abdominis taking the spine into flexion.

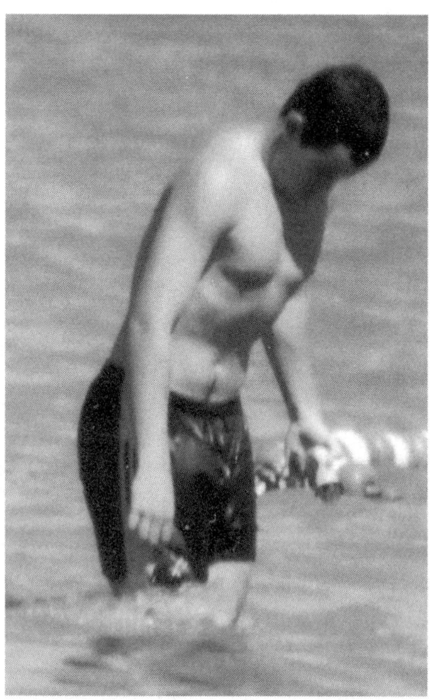
Figure 9.9 Chronic contraction of the external oblique muscles for postural support cinches and lifts the waist.

The transversus abdominis tends to co-contract with the perineal muscles of the pelvic floor (Figure 9.10). When the perineal muscles contract, they draw the sit bones together like purse strings. Co-contracting the perineum helps engage the lower fibers of the transversus abdominis independent of the obliques. This can be done by lightly drawing the sit bones together while lightly pulling the area above the pubic bone straight back, which will isolate the contraction below the navel.

The Psoas Major

The *iliopsoas muscle group* is made up of the *psoas major*, *psoas minor*, and *iliacus* (Figure 9.11). Anatomists tend to disagree about the primary function of the iliopsoas group and present evidence of many roles; a review of the literature on its function is contradictory. All do agree that the iliacus is slightly active during quiet sitting, standing, and hip rotation, and more active during hip flexion. Since the iliopsoas lies so close to the joints that it attaches to, it lacks a strong lever arm. Its contraction is more likely to contribute to the increase of axial compression on the front of the hip and lumbar spine. This, plus its slight activity

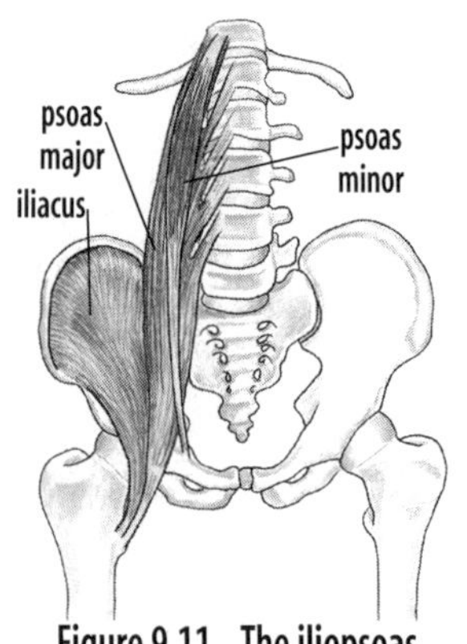

Figure 9.11 The iliopsoas muscle group

Patterning Exercise #86: Transversus Abdominis and Perineum

Figure out which position is easiest for you to feel tonic contractions of your transversus abdominis, and practice this exercise in that position.

1. *Feeling the hollow:* Lie on your back, pull your knees to your chest, and lightly draw your lower abdominal wall into your back, sensing the hollow shape this makes in your lower abdomen (PE Fig. 86a). Slowly lower your legs while keeping your abdomen in the hollow shape.

PE Fig. 86a

2. While sitting or standing, bend over, dropping your head below your knees. Lightly draw your lower abdominal wall into your back, sensing the hollow shape this makes in your lower abdomen (PE Fig. 86b). Slowly sit or stand back up while keeping your abdomen in a hollow shape.

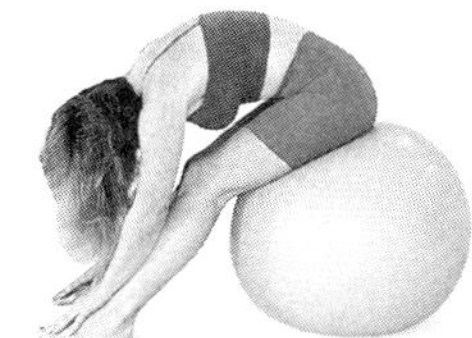

PE Fig. 86b

3. *Isolating transversus abdominis contraction:* While sitting in a chair, breathe in and out, then hold your exhalation and let your belly hang out to feel the transversus abdominis relax (PE Fig. 86c). Take several deep breaths with it relaxed so that you can differentiate between the sensations of relaxing and contracting it.

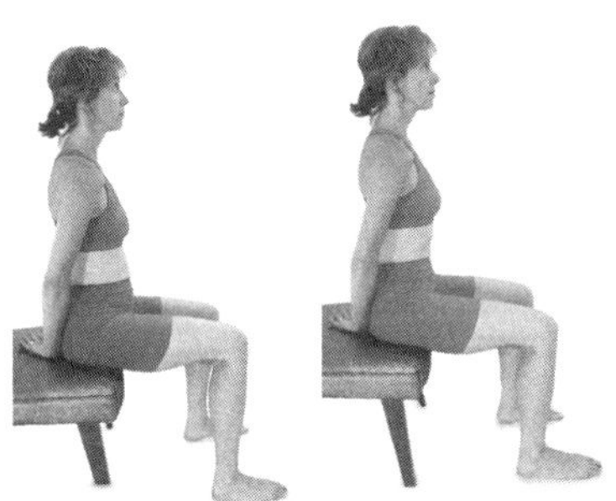

PE Fig. 86c PE Fig. 86d

4. Put your hands on your lower abdomen to monitor muscle tone. Then, slowly pull the lower abdominal wall straight back (PE Fig. 86d). If it moves up or down you are using the oblique muscles, so inhibit movement in either of these directions. Hold this contraction for about 10 seconds while breathing deeply, expanding your diaphragm and lower ribs as you inhale.
5. *Perineal contraction:* Slowly and lightly draw your sit bones together. Hold and breathe deeply into your lower ribs, then relax.
6. *In the quadruped position:* Let your abdominal wall relax completely and hang down, then take several deep breaths into your lower ribs (PE Fig. 86e).
7. Next, slowly and lightly lift your lower abdominal wall as though you were pulling it up away from a belt (PE Fig. 86f). Avoid lifting the upper abdominal wall. Hold it up while taking several deep breaths, then relax completely.

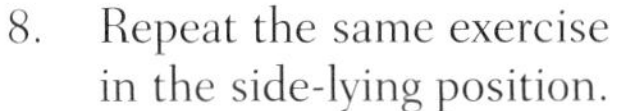

PE Fig. 86e

8. Repeat the same exercise in the side-lying position.
9. *In the standing position:* If you have difficulty inhibiting your oblique muscles, place one hand above your navel and the other below your navel to monitor your abdominal muscles. Then pull the lower abdominal wall straight back while keeping your upper abdominal wall relaxed. Make sure your abdominal wall moves straight back, not up or down, which indicates oblique muscle contraction.

PE Fig. 86f

during quiet sitting and standing, indicates that the iliopsoas has an important role as a primary hip and lumbar stabilizer.[132]

The psoas major and iliacus muscles share a common distal tendon that inserts on the *lesser trochanter* of the *femur*. Although they share a tendon, both muscles have a different origin, therefore they have somewhat different functions. Considering each muscle separately sheds light on their specific functions. It is commonly agreed that the iliacus is a hip flexor; it has been found to be active once past 30 degrees of hip flexion. The psoas minor is absent in 40 percent of the population and its function is unknown. The psoas major assists the iliacus in hip flexion after 30 to 40 degrees, and it is consistently recruited in a pattern of excessive lordotic lumbar curve.[133]

Of the three iliopsoas muscles, the psoas major has become popular in the burgeoning area of "core movement" in somatics and bodywork, particularly in Rolfing and Pilates. The psoas major lies behind the abdominal viscera along the front of the lumbar spine and, because of its depth, is a difficult muscle to study. Inserting the needles that are used to take electromyograph (EMG) readings of muscle activity in the psoas major is too painful for most research participants.

Although the psoas major is active during hip flexion, because it lies close to the joints to which it attaches, it does not have a long enough lever arm to flex the hip. Also, it has minimal extensibility; it lengthens only a fraction of an inch when relaxing.[134] Also, the anterior and posterior fibers of the psoas major have different functions. The anterior *fasciculi* (muscular slips) of the psoas major pull the head of the femur up into the hip socket in a movement so small its range is about the thickness of a matchbook. These anterior fibers contract when the body is in a slightly reclined position, along with the posterior fibers of the perineal muscles.[135]

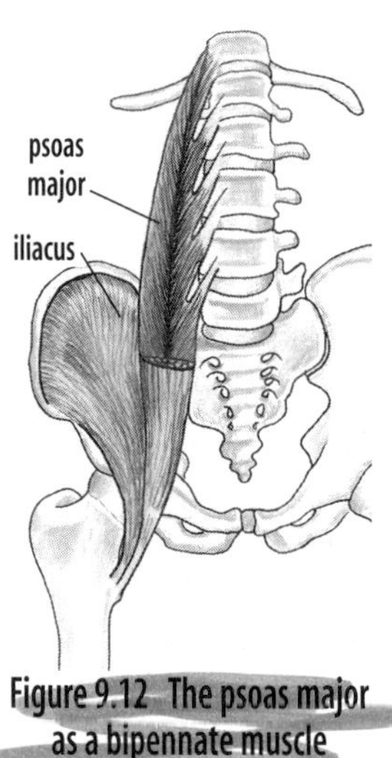

Figure 9.12 The psoas major as a bipennate muscle

Some anatomists have even found that the posterior fasciculi of the psoas major have a pennate shape, meaning that their short oblique fibers span only a few vertebral segments and attach to a central tendon (Figure 9.12).[136] Contractions of the short posterior fibers generate enough longitudinal force to increase axial compression along the front of the lumbar spine, pointing to the psoas major's primary role as a postural stabilizer. If the deep stabilizers along the back of the lumbar spine (the deep multifidus muscles) are inhibited and unable to counter the pull of the psoas major, its pull increases the lumbar lordosis.

The iliopsoas muscle group has been called a "hidden prankster" because dysfunction within it can lead to a number of chronic pain symptoms, including anterior groin pain, abdominal pain, and pain down the back of buttocks and thighs.[137] When dysfunctional, the iliopsoas can develop painful tender points that can be released with trigger point pressure (Figure 9.13). Holding these trigger points until they no longer hurt can release an enormous amount of pain generated by iliopsoas dysfunction.

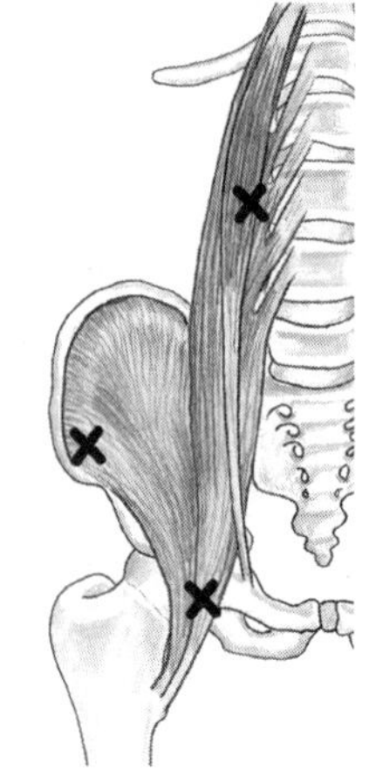
Figure 9.13 Trigger points in the iliopsoas

A psoas major contraction can be palpated in the groin area, about two to three inches lateral of the pubic bone, directly above the *inguinal fold*. Each segment of the psoas major is innervated separately; therefore, it is possible to learn segmental control over it. The value of doing this is that the chronically inhibited segments can be targeted and trained, although working with specific segments is an advanced skill and not necessary to gain the benefit of a general tonic contraction.

Patterning Exercise #87: Psoas Major

(Adapted from Kinetic Control.)

1. *Palpating the psoas major:* Lie on your back with both knees bent. Place your fingertips in the soft tissue area directly above your *inguinal ligament*, about two inches to the sides of your pubic bone (PE Fig. 87a). Although you need to contract the transversus abdominis muscle to stabilize the pelvis during leg movement, to be able to sink back far enough to palpate the psoas while it contracts, keep your extrinsic abdominal muscles relaxed as you lift one knee to your chest. You should feel the psoas tendon bulge under your hand (PE Fig. 87b). Repeat with the other leg.

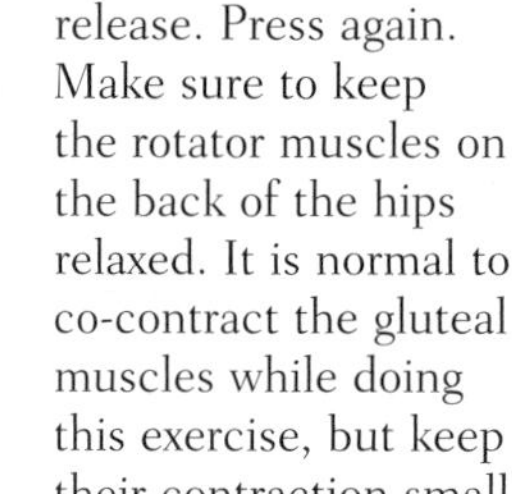
PE Fig. 87a

PE Fig. 87b

2. Straighten both legs and lie flat on your back. Begin rolling your legs in and out together as though your feet were windshield wipers. This movement tugs on the iliopsoas tendon, creating a pull right above the hip sockets on each side. It also helps to loosen your hip sockets.
3. *Contracting the psoas major:* Place the soles of your feet together, then lightly press them together, which should contract your psoas major muscles (PE Fig. 87c). This contraction of the psoas major will slightly pull and seat the heads of your femurs into the hip sockets. Hold for at least 10 seconds while breathing normally, then release. Press again. Make sure to keep the rotator muscles on the back of the hips relaxed. It is normal to co-contract the gluteal muscles while doing this exercise, but keep their contraction small.

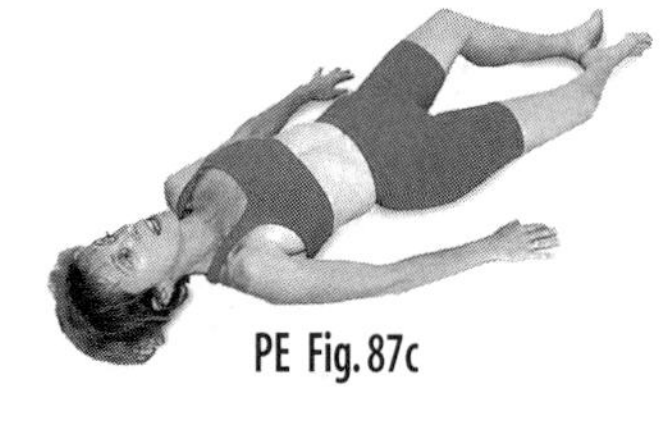
PE Fig. 87c

4. *To contract the psoas while sitting in a chair:* Sit upright, balanced over both sit bones, with both feet flat on the floor. Palpate your psoas tendons for feedback. Keeping your spine in neutral, raise one knee up and hold. You should feel the psoas on that side contract, creating a length and lift along the front of your lumbar spine. Keep it contracted as you lower the leg. Repeat on the other side.
5. Again, in an upright position, palpate your psoas tendons. Then lean back at your hips into a reclined posture (PE Fig. 87d). You should feel the psoas contract on both sides. Keep it contracted as you return to the upright position.
6. *To contract the psoas while lying prone on a table or bed:* Put one leg close to the edge and let it hang over the side just a little bit. Then lightly pull the leg up, pulling the hip into the socket. Hold for 10 seconds and breathe, then release. Do this several times, then repeat on the other side with the other leg.

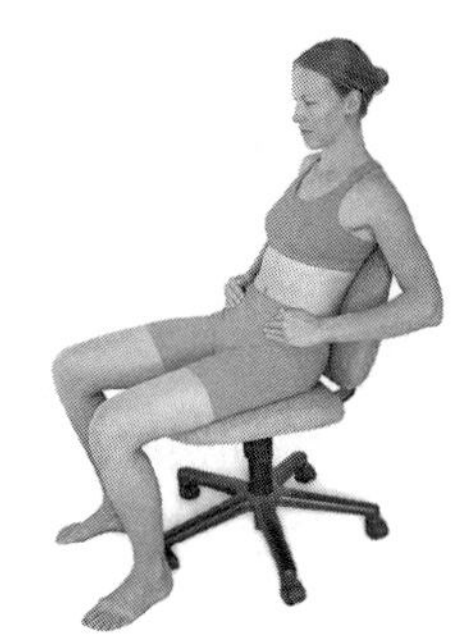
PE Fig. 87d

EMSPress.com

The Lumbar Multifidus

Like the psoas major, the lumbar multifidus muscle also has two layers—both deep fibers and superficial fibers. The deep oblique fibers of the multifidus are also short, about two to three centimeters long, attaching to the spinous process and inserting on the *transverse process* three vertebrae down. The multifidus arises from the *semispinalis muscles* that begin at the base of the skull. It spans the length of the entire spine in a herringbone pattern, ending at the sacrum. Its fibers are the thickest over the sacrum and lumbar spine, where they stabilize the lumbar vertebrae and the *lumbosacral junction*; its fibers are the thinnest in the thoracic spine.

The tonic contractions of the multifidus increase axial compression along the back of the lumbar spine, stiffening and stabilizing it. Its contractions can be felt in a bulge along the groove on either side of the lumbar spine, between the spinous and transverse processes (Figure 9.14). Several attributes of this primary lumbar stabilizer mirror the psoas major: it is a multi-segmental muscle with individually innervated fasciculi (muscle slips); therefore, one segment can be contracted while another is relaxed, and each segment can be controlled separately. Whereas the psoas major increases axial compression along the front of the lumbar spine, the multifidus increases it along the back.

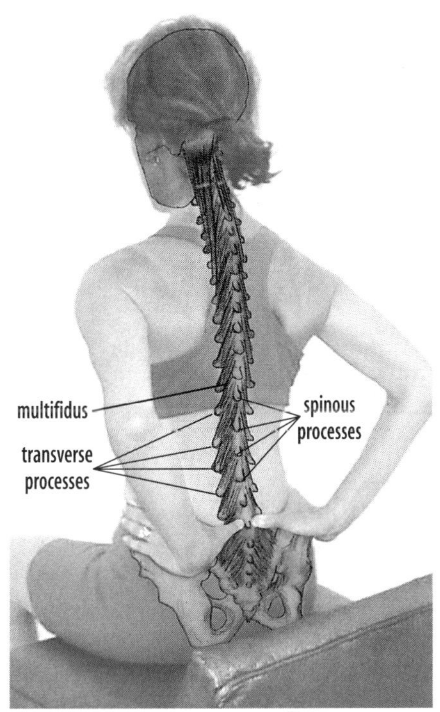

Figure 9.14 Palpating the lumbar multifidus muscle lateral to the spinous processes, in the lamina groove

The lumbar multifidus contracts bilaterally when a person leans forward from the hips as little as 30 degrees. It contracts contralaterally (on the opposite side) when a person raises one arm to shoulder level. And it contracts *ipsilaterally* (on the same side as the back leg) while taking a step forward.

The multifidus and psoas major work together to maintain and stiffen the normal lumbar curve in its posi-

Patterning Exercise #88: Lumbar Multifidus

(Adapted from Kinetic Control and Norris exercises.) Figure out which version of this exercise is easiest for you and practice this one first so that you will have a successful experience contracting this muscle. Once you learn to contract it at will, you can practice the other versions. Make sure to breathe during each exercise.

1. *Sitting comfortably:* Place your thumbs or fingertips close to both sides of the lumbar spine, between the spinous and transverse processes, in the lamina groove.
2. Keeping your spine straight, lean forward, bending at the hips. You should feel the lumbar multifidus muscles bulge under your fingers (PE Fig. 88a). If muscles lateral to your transverse processes bulge, you are contracting the larger erector muscles (PE Fig. 88b). Relax them to isolate the contraction to the multifidus. Keep the multifidus contracted as you lean back to your original position. Repeat several times.
3. *Standing:* Stand with both feet under your hips. Place your thumbs or fingertips on both sides of your lumbar spine, in the lamina groove to monitor the multifidus muscles.

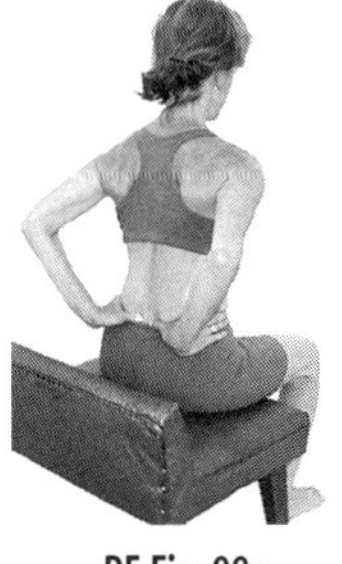
PE Fig. 88a

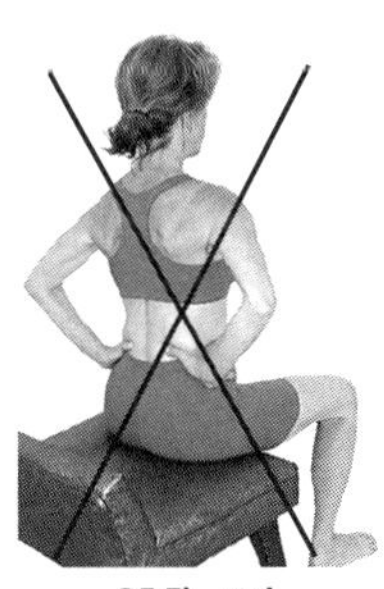
PE Fig. 88b

4. Step forward on one foot. The multifidus on the side of your back leg should contract and bulge (PE Fig. 88c).
5. Once it contracts, keep it contracted as your slowly step back on both feet. Repeat several times, then repeat the whole sequence on the other side.
6. *Arm movement:* Still standing, again place your fingertips along the spine to monitor the multifidus on one side. Raise your other arm to shoulder level and the multifidus should contract (PE Fig. 88d).
7. Lower your arm while keeping the multifidus contracted. Repeat several times, then repeat on the other side.
8. *Lying prone:* Lie on your belly with both legs straight. Again, place your fingertips on the multifidus. Keeping your legs straight, barely lift one leg until you feel the multifidus on that side contract. Hold it there and take several deep breaths. When it contracts it will lengthen your lumbar curve and subtly lifting it toward the ceiling. Slowly lower your leg while keeping the multifidus contracted. Repeat several times, then repeat on the other side.

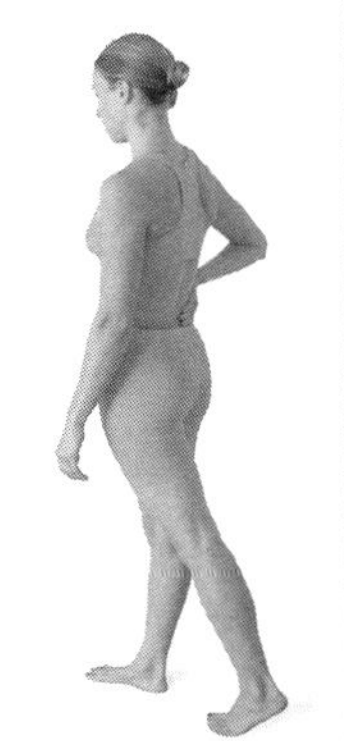
PE Fig. 88c

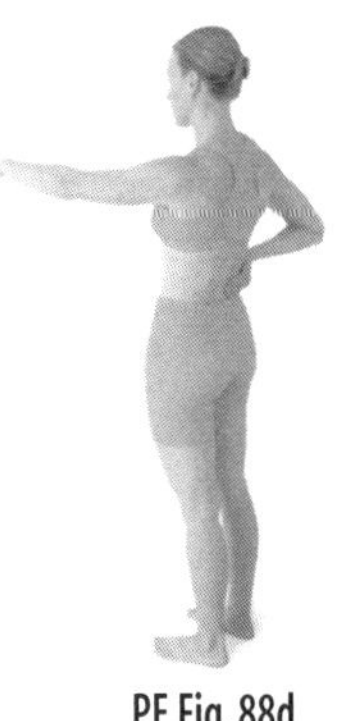
PE Fig. 88d

tion of maximal elongation, the multifidus along the back and the psoas major along the front (Figure 9.15). Many people try to solve the problems of an exaggerated lumbar curve by habitually flattening the lower back, which is problematic because this posture may inhibit and even overstretch the multifidus fibers and can eventually displace the lumbar discs backward. The tonic contractions of the lumbar multifidus can correct an exaggerated lumbar curve, pulling the lumbar spine straight back while elongating its curve.

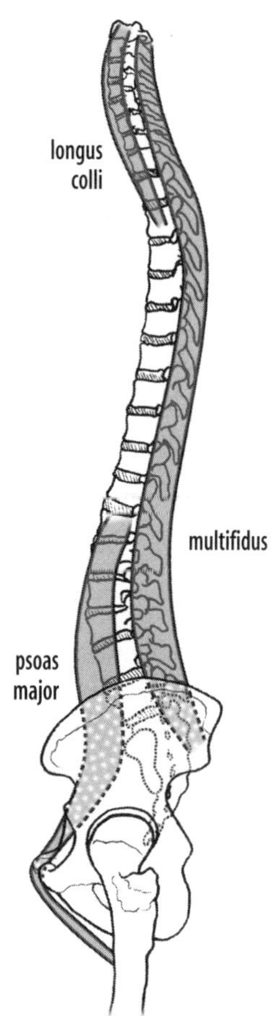

Figure 9.15 Intrinsic muscles that function as primary stabilizers along the spine

Ideally, a person can maintain a natural, elongated lumbar curve with the tonic co-contractions of the transversus abdominis, the perineum, the psoas major, and the lumbar multifidus. Together, these four stabilizers knit the pelvic bowl together and provide a lift to the lumbar spine, elongating its natural curve along both the front and the back.

The multifidus also contracts during any of the developmental movement patterns practiced from a prone position, such as the upper homologous push or optical righting exercises. Simple movements that initiate developmental patterns or reflexes can be practiced to develop the multifidus. For example, the optical righting exercise (see Patterning Exercise #3 titled "Optical Support and Optical Righting") and the initial phases of exploring the Landau reflex (see Patterning Exercise #60 titled "The Landau Reflex") engage both the lumbar and the cervical multifidus muscles as well as intrinsic muscles in the *suboccipital* region.

Like all the stabilizers, the multifidus should be firing whenever a person is upright and active. When it is inhibited, the larger *erector spinae muscles* lateral to it may overwork and hyperextend the lumbar spine into exaggerated lumbar curve (most people call this posture a "swayback"). When the erector muscles are chronically contracted, they create a large muscular bulge lateral to the transverse processes of the spine (see PE Fig. 88b). This muscular imbalance can indicate an inhibition of the multifidus muscle.

Postural Support and Scoliosis

This body story recounts patterning work the author did with a client who has scoliosis.

A young woman named Meg narrowly missed a complete spinal fusion as a teenager thanks to a concerned parent who cancelled the surgery at the last minute. Ten years later, Meg came to me for help in straightening out her scoliotic spinal curvature. She had sustained several injuries that left her with unstable lumbar and sacroiliac joints, and would spin into a pain cycle after the slightest bump or nudge. Meg wanted to become stronger, straighter, and most of all, more stable.

Initially, Meg's extrinsic muscles were so locked in asymmetrical muscle contractures that zig-zagged along her spine that she was unable to feel intrinsic sensations in her back. With stretching and subtle patterning exercises, Meg gradually learned to release her chronic contractures and strengthen her weak intrinsic muscles. She practiced intentionally asymmetrical exercises that pulled the spine back on line. Although her spine straightened out considerably, Meg was still susceptible to injury from the smallest impact, such as a friend hugging her too hard or bumping her heel on a curb.

Meg began practicing stability exercises, isolating specific postural muscles and learning to contract them. Although she was happy with her progress, she still suffered from the limitations of an unstable spine that restricted her to nonweight-bearing activities. So we switched to developmental patterning and began exploring reflexes that were weak. We found that the asymmetrical tonic neck reflex (ATNR), a reflex supporting hand-eye coordination, was strong on the right side and absent on the left. Conversely, the hand-mouth reflex was strong on the left side and absent on the right. Her ATNR took her spine into rotation with extension on one side of her body, whereas her hand-mouth reflex took her spine into rotation with flexion on the other side, and her spine compensated by twisting in the middle.

As Meg explored these patterns on the weak sides, her spinal muscles began to organize in a new way. Her chronic spinal muscle contractures began to relax on a much deeper level, while stubborn muscle fibers in previously inhibited and low tone areas began to fire, and her spinal curvatures visibly straightened within a single session. This was a great success. To date, Meg feels that working with developmental reflexes has straightened her spine more than any other approach, almost miraculously. She practices these reflexes as well as stabilization exercises daily, and is gradually adding weight-bearing exercises to her routine.

STABILIZERS OF SCAPULA NEUTRAL

Conscientious dance teachers who recognize the importance of proper body mechanics encourage modern dancers to "move with the arms on the back." This means that the shoulder blades need to stay connected to the trunk and anchored on the back during all arm movements. To maintain this connection, dancers use imagery (such as the scapula sliding down as the arm goes up) and sensory awareness of the scapulae to maintain this connection, although both these methods still leave the facilitation of the muscles that stabilize the scapulae up to chance.

An understanding of the functional anatomy of the scapulae and shoulder girdle can greatly enhance stabilization. The bony yoke of the shoulder girdle (made up of the scapulae and clavicles) is connected to the axial skeleton only through two small *sternoclavicular joints*. Therefore, the scapula relies on the tensional balance of muscular pulls to support its position (Figure 9.16). As with the spine, **scapula neutral** is the ideal neutral position of the scapulae maintained by the balanced pulls of numerous muscles connecting each scapula to the arm and trunk. When in neutral, its medial border lies about two and one-half inches from and parallel to the spine; the *acromion* is slightly higher than the *superior medial angle* of the scapula; and the scapula rests flat against the ribs and lies 15 to 30 degrees forward of the frontal plane (Figure 9.17a).[138] When unstable, the scapulae tend to "wing" (Figure 9.17b).

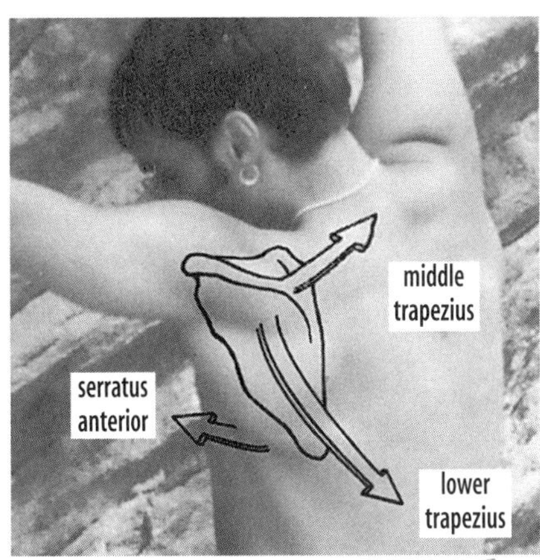

Figure 9.16 Muscular pulls on the scapula

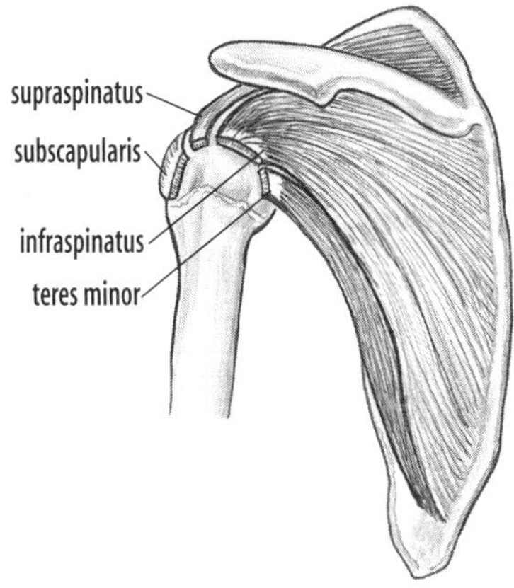

Figure 9.18 The rotator cuff muscles

Muscles attaching to the scapula act like guy ropes to stabilize it in neutral in the same way that the even pulls on a horse's reins keep the horse's head pointed straight ahead. The *glenoid fossa*, the most lateral aspect of the scapula, provides a socket for the *humerus* (upper arm). Tensional pulls of the four rotator cuff muscles around the shoulder socket stabilize the humerus and keep it centered in its socket (Figure 9.18). Due to the complexity of the shoulder muscles, only two major scapula stabilizers will be presented in this section: the trapezius and serratus anterior muscles. Both muscles are important in maintaining the neutral position of the scapulae, which greatly affects the dynamic balance of the shoulder girdle, the thoracic and cervical spines, and the arms.

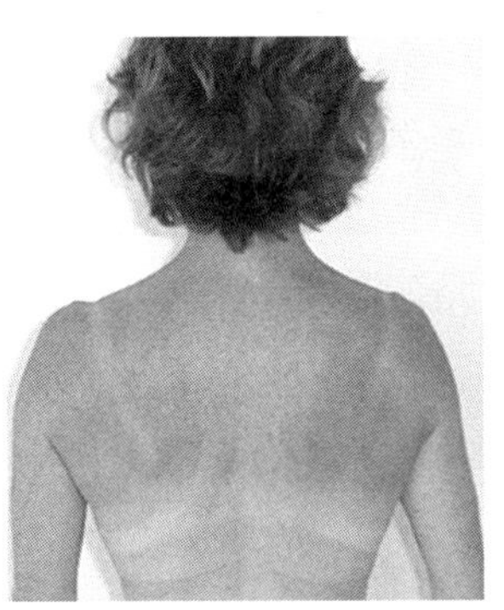
Figure 9.17a Scapulae in neutral reflect a balance of muscular pulls that maintain stability.

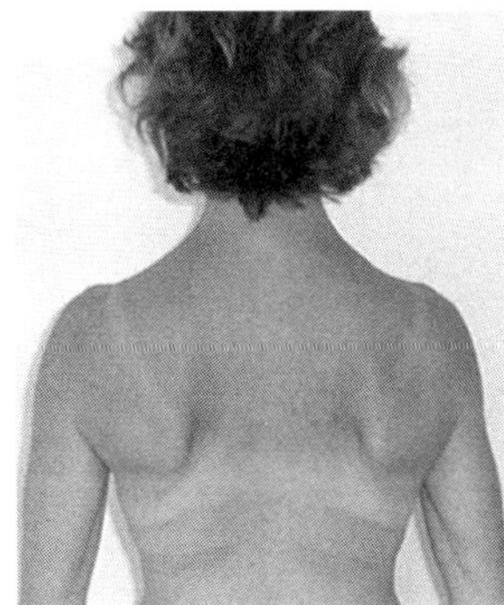
Figure 9.17b "Pseudo-winged" scapulae (not in neutral) indicate muscular weakness in the serratus anterior muscles.

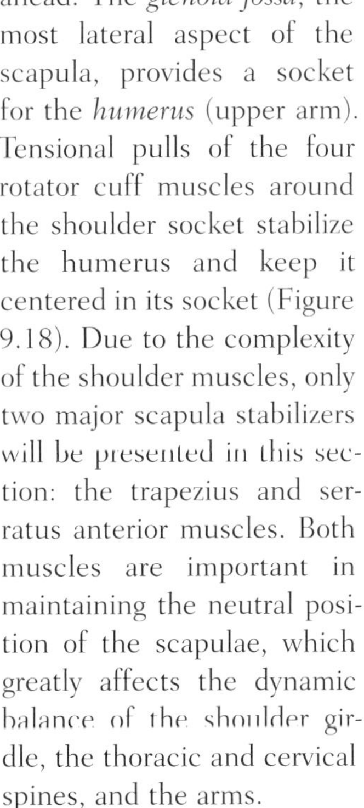

Since the *glenohumeral joint* is the most mobile joint in the body, any deviation from the neutral position of the scapula will reduce the efficiency of arm movement. Also, since the shoulders are supported and stabilized by the tensional pulls of myofascias attaching to the spine, unbalanced pulls in the scapulae and arms affect the alignment of the spine, particularly in the neck. This imbalance is obvious in rounded shoulders that put a downward drag on the neck and pull it forward into chronic hyperextension.

The Trapezius

The trapezius is a broad, flat, diamond-shaped muscle with a broad origin along the base of the *occiput* and along the spinous processes of the first cervical vertebra to the twelfth thoracic vertebra (Figure 9.19). It inserts along the spine of the scapula and the lateral third of the clavicle, draping over the shoulders like a shawl. The upper fasciculi of the trapezius suspend the scapulae and lateral end of the clavicles from the neck and upper spine; the middle and lower fasciculi anchor the bottom of the scapulae on the back without retracting them.

Since the upper and lower halves of the trapezius are innervated separately, they can contract independently of each other. This is significant in a common postural prob-

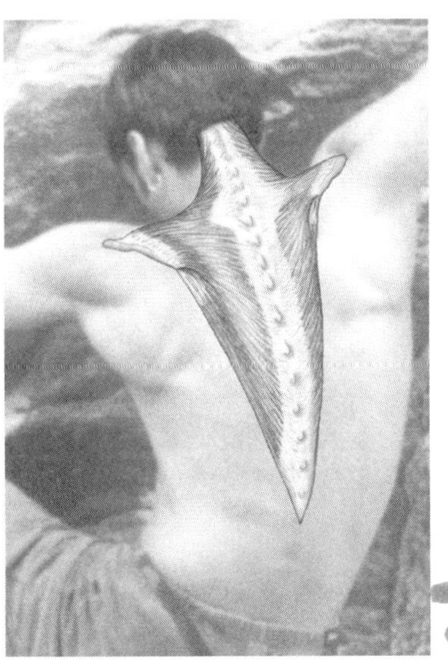
Figure 9.19 The trapezius muscle

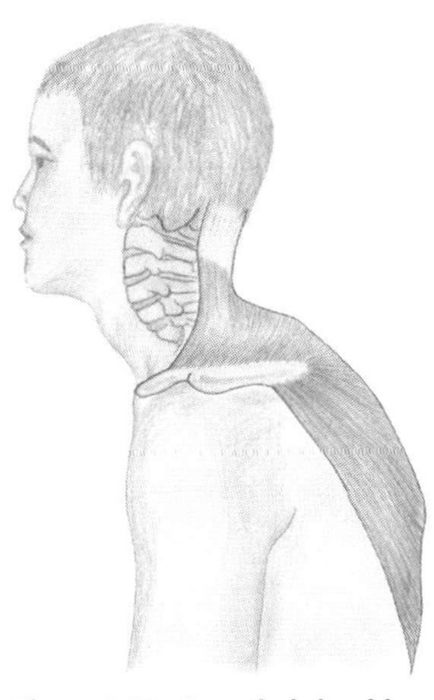
Figure 9.20 Rounded shoulders overextend the lower trapezius fibers while shortening the upper fibers

lem that occurs when the upper fibers become shortened from chronic contractions while the lower fibers overstretch, leading to hyperextension of the neck and rounding of the shoulders (Figure 9.20). Ideally, the middle and lower fibers of the trapezius work as a postural stabilizer for the scapulae: they have an abundance of slow oxidative fibers making them suitable for sustained tonic contractions. Since the trapezius muscle is connected to the base of the skull, any slack in the neck and cervical spine or chronic shortening in the upper trapezius fibers will interfere with the neutral position of both the scapulae and the upper half of the spine.

The Serratus Anterior

Up to now, only local stabilizers have been presented in detail, and a *local stabilizer* works regardless of whether or not the body is moving. A *global stabilizer* works during movement. The serratus anterior muscle functions as both a local and global stabilizer. Its contraction protracts the scapula and prevents its medial border from protruding or "winging," which indicates a weakness in this muscle (see Figure 9.17b). It also anchors the scapula against the ribcage during arm movement, allowing the scapula to glide along the ribs without winging.

Because its serrated slips resemble fingers on a hand wrapping around the sides of the ribs, the serratus anterior is nicknamed the "finger muscle" (Figure 9.21). It attaches along the anterior medial border of the scapula, inserts along the side of the upper eight ribs, and can be palpated by pressing against the ribs in the armpit. It is an antagonist of the rhomboid muscle, whose contraction retracts the scapula. It is a crucial stabilizer for the scapula during all movements of the arm.

Finding Scapula Neutral

To place the scapulae in a neutral position and maintain this posture, a person needs to be able to recognize what scapula neutral feels like. Most people overwork when putting their shoulders in what they feel is a correct position. As a result of these extraneous efforts, they contract extrinsic muscles that actually pull the scapulae off neutral by pinch-

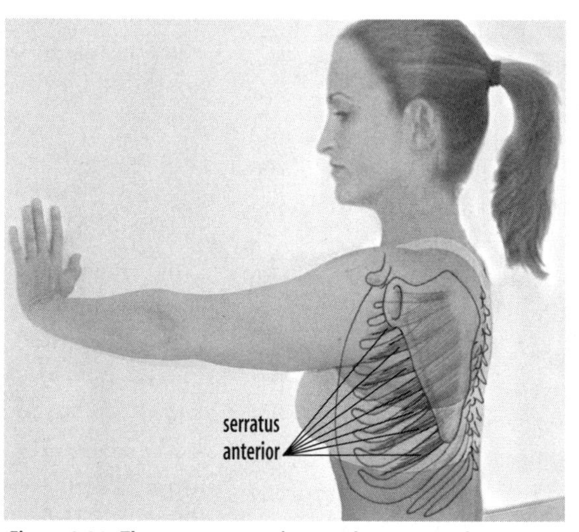

Figure 9.21 The serratus anterior muscle protracts the scapula, working concentrically in a pushing movement.

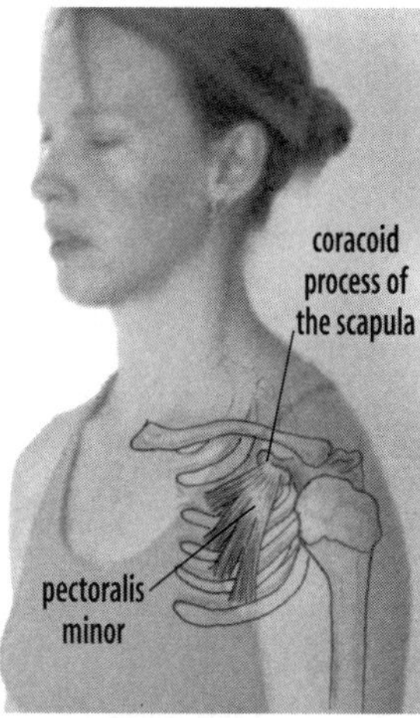

Figure 9.22 The pectoralis minor muscle lifts the ribs up toward the top the shoulder.

Patterning Exercise #89: Middle and Lower Trapezius

1. While lying prone, put one hand between your lower scapula and your spine to locate and monitor contractions of the lower trapezius muscle. (If you cannot reach this area, have a friend monitor it or do the exercise without feedback.) Place the other arm overhead, then lift it several inches off the ground (PE Fig. 89a). Your lower trapezius should contract under your fingers. Repeat on the other side, again feeling the contraction of the lower trapezius.

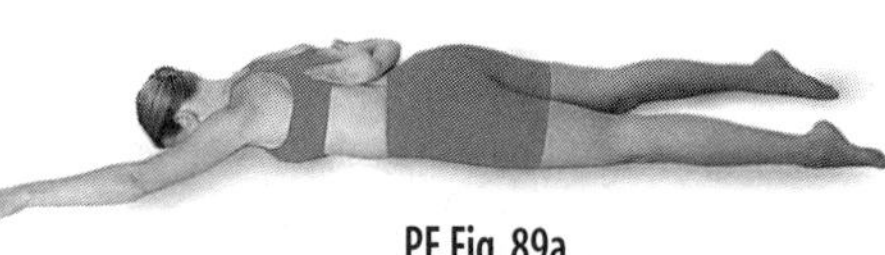

PE Fig. 89a

2. Still lying prone, with your arms at your sides, externally rotate your shoulders to relax the pectoralis muscles on the front. Then lift the corner of one shoulder about one inch, using the middle and lower "traps" to place the scapula in neutral. Hold for about 10 to 20 seconds (PE Fig. 89b). If you are using the right muscles, it will be easy to hold. Make sure to lift straight up. Avoid pulling your scapula down, or pinching your shoulder blades together. Breathe as you hold it, then relax. Repeat on the other side.

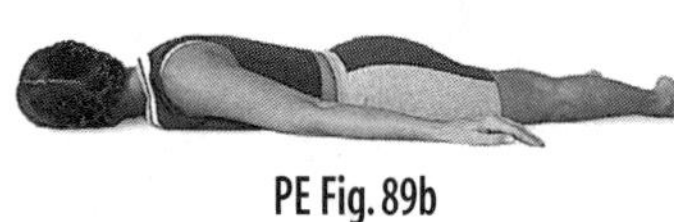

PE Fig. 89b

3. Once you are comfortable lifting the corner of your shoulder, then lift your entire arm about one inch off the ground and hold (PE Fig. 89c). Take several deep breaths. Then relax. Repeat on the other side.

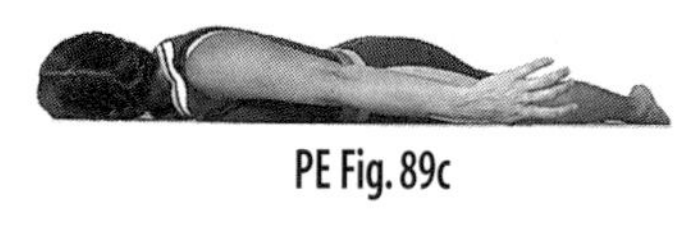

PE Fig. 89c

4. Stabilize your lower back by pulling your lower abdomen in. Then progress to simultaneously lifting both arms and your head (PE Fig. 89d).

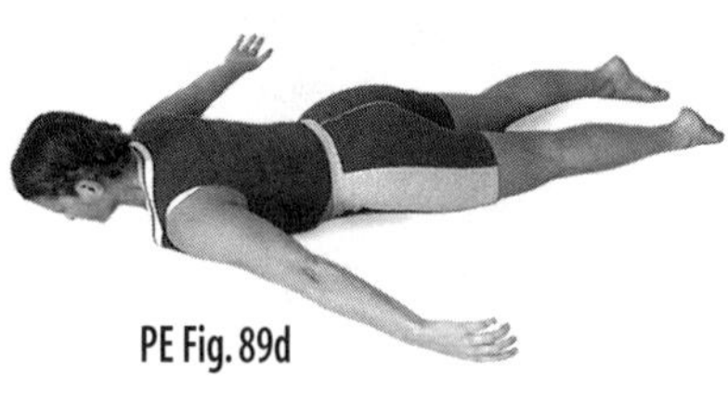

PE Fig. 89d

EMSPress.com

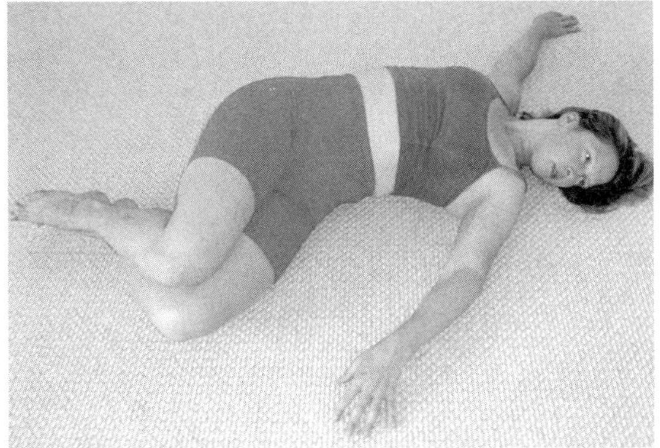

Figure 9.23 Stretching the pectoralis muscles

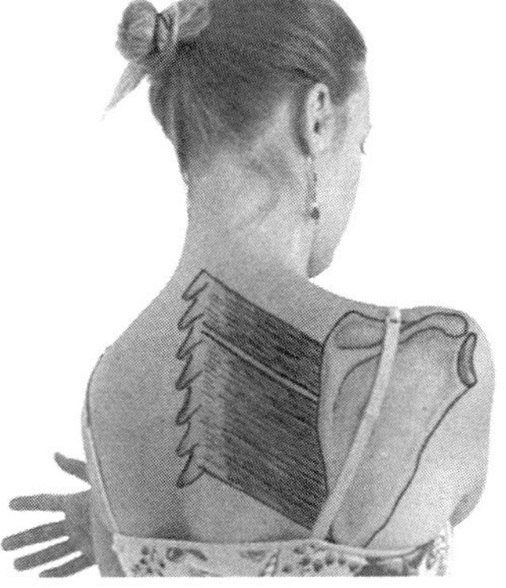

Figure 9.24 Stretching rhomboid muscles

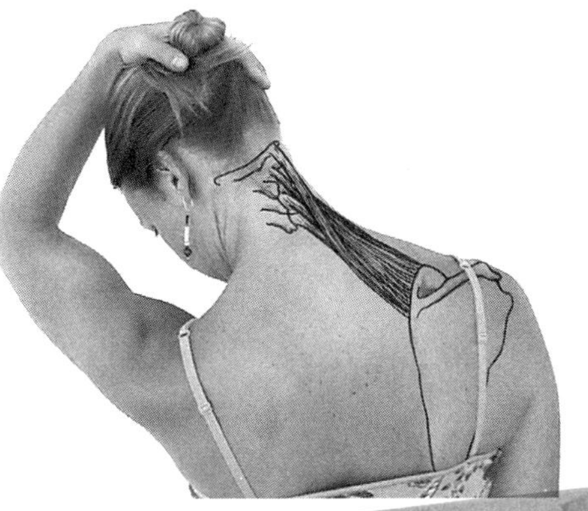

Figure 9.25 Stretching the levator scapula muscle

ing the shoulder blades together, hiking the shoulders, or even rounding the shoulders.

Several muscle groups are primary culprits in chronically pulling the scapulae off neutral and may need to be stretched before a neutral position can be achieved. If the shoulders are rounded, the *pectoralis minor muscles*, which connect the *coracoid process* of the scapulae to the upper ribs, probably need stretching. Ideally, the "pec" minor lifts the front of the upper ribs (Figure 9.22). However, when the pectoralis minor is tight, it pulls the coracoid process down, tilts the scapula, and rounds the shoulders. It is a difficult muscle to stretch because it requires depressing the scapula down the back away from the anterior ribs, an action that has a short range. To stretch the general pectoralis area, a person can lie on the side, with the knees together and open one arm behind the body while simultaneously depressing the scapula on that side. In this position, the weight of the arm creates a diagonal pull that stretches the pectoralis muscle group (Figure 9.23).

If the scapulae tend to retract and pinch the shoulder blades together, the rhomboid muscles between the shoulders are probably tight and need stretching. To stretch the rhomboids, a person can pull the arms across the body (Figure 9.24). If the shoulders tend to chronically hike, the upper trapezius and *levator scapulae muscles* probably need to be stretched. This can be done by pulling the head diagonally toward one knee and simultaneously away from the opposite shoulder (Figure 9.25).

Finding scapula neutral requires refined sensory feedback. To get accurate feedback, a person can place the hand on the medial (inner) scapular border to feel where it rests and when it rests in neutral in a flat position. Also, a person can place the fingertips on the important bony landmarks of the scapula and direct them toward neutral. For instance, the coracoid process in the hollow space at the front corner of the shoulder usually lifts a bit as the scapula moves to neutral. In the back, the scapula is a triangular bone with three angles. As the scapula moves to neutral, all three angles move simultaneously like three hands turning on a triangular wheel. The lower angle moves down, the lateral angle lifts, and the medial angle moves in.

It also helps to have an experienced person place a learner's scapula in neutral to position it, then have the learner find scapula neutral by recreating the sensation of neutral without the teacher's help (Figure 9.26a). To do so, first the teacher can place the learner's scapula in the neutral position described earlier and hold it there until the learner can contract the right muscles to maintain this position. The teacher can also palpate the learner's lower trapezius muscle to help him feel the muscle and then encourage him to contract it. Once contracted, the scapula can be released slowly as the learner holds it in neutral (Figure 9.26b).

It should be noted that it is difficult to find scapula neutral without already having a neutral posture in the spine, particularly the neck. This can be achieved by reaching the top of the head toward the ceiling, which lengthens the extrinsic muscles of the neck, particularly the upper trapezius muscle. Other directional hints for finding scapula neutral include:

- simultaneously widening the front and back of the chest,
- letting the arms hang without effort or holding,
- slightly lifting the lateral portion of the clavicle,
- and pointing the corners of the shoulders out to the sides.

Lastly, since the shoulder girdle is a hanging yoke, a person should practice finding scapula neutral while standing, where the body is under tensional and habitual myofascial pulls.

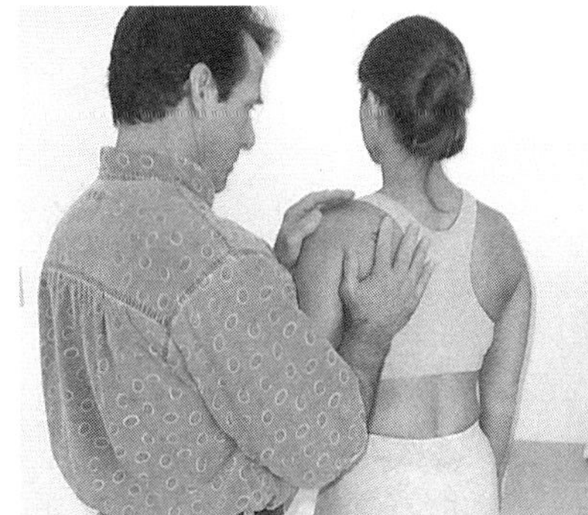

Figure 9.26a Putting the scapula in neutral

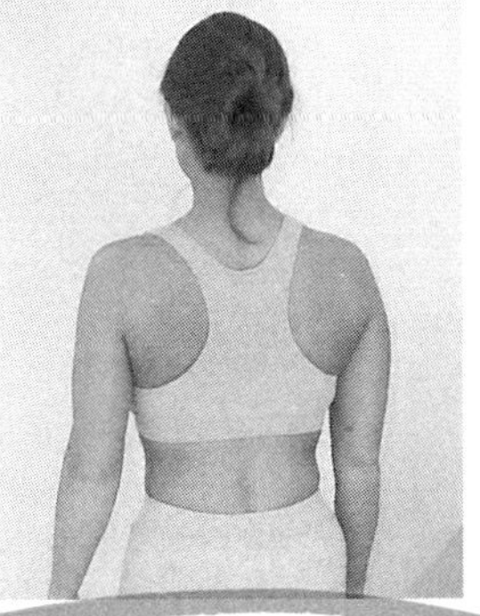

Figure 9.26b The results

Patterning Exercise #90: Finding and Moving in Scapula Neutral

1. *With a partner:* Have your partner lie prone on the floor. Reach under her scapula to palpate her pectoralis muscles and give her feedback about whether or not they are relaxed. Next, stretch the pectoralis muscles by externally rotating to shoulder joint, pulling the corner of the shoulder over, out, and up.

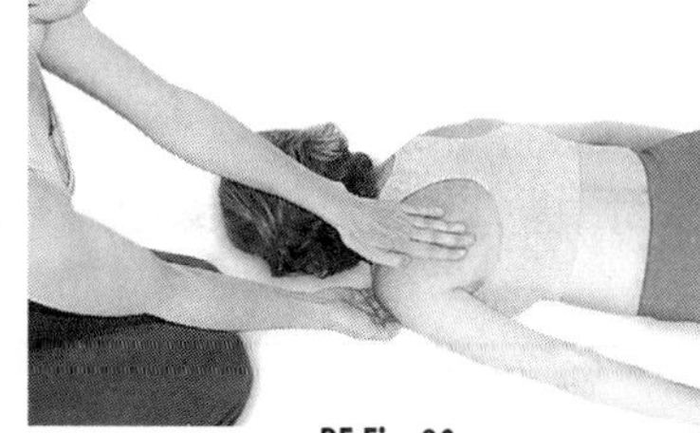

PE Fig. 90a

2. With one hand, gently lift the corner of your partner's shoulder slightly off the floor while using your other hand to seat her lower scapula against the ribs (PE Fig. 90a). This should place her scapula in neutral. Then ask her to hold it there without moving while you slowly let go. If she is in neutral, her shoulder will remain in the position you put it in. If she moves out of neutral, start over. Repeat the whole process of placing her scapula in neutral, then slowly letting go.
3. Have her lower her scapula and rest, then compare the two sides. After comparing, repeat steps 1-2 on the other side.
4. *Using a wall for feedback:* Stand with your back against a wall and sense how your shoulders make contact with the wall. Gently reposition your shoulders so that the medial borders of your scapulae lie against your ribs and the wall (PE Fig. 90b). Reach through the top of your head, widen the shoulders across the front and back, then ever so slightly lift the corner of your shoulders up, out, and over. Avoid contracting the upper trapezius by not hiking the shoulders. Avoid contracting the rhomboids by keeping the space between the scapulae wide. Avoid contracting the pectoralis muscles by staying wide across the chest and gently pulling the corners of your shoulders out and up. Hold for 10 seconds and sense the position.

PE Fig. 90b

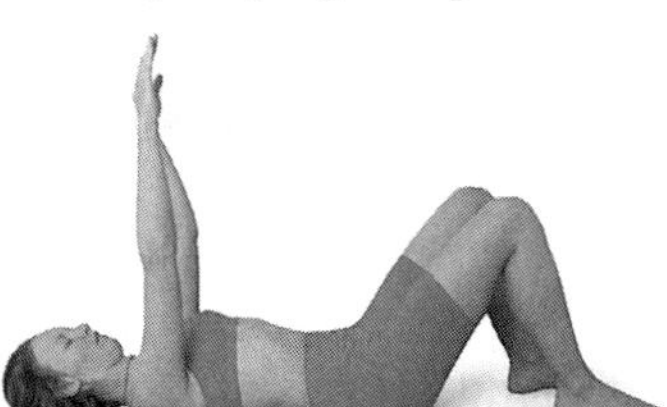

PE Fig. 90c

5. Relax and return to your original posture. Move between the old and new position to become get used to adjusting your scapulae to neutral during the course of daily activities.

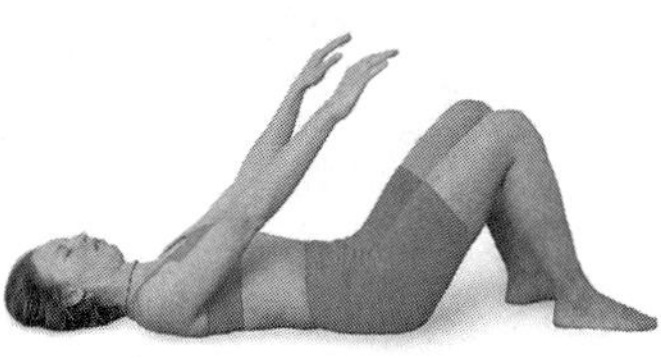

PE Fig. 90d

6. *Using the floor for feedback:* Lie on your back. Reach through the top of your head to lengthen your neck. Relax your pectoralis muscles and lightly press the corners of your shoulders into the floor. Widen between your scapulae. Lightly contract your middle and lower trapezius muscles. Feel the medial scapulae borders flatten on the floor. sense the bottom of the scapulae moving down your back. Slowly move your arms while keeping your scapulae connected to the floor, with the medial borders flat against the ribs (PE Fig. 90c-d).
7. *Serratus anterior contraction:* Stand an arm's length from a wall, facing it, and place your right hand on it. Put your left hand around the front and under your right armpit to monitor your serratus anterior. Slowly press into the wall to contract the serratus anterior muscle. Release the pressure but keep the serratus contracted.

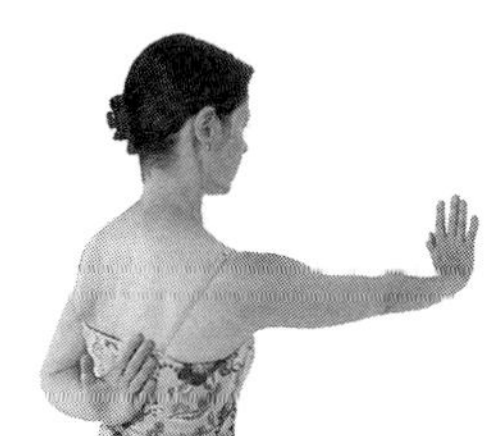

PE Fig. 90e

8. *Keeping the scapula flat while moving:* If you can, place your left hand on the medial border of your right scapula to monitor it as you move (PE Fig. 90e). It should lie flat against your ribcage. If you can't reach it, have a partner put his hand over it to give you feedback as you move. Now, with your right hand still on the wall, slowly open your body away from the wall while keeping your scapula flat as it slides along your ribcage (PE Fig. 90f). You will feel the scapula slide around the ribs in the horizontal plane. Avoid lifting it or winging its medial border.

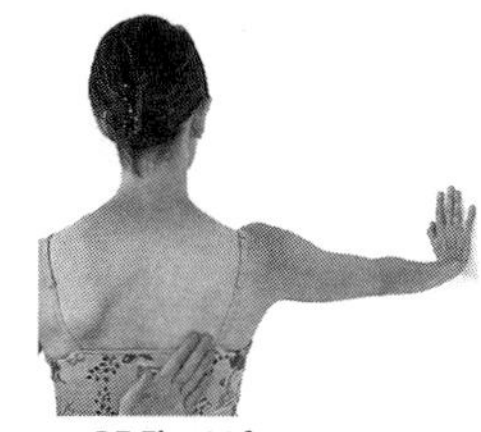

PE Fig. 90f

9. Reverse the movement and return to your original position facing the wall, again keeping your scapula flat against your ribcage as it slides across the ribs. Repeat several times until you sense the role of the serratus anterior in stabilizing the scapula during movement. Then repeat the entire routine with the other arm.
10. *Stabilizing the scapula while bearing weight with the arm:* Get in the quadruped position. Then isometrically push both arms into the floor to engage the serratus anterior and lower trapezius, flattening the scapulae against the ribs (PE Fig. 90g). Practice slowly lifting one arm to the side while keeping the supporting shoulder in a neutral position (PE Fig. 90h). Then practice on the other side.

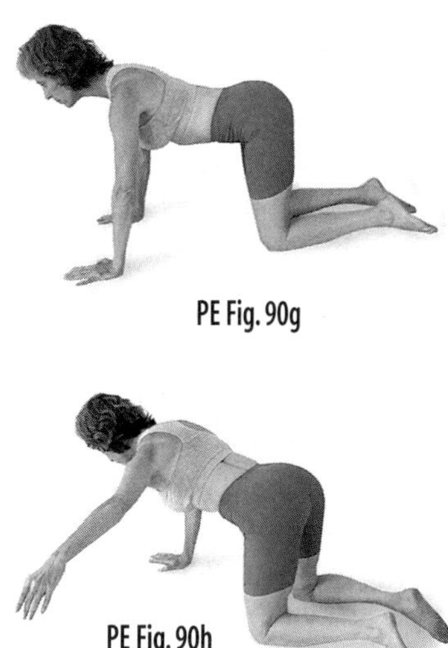

PE Fig. 90g

PE Fig. 90h

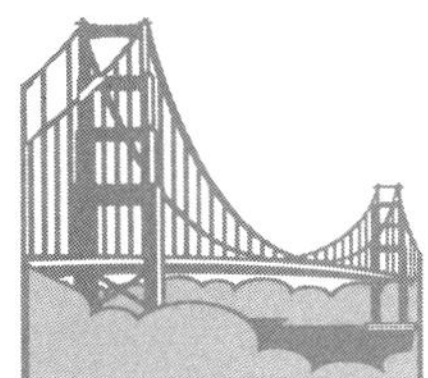

Bridge to Practice

Placing the Client's Scapula in Neutral

There are several steps in helping a client find "scap" neutral. Begin by tracing the bony landmarks of your client's scapulae so that he can sense them more easily. Then help him release extraneous muscular tension around the scapulae, especially if he tends to hike or round his shoulders. Stand behind him, place your hands under his shoulders, and lift them up. Hold his shoulders up until he can yield their weight into your hands, then gradually lower them down and release your hold. This will give your client a sense of letting his shoulder girdle rest down on his rib cage so that his arms can hang without extraneous effort. You can also stretch tight muscles that prevent his shoulders from resting in neutral, such as the pectoralis minor, levator scapula, upper trapezius, or rhomboid muscles.

Most importantly, help him recognize the what it feels like to have his scapulae in neutral. Place one of his scapula in the correct position and hold it there until your client can hold it there on his own. If he is unable to do this, palpate his lower trapezius and have him contract it, giving him verbal and tactile feedback about when it is contracting. Once he has found it and can hold his scapula in neutral, slowly release it. If he loses neutral, reposition his scapula and start over. If he can find it on one side, the sensation of the neutral position will probably contrast with his other side, which will give him a good perception of where the optimal position is.

This educational process can be slow because it takes time to place a scapula in neutral, and it takes time for your client to accurately sense scap neutral. Once he can feel the neutral position in a standing posture, he will be able to recreate it. If you create a clear enough experience of scap neutral, he will eventually be able to recreate it on his own.

Different clients are able to work at different levels, depending upon their initial posture. If your client's scapulae are extremely out of balance (off neutral) and held by chronic muscular holding, you may need to apply deep tissue stretching and trigger point work to release tight myofascia before helping your client find neutral. Since you want your client to have a successful experience, make minor adjustments toward neutral, such as helping the client widen between the shoulders to flatten the medial border. Don't give a lot of feedback at first or your client might become frustrated. Make sure your directives are within his reach, something he can easily accomplish.

STABILIZERS OF THE CERVICAL SPINE

Recall from Chapter 7 that neuromotor development begins in the head and progresses down the spine, and that the balance and movement of the head sets the tone for the whole body. Ideally, the cervical spine elongates in one normal and natural curve. But like the lumbar spine, the cervical spine can flatten and lose its natural curve, or can become chronically hyperextended. For example, ballerinas often have straight or reversed cervical curves from the excessive vertical tensions they put on their necks, and computer operators tend to thrust the head forward and hyperextend the neck, bending the neck in the middle.

Given that the vital blood and nerve supply to the brain passes through the small spaces from the head and the neck, and that the vestibular system in the inner ear sets up equilibrium for our entire posture, head and neck alignment is crucial for healthy function.[139] In an ideal posture, the back of the head rests about one inch anterior to the back of the thorax, the cervical spine is at its maximum length with a gentle lordotic curve, being supported and stabilized by the intrinsic muscles of the neck. If these deep muscles are doing their job, the extrinsic muscles will be relaxed while a person is in a neutral posture and during the continuous subtle head adjustments initiated by the perceptual organs.

The primary neck stabilizers are the *longus colli, longus capitis,* and *anterior suboccipital muscles* along the front of the spine; and the *posterior suboccipital muscles* and *semispinalis capitis muscle* along the back of the spine (Figure

Links to Practical Applications

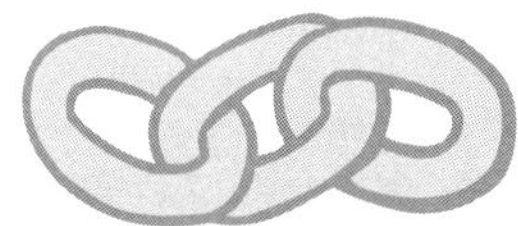

Dealing with Chronic Neck Pain

People with chronic neck pain tend to have stiff, tight neck muscles because pain inhibits intrinsic muscles while triggering protective spasms in the extrinsic muscles. For this reason, it can be difficult to facilitate the intrinsic cervical muscles if you have chronic pain and stiffness in your neck. Start by relaxing the extrinsic muscles with heat and massage, and then stretch them on a regular basis.

Also, if you receive massage and your extrinsic neck muscles become relaxed, make sure to do some subtle, small movements before you sit up to engage your intrinsic muscles. The reason this is necessary is that if the intrinsics are inhibited, the extrinsics will take over their stabilizing function. But if you remove this support by releasing the extrinsics and sit up without intrinsic support, the extrinsics may spasm to protect your neck. To prevent this, before sitting up after a massage or bodywork session, subtly rock and nod your head, and reach through the top of your head to facilitate intrinsic muscular support.

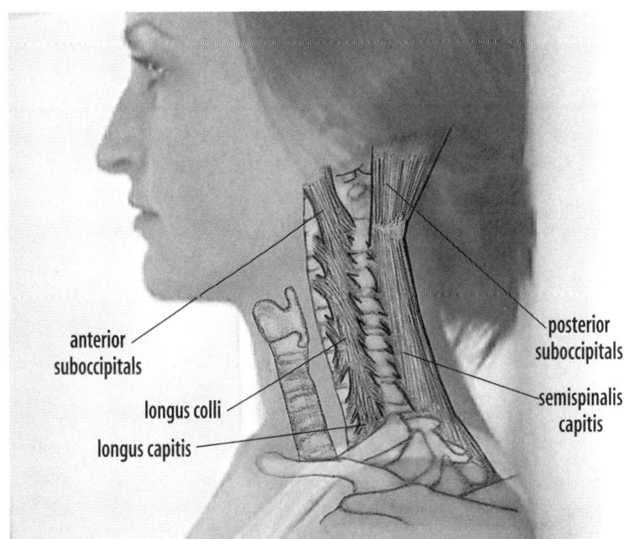

Figure 9.27 Intrinsic muscles of the neck that function as stabilizers

Patterning Exercise #91: Stretching the Back of the Neck

This stretch can help you feel each cervical vertebra move individually and can also give you a deep stretch along the upper spine and between the shoulder blades.

Caution: If your upper cervical spine is unstable, do not attempt this stretch.

1. Stand or sit in a comfortable position. Reach through the top of your head to lengthen your neck.
2. Making a very small movement, lift your hyoid bone up and back toward your ears. Then subtly roll your head forward, isolating flexion between your skull and first cervical vertebra.
3. Continue to flex your neck, curling it like a seahorse, rolling forward one vertebra at a time, until your chin is resting on your upper chest (PE Fig. 91). If your cervical spine is restricted at any one segment, you will not be flexible enough to stretch this far at first, but should be able to with regular practice.

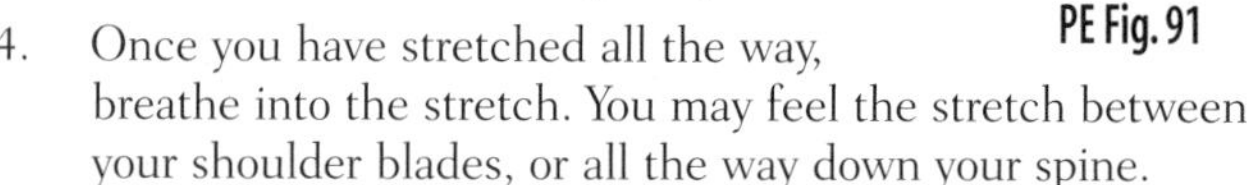

PE Fig. 91

4. Once you have stretched all the way, breathe into the stretch. You may feel the stretch between your shoulder blades, or all the way down your spine.
5. Unroll and return to neutral in one slow, smooth motion.

EMSPress.com

9.27). If we could look behind the throat and esophagus, we would find the longus colli and longus capitis, a chain of muscles plastered along the front of the vertebral bodies and discs in the cervical spine.

On the back, the semispinalis capitis muscles lie under several layers of more extrinsic muscles, insert along the base of the occiput, and blend into the multifidus muscles at the top of the ribs. The suboccipitals are even deeper. In the back of the neck they are buried under two to three inches of thick myofascia and are therefore difficult to palpate. Their short oblique fasciculi attach from the base of the skull to the transverse and spinous processes on the first and second cervical vertebrae. They control the small, refined movements of the head we continually make during perceptual shifts to sights and sounds, and subtle head righting adjustments. They contract as we speak, chew, and make small eye movements, activities that are constant during waking hours. A person can sense the deep and subtle movements the neck intrinsics generate with the oscillating rocking of the head, and during sucking or chewing.

It is important while patterning the postural stabilizers in the neck to inhibit contractions in the extrinsic musculature. A person can monitor the extrinsic muscles of the neck when engaging the intrinsics (see Patterning Exercise #92) to get feedback about whether or not the extrinsic muscles are relaxed (Figure 9.28).

Figure 9.28 Monitoring the sternocleidomastoid muscles while patterning the intrinsics

Neck pain tends to inhibit the intrinsic, stabilizing muscles, which triggers chronic contractions and perhaps even spasms in the extrinsic muscles that fire to stabilize and support the neck. Contractions or spasms in the extrinsic muscles can usually be observed in muscular cords that pop out on either side of the neck or at the base of the skull. Recall from Chapter 2 that when the larger muscles of the neck become chronically contracted, they tend to bend and shear the vertebrae and displace them from their neutral zone (Figure 9.29). Since the cervical

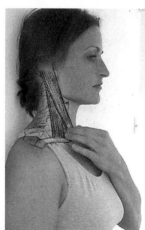

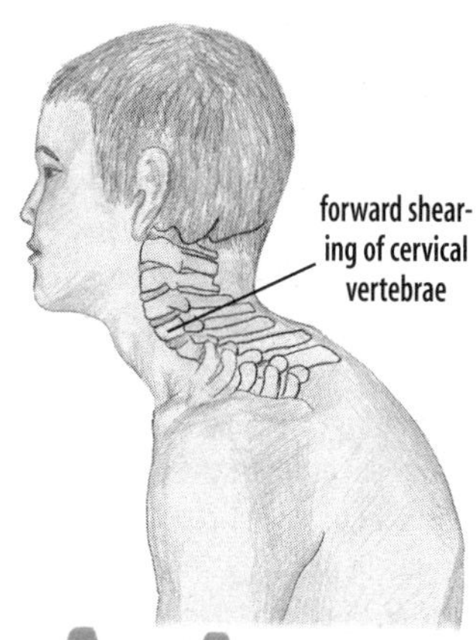

Figure 9.29 A collapsed neck puts undue stress on the spine, causing shearing between vertebrae.

Patterning Intrinsic Motion at the AO Joints

Clients with neck tension tend to overwork the superficial, extrinsic muscles in the neck. When this occurs, help your client engage the intrinsic muscles through subtle movement at the top cervical joints, the *atlanto-occipital (AO) joints*. To approximate the axis of these joints, lightly place your index fingers in the hollow below the ear on the transverse process of C-1. Have your client sense the axis between your fingers, then gently nod her head up and down in the "yes" gesture to clarify movement along this axis. The smaller the movement, the more the intrinsic muscles will become active.

For clients who use excessive effort, direct them by saying something like, "Feel the circular dimension of the base of your head. Imagine the center of this ring. Move right in the center of the ring. Make your movement so small that you can barely feel it, as though you are just imagining movement there," or "Relax completely, then nod your head, using about 10 percent of the previous effort you were using."

Patterning Exercise #92: Postural Stabilization for the Head and Neck

Caution: Be careful not to use too much effort. Most people, particularly those with tight neck muscles, tend to overwork in this exercise, which can make you even tighter. If you feel pain or dizziness while doing this exercise, you may have a muscular restriction that is cutting off circulation when you move. If so, you need to see a specialist who can realign your cervical spine as soon as possible.

1. *With a partner:* Stand beside your partner and lightly cup her chin and occiput, placing your fingertips lightly on the mastoid processes. Ask her to let her neck relax into your hands (PE Fig. 92a). If she has a collapsed posture her neck may drop down.

PE Fig. 92a

2. Then give your partner a gentle lift under the chin and occiput, and subtly lift your head toward the ceiling (PE Fig. 90b). The touch should be light enough to just suggest where the head needs to go. If she follows your hands and lifts her head, apply more pressure to lift her head and stretch her neck.

PE Fig. 92b

3. *Sitting or standing:* Sit or stand with your shoulders against a wall, your knees slightly bent. You may need to slip a small piece of one-inch thick foam behind your head to feel the wall behind your head.
4. Place your hands lightly on the front of your neck to monitor tension or relaxation in the extrinsic muscles (PE Fig. 92c). Subtly rock your head on your neck, as if you were nodding "yes," isolating the movement in the top joints. As you do this, energetically reach the top of your head toward the ceiling. Imagine your neck ratcheting up a notch on each rock (PE Fig. 92d). Breathe into the width of your lower ribs. Feel your neck lengthens and scapulae reposition as the upper trapezius muscles lengthens.
5. Relax completely, letting the weight of your head down into your neck and thorax. Take several deep breaths.
6. Next, using minimal effort, lift the back of your head toward the ceiling without lowering your chin and hold for 10 seconds. Then relax completely. If your neck becomes tight while doing this, you are working too hard. To use less effort, simply visualize the back of your head lifting.

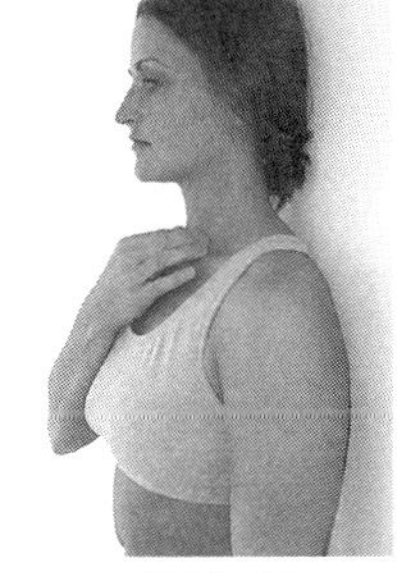

PE Fig. 92c

Feedback: When you engage the intrinsic stabilizers of your neck, you might feel a stretch between your shoulder blades, or even feel pain. Lift only to the edge of the stretch or pain. Avoid lifting too hard and overstretching. This action should feel pretty easy. If you find you are working too hard and cannot relax, try the same exercise while lying on your back.

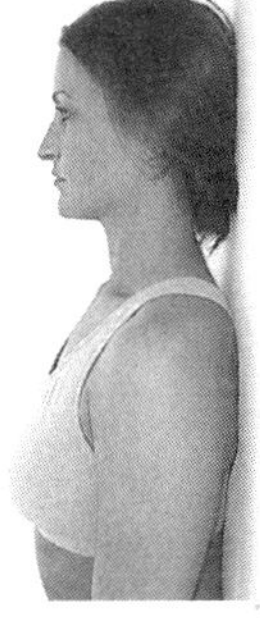

PE Fig. 92d

7. *Lying supine:* Find a comfortable resting position. Reach through the top of your head and let your scapulae widen and sink. Place your fingertips lightly at the base of your skull to monitor and relax the extrinsic muscles there as you move. Then slowly and subtly rock your head at the place where your head meets your neck. Sense your intrinsic muscles working while actively relaxing the extrinsic muscles. As you rock, keep your shoulders wide and relaxed, and slowly lengthen your neck along both the front and back sides.

arteries thread through small foramen in each vertebra, spasms can disturb the delicate alignment of the cervical spine and restrict blood flow to the brain. This can lead to a parade of symptoms, such as vascular headaches, fatigue, dizziness, mental confusion, and, in extreme cases, fainting.

The seven vertebrae of the cervical spine move in two functional units, from the second vertebra up, and from the third vertebra down to the seventh. Holding patterns can affect the upper or lower cervical spine separately, so the alignment of each unit needs to be addressed separately. For example, both the upper and lower cervical spine can hyperextend or chronically flex (which will flatten the neck). The upper cervical spine can become fixed in chronic flexion with the lower cervical spine in hyperextension. To further complicate the matter, any of the cervical vertebrae can become fixed in a twisted position. Keep in mind that all of these misalignments are caused by chronic contraction of the extrinsic neck muscles, a condition that can be alleviated with patterning exercises and myofascial release work.

People with extreme instability in the upper cervical spine often comment that their heads feel wobbly, as though they might fall off, and they experience pain during and after head flexion. They also tend to brace the neck to hold it stable and comment that they have difficulty finding a position in which their head rests on top. Instability in the lower cervical spine usually causes a forward shear at the fifth cervical vertebra, which can be observed in a fold in the middle of the back of the neck.

Obviously, good posture in the head and neck is crucial. Probably the single most effective way to keep the head and neck aligned without becoming rigid is to facili-

Patterning Exercise #93: Co-contracting the Postural Stabilizers

1. *Setting up a feedback loop:* Lie on your back and sense the places where your back makes contact with the floor. Then take several deep breaths. On each exhalation, let the various parts of your back relax and sink into the floor.
2. Slowly and lightly pull your lower abdominal wall straight back and hollow your lower abdomen.
3. Slowly and lightly pull your sit bones together.
4. Slowly contract the muscles along either side of the back of your lumbar spine. (If your lower back is flat, it should lift and slightly arch. If your lower back is overarched, the arch should flatten somewhat, but not all the way.)
5. Slowly pull both of your thighs into their sockets and contract the muscles along the front of your lumbar spine.
6. Widen your shoulders in the front and back, slightly externally rotate your upper arms, then lightly anchor your shoulder blades down to your back.
7. Reach through the top of your head, lengthening your neck while still keeping a curve in your neck. Avoid shortening the front of your neck to lengthen the back.
8. Hold all of these tonic contractions while you breathe into the width of your lower ribs.
9. *Integrating spinal stability with movement:* Explore tiny micromovements while you keep your trunk and head stable yet relaxed. For example, slowly nod your head, point and flex your ankles, raise and lower a knee, tilt and untilt your pelvis, or raise and lower an arm.

EMSPress.com

tate tonic contractions in the intrinsic muscles. There are simple ways to do this, such as by practicing reaching the top of the head up, by isolating small movements at the base of the skull such as nodding or the sucking pattern mentioned earlier, and by keeping the head aligned over the body through practiced awareness. Simply remembering to reach the top of the head up toward the ceiling now and then during the course of the day will go a long way in helping a person develop control over the intrinsic muscles. Also, a person can do a subtle rocking motion of the head at the top joint to engage the intrinsic muscles of the neck while relaxing the extrinsics. The benefits of doing this not only include better posture but better blood flow to the brain, which can help a person stay alert yet relaxed.

THE CO-CONTRACTION OF SPINAL STABILIZERS

A point that can't be emphasized too strongly is that *it is impossible to achieve good alignment and stability in the neck without having it along the entire spine and shoulder girdle.* Even though the stability exercises have been presented in parts, all the parts are inextricably connected and must work together. This means that all the stabilizers along the spine need to co-contract as a team.

Training is progressive. First one postural stabilizer is brought under control, then another, then the whole group. Although this may sound complicated, it is quite simple once a person can control individual muscles in the stabilizer group. A person merely goes through a mental checklist, such as "pull the lower abdomen back, pull the pelvic floor in, lift along the front of the lumbar spine, and then lift along the back." Once this is achieved, the neck and scapula stabilizers can be added with mental directives such as "lift out the top of the head, widen the shoulders, and place the scapulae in neutral."

It is helpful to go through this checklist while sitting or resting at first, then to begin using it during the course of daily activities. Images are also helpful. For instance, when walking a person can imagine the head floating, wind blowing the lower abdomen back against the spine, and small sandbags anchoring the scapulae down on the back. People need to be creative and to find images that work for them, though images are generally more effective if they are based on anatomical structures. Or a person can call up a clear mental picture of the muscles and bones to engage postural muscles during the course of the day. Recognizing the sensations of good postural alignment also helps a person recreate this alignment.

SUMMARY

An understanding of how muscles work as postural stabilizers and precisely which muscles stabilize which joints is essential to anyone working to improve posture and alignment, particularly practitioners. Generally, stabilization has been approached in the somatic field as a balance between intrinsic and extrinsic muscles. This is somewhat accurate, yet to be more precise, stabilization involves the recruitment order of muscles, specifically of tonic contractions in stabilizers prior to phasic contractions in mobilizers.

As with any kind of training, postural stabilization builds with increasingly more complex motor challenges, beginning with isometrics done in place; and progressing to simple movements such as hip flexion and extension being added on top of simple stabilization exercises. This chapter presents an introduction to postural stabilization but does not go into the complexities of this approach nor the subsequent levels of training. In more comprehensive stabilization training, a person would next learn to train the global stabilizers,

Patterning Exercise #94: Stabilizing the Trunk during Leg Movement

1. *Finding the hollow:* Lie on your back and lightly pull your abdominal wall toward your lower back to engage your transversus abdominis.
2. *Stabilizing during hip flexion:* Straighten one leg. Then lightly contract the oblique muscles around your waist. Now lift that leg about one inch off the floor and hold (PE Fig. 94a). Keep your pelvis and spine stable as your hold your leg.

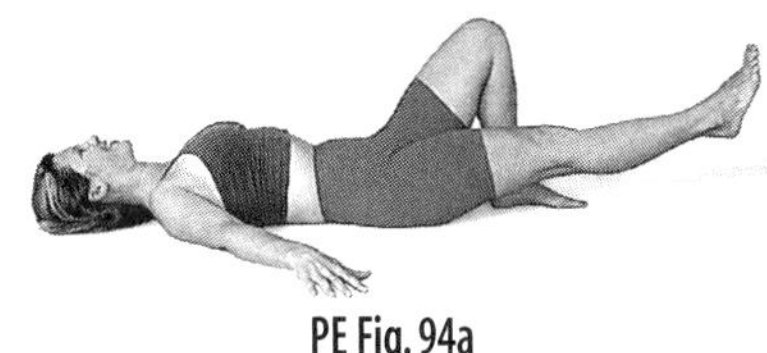

PE Fig. 94a

3. Relax and repeat with the other leg.
4. *Stabilizing during leg flexion and extension:* Lie on your back with both legs bent and parallel, feet flat on the floor. Stabilize your trunk by co-contracting the stabilizers along the spine (see Patterning Exercise # 93 titled "Co-contracting the Postural Stabilizers"). Using the least amount of effort possible while keeping your pelvis and trunk stable and still, slide one heel down along the floor and extend that leg (PE Fig. 94b). Reverse the movement by sliding that same heel back along the floor and bringing the knee to a flexed position.
5. Flex and extend one leg several times, then rest and compare your two sides. Is that side more relaxed? Repeat on the other side.
6. *Stabilizing in a sidelying position:* Lie on your side with both legs straight, one on top of the other. Engage your trunk stabilizers, then slowly raise your top leg and hold it in a stable position (PE Fig. 94c). Keep your pelvis level and your spine stable as you raise your leg. Avoid hiking your hip (PE Fig. 94d). Repeat several times with one leg, then switch sides and repeat several times on the other side.

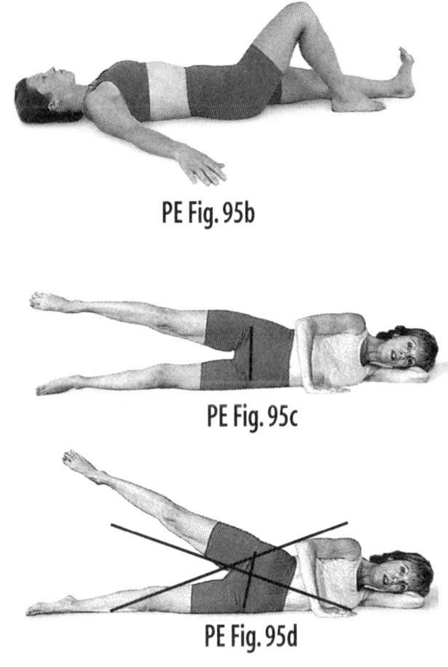

PE Fig. 95b

PE Fig. 95c

PE Fig. 95d

EMSPress.com

which control the range of motion. This term is discussed under "Stability Rehabilitation" in Chapter 12. Several of these muscles have been referred to throughout the text. For example, the oblique muscles control rotation of the trunk; and the gluteal muscles function as local stabilizers in standing, as global stabilizers to control trunk flexion, and as prime movers in actions such as climbing and sprinting. More advanced levels of training involve stabilizing during weight-bearing and cardiovascular exercise.

The reader is encouraged to integrate postural stabilization isometrics into each of the patterning exercises in the next chapter on fundamental movement patterns. Although this integration will not be stressed in Chapter 10, Patterning Exercise #94 titled "Stabilizing the Trunk during Leg Movement" is a sample of how to integrate stabilization isometrics with fundamental movements.

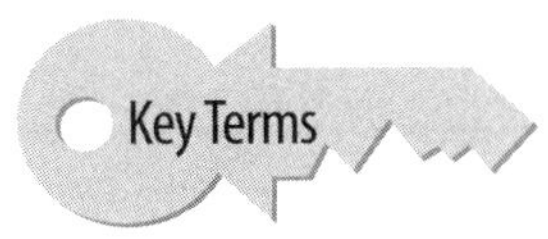

dissociation of movement **scapula neutral** **substitution pattern**

OVERVIEW OF CHAPTER 10

Fundamental Movement Patterns

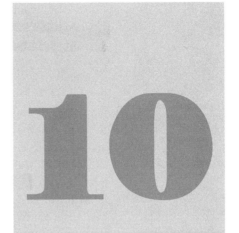

Nothing is more revealing than movement.

—*Martha Graham*

This chapter presents what will be referred to as the **fundamental movement patterns** of flexion, extension, and rotation of the limbs and spine, as well as weight shifts and gait patterns, all patterns that can be found in any kinesiology text. Rather than taking the traditional approach, which involves the study of each joint and muscle in the body, this approach is based on a balance between cognitive and experiential learning and also on the integration of the movement of each body part into a full-body pattern.

Each fundamental movement pattern will be explored here through images and analogies. Also, a basic discussion of joint structure and body mechanics in each major part of the body is offered as a guide for practicing the movement exercises. For example, the arms and legs attach to the body at ball-and-socket joints that swing like pendulums. A person can loosen these joints by swinging them back and forth, and can then integrate this swinging action into walking and lifting to bring ease to these actions.

This chapter was inspired by dancer and physical therapist Irmgaard Bartenieff, who developed the study of Laban Movement Analysis in America and founded the Laban Institute of Movement Studies (LIMS) in New York City (see Chapter 11). Bartenieff enlivened the experiential study of movement with her approach to integrated, full-body patterns that stressed an upper-lower body connection. She not only inspired her students to explore basic patterns using lively effort qualities and clear spatial intent, but she also made the study of kinesiology more easily understood and practical by identifying six fundamental patterns through which all movement can be analyzed. These patterns—the *thigh lift*, *forward pelvic shift*, *lateral shift*, *body half*, *arm circle*, and *condensation patterns*—make up the Bartenieff Movement Fundamentals (see Figure 11.6). Although this chapter is not about the Bartenieff Movement Fundamentals per se, since there are only so many fundamental movement patterns of the human body, there will certainly be overlap.

STANDARD TERMS TO DESCRIBE MOVEMENT

Before delving into the fundamental movement patterns, a few kinesiological terms previously mentioned will be reviewed and new ones introduced. Also, it is important to note that every movement is relative to the anatomical position—a neutral standing posture in which both legs and spine are vertically aligned in extension, the arms are resting beside the body, and the knees and toes are facing forward.

Recall from Chapter 2 that *flexion* is a movement that decreases the angle of a joint, while *extension* is a return from flexion. The hip flexes when we lift the thigh in front of the body; it extends when we reverse the movement and lower the thigh below the pelvis. *Hyperextension* is any movement that extends a joint behind the frontal plane. We hyperextend the hip by extending the lower limb behind the body; we hyperextend the spine when we arch over backward. Since neither the knee nor elbow can move past an extended range, hyperextension in either of these joints, which has been referred to as "locking," should be avoided because it can overstretch and even damage the joint capsule (Figure 10.1).

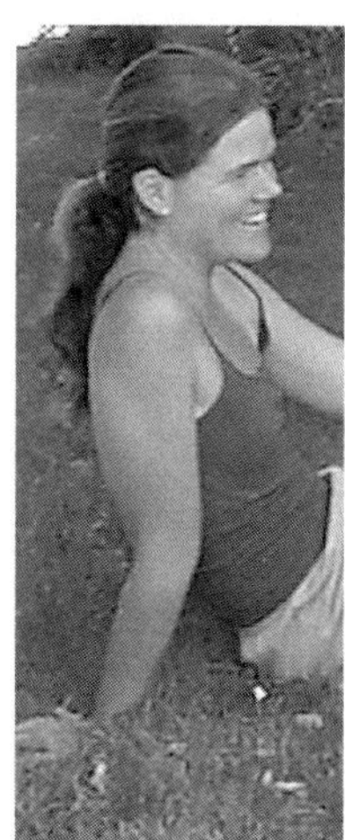

Figure 10.1
Hyperextension

Adduction is movement toward midline; we adduct the legs or arms when we return them to midline from an abducted position (Figure 10.2a). **Abduction** is movement away from the midline; we abduct the legs or arms when we lift them to the sides (Figure 10.2b). Likewise, to abduct the fingers is to spread them apart; bringing the fingers closer together adducts them. An easy way to remember the difference is that adduction, which begins with the letters "add," *adds* to the midline.

Outward rotation (also called "lateral" rotation) turns a limb so that the knee or the crease of the elbow is facing away from the trunk; **inward rotation** (also called "medial" rotation) turns a limb so that the knee or the crease of the elbow is facing toward the trunk (Figure 10.3a-d). When the legs are held in a chronically outwardly rotated position, a person usually has a toed-out gait. When the legs are held in a chronically inwardly rotated position, a person usually has what is commonly known as a pigeon-toed gait.

The scapulae have a unique range of motion. **Elevation** raise the scapulae; **depression** lower the scapulae (Figure 10.4a-b). **Retraction** draw the scapulae together in back; **protraction** pull them around to the front (Figure 10.4c-d). Young teenage girls often protract the scapulae and fold the chest to hide their budding breasts, whereas soldiers retract the scapulae to push the chest out with pride. An *upward rotation* simultaneously elevates and protracts the scapulae when we give someone taller than us a hug. An *upward tilt* of the scapulae occurs when we grasp the hands together behind the hips.

The hands and feet also have a unique range of motion. Turning the palms up takes the hands into **supination**, while turning the palms down takes them into **pronation** (Figure 10.5a-b). Likewise, lifting the medial arch on the inner edge of the foot is an action called **inversion**; lifting the lateral arch on the outer edge of the foot is an action called **eversion** (Figure 10.6a-b). We evert the foot when we push a door open with its outside edge and invert the foot when we turn it and lift its inner edge to scratch an itch on the sole. Pointing the toes or standing on the tip-toes takes the ankles into **plantar flexion,** commonly referred to as "ankle extension." Lowering the heel from a tip-toed position to the ground or lifting the toes toward the shin takes the ankle into **dorsiflexion,** commonly referred to as "ankle flexion" (Figure 10.7a-b).

THE SPINE

Numerous patterns of spinal movement have already been covered. Chapter 5 introduced the subtle and constant physiological flexion and extension that the breath creates along the spine, and how the special senses of the head initiate an

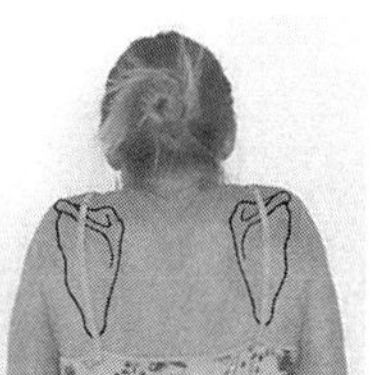

Figure 10.4a
Elevation

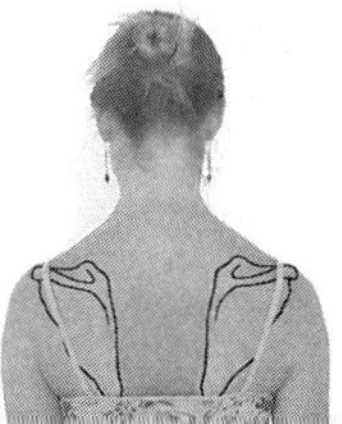

Figure 10.4b
Depression

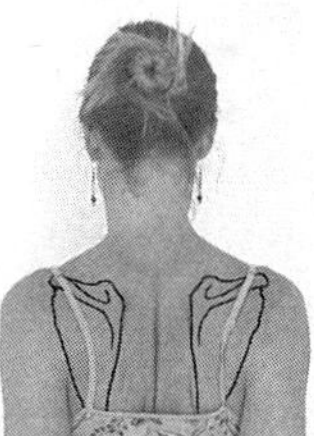

Figure 10.4c
Retraction

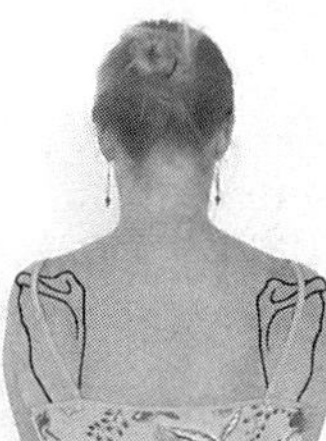

Figure 10.4d
Protraction

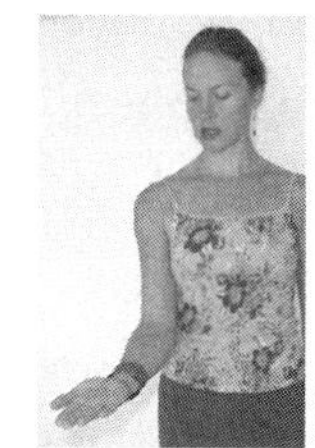

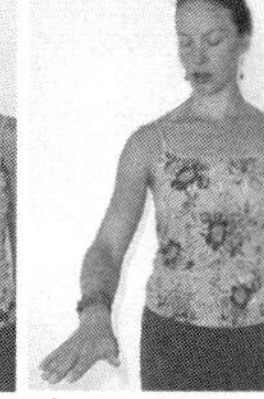

Figure 10.5a
Supination

Figure 10.5b
Pronation

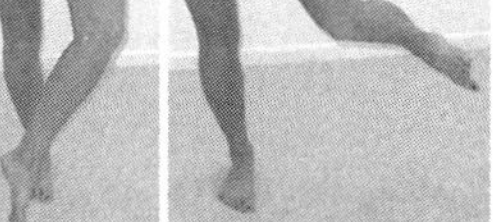

Figure 10.6a
Inversion

Figure 10.6b
Eversion

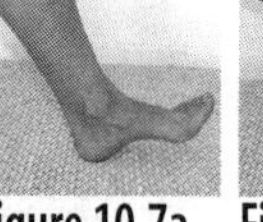

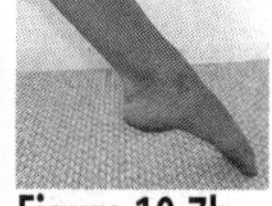

Figure 10.7a
Dorsiflexion

Figure 10.7b
Plantarflexion

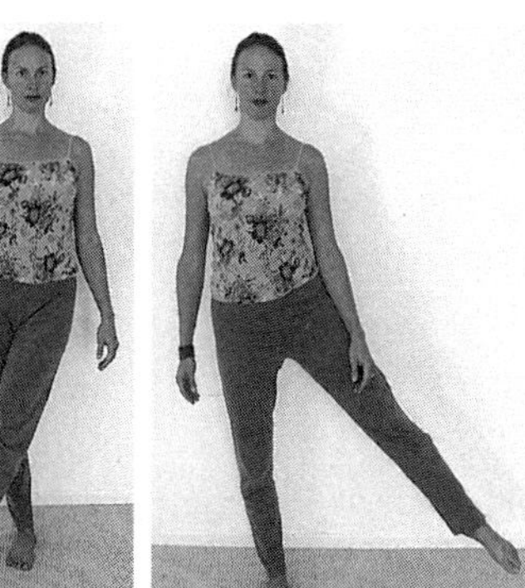

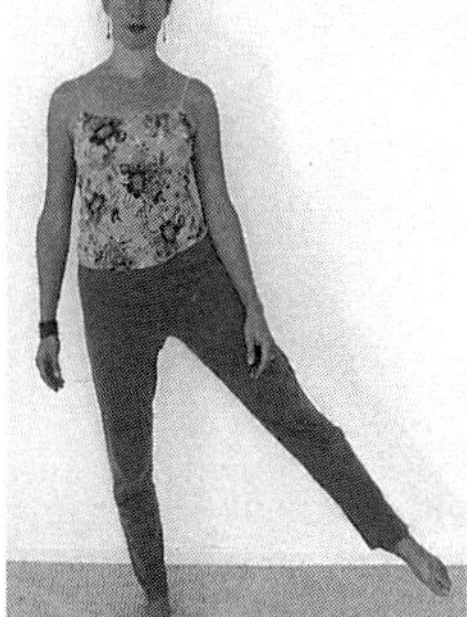

Figure 10.2a
Adduction

Figure 10.2b
Abduction

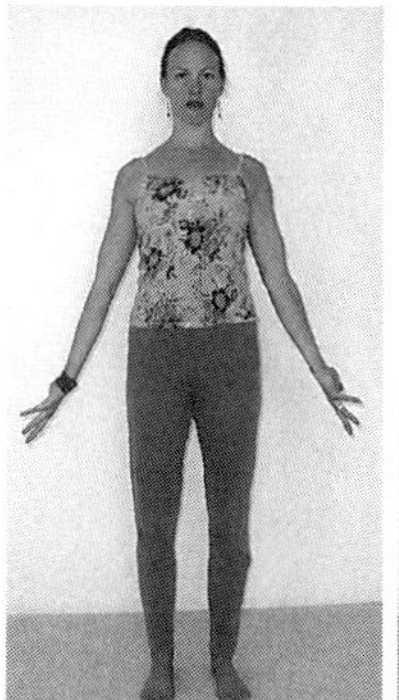

Figure 10.3a
Outward rotation of arms

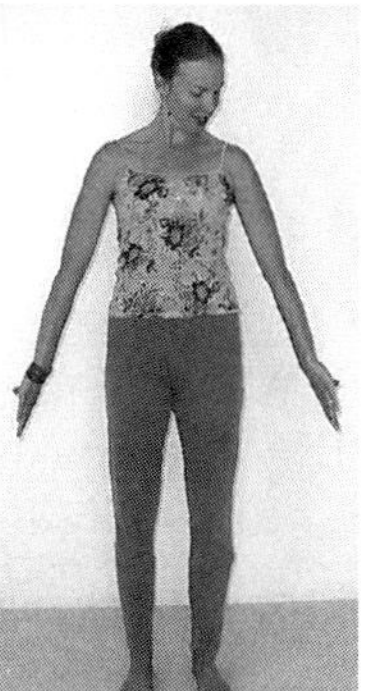

Figure 10.3b
Inward rotation of arms

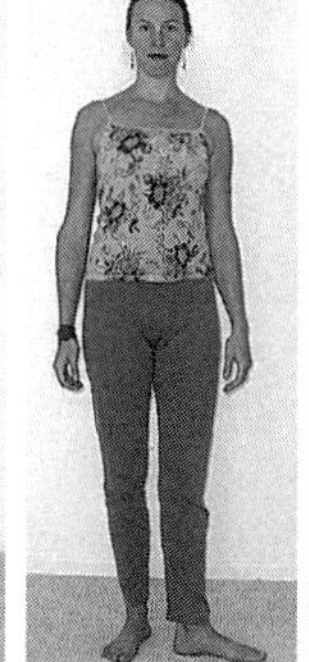

Figure 10.3c
Outward rotation

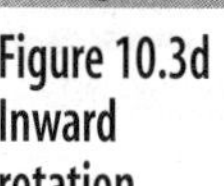

Figure 10.3d
Inward rotation

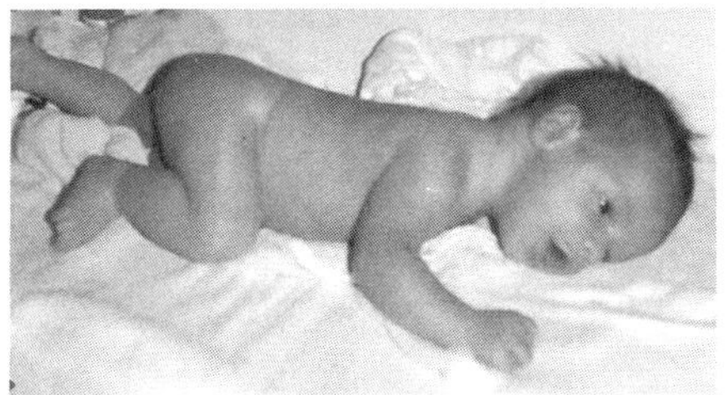

Figure 10.8a The cervical curve develops as this six-week-old infant lifts his head.

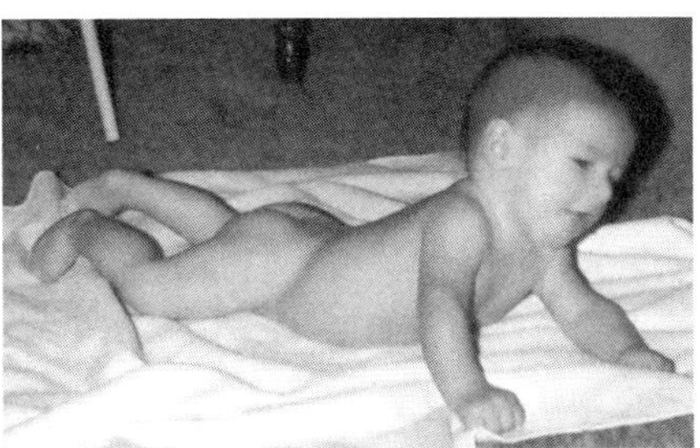

Figure 10.8b The lumbar curve develops as this three-month-old baby lifts his head and chest (photos courtesy of L. Bright).

ongoing progression of movement impulses in the spine during the actions of looking, listening, talking, eating, and expressing emotion. Chapter 6 explored the influence of the circulatory patterns on physiological and organic spinal responsiveness. Chapter 7 covered the developmental patterns and reflexes that lay down the neuromotor pathways for basic spinal patterns. And Chapter 9 examined the system of anti-gravity muscles that work as postural stabilizers for the spine. This chapter concludes spinal patterns with a look at the functional anatomy of the vertebral column and how it affects spinal movement.

Most people tend to think that the spinal column is located on the back of the body because that is where they feel it, but the spine is actually inside the torso. When viewed from the side, the average spine fills one third to one half of the trunk from the middle of the body to back. The spine has three sections: a front, middle and back. The front of this bony column is made up of a stack of fibrous gel-filled discs and spongy vertebral bodies that are firmly attached by five longitudinal layers of ligaments. Several layers cover the column from top to bottom like strong strapping tape. The middle of each vertebra has a *foramen* (opening) through which the spinal cord runs. The back of the spine is made up of a series of bony knobs that serve as attachment sites for muscles.

The human spinal column has four functional curves: two **lordotic curves** (*convex* toward the front) in the cervical and lumbar areas, and two **kyphotic curves** (*concave* toward the front) in the thoracic and sacral areas. An infant comes into the world curled in flexion with one primary C-shaped kyphotic curve. The secondary curves develop through movement. The cervical curve gradually forms as the infant lifts his head to do such things as nurse or look around (Figure 10.8a). The lumbar curve gradually forms as he learns to push up to sitting and standing (Figure 10.8b).

The spine is a multi-segmented and relatively stiff column that provides a central axis of support for the body, yet is flexible enough to bend and twist as we move. The spinal curves create a sturdy yet resilient column because a bowed column is much stronger than a straight column. For example, imagine the difference between jumping on a straight wooden board and jumping on an upwardly bowed wooden board. The straight board would probably break whereas the bowed board would probably bend and then spring back. Likewise, the combined flexibility of the spinal curves gives the backbone a high degree of resiliency and ability to absorb shock. When each curve is in a position of maximal elongation without being flattened, the spine can move from an aligned posture that has maximal support (Figure 10.9a). (Recall from Chapter 9 that elongation is maintained by the isometric contractions of postural stabilizers. Also, the forces of weight and movement pass more efficiently through the spine if the three body masses of the head, thorax, and pelvis move in an aligned relationship.)

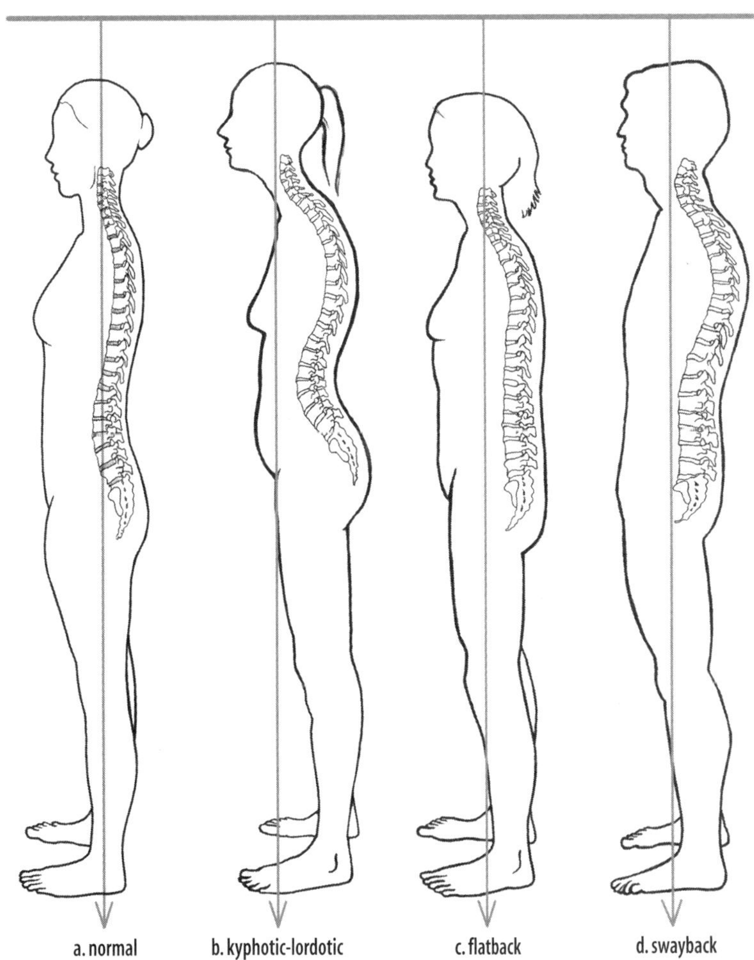

Figure 10.9a-d Different types of spinal curves

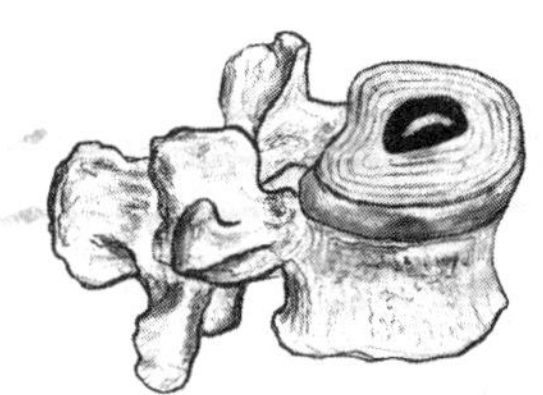

Figure 10.10 The disc functions like a ball-bearing for the adjacent disc to pivot upon.

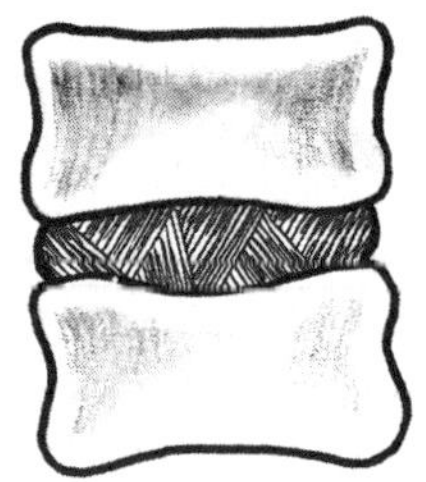

Figure 10.11 Oblique fibers in and around the vertebral discs transfer forces between vertebrae.

Spinal alignment varies with structural differences in the shape and size of the vertebrae and the surrounding muscles. The orientation of the sacrum also affects the alignment of the entire column: a horizontally oriented sacrum predisposes a person to pronounced curves, whereas a vertically oriented sacrum predisposes a person to nearly flat curves (a type of alignment advocated by Ida Rolf, whose work in Rolfing is discussed in Chapter 12). Most spines have curvatures somewhere in between.[140] The shape of an individual's spine is determined both by genetic predisposition and by postural habits. There are several types of deviation in spinal alignment that compress and bend spinal curves, flatten or twist them, or flatten one while bending another (Figure 10.9b-d).[141]

What happens to the intervertebral discs when the body's weight is habitually held behind the center of gravity?

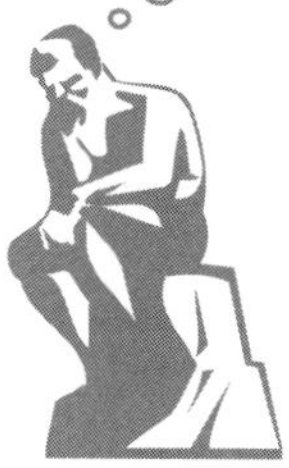

The Front of the Spine

The stack of vertebral bodies and discs in the front of the spine serves as both a stiffening rod and shock absorber. Each vertebral disc has a nucleus filled with a colloidal gel composed of about 88 percent fluid that functions like a ball-bearing upon which the adjacent vertebral bodies swivel (Figure 10.10).[142] The nucleus is surrounded by layered rings of crisscrossed oblique fibers that blend into the surrounding ligaments and tendons and transfer rotational forces between the spinal muscles and the vertebral column (Figure 10.11). During the course of the day, the combined forces of movement and weight-bearing increase axial compression along the spine, squeezing fluid toward the sides of the spongy discs and somewhat flattening each disc. The column returns to a neutral alignment during sleep when the fluid gradually seeps back into the center of the discs, which is why a person is slightly taller in the morning than at night. The proportion of fluid in the disc decreases with injury, disease, or dehydration from aging.

The discs absorb impact and, if hydrated, create a hydraulic lift that pushes the vertebrae apart and pulls the surrounding ligaments taut. This action is similar to the support a person gets sitting on an inflated beach ball; the weight of the body makes the ball firmer, increasing the tensional forces in the ball to meet the compressional forces of the body, thereby providing more support.

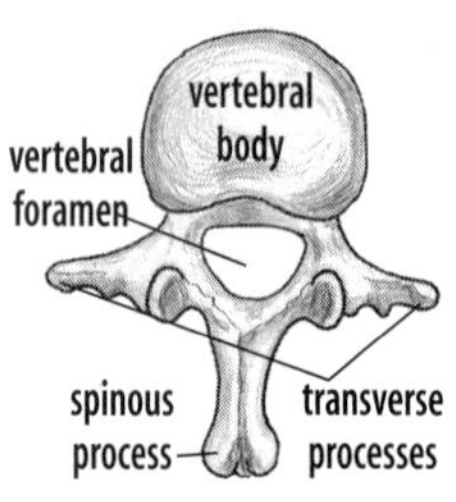

Figure 10.13 Schematic of a typical vertebra

In his book *The Alexander Technique: Body Awareness in Action,* Alexander teacher Franklin Jones describes the postural mechanism initiated in the head and neck while the Alexander practitioner lightly guides the student's head (Figure 10.12a-b).[143] During **head righting reactions**, the head reflexively lifts and rights over the body, taking the slack out of the longitudinal ligaments along the spine. The head righting reaction pattern can be observed when a horse falls and its head pops up to vertical, then its body follows and also pops up to standing. When the head rights and lifts, the ligaments along the spine become more taut from the lift and the spine becomes longer and more stable. When the ligaments elongate, they press laterally into the sides of the *intervertebral discs* and lengthen the spine. The lateral pressure also pushes fluid toward the center of the discs, making them more buoyant and further elongating the spine.

Jones speculates that the lift in the cervical spine pulls slack out of the entire spinal column, lengthening the span of ligaments and muscles all along it. Most people describe this experience as creating a pleasant, almost magical decompression through the entire trunk, often one of relief if compression was causing back pain. The Alexander Technique has a reputation for being effective in relieving chronic neck and back pain, perhaps because of this normalizing mechanism on the spine.

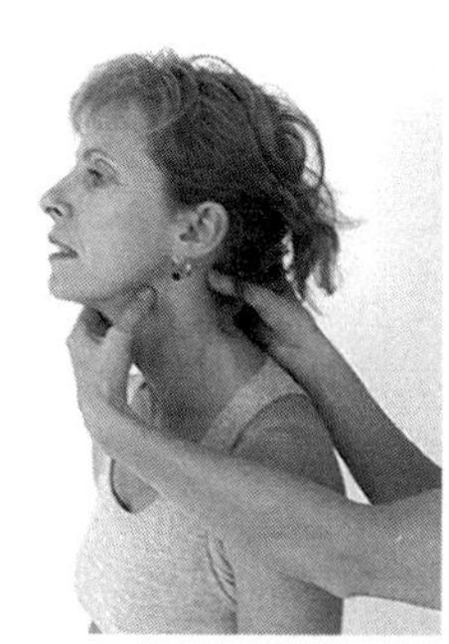

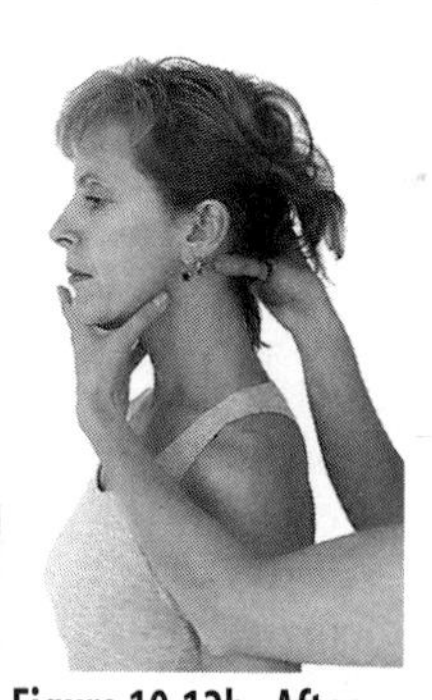

Figure 10.12a Before assisted head righting

Figure 10.12b After assisted head righting

The Back of the Spine

Each vertebra has a *spinous process* in the center of the back and two *transverse processes* on each side (Figure 10.13). The spinous process and transverse processes provide attachment sites for a complex array of tendons and ligaments. Each vertebra has four bilateral articular surfaces about the size of a fingernail that connect with articular surfaces in vertebrae above and below it to form *facet joints*—small synovial joints that span the length of the entire column. There are two facet joints connecting each pair of adjacent vertebra, adding up to

48 vertebral facet joints along the back of the spine. Each thoracic vertebra also shares three small facet joints with each adjacent rib (only two at the first rib pair), for a total of 68 *costovertebral joints*, adding up to 82 facet joints along the thoracic spine alone. The combined movement along the facet joints and vertebral segments gives the spine the capacity for sinuous, snake-like undulations, a prespinal quality seen in hula and belly dance (Figure 10.14).

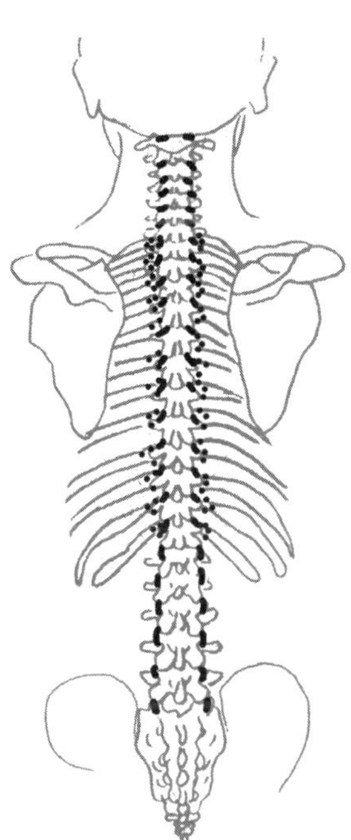

Figure 10.14 A schematic of the facet joints along the spine

All spinal movements involve some combination of flexion, extension, and rotation that moves the spine in all three planes (Figure 10.15). The plane in which the articular surfaces of the facet joints lie determines the range of motion inherent to that part of the spine alone (Figure 10.16). Since the lumbar facets are vertically oriented in the sagittal plane, the lumbar spine favors flexion and extension but limits rotation and lateral flexion (side-bending). Since the thoracic facets are oriented at about 60-degree angles in the frontal plane, the thoracic spine favors rotation but limits flexion and extension. Since the cervical facets are oriented at 45 degrees and are nearly horizontal, the cervical spine has the broadest range of motion in all three planes.

Although each facet joint has a small range of motion, the combined movement of all the facet joints allows the spinal column a fair degree of flexibility. Ideally, each facet is mobile within its physiological range, and there is a continuity of mobility throughout the spine. In

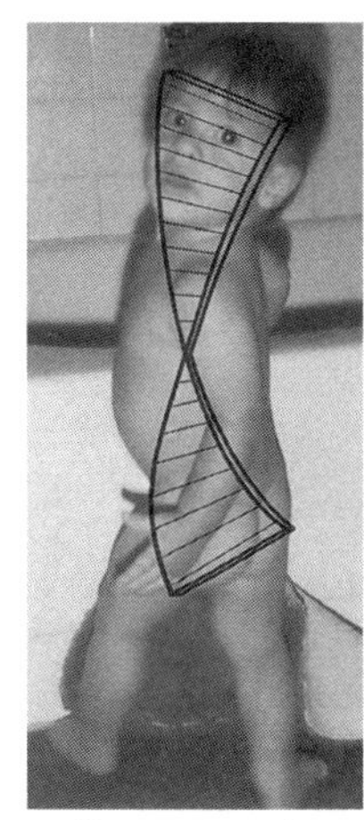

Figure 10.15 An illustration of spinal movement in all 3 planes during extension with rotation (photo courtesy of L. Bright).

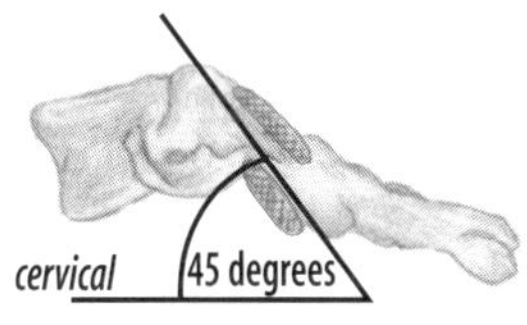

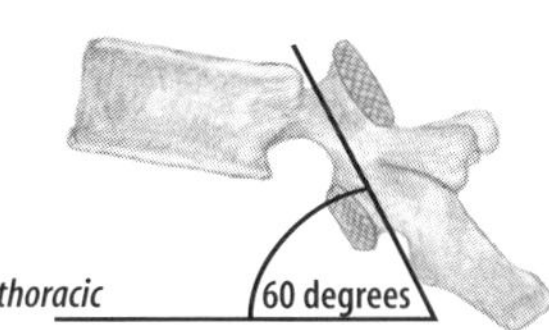

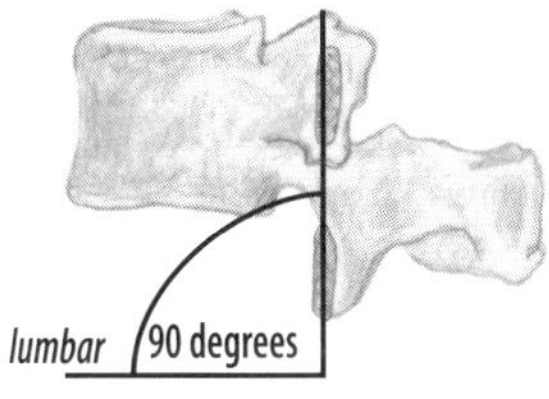

Figure 10.16 The angle of facet joints in each type of vertebra reflect the direction of movement in that part of the spine.

Patterning Exercise #95: Contrasting the Front and Back of the Spine

1. *Absorbing impact through the discs:* Sit on a physioball or a springy couch and gently bounce. Experiment with your position, leaning slightly forward and back to sense the place where you feel the impact being absorbed by the discs along the front of your spine (PE Fig. 95a).

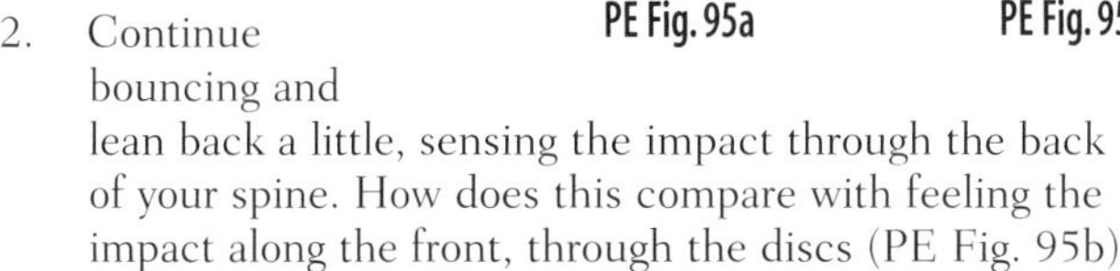

PE Fig. 95a PE Fig. 95b

2. Continue bouncing and lean back a little, sensing the impact through the back of your spine. How does this compare with feeling the impact along the front, through the discs (PE Fig. 95b)?
3. *Contrasting moving with a focus on the front or the back:* Lying on your back, alternately flex and extend your spine using small, subtle motions, first with a focus along the front of the spine, moving the discs and organs while relaxing your back against the floor (PE Fig. 95c).

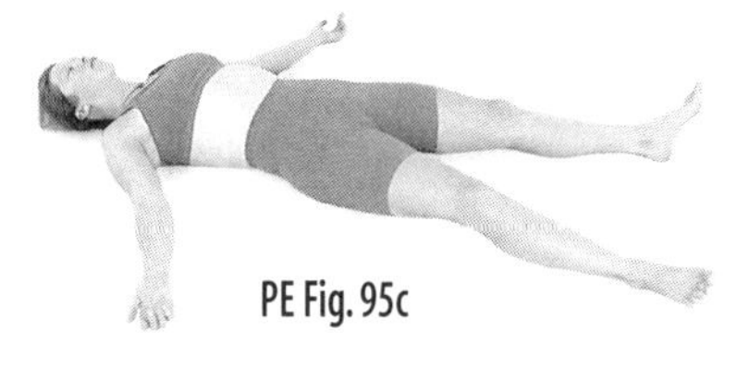

PE Fig. 95c

4. Switch your focus, and sense how flexion and extension affect the back of your spine. How is the quality of movement different from focusing on the front of the spine?
5. Now flex and extend with a focus on both the front and back to integrate the two.
6. Turn over to a prone position and explore steps 3 and 4 (PE Fig. 95d). Again, contrast moving with a focus on the front of the spine, then the back, then on both.

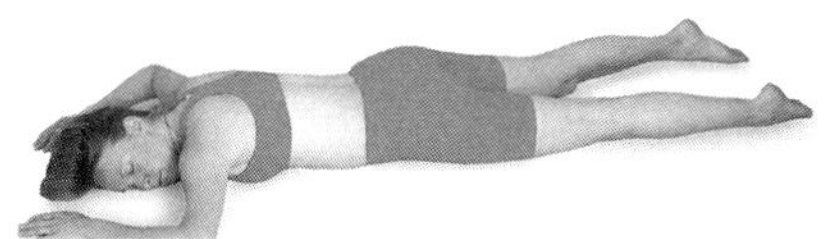

PE Fig. 95d

EMSPress.com

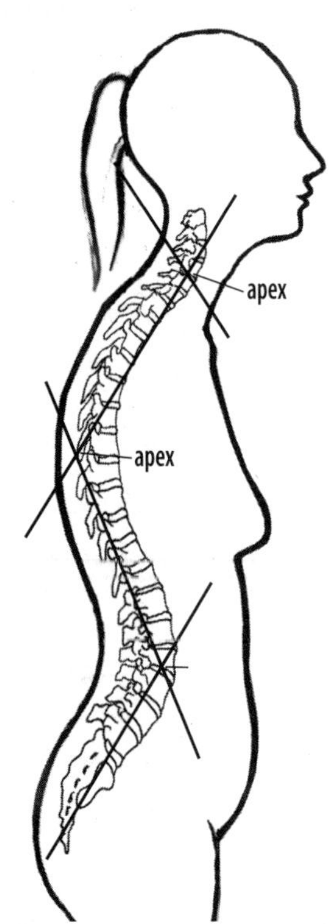

Figure 10.17 Common areas of instability in a kyphotic-lordotic "zig-zag" spine are at the apex of the curves.

most spinal holding patterns, it is common for facet joints in areas that lack mobility to become rigid while facet joints in hypermobile areas become unstable and bend. A dysfunctional facet is usually sore to palpate. If rigid, it can be mobilized with a pointed, intermittent pressure. The most common areas of instability occur in the middle of each curve, obvious in a crease in the back of the neck, a hunchback posture, or an excessive sway of the lower back (Figure 10.17).

The lumbar spine has minimal rotation when a person is sitting or standing in a neutral posture, but lumbar rotation increases fourfold during flexion because the facet joints glide open.[144] This makes the lumbar spine vulnerable to injuries from excessive rotation during flexion: a common lower-back injury occurs when a person lifts something heavy while bending over and twisting.

Integrating Spinal Movement through Arcing

During normal spinal flexion, the cervical and lumbar curves flatten, and the kyphotic curve in the thoracic spine increases (Figure 10.18a). During normal spinal hyperextension, the cervical and lumbar curves increase, and the thoracic curve flattens (Figure 10.18b).[145]

In what activities do you move your spine with an undulating quality?

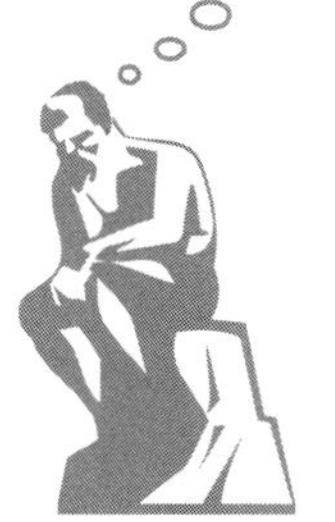

The segmented spine of a snake bends in smooth curves and arcs because each segment contributes its respective range to the overall motion. Likewise, if each segment in the human spine can move within its capacity, the overall range of motion will be greater and more congruent. Also, the spine will move like a single limb in a graceful curvilinear arc that is flexible yet connected. For the spine to move in an integrated arc, the five curves—head, neck, thorax, low back, and sacrum—must move in synchrony. If any segment or group of segments is rigid or unstable, the shape of the movement will lose its smooth arc, moving like a block at the rigid segments and bending like a hinge at the weak segments. By observing the shape of the spine during movement, the level of synchrony among the curves can be assessed. Breaks in the curves from compression, shearing, or bending forces will create a zig-zag shape.

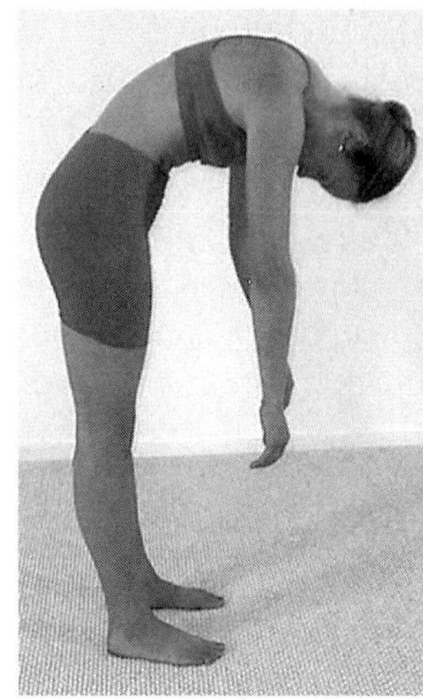

Figure 10.18a During normal spinal flexion, the lumbar and cervical curves flatten, and the thoracic curve increases.

To help a motion sequence through the entire spine, from one end to the other, it helps to initiate the movement at either the head or tail during patterning. If movement habitually initiates somewhere in between, it usually sequences in only one direction rather than through the entire spine. Recall the analogy of whipping a rope from Chapter 5. If a person holds the rope at the end, the whipping motion will travel through the whole rope. But if a person whips the rope from the middle, the sequence will be more erratic; the whipping motion will travel one direction or the other, but not along the entire rope.

To help a person learn how to flex and extend the whole spine in an integrated pattern, Judith Aston, the founder of Aston Patterning (see Chapter 12), created a patterning exercise called "arcing." **Arcing** coordinates the movement between the many spinal segments so that flexion and extension initiating in the head or tail sequences through each vertebra like the teeth of a well-oiled zipper. Arcing also establishes a relaxed neutral posture from which a person can move in any direction. It cultivates a fluidity, ease, and responsiveness in the spine so that even small movements ripple effortlessly from one end to the other.

To learn arcing, a person practices initiating flexion and extension at the head or tail, sequencing through each segment until the movement reaches the other end, bowing the whole column as one integrated limb. This is extremely helpful for people who tend to move one part of the spine against the rigidity of another, thereby blocking the flow of movement through the entire column and stressing hyperflexible segments.

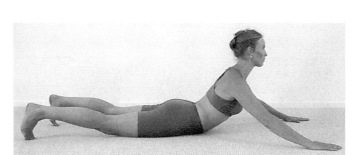

Figure 10.18b During normal spinal hyperextension, the lumbar and cervical curves increase, and the thoracic curve flattens.

Patterning Exercise #96: Arcing: Flexing and Extending the Spine

(This exercise is adapted from Rolfing Movement.) Read the entire exercise before practicing it. Better yet, have someone read it to you as you practice it. Explore arcing slowly at first, then speed it up to make the action more fluid and less controlled.

1. *Isolating flexion and extension at the tail:* Sit in a neutral posture on top of both your sit bones. Take several deep breaths. As you exhale, flex your tail and pelvic floor. To initiate spinal movement at the tail, put your fingertips on your coccyx for feedback. Then explore turning your tail under, then extending it to get a sense of isolating movement this low. (These will be very small movements.) Imagine rocking a hinge between your coccyx and sacrum, or imagine your tail reaching the floor and first pointing toward your heels, then toward the floor behind you.
2. *Flexing:* Begin in a neutral posture (PE Fig. 96a). Breathe in and out. As you exhale, begin flexion in your tail and pelvic floor and allow it to sequence through your entire spine, rounding you over in a C-curve shape (PE Fig. 96b). Make sure that your shoulders are over your hips and that your shoulders remain wide. Avoid folding your chest or rounding your shoulders. Take several deep breaths in the flexed position, letting weight sink through the back of your waist as you exhale.
3. *Extending:* Inhale and extend your tail. Allow the extension to sequence up the front of your spine as though you were unzipping a zipper. Feel the inhalation fill and lengthen your spine as you arc over backward (PE. Fig. 96c). Avoid collapsing anywhere along your spine. Keep your neck long and supported, as though an invisible hand were lifting the back of your head. Do not let your neck bend in the middle causing your head to drop behind you (PE Fig. 96d). Your head should be over your pelvis and entire spine extended in a graceful arc.
4. *Return to neutral:* As you exhale, relax your jaw; then bring the top of your head back to neutral (PE Fig. 96e). Then sequentially return your entire spine, moving one segment at a time from the head down, to your neutral starting position. Rest here and take several deep breaths. Your head should be balanced over the ribcage, and your ribcage balanced over your pelvis. You have just moved through one arcing cycle.
5. Repeat the arcing movement several times using a fluid, smooth motion. Sequentially bend each spinal segment one at a time. Also, use the support of your breath. Imagine your trunk as tubular balloon that fills and lifts as you inhale, drains and collapses as your exhale.

Feedback: Sit sideways to a mirror and watch yourself arc. Which segments of your spine do you tend to skip over and which segments are hypermobile? Focus on getting movement to sequence through rigid segments and to stabilize loose segments.

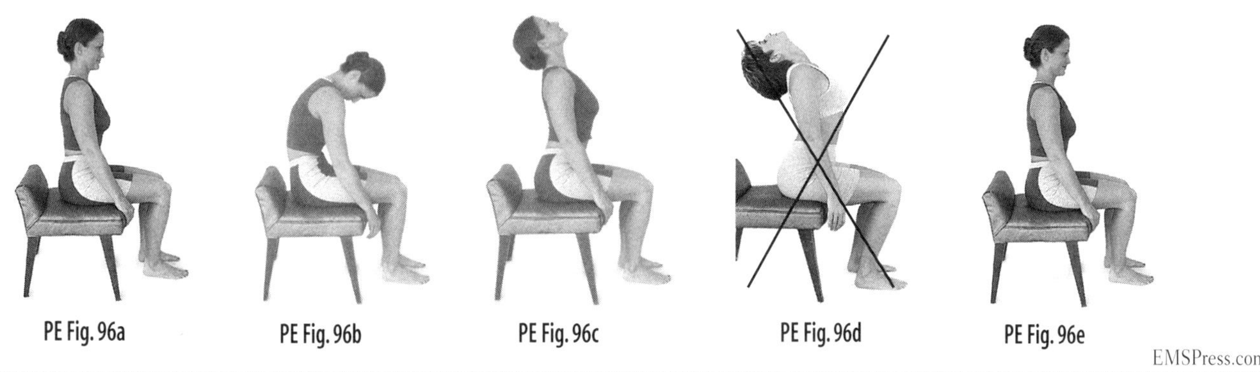

PE Fig. 96a PE Fig. 96b PE Fig. 96c PE Fig. 96d PE Fig. 96e

EMSPress.com

COMPARING UPPER AND LOWER LIMB MOVEMENT

How many times do you use a swinging motion in your arms during the course of your daily activities? During which activities?

The upper and lower limbs have similarities and differences in their structures that are important to consider when patterning them. Both the hips and shoulders have ball-and-socket joints called *proximal joints*, which allow them to rotate in all three planes and swing like pendulums. Whereas the legs swing under the body during walking or running, the arms swing at the sides. This may seem like an overly simplistic point, yet many imbalances occur when the legs swing or paddle off to the sides while walking. The same is true of the arms. They hang at the sides when a person is in a neutral posture. Yet chronic holding in the shoulder muscles can restrict the range of motion in the arms or pull them in front of or behind the sides of the body.

Although the arms and legs have many mechanical similarities, some major structural differences distinguish them from each other. The most obvious difference is that the arms are hanging structures suspended from the shoulders at our sides while the legs are buttressed columns of support beneath us. The arms generally move in an open kinematic chain, unless we use them to bear weight, to push, or to walk on our hands. The legs generally move as a closed kinematic chain against the external resistance of the floor. During locomotion,

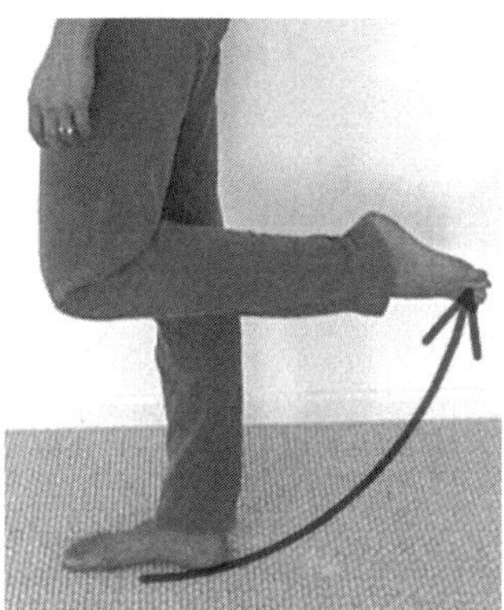

Figure 10.19a The knee flexes and extends primarily in the sagittal plane.

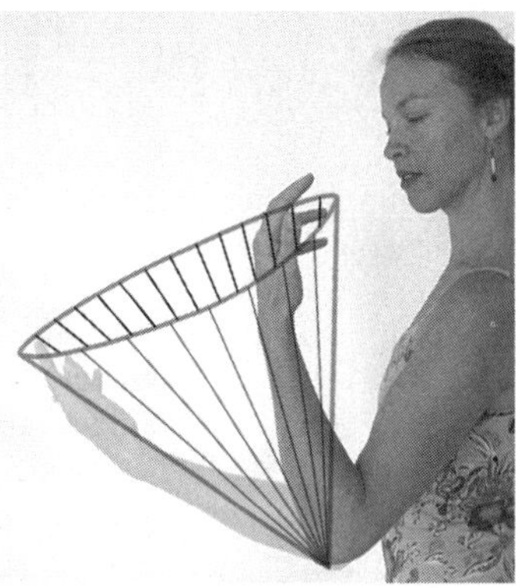

Figure 10.19b The elbow flexes and extends in a conical range made possible by rotation in the shoulder.

the legs alternate between open- and closed-chain functions, alternately bearing weight and swinging as a free limb.

A second difference is that the hip and knee flex in opposite directions of the same plane, whereas the elbow and shoulder flex in the same direction in the same plane. The angle of the knee closes behind the body during flexion whereas the angle of the elbow closes in front of and toward the body during flexion. Also, the knee flexes and extends primarily in one plane while the elbow can transcribe a circle in a wide conical range due to the rotational flexibility of the shoulder (Figure 10.19a-b).

A third difference is in the range of motion allowed by the shallowness of the shoulder socket and the depth of the hip socket. The hip socket covers three-fourths of the globe of the femur, restricting the range of rotation in the legs. Since the legs and hips evolved for weight-bearing, the depth of the socket makes the hip joint more stable than the shoulder joint. In contrast, the shoulder socket—made up of the *humerus* and *glenoid fossa* of the scapula and therefore called the *glenohumeral joint*—is shallow (being more like a saddle than a ball-and-socket joint), allowing the arms a much greater range of motion yet decreasing their stability. The hands can reach all around the body whereas our feet are restricted primarily to movement in front of, below, beside, and behind the body.

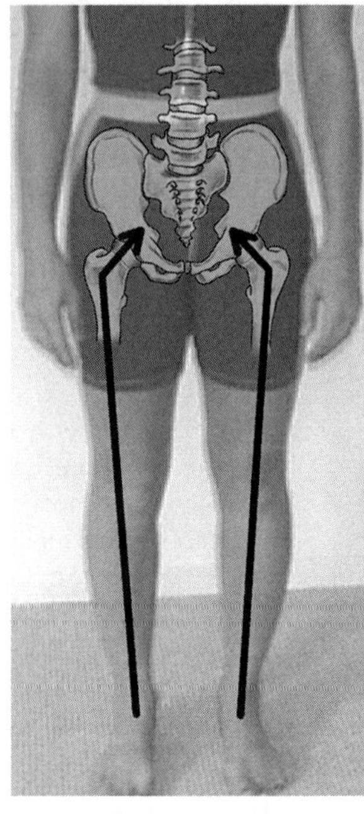

Figure 10.20 The line of thrust between the legs and the pelvis

The distance between the *coxofemoral joints*, two hip sockets, is approximately the distance from the fingers to the wrist. However, most people think of their hip sockets as being on the outsides of their thighs, though this is the

Patterning Exercise #97: Arm and Leg Swings

Caution: Swing your arms and legs only within a range that is comfortable to you. It is possible to hurt yourself by using too much effort and going beyond your range of motion.

1. Stand in a comfortable position with both feet firmly planted on the ground, one foot in front of the other.
2. *Arms:* Swing one arm forward and back like a pendulum, moving through a half arc. Increase the range and make a full circle (PE Fig. 97a-b). Then reverse directions. Repeat with the other arm.

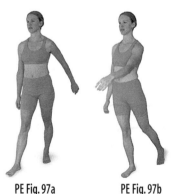

PE Fig. 97a

PE Fig. 97b

3. Now explore swinging both arms together in the same direction, then swinging them in opposition. Swing them with a free flow movement, like you were going to toss a ball. Feel weight in your hands as you move.
4. Explore swinging your arms across your body or around your head as though you were swinging a lasso.
5. *Legs:* Stand on one leg and swing the other leg back and forth in a free flowing movement (PE Fig. 97c-d). (You may need to hold onto a wall or doorknob to balance.) Use the swinging motion to loosen up your hip. Repeat on the other side.
6. Lie on your side and swing the top leg in an arc that goes in front of you and slightly behind you. Make sure to stabilize your spine when you swing your leg behind you to avoid hyperextending your lower back. Repeat on the other side.

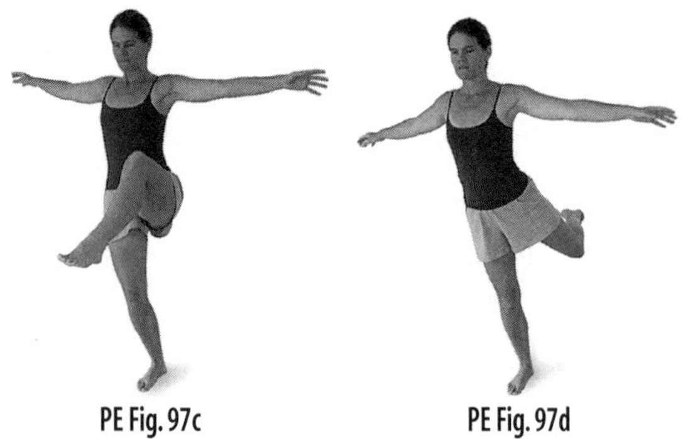

PE Fig. 97c

PE Fig. 97d

location of the *greater trochanter.* The narrow orientation of the hip sockets establishes a line of thrust from the legs into the hips that is close to midline and therefore more stable (Figure 10.20). In contrast, the width of the shoulder girdle orients the arms for a broad range of mobility, although the transfer of forces from the hands to the trunk is less stable.

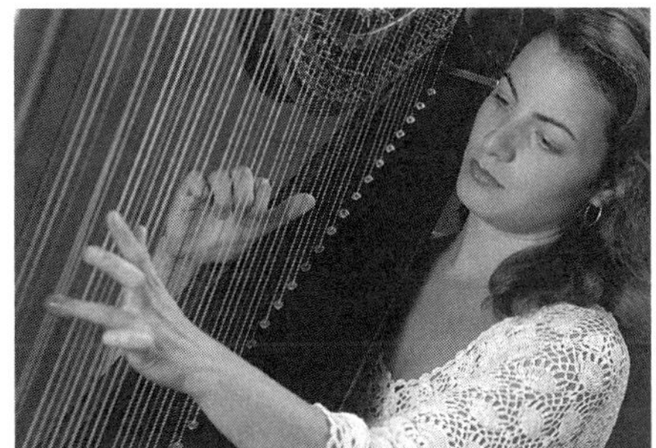

Figure 10.21 The refined dexterity of the hands

A similarity between the lower and upper limbs is that each limb moves in a coordinated ratio to the pelvis or shoulders. For example, bending over involves a coordinated action between flexion of the lumbar spine and flexion of the hips. Raising a leg also involves coordination between hip flexion and a posterior pelvic tilt, just as lifting an arm involves a coordinated movement between the arm and scapula. These coordinations, known respectively as the *lumbar-pelvic rhythm* and *scapulohumeral rhythm*, will both be described in detail later in the chapter.

Dexterity of the Upper Limbs

Observe any cat or dog throughout a day and it becomes obvious how these mammals navigate their worlds through the channels of smells and sounds. In comparison, the neuromotor programs of humans have evolved in the world of ideas through which we navigate via the primary channels of language and human expression. On a functional level, this translates into a large area of our motor cortex devoted to the hands, mouth, and tongue, the primary organs of human expression (see Figure 1.11). Consequently, the arms and shoulders function in subordination to the movement demands of the hands, whose diverse prehensile abilities evolved as a direct outgrowth of our uniquely human cortex.

The refined dexterity of the hands, made possible by opposable thumbs, allows for a seemingly boundless range of prehensile abilities, from the precise dexterity of a surgeon to the creative proficiency of a painter or musician (Figure 10.21). To carry out the broad repertoire of prehensile capacities in the hands, our shoulder girdles have evolved free of weight-bearing functions and are highly mobile in any direction.

In the first chapter, we discussed the paradox of the human movement potential and how our unique ability to be aware of awareness can actually impede our instinctive responses. On a parallel note, as the modern prehensile tasks of humans become more refined, the range of movement in the highly mobile arms narrows. A person working at a computer or drafting table all day is highly unlikely to go through the range of arm motion required of a carpenter or gardener. To counter this tendency, we need to take our arms and shoulders through a full range of motion on a regular basis.

Hand-Eye Coordination

Not only is a huge part of our motor cortex devoted to the fine motor control of the hands, it is also devoted to the movement of the mouth and eyes. In fact, the majority of the movements made with the hands involve some kind of hand-mouth or hand-eye coordination (see Chapter 7). Whenever we use our hands, we instinctively rotate the head and neck so that the eyes can track what the hands are doing. Eye tracking coordinates neuromotor pathways between the arms and torso. By watching the hands during arm movement, we not only strengthen the connection between the hands and eyes, but we pattern the movement of the upper spine as well.

Hand Movement

Arm movement initiated in the hand is much more articulate and refined than arm movement initiated in the shoulder. Compare lifting the arm from the shoulder muscles with lifting the arm by reaching through the fingers. The first movement will probably be more cumbersome because the small muscles of the hand are left out of the sequence.

The muscles of the hand have evolved for fine motor control, so they have fewer fibers per motor unit; some have as few as 50. In contrast, the large muscles of the shoulders have evolved to generate strong, large actions, and therefore have many more fibers per motor unit, as many as 1,000. Most functional movements of the arms initiate in the hands, sequencing from the smaller to larger muscles. (The same is true of the spine: most functional movements initiate in the head or tail, particularly in the sense organs of the eyes, nose, mouth and ears, as described in Chapter 5.) Therefore, to pattern functional shoulder movement that can be integrated into common daily activities, it helps to initiate the chain of action in the fingers.

The range of movement of hands and fingers is broad yet intricate. The movement of each finger triggers a slightly

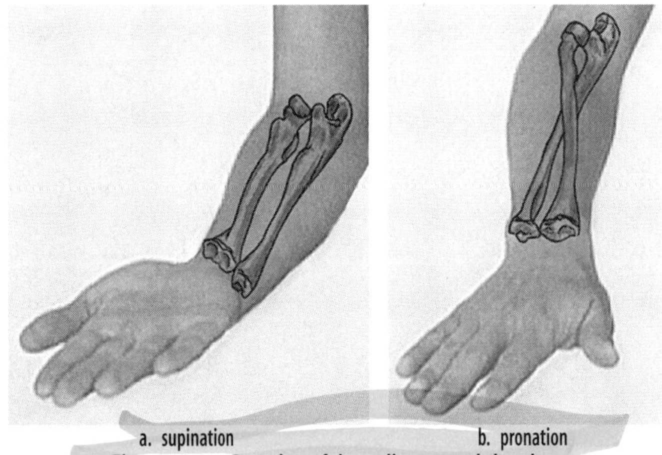

a. supination b. pronation

Figure 10.22 Rotation of the radius around the ulna

Patterning Exercise #98: Hand-eye Coordination

1. While sitting or standing, explore hand-eye coordination by slowly reaching your hand through various pathways in space around your body. Watch your hand on each point along the pathway of motion (PE Fig. 98a). Keep your elbow relaxed as you move. Imagine the elbow and shoulder as a hollow tunnel through which energy can flow between the body and the hand. Reach in front of, above, below, and behind yourself. Notice how your entire spine rotates to follow your hand as you watch it move behind you. Spend extra time moving through the areas where you lose the connection between your hand and eyes or feel the movement restricted by muscular tension.

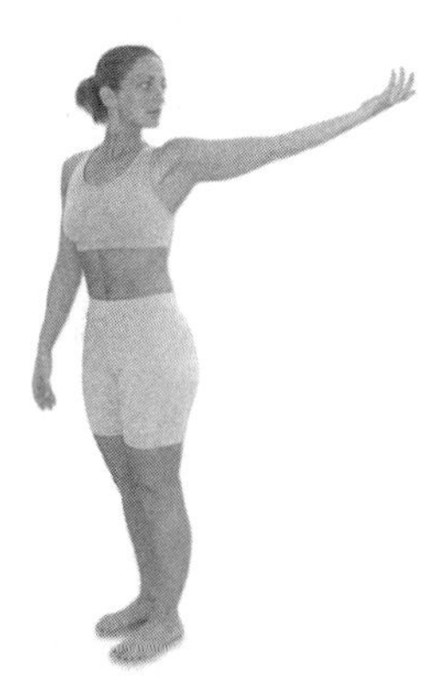

PE Fig. 98a

2. Lie on your back or your side and explore hand-eye coordination by drawing large circles around your body (PE Fig. 98b-c). Go both ways by reversing the circle. As you move, let the weight of your head and spine sink into the floor, even when you are on your side.

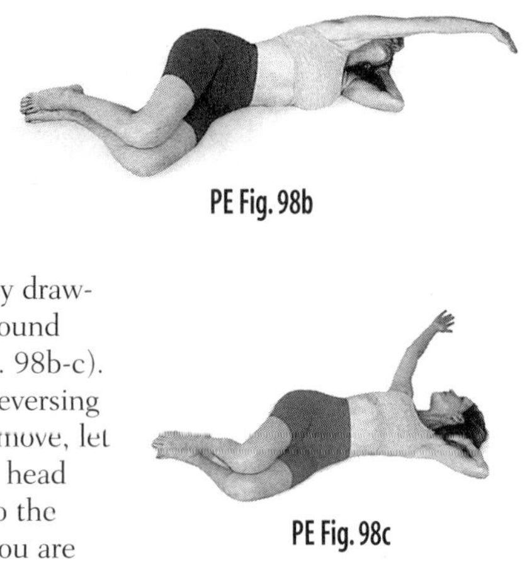

PE Fig. 98b

PE Fig. 98c

EMSPress.com

different movement sequence in the forearm. Each finger can flex, extend, abduct (spread the fingers apart), adduct (draw the fingers together), and *circumduct* (draw a circle). The ten fingers can move individually or together in a vast array of combinations. The hands can also supinate, turning the palms up, or pronate, turning the palms down, in rotations that twist the *radius* around the *ulna* (Figure 10.22). Since the wrists and shoulders have a range of motion similar to that of the fingers, the various combinations of this chain of joints can produce countless gestures and prehensile patterns.

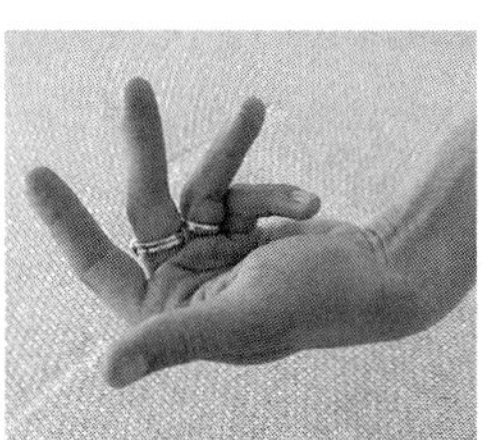

Figure 10.23 A progressive fanning of the fingers

A progressive fanning of the fingers can initiate a full range of rotation in the arm (Figure 10.23). The movement of each finger sequences along a specific pathway into the arm and shoulder. Thumb movement sequences along the inside of the arm into the front of the shoulder, middle finger movement through the center of the arm into the shoulder socket, and little finger movement along the outside of the arm into the scapula. Movement initiated by the subtle articulations of the fingers not only brings more articulation and refinement to the range of the arms, but it also gives them an expressive quality. Consider the sweeping arm gestures of an orator, the Shiva-like twists and turns of an East Indian dancer, or the spirals and swirls a conductor's hands carve in space. Also, the limb rotations that gymnasts initiate in the subtle articulations of the fingers and toes produce powerful yet precise connections into the trunk (Figure 10.24).

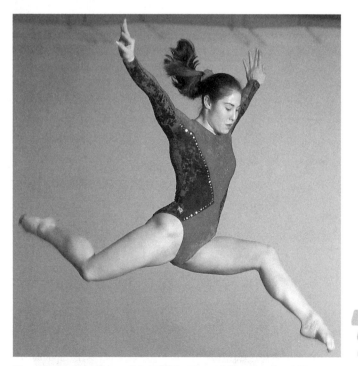

Figure 10.24 Note the precision of this gymnast's fingers and toes.

The Shoulder Girdle

As discussed in Chapter 9, the shoulder girdle—made up of the clavicles, scapulae, and arms—sits like a yoke on top of the rib cage. The entire girdle has only one joint that attaches it

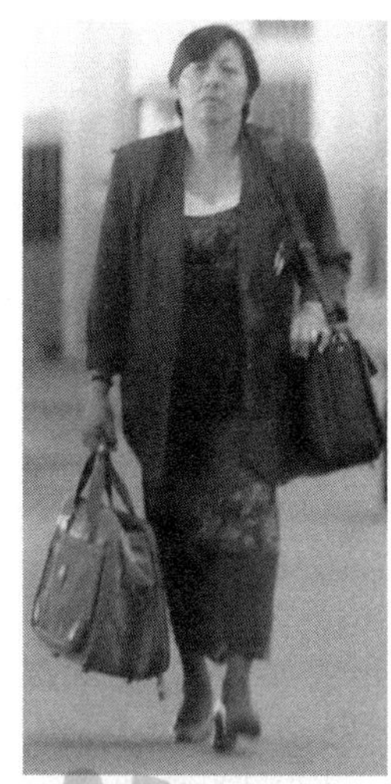

Figure 10.25 The shoulder yoke transfers weight from the arms to the spine.

Patterning Exercise #99: Initiating Arm Movement with the Fingers

Movement initiated by different fingers sequence into the shoulder along slightly different pathways.

1. Initiate arm rotations with your hands by carving a figure-eight shape leading with the thumb side of your hands (PE Fig. 99a). Sense how the movement of your hand sequences from the thumbs along the top of the arms and shoulders.

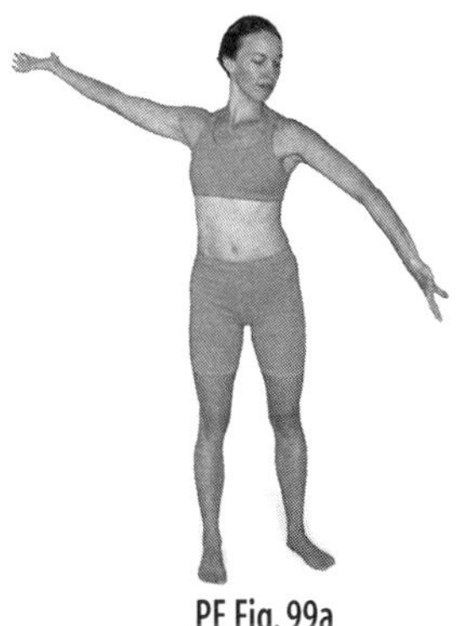

PE Fig. 99a

2. Now carve figure-eight shapes leading with the little finger side of your hands (PE Fig. 99b). Sense how the movement sequences from your little fingers along the underside of the arms and shoulders.

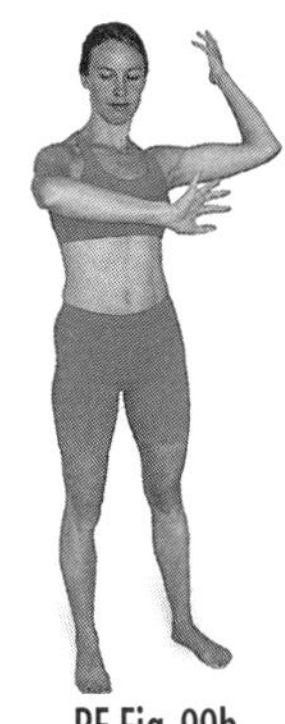

PE Fig. 99b

EMSPress.com

Links to Practical Applications

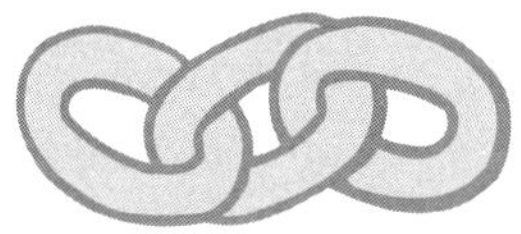

Observing Shoulder Patterns

Go to a park, mall, or airport to watch people walking or running. Notice how freely their arms swing. When you notice the natural swing is restricted, what restricts the motion? Where are the shoulder muscles chronically contracted? Also, notice if their arms hang beside, in front of, or behind the body, or if the shoulders are elevated or depressed. This will give you a clue about where the muscles are chronically held.

to the axial skeleton—the small sternoclavicular joint between the clavicles and the sternum. All one joint that attaches it to the axial skeleton— the small *sternoclavicular joint* between the clavicles and the sternum. All other attachments come from the tensional support of numerous shoulder muscles, tendons, and ligaments that secure the arms to the trunk. This highly mobile girdle is also suspended from numerous neck muscles.

The weight of the arms creates a horizontal tension across the girdle that balances the yoke in a manner comparable to the way a coat balances on a hanger. Arm weight pulls the lateral ends of the clavicles down while levering their medial ends up. In the same manner that a yoke allows weight carried on the shoulders to be borne through the trunk, the shoulder girdle converts the side load of the arms into a top load carried by the sternum, ribs, and spine (Figure 10.25).

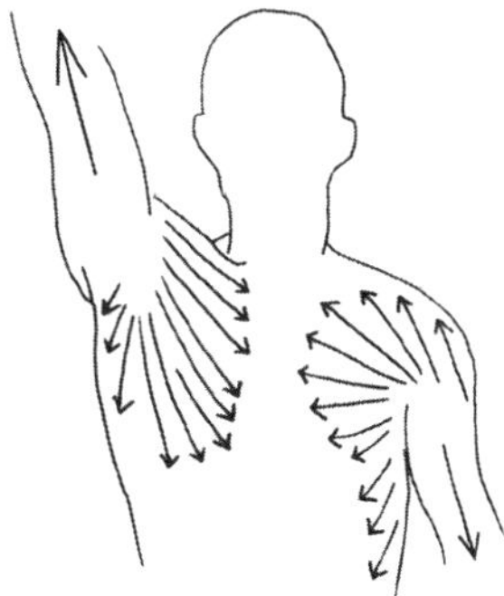

Figure 10.26 Tensional pulls on the arm from shoulder muscles

The strength and stability of the highly mobile glenohumeral joint are secured by the combination of a strong joint capsule and the tendons from which the arms literally hang. The tensional pulls of the rotator cuff muscles and tendons—the *infraspinatus, subscapularis, supraspinatus,* and *teres minor muscles*—when balanced, are arranged with the symmetry of the spokes of a wheel (Figure 10.26). As a group, their tendons seat the humerus in the center of the socket and reinforce the joint capsule (see Figure 9.18). The muscles around the shoulder could be compared to tensional reins on a circular harness; they work in coupled pairs to move the scapulae and upper arms. For example, the serratus anterior and trapezius muscles work together to rotate the scapula, one pulling down while the other pulls up at the opposite corner (see Figure 9.18). Likewise, the infraspinatus muscle attaches to the back of the scapula and glenohumeral joint and externally rotates the humerus. Its antagonist, the subscapularis muscle, attaches to the front of the scapula and glenohumeral joint and internally rotates the scapula.

The way the arms are held or hang affects the transmission of pushing or pulling forces from the arms into the body. Ideally, lines of force transfer through the center of the arms into the shoulders and down the spine, but this occurs only when the yoke is balanced and symmetrical. If a person hikes the shoulders, the forces will travel into the neck, tightening and stressing the cervical spine (Figure 10.27). Many holding patterns of the shoulder girdle interfere with the natural swinging motion of the arms during walking or running by pulling the yoke off its optimal balance. If the shoulders are twisted, movement of the arms can also chronically twist the lower cervical or upper thoracic vertebrae. If the shoulders do hike, retract, or slump, the delicate balance of the yoke is disturbed.

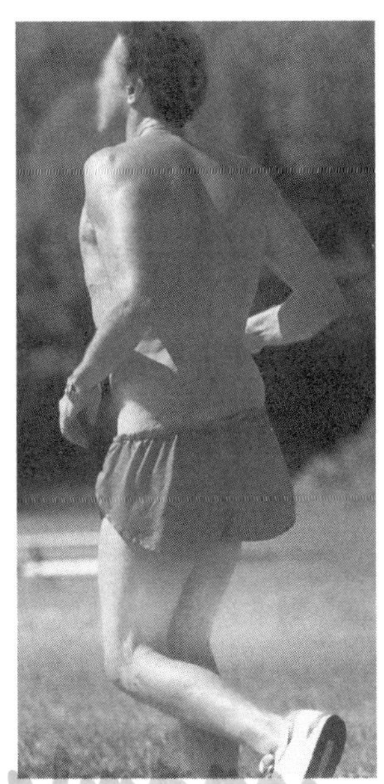

Figure 10.27 Hiked shoulders and held elbows compress the neck and inhibit the arm swing.

Rotation and Circumduction

The remarkably broad range of arm motion is made possible by the combined range of movement in the many joints linking the fingers to the shoulder. Each of the fingers, the wrist, and the shoulder move within a range of **circumduction,** a motion that describes a cone (see Figure 10.19b). The wrist moves in circumduction during a stirring motion whose circumference can be enlarged with the addition of the hinge-like flexion and extension range of the elbow. Flexion of the elbow allows the arm to fold so that the hand can touch the face.

Pathways of circumduction are as numerous as the locations the hand can reach in the space around the body. During circumduction of the shoulder, the hand moves in a large circle around the body like the pencil of a compass with the shoulder socket functioning much like the point of the compass (Figure 10.28). The shallow ball-and-socket of the glenohumeral joint allows the arms to circumduct in all planes, from winding up a baseball pitch (sagittal plane) to circling a lasso overhead (horizontal plane) or drawing a large circle on a wall (frontal plane).

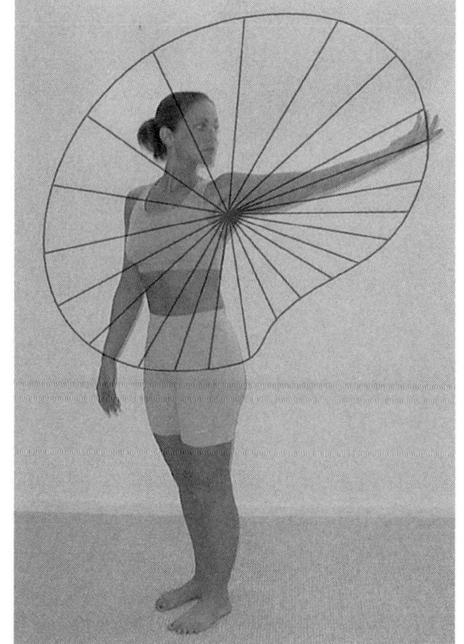

Figure 10.28 The range of arm circumduction

In her Movement Fundamentals, Bartenieff refined the coordination between the forearm and upper arm during circumduction using her concept of **gradation with rotation.**[146] During the "arm circle" (one of the six Bartenieff Fundamentals), both the rotation of the shoulder and the elbow are gradated or spread out over the entire circumference of circumduction. By gradating the internal and external rotation of the arm, the ball of the humerus turns smoothly and

Patterning Exercise #100: Arm Rotations and Circumduction

(Adapted from Bartenieff's arm circle.)

1. *Differentiating rotation of the upper and lower arm:* Lie on your back with your hands resting about one foot from your hips. Rotate just your lower arm by turning your palm up and down while keeping your upper arm stationary. Then, without rotating your lower arm, rotate just at the shoulder socket, turning your upper arm back and forth like a rolling pin.
2. *Circumduction:* While sitting or standing, draw a large circle around you from one side to the other with one arm. Reach through your fingertips to take the slack out of your arm as you move (PE Fig. 100a-c). Watch your hand during the entire circumference of the circle to coordinate the arm, head, and neck rotation. Do a series of arm circles in one direction, then reverse the motion. Feel the movement of these rotations pulling through your waist.

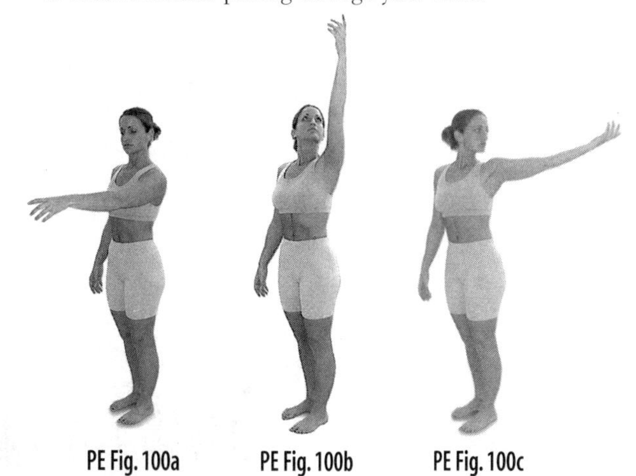

PE Fig. 100a PE Fig. 100b PE Fig. 100c

Pointers: Keep the circumference of the circle you draw round and even. Avoid jerky movement. Avoid flipping your hand over by gradually turning your palm up (supinating it) during one-half of the circle, and gradually turning it down (pronating it) during the other half of the circle. Also, keep your elbow slightly bent to avoid locking it.

3. Repeat with the other arm.
4. Lie on the floor on your back. Draw a large circle on the floor around your body with your hand. Relax the weight of your back into the floor as you move. Move in both directions, then switch arms. You'll be unable to see your hand when it's moving over your head, but still keep it in your peripheral vision. Feel the movement of your arm stretching down to your lower body (PE Fig. 100d).

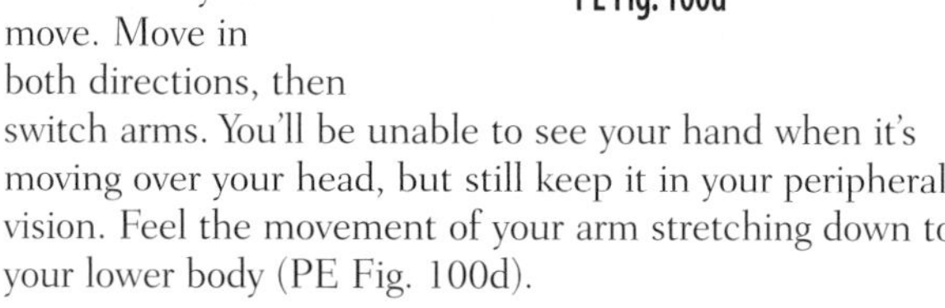

PE Fig. 100d

5. Now lie on your side. Draw an arm circle on the floor around you. Be sure to watch your hand along the entire pathway of movement although there will be places over your head and behind you where you will not be able to see it. Go in both directions.
6. Then roll over and repeat on the other side with your other arm.

evenly in the socket, being pulled along by shoulder and arm muscles that fire in an orderly consecutive sequence. Without gradation, the movement might be jerky, the hand might suddenly flip, or the elbow might become locked and stiff. Conversely, circumducting the arms with a hyperextended and locked elbow will limit gradation with rotation.

Bartenieff also used spatial intent to elicit the expressive movements of the arm with finely gradated rotations, encouraging students to carve and shape the space around them by scooping then scattering imaginary sand. She stressed the importance of carving a round circle in the space around the body and of an upper-lower body connection during arm circles by allowing arm rotation to pull through the *oblique muscles* of the waist along a changing series of diagonal pathways (see Figure 8.38). Also, each finger leads during various parts of the movement to access the subtle articulations initiated in the more refined and expressive movement of the hands. During one part of the circle, a person leads the rotation with the thumb, then leads by reaching through the central axis of the middle finger, then twists the arms in the opposite direction by leading with the little finger.

The Scapulohumeral Rhythm

The ratio of movement between the humerus and scapula is called the **scapulohumeral rhythm**.[147] The scapula remains stable as a supporting base for the humerus during the first part of an arm movement. Recall from Chapter 9 that the neutral position of the scapula is maintained by the tonic contractions of stabilizer muscles. Once the humerus reaches a certain range of motion, the scapula begins to move, distributing movement proportionally between the humerus and scapula at about a two-to-one ratio (Figure 10.29).

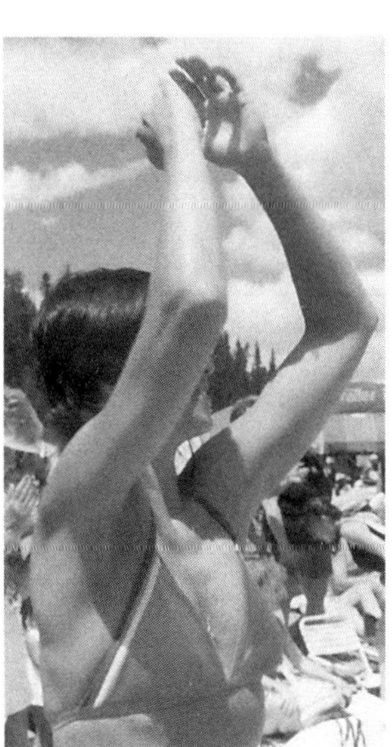

Figure 10.29 The scapulaw moves with the arm when the arm is above horizontal (photo courtesy of L. Bright).

For approximately every 2-degrees of arm movement, the scapula moves 1-degree. For example, if the arm is raised beside the body in abduction, the humerus moves without the scapula during the first 60-degrees. Above this point, the scapula begins to externally rotate and glide across the ribs. Likewise, when the arm is raised in front of the body in flexion, the scapula remains stable until the arm reaches the height of the shoulder. Above that point, the scapula externally rotates and moves 1-degree for every 2-degrees of arm motion (Figure 10.30). This two-to-one ratio is approximate and not exactly true for every motion. At the upper range of the movement when the arm is overhead, the humerus and scapula rotate at a more even ratio.

The space between the scapulae and ribcage, where the shoulder blade glides over the ribs, is considered a functional joint called the *scapulothoracic joint*. The distribution of motion between the glenohumeral joint and the scapulothoracic joint in the scapulohumeral rhythm increases the range of shoulder motion. The scapulohumeral rhythm also helps maintain the glenohumeral joint in an optimal position to reduce excessive shearing and ensures that the shoulder muscles work within their ideal range. Conversely, if either the glenohumeral joint or the scapulothoracic joint are restricted, the other joint will compensate by becoming hypermobile and even unstable.

To feel the scapulohumeral rhythm, a person can stand against a wall, using the wall for feedback from the scapular motion, and slowly raise the arms in front of the body. The scapulae should remain stationary until the arms reach shoulder height. As the arms continue rising and

Links to
Practical Applications

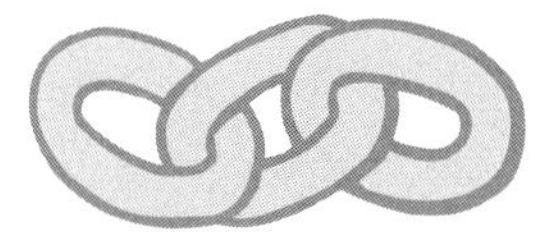

Letting Hiked Shoulders Hang

Since the shoulders are a hanging structure, if you tend to habitually hike your shoulders and then suddenly start to relax them, the weight of your arms will begin to stretch the myofascias of your neck and shoulders, which may cause discomfort. It may take days or even weeks for these soft tissues to completely stretch and normalize, so don't be alarmed by the discomfort the stretch creates. It is only temporary because eventually your tissues will reach their optimum resting length. In the meantime, just let your shoulders relax and your muscles will gradually readjust.

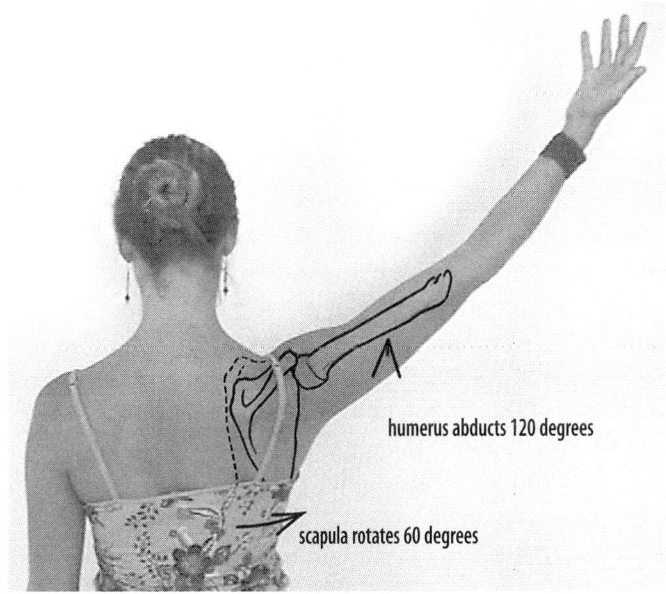

Figure 10.30 Schematic of the scapulohumeral rhythm in a 2-to-1 ratio

Patterning Exercise #101: Scapulohumeral Rhythm

To find the scapulohumeral rhythm, you need to begin with both scapulae in the ideal neutral position. To find this position, see Patterning Exercises #89 and #90.

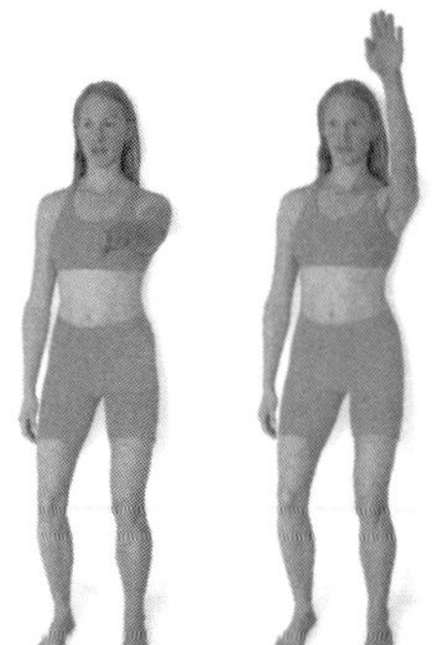

PE Fig. 101a PE Fig. 101b

1. Have a partner stand behind you and place her hands on both of your scapulae to give you feedback about when, during arm motion, the scapulae move. If you do not have a partner, stand against a wall or lie on the floor, using the pressure of your scapulae against the wall or floor for feedback.
2. *Arm flexion and extension:* Slowly raise your arm in front of your body. At what point does your scapula move? Movement at 90-degrees is normal. Lower your arm to the side.
3. This time keep your scapula stable as you slowly raise your arm in front of the body to shoulder height (PE Fig. 101a). Then continue raising your arm overhead while allowing your scapula move (PE Fig. 101b).
4. Return to your starting position by reversing the motion, slowly lowering your arm to shoulder height while allowing your scapula to return to neutral. Then stabilize your scapula as you lower your arm to your side.
5. *Abduction and adduction:* Stand against a wall so that you can feel your scapula move along the wall. Slowly raise your arm to the side (PE Fig. 101c). At what point does your scapula move? Movement at 60-degrees is normal. Lower your arm.
6. This time keep your scapula stabilized while you slowly raise your arm out to the side to about chest height. After this point, allow your scapula to externally rotate as you continue raising your arm overhead (PE Fig. 101d).
7. Return to your starting position by reversing the movement, lowering your arm to breast height while returning your scapula to its ideal neutral position. Then stabilize your scapula as you lower your arm.
8. Repeat steps 2 to 8 with both arms moving together.

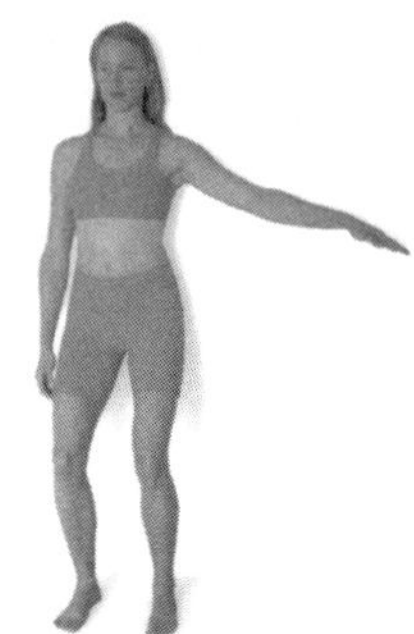

PE Fig. 101c

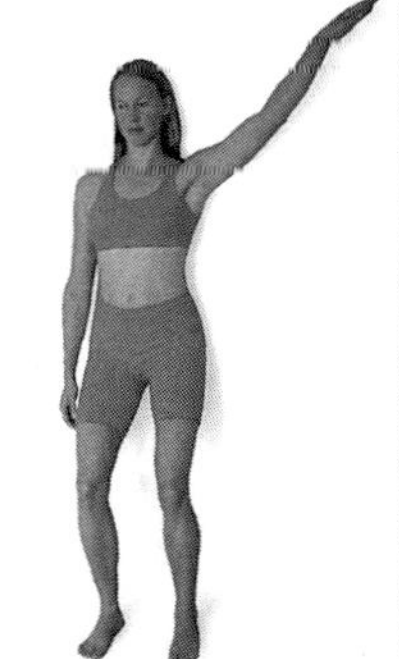

PE Fig. 101d

EMSPress.com

the hands move toward the ceiling, the scapulae adduct, elevate slightly, and upwardly rotate. When the movement is reversed, the rhythm reverses. The scapulae rotate back to neutral as the hands are lowered to shoulder height, after which point they remain stationary while the arms are lowered. The same description applies if the arms are raised to the sides, only now the scapulae begin rotating when the arms have reached 60 degrees.

Movement of the scapulae is a combination of abduction or adduction, during which each scapula slides sideways in a horizontal orientation, plus slight elevation or depression with upward or downward rotation. Ideally, the horizontal range of the scapula is stronger than the vertical range so that the forces of movement generated by the arms can sequence from the scapulae into the thoracic spine rather than up into the neck. To avoid elevating the shoulder girdle when reaching overhead, the arm needs to externally rotate so that the *greater tubercle* on the humerus (a small bony knob that provides an attachment site for muscles) can clear the *acromion process* (Figures 10.31a-b).

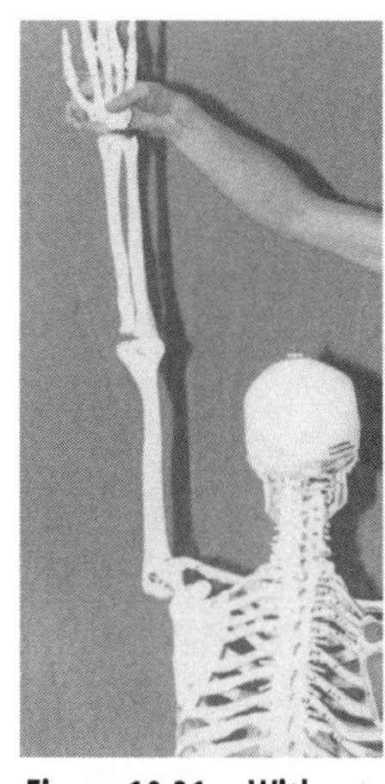

Figure 10.31a Without rotation, the arm elevates the shoulder.

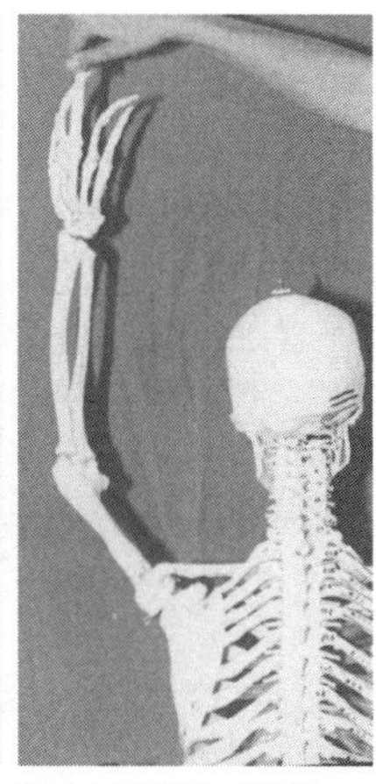

Figure 10.31b With rotation, the shoulder girdle remains stable.

Several conditions restrict the scapulohumeral rhythm, thereby limiting the range of motion in the shoulder. These include myofascial adhesions that limit rotation, instability in the scapulae that results in premature motion, and disturbances in the neutral position of the scapula from chronic and habitual postural deviations. Also, movement restrictions in the glenohumeral joint may occur due to faulty postures such as chronically rounded, elevated, or retracted shoulders; joint stiffness and rigidity; or instability in the joint. Short of structural or neurological damage, muscular imbalances and poor coordination usually cause these problems, both conditions that can be improved with patterning exercises.

The Pelvis

The pelvis is a bony basin often compared to a bowl-like container for the lower abdominal organs. It transfers weight and the forces of movement between the body and the legs, and provides sockets for the hip joints. As mentioned in Chapter 8, the pelvis has similar architectural features to a buttressed arch made up of five stones. The legs buttress into the pelvic bones, which in turn buttress into the sacrum, the

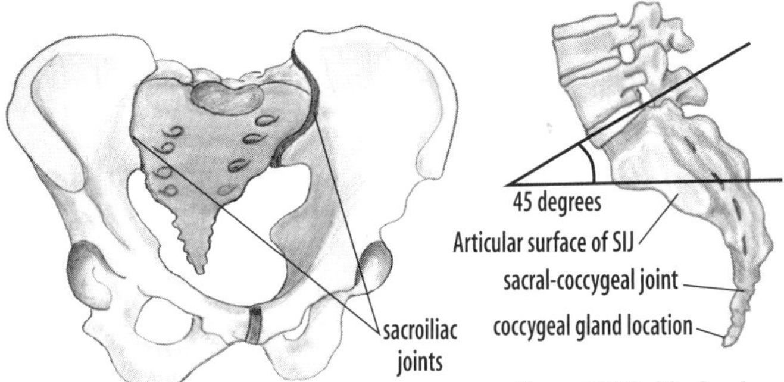

Figure 10.32 The sacroiliac joints (SIJ's)

Figure 10.33 The lumbosacral junction

keystone of the arch. The sacrum is wedged in between the two pelvic halves at the *sacroiliac joints (SIJs)*, two unusual joints that kinesiologists have trouble classifying because of a long-standing debate about their range of movement (Figure 10.32). It is generally agreed that these kidney-shaped joints are semi-movable and considered part synovial, part fibrous.

To visualize this wedged structure, imagine a book with a wide spine opening at a 45-degree angle on each side. The spine of the book is analogous to the sacrum, the front and back covers analogous to the two hips. As the book closes, its covers press in on the sacrum in a self-locking system of force closure. In the same way that the spine of a book can become sprung when opened too far, the hips can also flare out if the SI joints are too loose, a problem usually associated with joint instability and weak lower abdominal muscle control.

The pelvis articulates with the spine at the *lumbosacral junction*, the joint between the fifth lumbar vertebra and the top of the sacrum (Figure 10.33). This joint is highly vulnerable because it bears the bulk of the body's weight at a 45-degree angle. Its disc is wedge-shaped in contrast to the other lumbar discs, which have parallel surfaces. Also, 75 percent of lumbar spine flexion occurs at this segment, a range that will be revisited in the discussion on the lumbar-pelvic rhythm.[148]

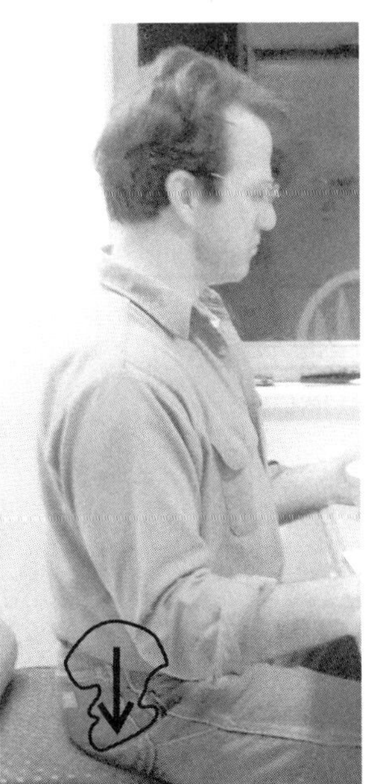

Figure 10.34 Sitting on top of the sit bones

The bony protuberances at the bottom of the pelvis, the *ischial tuberosities*, are better known by their slang name as the "sit bones," referring to the bony protuberances upon which we sit. The sit bones provide a base of support for sitting. The same way that we need feet under us for optimal support while standing, we need our sit bones directly under us for optimal support while sitting (Figure 10.34). If a person sits with the body's weight too far behind the sit bones, this posture will compress the sacroiliac joints and lumbar spine as well as compress vital nerves and organs. If the body's weight rests too far in front of the sit bones, the lumbar spine will tend to hyperextend, the erector spinae muscles along the spine will overwork, and the abdominal viscera may even spill forward.

Links to Practical Applications

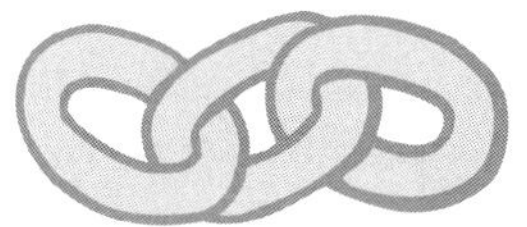

Finding Support while Sitting

Your sit bones are like feet when you are sitting because they provide a base of support. To feel the place where your body is directly over them, rock back and forth on them and sense where your body feels centered on them. During the course of your day, reestablish your awareness of their support by rocking on them.

Movement of the Sacrum and Pelvis

The sacrum, derived from the word "sacred," is actually five individual bones at birth that eventually fuse into one. The top of the sacrum provides a base of support for the spine and is wider than the bottom. Its triangular shape makes a natural keystone for a three-point intersection that transmits ground reaction forces from the legs into the pelvis and spine, and transmits weight from the spine through the pelvis into the legs (see Figure 8.9). The SI joints allow the sacrum a few degrees of flexion and extension in a nodding motion called *nutation* and *counter-nutation*. This range allows about 3-degrees of give in the SI joints during subtle anterior and posterior pelvic tilts that occur with hip flexion and extension.

The sacrum tapers to a point in a remnant of a vestigial tail called the *coccyx*—a tiny bone made up of approximately three to five fused vertebrae. Since the coccyx hangs from the sacrum like a plumb bob, it can be used like a "rudder" on the bottom of the spine to direct movements such as reach with the tail, pelvic tilts, and pelvic rotations.

The pelvic bones tilt on the legs during many actions. If the pelvis is visualized as a bowl of water, an **anterior**

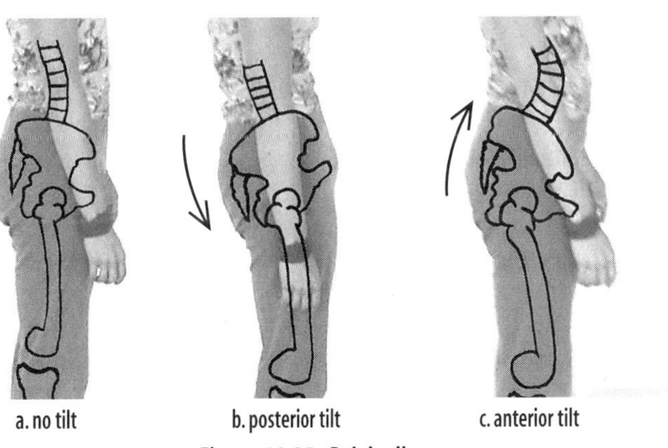

Figure 10.35 Pelvic tilts

tilt spills water out the front, while a **posterior tilt** spills water out the back (Figure 10.35a-c). When a seated person reaches across a table, the body rocks forward over the sit bones in an anterior tilt; when that person leans back, the body rocks backward over the sit bones in a posterior tilt.

Sometimes a person will chronically tilt the pelvis in a habitual posture, either tucking in a posterior tilt, or tipping the top of the pelvis forward in an anterior tilt. Recall from earlier discussions that when a person is aligned chronically off-center, the off-center posture will eventually begin to feel normal. Because of this perceptual distortion, a person stuck in a tucked position will feel as though he is sticking his behind out quite far when he tips it the other way. Likewise, a person stuck in an anterior tilt will feel as though she is tucking quite far when she tips it under to a level position.

A pelvic tilt takes the pelvic girdle into an anterior and posterior rotations in the sagittal plane. The pelvis also moves in **forward rotation** and **backward rotation** when one hip shifts forward while the other hip simultaneously shifts back. If the pelvis is compared to a bowl, rotation turns the bowl in the horizontal plane.

The pelvis can also rotate laterally in a small range. **Lateral rotation** spills water out the sides of the pelvic bowl; it occurs in the frontal plane as one hip is hiked. By clarifying the range of motion in the pelvis, a person can find the pelvis's ideal neutral balance and can increase coordination and control of movement in the pelvis.

The Coccyx and Pelvic Floor

Strong athletic movements usually involve action coordinated between the legs and the torso through the perineal muscles, also called the pelvic floor (Figure 10.36a-b). The pubic bone, coccyx, and sit bones border the diamond-shaped pelvic floor. They provide bony attachment sites for the perineal muscles that span the bottom of the pelvis like a muscular hammock, providing a base upon which the abdominal organs sit. Although associations with the perineum are often limited to sexual or bathroom functions, this muscular

Patterning Exercise #102: Pelvic Tilts and Lifts

1. *Pelvic tilt:* Lie on your back with both knees bent and feet parallel (PE Fig. 102a). Tilt your pelvis by turning your tail toward the back of your knees. Keep your torso on the ground and your spine long. To elongate your spine, reach through the top of your head as you tilt your pelvis. Keep tilting, gently pressing the back of your hips and waist into the ground, tipping your abdominal viscera from the bottom of your pelvic bowl into the back of your waist (PE Fig. 102b). Your lower abdomen should sink into your lower back and be hollowed out. Avoid bulging your abdomen or squeezing your buttocks together.

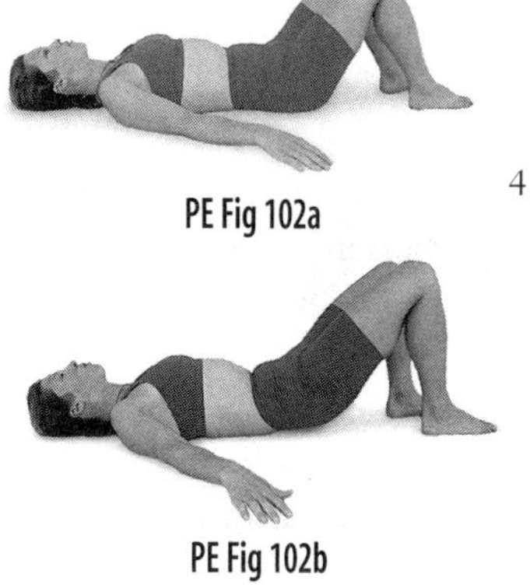

PE Fig 102a

PE Fig 102b

2. Hold the tilted position and breathe gently into your diaphragm, expanding your lower ribs on each inhalation and feeling weight sink into your back on each exhalation.

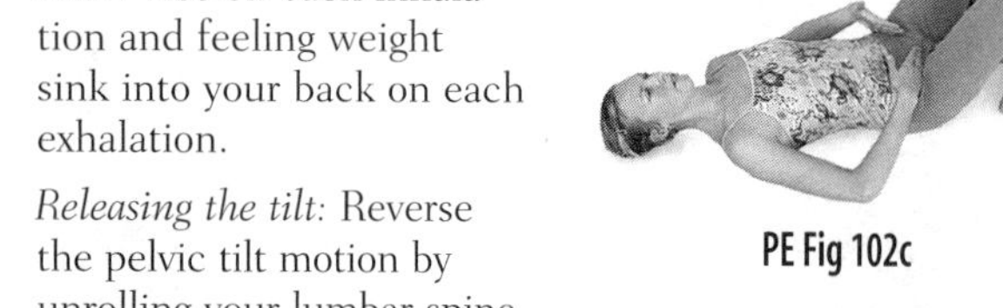

PE Fig 102c

3. *Releasing the tilt:* Reverse the pelvic tilt motion by unrolling your lumbar spine, sacrum, and coccyx toward your feet. (If you have an exaggerated lumbar curve, to correct it keep your lower back close to the floor as you release the tilt.) As you release the tilt, your pubic bone should move toward your heels, allowing weight to roll from your lower back toward your tail. Focus on sinking into the *inguinal crease* in the front of your hip sockets (PE Fig. 102c).

4. *Tilting while standing against a wall:* Stand with your back against a wall and your knees slightly bent. Reach through the top of your head to elongate your spine. Then tilt your pelvis and press your lumbar spine into the wall, again using the least amount of effort possible. Hold and take several deep breaths, then release.

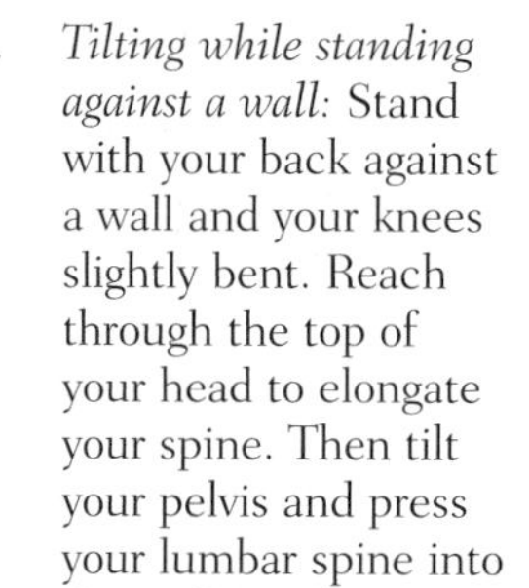

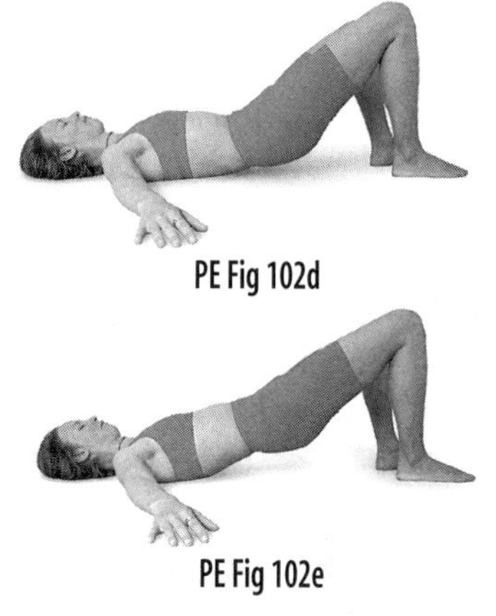

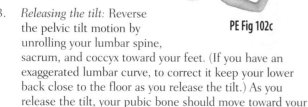

PE Fig 102d

PE Fig 102e

5. *Pelvic lift:* Lie on the floor again with both knees bent, legs parallel. Imagine your spine from tail to head like a string of 32 pearls (7 in the sacrum and coccyx). Slowly peel one pearl at time off the floor, starting at your tail (point your tail toward the back of your knees), then your sacrum and lumbar spine (PE Fig. 102d). Your body weight should be resting between your feet and the back of your lower ribs (PE Fig. 102e). Keep your upper body wide and your neck long yet naturally curved.

6. *Releasing the pelvic lift:* Now reverse the action by placing one segment or pearl on the floor at a time. Your weight will sink from your lower ribs through your lumbar spine, sacrum, and into your tail and hips. End with weight resting in both hips sockets, lengthening your sit bones toward your feet, without letting your lumbar spine hyperextend (the lumbars will come off the floor a little bit because of its natural lordotic curve).

Patterning Exercise #103: Pelvic Rotations

1. Place your hands on your hips while you look at yourself in a full-length mirror. Are your hips level and symmetrical? Rotate your pelvis several times forward and backward, then in an anterior and posterior tilt, then alternate hiking your right and your left hip (which will take your pelvis into lateral rotation). Keep your hands on your hips to monitor symmetry. Are your hips symmetrical as you move? In which direction do they have greater range?

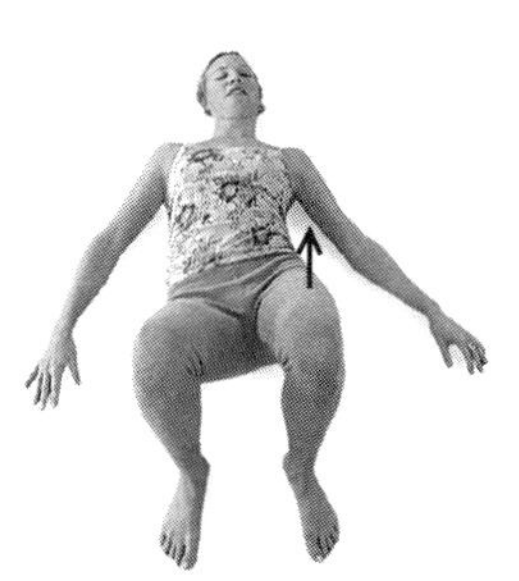

PE Fig. 103a

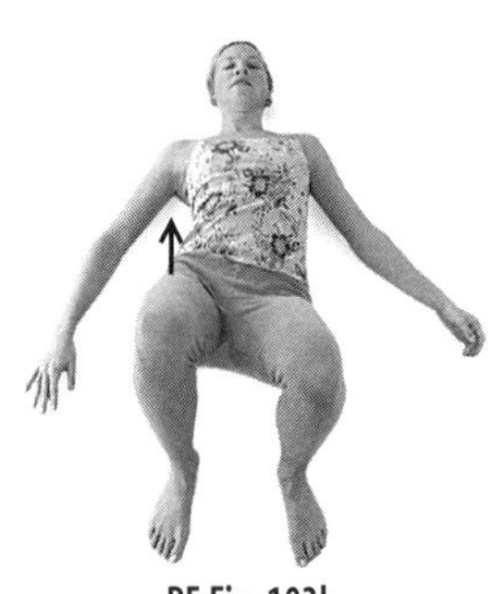

PE Fig. 103b

2. *Lateral rotation:* Lie on your back. (You might put your hands on your hips to monitor symmetry in your pelvis as you move.) Without twisting your hips or raising one side toward the ceiling, hike one hip by pulling that hip straight up toward the shoulder on the same side (PE Fig. 103a). This will be a small movement. Then lower it back to neutral. Repeat on the other side (PE Fig. 103b). Can you do this without lifting your pelvis? Does one side hike higher than the other? Alternate sides until they feel even and you can control the action.

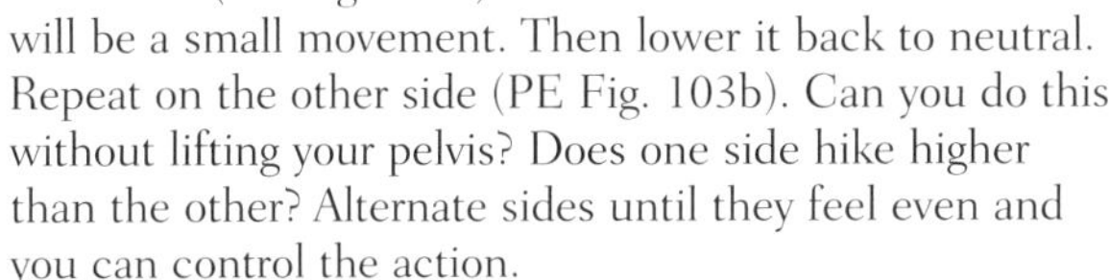

3. *Forward and backward rotation:* Again, lie on your back. Using a small movement, raise one hip straight toward the ceiling without lifting that shoulder from the ground (PE Fig. 103c), then lower your hip. Repeat on the other side (PE Fig. 103d). How far can you move in this direction? (This will be a small movement.) Again, alternate sides until they feel even and you can control the action.

PE Fig. 103c

4. *Pelvic clock* (adapted from a Feldenkrais lesson): Lie on your back with your knees bent, feet flat, and legs parallel. Imagine that you have a round clock on the back of your pelvis and sacrum. Mentally locate six o'clock at your tailbone, twelve o'clock near the back of your waist, nine and three o'clock out to each side.

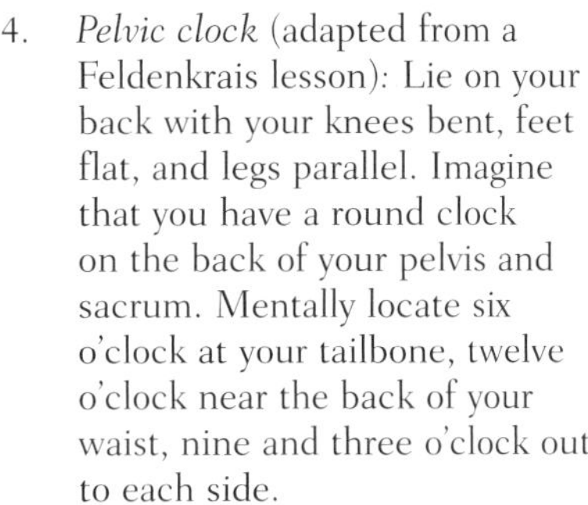

5. Slowly roll around the numbers of the clock, one number at a time. Notice which areas of your imaginary clock are easy to move through and which are not. Go in any direction you choose. Cut across the center of the clock in any pathway along which you want more freedom of motion.

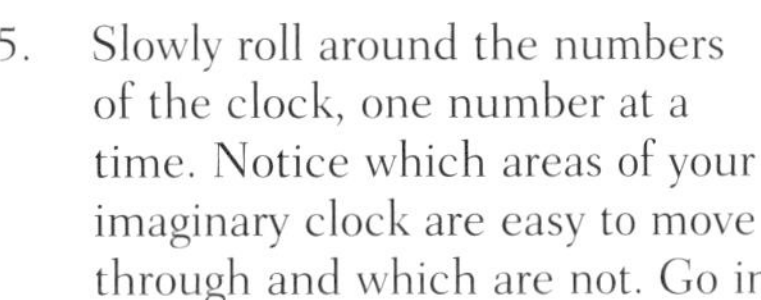

PE Fig. 103d

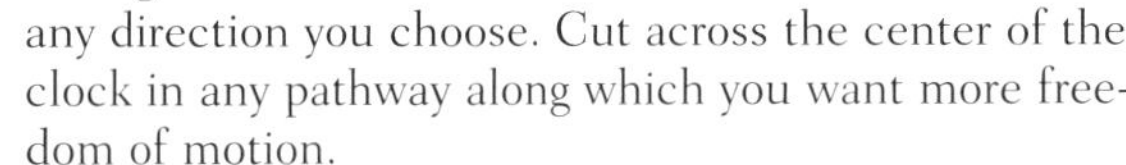

6. Smooth out any bumpy areas in your clock. Allow the back of the hips to sink and widen as you move. Keep your abdominal wall dropped back toward the spine. The smaller the motion, the more active the intrinsic muscles, the more refined the control over pelvic motion.

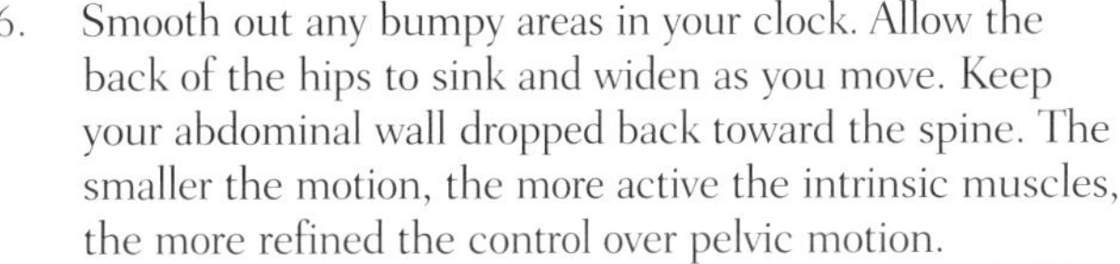

sheath is an important stabilizer muscle. The pelvic floor muscles are also responsive to respiratory rhythms; in fact, these muscles are referred to as the "pelvic diaphragm" because they rise and lower slightly on each breath cycle. Tone in the pelvic floor helps increases intra-abdominal pressure during respiration and can help with bladder control. Having control over the perineal muscles also gives the movement of the pelvis more articulation and can help release muscular holding in the lower back and around the hips.

The small joint between the sacrum and coccyx, the *sacro-coccygeal joint,* has a slight passive range of motion that extends the coccyx during defecation and childbirthing labor, and can be damaged by a hard fall on the derriere. A small glandular body about the size of a pea, called the *coccygeal gland,* is located on the anterior side of the coccyx (see Figure 10.33).[149] Some somatic teachers, including Ida Rolf, feel that the unknown function of this glandular body could involve the movement of "kundalini," a life-force energy that is believed by some to travel along the spine. When people first feel kundalini release, they often describe it as an exhilarating rush of energy surging from the base of the spine toward the head. Many practitioners of both yoga and somatic therapies recognize the

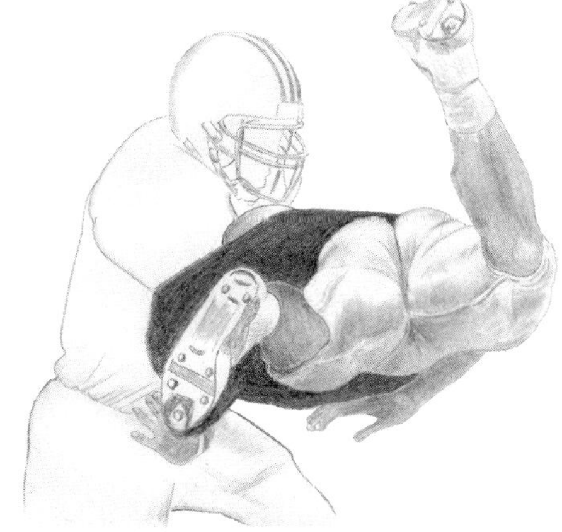

Figure 10.36a Muscular power involves the integrated action of the pelvic floor with the legs.

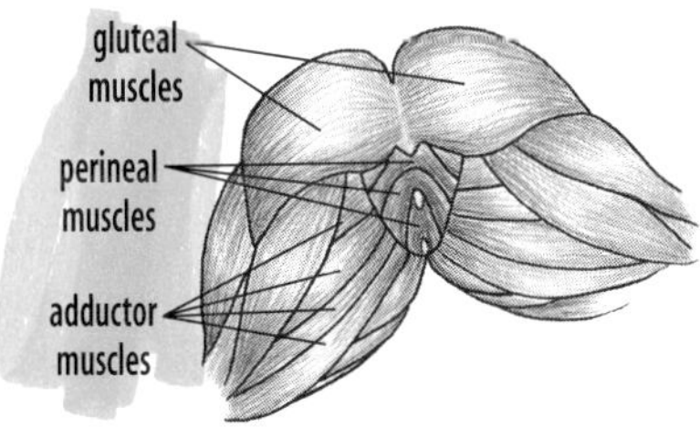

Figure 10.36b The gluteal and adductor muscles meet at the perineal muscles of the pelvic floor.

Patterning Exercise #104: Isolating Movement in the Pelvic Floor

1. Lie on your back and pull your knees to your chest (PE Fig. 104a). Lightly contract your lower abdominal muscles and pull them into the lower back to hollow out the lower abdomen.
2. Breathe into your coccyx to relax and open the pelvic floor muscles. If this is difficult, imagine your coccyx like a balloon. Breathe into it, expanding the muscles of the pelvic floor (also called the pelvic diaphragm) during each inhalation. Allow this expansion to lengthen your lower back and entire torso. Slowly lower each foot to the floor while keeping your pelvis stable.

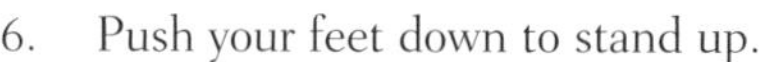

PE Fig. 104a

3. Next, imagine your coccyx like a flashlight. Shine its light toward the back of your knees, then down toward the floor, then toward one heel, then the other. Sense the subtle pelvic tilts and rotations this creates.
4. Contract your pelvic floor by pulling your sit bones together. Then relax it. Contract and relax several times until you feel you have control over your perineal muscles.
5. *Squatting:* Find a squatting position that is comfortable (PE Fig. 104b). You might need to use your hands to balance. Breathe into your coccyx in this position.
6. Push your feet down to stand up.
7. While standing, slightly bend both knees. Again, use an imaginary flashlight on your tail to draw figure eights on the floor. Sense the motion across your pelvic floor and through your hip sockets. Then reverse the action and move in the opposite direction.

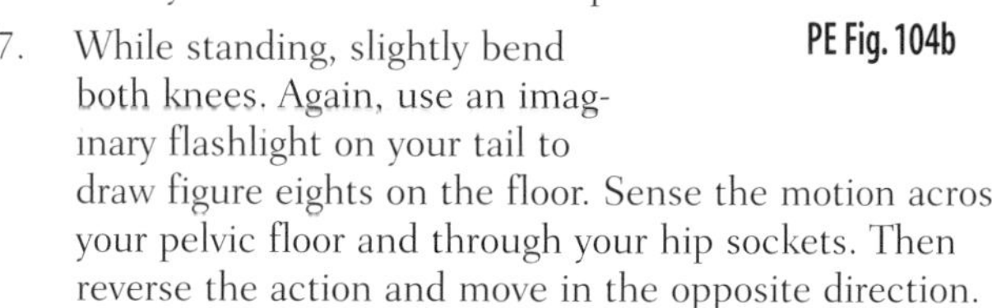

PE Fig. 104b

EMSPress.com

importance of the coccyx as an energetic center at the bottom of the spine. They use techniques such as breathing into the tail to access the vitality of energy believed to be stored in the coccygeal body.

Squatting stretches the area around the coccyx and opens the pelvic floor, creating an ideal position for elimination and childbirth. Women have traditionally birthed in this position, sometimes on squatting stools. A number of Asian cultures still commonly sit in a squatting position, which lengthens the lower back and may even relieve tension in it. It is also a useful position to assume occasionally to maintain flexibility in the hips and stretch the tissues around the tailbone. Squatting drops the abdominal organs into the back bottom of the pelvic bowl, giving the person more room to contract the lower abdominal muscles and hollow the lower abdomen. This can be helpful for people who have trouble sensing or controlling muscles in the area below the navel. Also, finding the subtle movements of the tail can help a person develop more articulation in the pelvic floor, which can release tension in the hips.

The Hips and Legs

The lower limb is made up of the foot, leg (below the knee), and thigh. Our legs have two seemingly contradictory roles—support and mobility. These two roles require that each joint in the lower limb be aligned and move within its physiological range. This means the curvilinear articulations of the foot, ankle, knee, and hip must be aligned and move in synchrony within the sagittal plane (Figure 10.37). In an oversimplistic analogy, alignment of the joints in the legs could be compared to the balance of tires on a car. The tires must be pointing straight ahead for the car to stay on the road. Likewise, the hip, knee, and ankle joints need to move in alignment for efficient support and gait patterns. This means that the knee is under the hip and in alignment with the toes, even when the leg is rotated.

When the legs bear weight, they function in a closed kinematic chain—a system of articulations joined by external resistance.[150] Resistance comes from a combination of the compressive forces of body weight coupled with ground forces. Muscles working in a closed chain create a rotary effect on all the joints in the limb, whether the muscles are directly attached to those joints or not. Resistance passes through the natural rotations of the hip, knee, and ankle joints during movement and, ideally, these rotations conform to the physiological range of movement within each joint.

Imbalance in alignment or restriction in the motion of any one joint in the lower limb can affect the balance of the entire chain. For example, if the knee is stiff, a person will have to exaggerate the forward swing of the hip and

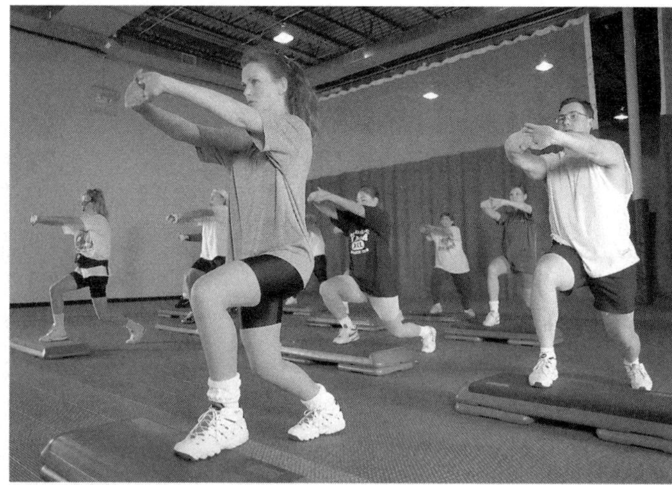

Figure 10.37 Notice whether the hip, knee, ankle, and foot are in alignment.

pelvis to be able to walk. Or if the knee is twisted, its torsion usually translates into other joints, creating twists in the ankle, hip, or spine. Therefore it is of the utmost importance that each joint of the lower limb move with its maximal mobility from an aligned neutral position to avoid stressing other joints along the chain.

Flexion and Extension of the Lower Limb

Ideally, hip flexion and extension during walking begins from a neutral position. In a neutral standing posture, the center of gravity of the pelvis lies in front of the sacrum, the distal end of the femur (near the knee) is internally rotated, and the thigh muscles spiral in from the hip to the knee. During hip flexion, the knee draws toward the chest, gliding the head of the femur in the socket; extension reverses the action. The socket can also glide around the head of the femur, in movement such as a forward bending that turns the pelvis on top of the legs. Usually hip flexion occurs with a small posterior tilt of the pelvis, and hip extension with a small anterior tilt of the pelvis.

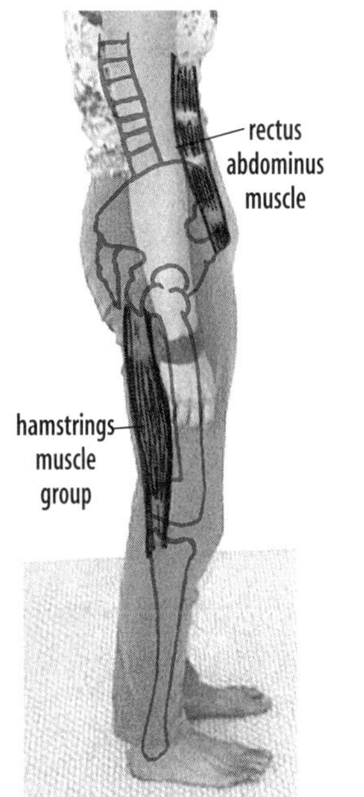

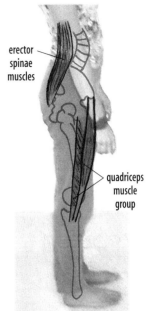

Figure 10.38a Posterior tilt

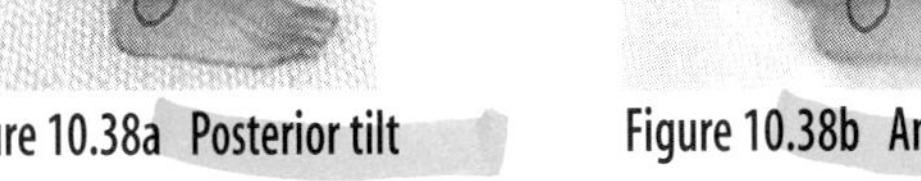

Figure 10.38b Anterior tilt

A balance of flexor and extensor tone in the muscles of the thigh, pelvis, and waist keeps the pelvic bowl level in a neutral posture. If the hamstrings and/or rectus abdominis muscles are tight and short, the pelvis will tend to tilt under or backward in a standing posture (Figure 10.38a). If the quadriceps muscles on the front of the thigh and/or the large erector spinae muscles are tight, the pelvis will tend to tilt forward (Figure 10.38b).

Patterning Exercise #105: Lower Limb Flexion and Extension

1. *Hip flexion and extension:* Lie on your back with both knees bent, feet flat, and legs parallel. Maintain the same angle of your knees during the entire movement. Keeping your pelvis stable, slowly flex one hip and let your shin float up toward the ceiling (PE Fig. 105a). Sense the weight of that leg sinking into the hip socket, deepening the crease in your groin. Your abdominal wall should sink toward your spine; you are working too hard if your rectus abdominis contracts and bulges out. Sense your upper back widening and allow it to be cradled by your shoulder blades. Imagine your hip opening and closing with the precision of a jackknife.

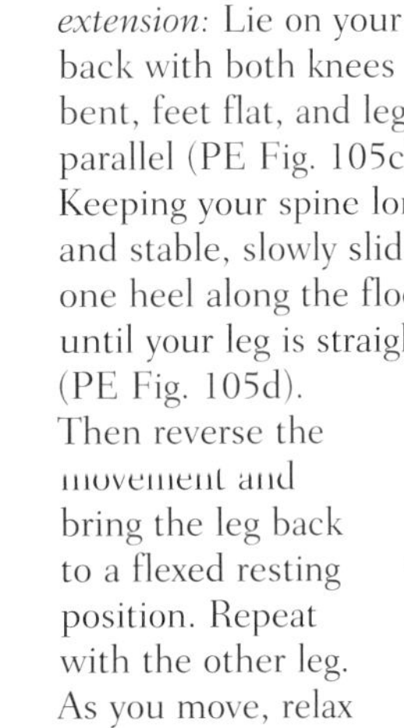

PE Fig. 105a

2. Slowly lower your leg and return your foot to the floor. Move with the least amount of effort possible while keeping your pelvis stable (PE Fig. 105b).

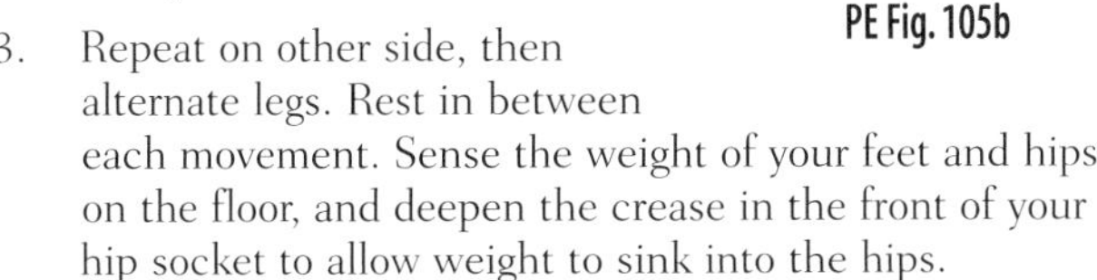

PE Fig. 105b

3. Repeat on other side, then alternate legs. Rest in between each movement. Sense the weight of your feet and hips on the floor, and deepen the crease in the front of your hip socket to allow weight to sink into the hips.
4. *Lower limb flexion and extension:* Lie on your back with both knees bent, feet flat, and legs parallel (PE Fig. 105c). Keeping your spine long and stable, slowly slide one heel along the floor until your leg is straight (PE Fig. 105d). Then reverse the movement and bring the leg back to a flexed resting position. Repeat with the other leg. As you move, relax any part of your body that is tight and release any extraneous work. Allow your trunk and leg to be weighted to teach yourself to keep your spine long while moving your leg.

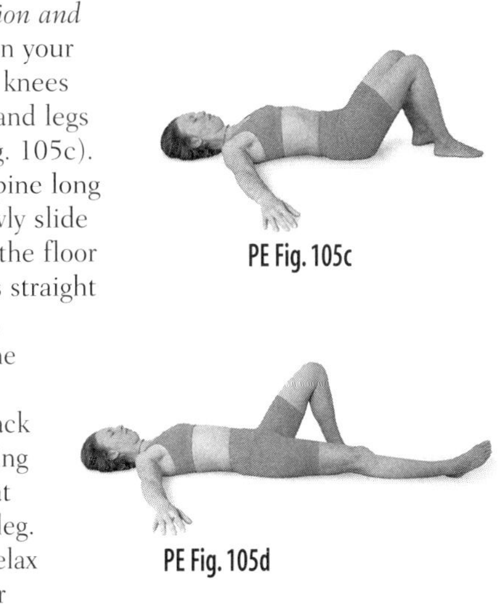

PE Fig. 105c

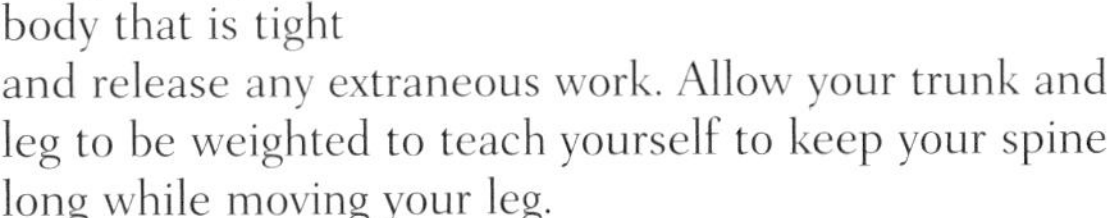

PE Fig. 105d

5. *Lower limb flexion and extension while standing:* Stand with your back flat against a wall, using the wall for feedback about your pelvic alignment. Slowly lift one knee keeping your pelvis level and your spine stable. Avoid hiking or twisting your hips. How far can you lift it before your pelvis starts to tilt?
6. Repeat with the other leg.

Rotation of the Lower Limb

The highly mobile ball-and-socket joint of the hip allows motion in all three planes. The legs swing in flexion and extension under the body during walking. They also turn in or out during rotation, an action we use to make changes in direction. Like that of the shoulders, the full rotational capacity of the hip sockets may rarely be used unless a person is involved in a sport, dance, or work activity that calls for this range of motion. To keep this range intact, a person is encouraged to take the hips through their full range of rotations on a regular basis. Recall that movement of a joint spreads synovial fluid in it, therefore circular movements can lubricate and nourish the hip sockets.

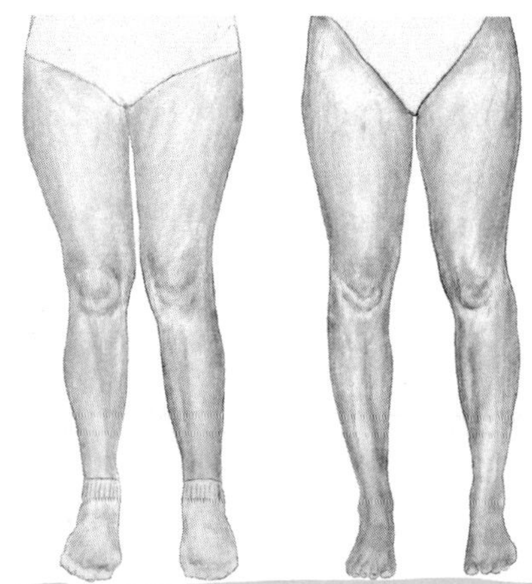

Figure 10.39a Valgus Figure 10.39b Vagus

Rotation of the pelvis occurs in the waist, while rotation of the lower limbs occurs at the hip sockets. Ideally, the legs align under the body in the sagittal plane when a person is standing in a neutral posture, being neither internally nor externally rotated. Any rotations in a neutral posture will point the toes and knees in or out and interfere with normal flexion and extension during walking or running. Chronic contractions in the muscles around the hips can create chronic rotations in the legs and pelvis. External rotation of the lower limb is usually caused by chronic contractions in the rotator muscles on the back of the buttocks; internal rotation of the lower limb is usually caused by chronic contractions of adductor muscles of the hip

Patterning Exercise #106: Leg Rotation

1. *Leg rotation:* Lie on your back with both legs bent, feet flat, and legs parallel. Slowly lower both legs to one side (PE Fig. 106a). Keep several inches in between your knees so that your bottom thigh externally rotates and your upper thigh internally rotates. When the rotation of your thighs reaches end range, your pelvis and spine will begin to twist in the direction of your knees.

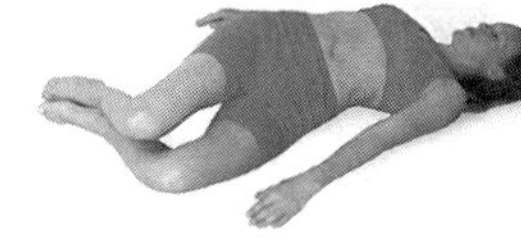

PE Fig. 106a

2. Return to neutral by reversing the movement and pressing both feet back to their original position.
3. Next, lower the legs to the other side and repeat the whole sequence.
4. Now, keep your knees together as you lower both legs to the left side (PE Fig. 106b). Feel how this limits rotation in the thighs, which creates more rotation in the spine. Return to neutral and repeat on the other side.
5. *Stabilizing leg rotation:* Start on your back with both legs bent, feet flat, and legs parallel. Lightly contract and pull your lower abdominal muscles straight back toward your spine. Also contract the oblique muscles of your waist.

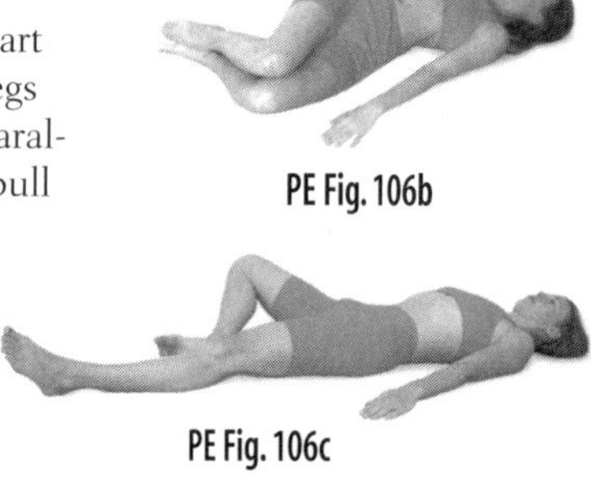

PE Fig. 106b

PE Fig. 106c

6. Slowly lower one knee to the floor, stabilizing your pelvis with the obliques (PE Fig.106c). Move only as far as you are able while keeping your pelvis stable. If your hips start to twist, stop there. Return to your starting position. Repeat on the other side.
7. *External rotation:* (This exercise corrects chronic internal rotation of the thighs.) Lie on your side with your knees bent and legs together. To feel abduction without rotation, lift your leg toward the ceiling (PE Fig. 106d). Then lift your knee toward the ceiling while keeping your ankle in the same place (PE Fig. 106e). This will externally rotate your thigh. Sense the rotator muscles in the buttocks working to lift the knee, or reach back and feel them bulge as they work.
8. Now slowly lower your knee with control. Roll over and repeat with the other leg.
9. *Internal rotation:* (This exercise corrects chronic external rotation of the thighs.) First lift your leg up without rotation (PE Fig. 106d). Then keep your knee in the same place and lift your top ankle toward the ceiling (PE Fig. 106f). Sense the internal rotators working on the front of the hip and the inside of the thigh to lift the ankle.

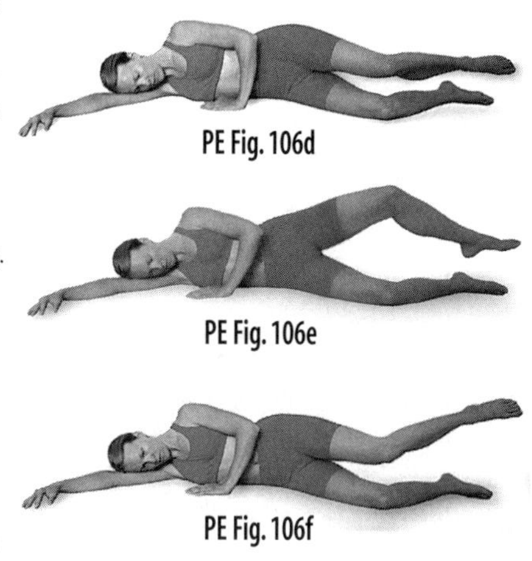

PE Fig. 106d

PE Fig. 106e

PE Fig. 106f

10. Slowly lower your ankle with control. Roll over and repeat steps 7–9 with the other leg.

EMSPress.com

and inner thigh. These patterns place torsion stresses on the sacroiliac joints and may even translate into undue torsion in the joints of the knees, ankles, or spine.

To keep the legs aligned and release rotations, a person could imagine having headlights on the hip sockets and knees that shine straight ahead while standing, walking, or running. If the legs are outwardly rotated, as in a toed-out gait, a person can learn to control and strengthen the internal rotators. Chronic inward rotations are less common and create a toed-in gait and a pigeon-toed stance.

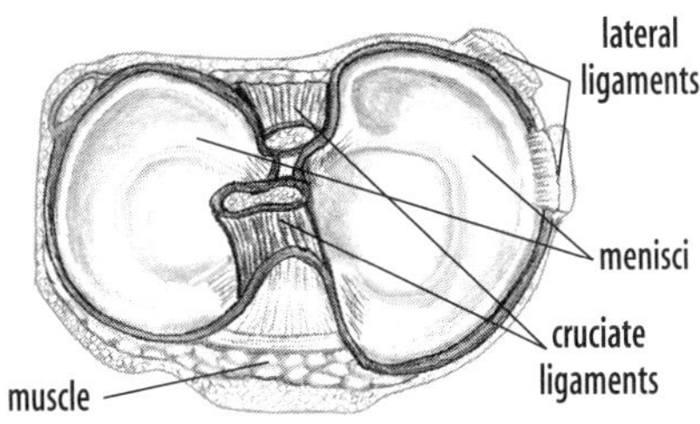

Figure 10.40 Cross section of the knee looking down on the menisci

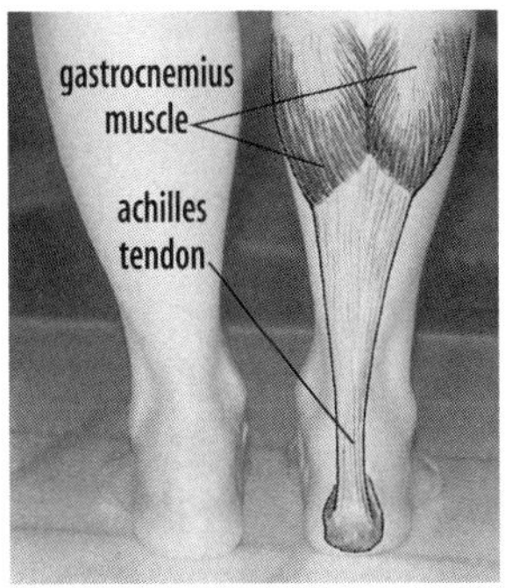

Figure 10.41 The achilles tendon is oriented vertically.

Chronic rotations in the legs may be rooted in developmental processes. A preborn's legs are tightly folded in flexion and external rotation in the womb, a pattern that is still strong in a newborn. Gradually, as a baby pushes and reaches through her feet, she learns to bear weight on the legs. Ideally, the push sequences through all five digits, from the big toe to the little toe, gradually internally rotating and straightening the legs so that by the time a baby stands on them, they are aligned in the sagittal plane under her body. There are many cases where the legs and feet fail to align during early motor development, resulting in knock-kneed, pigeon-toed (*valgus*) or bowlegged (*vagus*) patterns (Figure 10.39a-b). Recall from Chapter 2 that a baby who is made to stand before she pushes up on her own might learn to brace her body on locked knees in a toed-out or toed-in posture. The orthopedist Arthur Michelle claims that 30 percent of babies are born with tibial torsion, a combination of bowing and extreme rotation of the lower leg.[151] Push patterns should straighten the tibia if the baby's motor development proceeds normally. If not, a person can always learn patterning exercises to help align the joints in the legs later in life.

The Knee and Sagittal Tracking

The knee joint is the most complex joint in the body. It functions as a shock absorber between the lower leg and thigh. Two menisci shaped like horseshoes and made of cartilage pad each knee (Figure 10.40). Both menisci rest on top of the *tibia*, the sturdy, pillar-like bone most people know as the shin. The top of the tibia is a horizontal-articulating surface appropriately named the *tibial plateau*. In a balanced body, the tibia is the most vertically oriented bone in the body. Its degree of verticality can be gauged by looking at the *Achilles tendon* of the *gastrocnemius muscle* that rises from the heel: it should be straight up and down (Figure 10.41). The tibia transmits body weight from the thigh to the foot and transmits ground forces from the foot to the thigh.

The *femoral condyles* move the menisci backward and forward during knee flexion and extension like a pestle moving grain in a mortar. When the knee flexes, the condyles press the menisci backward on the tibia plateau. When the knee extends, the action reverses and the condyles press the menisci forward on the tibial plateau (Figure 10.42).

A small bone on the side of the foreleg, the *fibula*, attaches to the tibia by a thick, *interosseous membrane*. The distal end of these two bones form the *malleoli*, the bony knobs on the sides of the ankle. When a person flexes the ankle, the fibula slides down slightly. If the ankle is stiff and the muscles of the lower leg chronically contracted, jumping can create minor tears in this membrane that are called "shin splints" (Figure 10.43). To avoid shin splints, a person needs to be able to flex and extend the ankle freely and jump with a spring in the arches.

During hip and knee flexion, the femur externally rotates against a slight internal rotation of the tibia. When the knee is in full extension, no rotation is possible. The knees take a beating from the rotational demands of sports such as skiing or tennis, from the impact of sports such as running, and even from a gait pattern marked by a hard heel strike. People often injure the knee when they rotate the leg with the foot in a fixed position. For example, if a person turns his body while his foot is adhered to the floor (a common occurrence between sneak-

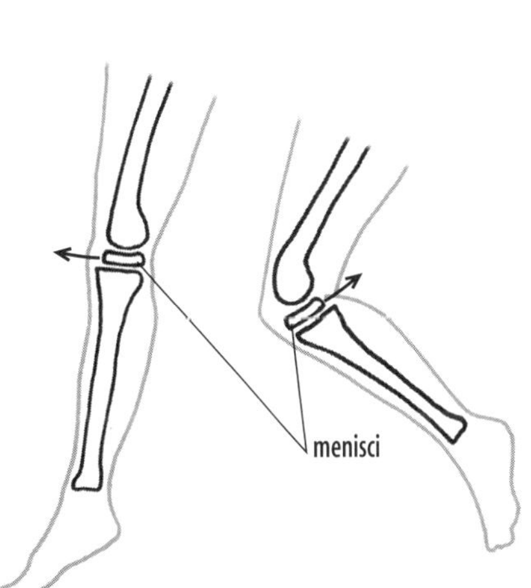

Figure 10.42 As the knee extends and flexes, the menisci move forward and backward.

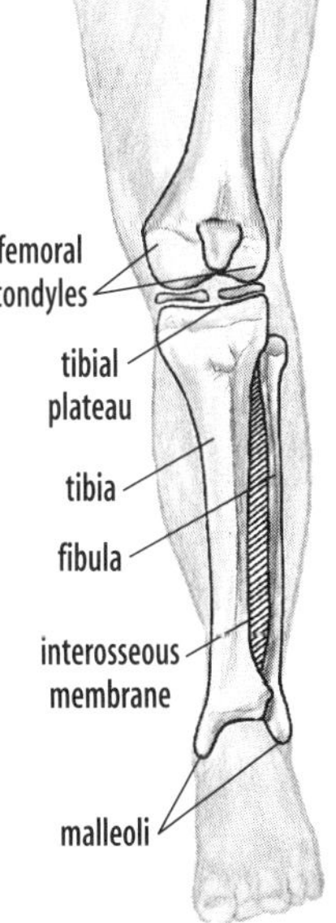

Figure 10.43 Shin splints tear the interosseous membrane.

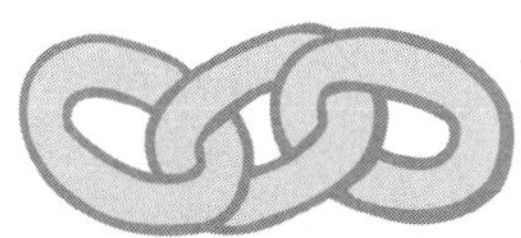

Links to Practical Applications

Checking Ankle Flexibility

To check the flexibility of your ankles, stand in front of a mirror and bend your knees, making sure that your knees are under your hips and aligned with your second toes during the entire movement. Your heels should remain on the ground, the tendons in the crease of your ankles should stay relaxed, and your toes should stay extended and flat on the floor. If your heels tend to pop up, you may need to stretch the muscles in your calves. If the tendons in the crease of your ankles pop out, relax them. If your toes flex and grip the floor, learn how to extend your toes and flatten them while standing.

ers and non-slip surfaces), he will twist the knee past its limited range of rotation. Ideally, the feet, ankles, and knees stay aligned in the sagittal plane during movement, and rotation occurs primarily in the hip socket. To keep this alignment, a person needs to always keep the knee over the second toe, even when the hip rotates in or out to change directions.

The Feet

The feet tell the story of the whole body. When the feet hurt, the entire body suffers. When feet are energized and springy, the whole body feels good. Any imbalance in the feet can throw off the entire body. For example, a person who walks on her heels probably leans back, creating tension along the back of the body. A person who walks on the outside of the feet probably drops weight along the outside of the legs and hips, which can stress the ankles, knees, and sacroiliac joints. And a person with pigeon-toed feet probably has compensatory twists in the knees and hips, which may even translate all the way up the spine.

Each foot is a complex and intricate structure of 26 tarsal bones and approximately 104 ligaments. Multiple articulations between the many tarsal bones make our feet adaptable to the changing contours of irregular surfaces. The feet have three primary roles: weight-bearing, shock absorption, and propulsion.

Each foot has three arches that connect to form a tripod. The three points of support in a tripod make a more mobile base than a four-point, quadruped support, and a more stable base than a bipedal, two-point support. Together the arches form an architectural vault that functions like an elastic spring, absorbing shock and levering the foot forward on each step (Figure 10.44).

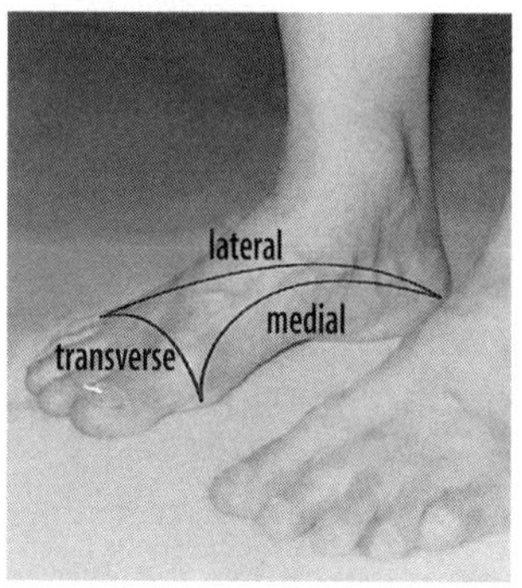

Figure 10.44 The three arches of the foot form an architectural vault.

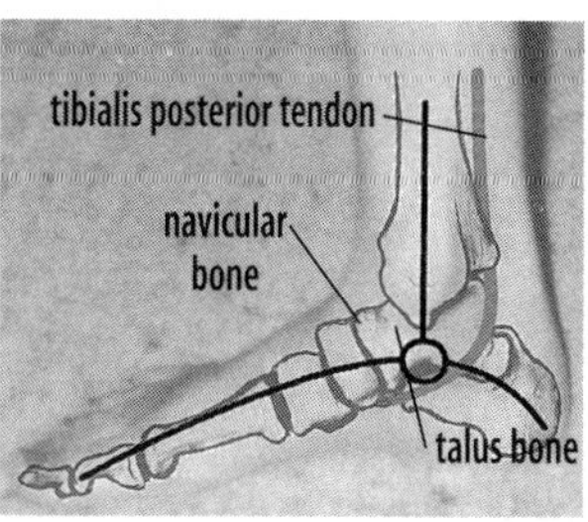

Figure 10.45 The medial arch

Each arch is oriented along an axis of motion: the lateral, medial, and transverse arch. The *lateral arch* runs along the outside edge of the foot from heel to little toe; it is lower and more rigid than the other two arches to effectively transmit the thrust of forward propulsion. The *medial arch* runs along the inside edge of the foot from heel to big toe; it is higher and more flexible than the lateral arch. The *navicular bone* is the keystone of the medial arch, and the *tibialis posterior tendon* acts as a sling for the navicular bone, stabilizing

Patterning Exercise #107: Sagittal Tracking with "Toes Up, Toes Down"

(Adapted from a Rolfing Movement exercise to improve the sagittal alignment between the toes, ankle, knee, and hip.)

1. Sit in a chair with your shoes off, both feet on the ground, and legs parallel to each other. Make sure you are sitting in a neutral posture with your body weight over both sit bones. Put your feet as far apart as your sit bones (PE Fig. 107a).
2. Starting with one foot, raise all five toes while keeping the bottom of the foot on the ground (PE Fig. 107b). You should feel your arches stretch. Lower your toes and raise them again. Watch them to make sure they all come up together; it's typical for the big toe or little toe to lead.
3. Next, raise your whole foot except the heel by flexing your ankle (PE Fig. 107c). Make sure to keep your heel on the ground. Feel the back of your lower leg elongate; you may even feel your hamstrings stretch slightly.
4. Leave your toes up and put your ankle down, then put your toes down.
5. Practice this movement—toes up, ankle up, ankle down, toes down—several times on one foot. Make sure to keep your hip, knee, and foot in the same plane, as though your foot and leg were sandwiched between two narrow walls.

PE Fig. 107a

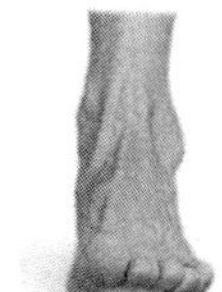

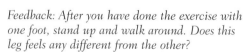

PE Fig. 107b

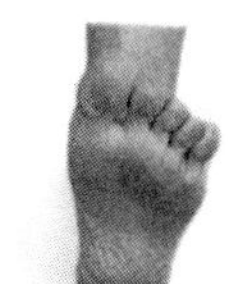

PE Fig. 107c

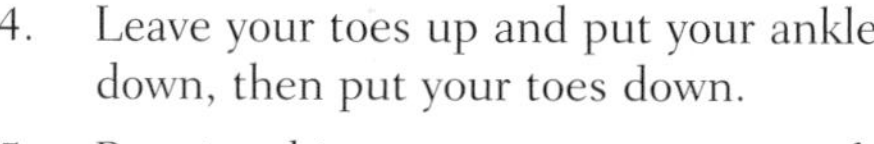

Feedback: After you have done the exercise with one foot, stand up and walk around. Does this leg feels any different from the other?

6. Repeat the entire exercise with the other foot. Then get up and walk around to sense any changes in your gait.

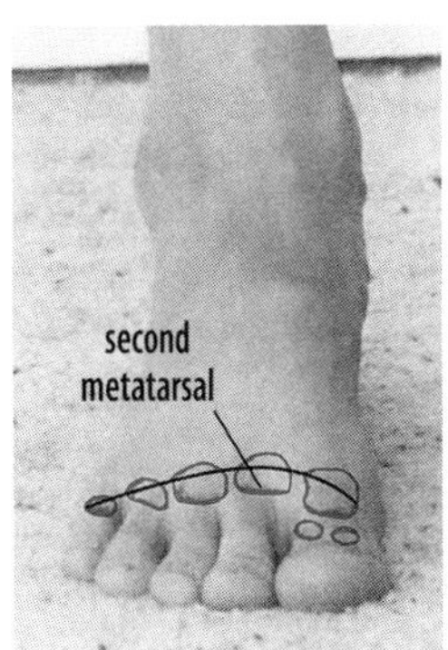

Figure 10.46 The transverse arch

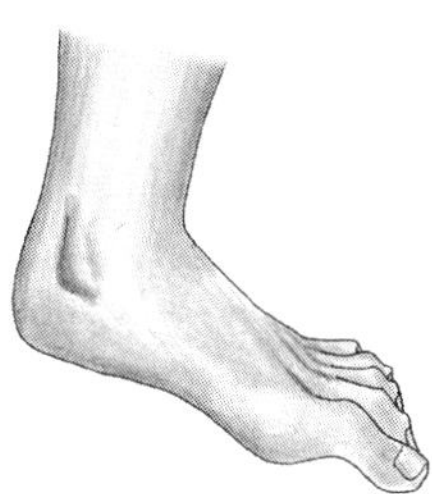

Figure 10.47 Clawfoot

the medial arch to keep it from falling (Figure 10.45). The *transverse arch* runs across the ball of the foot, with its highest point and keystone being at the *second metatarsal* (Figure 10.46). It flattens when we roll through the toe hinge while walking.

The arches present an intricately balanced architecture. They create a series of triangular relationships that work together as a unified spring to allow the foot to absorb shock on each step. The arches redirect the impact of heel strikes into the energy needed to thrust the legs off the ground and propel them forward. They must be strong yet pliable to be able to move the lower limb through full cycles of flexion and extension during walking.

Numerous small muscles in the foot, many arising from the tendons of calf muscles, help with the subtle motions of the feet. The keystone of the ankle, the *talus bone*, is called the "caged bone" because it is surrounded and supported solely by fourteen tendons of the lower leg muscles; it does not have a single muscle attached to it (see Figure 10.45).[152] For this reason, it is of prime importance that the muscles of the lower leg function in a balanced manner to keep the talus centered.

The arches stretch as we step onto the foot and roll from the heel to the toes. As the arches flatten, tendons from the muscles of the lower leg stretch. This stretch builds elastic energy that triggers the next cycle of muscular contractions in the lower leg and foot and propels the gait cycle. Ideally, the toes flatten and press against the floor to balance the body, leaving the arches free to uncoil and recoil in a spring-like action. If the toes grip in a clawfoot or hammertoe pattern, this tendency disturbs the coordinated movement of the entire foot (Figure 10.47). This gripping of the toes indicates a dysfunction in one peculiar muscle group called the *lumbricals*. They arise from the tendons of the *flexor digitorum longus muscle* of the lower leg. When

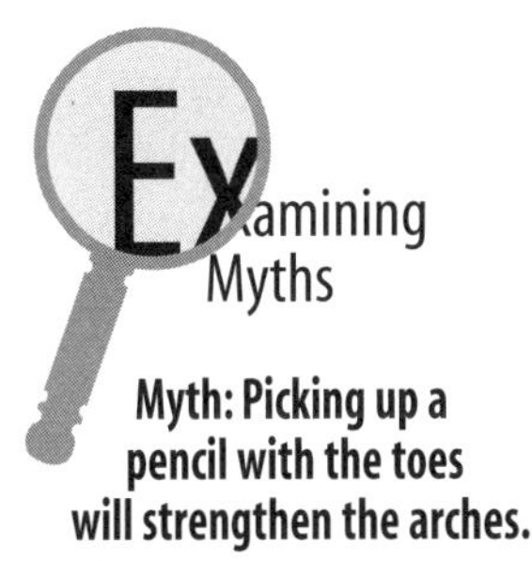

Myth: Picking up a pencil with the toes will strengthen the arches.

Although this exercise will strengthen the flexors of your toes, it may or may not strengthen the arches. The muscles that lift the arches, the lumbricals, also extend the toes; therefore, picking up a pencil with your toes, which flexes the toes, will bypass the lumbricals completely and fail to strengthen the arches. More likely, this exercise will reinforce bad habits of gripping the toes, and the toes need to remain flat and extended while standing for balance and to maintain tone in the arches.

Patterning Exercise #108: Strengthening the Arches

1. Sit comfortably in a chair in a neutral posture. Remove your shoes and socks so that you can watch your feet. Move one foot at a time.
2. Keeping the foot on the floor, lift your arches as though the bottom of your foot were a suction cup pulling up (PE Fig. 108a). Keep your toes extended and flat as you pull the arches up.

PE Fig. 108a

3. Then open your arches as though the bottom of your foot were yawning, and lower your instep.
4. Repeat several times until you can easily move your instep up and down without gripping or flexing your toes.
5. Then get up and walk around. Does that foot feel any different from your other one? It will probably be more supple and energized.
6. Repeat the entire exercise with the other foot.
7. If your feet are stiff and you cannot lift your arches, roll your feet on a tennis ball to stimulate reflexes in your feet and loosen myofascia on the soles of your feet.
8. *Inchworm:* Slowly walk your foot forward along the floor, moving it like an inchworm by drawing your heel toward your toes while keeping your toes stationary, then extend and flatten your toes (PE Fig. 108b-c).
9. Now reverse the movement and inch your foot backward by drawing your toes toward your heel while keeping your heel stationary, then lifting and extending your heel back.
10. Repeat forward and backward several times, then repeat with the other foot. This will help make your arches more supple and articulate.

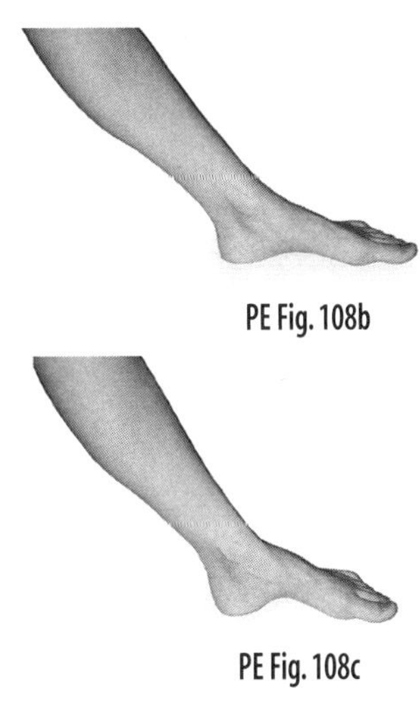

PE Fig. 108b

PE Fig. 108c

Patterning Exercise #109: Initiating Hip and Leg Rotation in the Feet

1. While standing with both knees bent or sitting at the edge of a chair, draw a figure eight on the floor with one foot. Allow the rotation to sequence all the way into your hip. Let your toes lead the movement, and let the movement be fluid and supple. After you have gone over the pattern several times, reverse directions. Then repeat with the other leg.
2. Stand or sit in a comfortable position. Scoop one foot across your body in an arcing motion, leading with your medial arch (PE Fig. 109a). Let the foot lead, sensing how your knee and hip follow.
3. Now press your lateral arch out to your side in an arcing motion (PE Fig. 109b). Let your whole leg follow your foot.

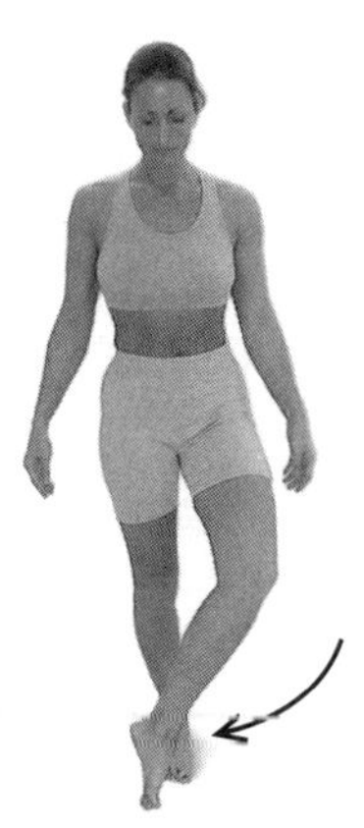

PE Fig. 109a

4. Scoop and press your foot back and forth several times until the action is smooth and easy. Repeat with the other foot.
5. Now lie on your back and repeat the same motions. With your foot above you and your knee slightly bent, draw a figure eight in the air with your foot. Go several times in both directions, then switch legs and repeat.
6. Next, scoop an arc with your inner arch, then your outer arch, taking your foot and leg back and forth across your body. Make sure to do both legs.

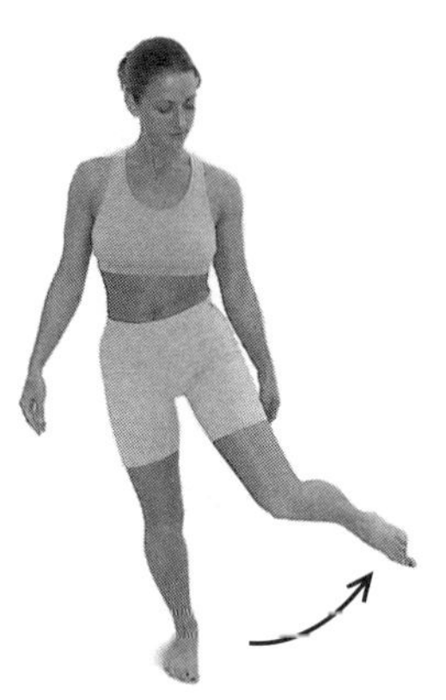

PE Fig. 109b

EMSPress.com

they contract, the lumbricals lift the vault of the arches while extending the toes and pressing them against the floor (see PE Fig. 108a).

The lumbricals are the only muscles in the body attached to both the plantar and dorsal surfaces. Joint physiologist I. A. Kapandji describes the action of the lumbricals as similar to a two-way transistor, translating motion from one side of the foot and leg to the other through the combined action of flexion and extension.[153] By being both flexors and extensors, attached to both the plantar and dorsal surfaces of the foot, the lumbricals help to coordinate the alternating sequence of flexor and extensor activity in the lower leg and foot.

In the same way that arm movements are made more articulate by initiating them with the fingertips, lower limb movement can also be refined by initiating it with the toes and arches. Movement initiated by the big toe sequences along the inside of the leg into the groin and the front of the pelvis. Movement initiated in the middle toe sequences through the center of the leg into the hip socket. Movement initiated in the little toe sequences along the outside of the leg into the back of the pelvis. Ideally, when we step off the foot during walking, we roll evenly through all five toes. If we tend to favor one side of the foot or the other, we will limit the chain of action to that side of the leg and hip.

The Lumbar-Pelvic Rhythm

Forward bending is a combination of trunk and hip flexion. Cailliett describes this combination as the **lumbar-pelvic rhythm,** which increases the range of motion in trunk and hip flexion by distributing the movement between the lower back and the pelvis.[154] This rhythm, similar to the scapulohumeral rhythm, occurs during forward bending of the trunk in two stages. In the first stage, the lumbar spine flexes, moving from concave to flat to convex, with 75 percent of the flexion occurring at the *lumbosacral junction* (Figure 10.48a.). In the second stage, the pelvis rotates on the legs, increasing the range of trunk and hip flexion (Figure 10.48b.). The sequence reverses as a person stands back up: first the pelvis rotates on the legs; then the lumbar spine extends.

If either lumbar flexion or pelvic rotation is restricted, the range of the overall flexion will be limited. If hip flexion is restricted, the lumbar spine will overcompensate and flex too much. This pattern is common in men who have trouble touching their toes; they have restricted hip

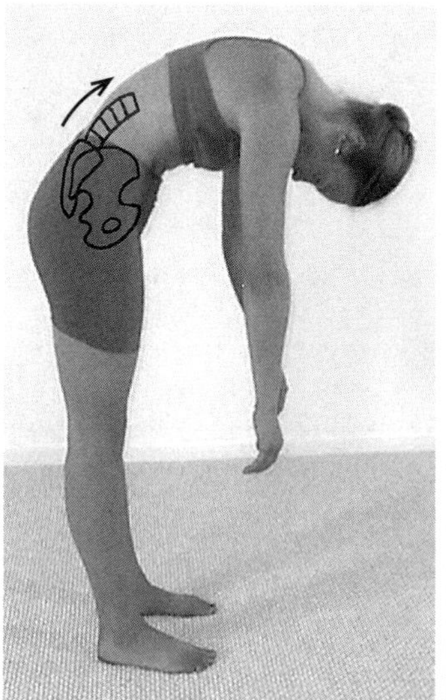

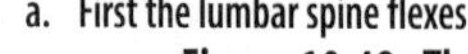

a. First the lumbar spine flexes

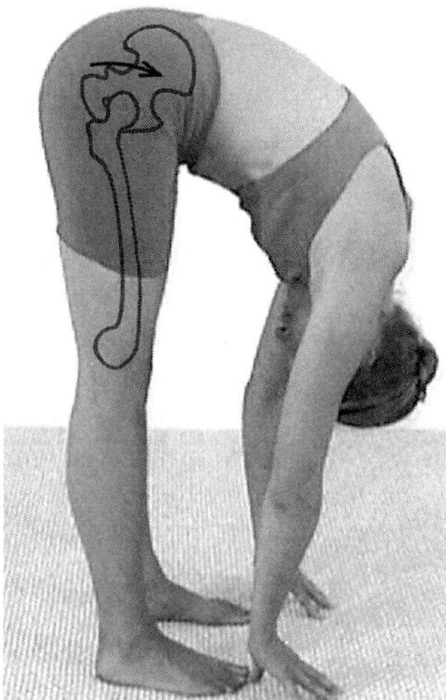

b. Then the pelvis rotates on the hip

Figure 10.48 The two phases of the lumbar-pelvic rhythm

Patterning Exercise #110: Feeling the Lumbar-Pelvic Rhythm

1. *Lumbar flexion:* Stand sideways to a mirror and watch yourself bend over. Does your lumbar spine flex first? To what degree? At what point does your pelvis rotate on your hips?
2. Bend your trunk forward by isolating flexion in your lower back.
3. Once your lumbar spine is flexed, anteriorly tilt your pelvis at the hips and bend over and touch your toes.
4. Reverse the action to return to standing. First posteriorly tilt your pelvis on your legs, then extend your lower back and return to standing.
5. *Hip flexion:* Lie on your back with both legs bent, feet flat, and legs parallel. Slowly flex one hip, lifting your foreleg toward the ceiling and then toward your head (PE Fig. 110a). Sense the point in the movement in which your pelvis begins to rotate and the weight of your leg shifts from your hip socket into your sacrum, then into your lumbar spine (PE Fig. 110b).
6. Slowly reverse the movement and aim your foot back to its original starting place. Sense the weight shift from the lumbar spine into the sacrum, then into the hips as you lower your foreleg to the ground.
7. Repeat with the other leg. Do your legs move symmetrically?

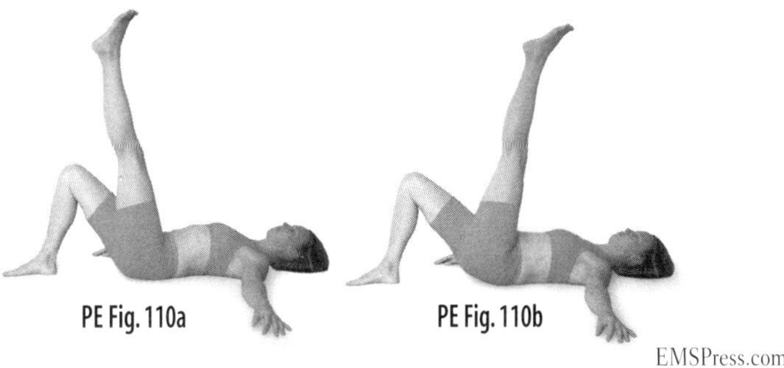

flexion and excessive lumbar flexion. Another common pattern is chronic anterior tilt of the pelvis and chronic hyperextension of the lower back that restricts lumbar flexion. When the lower back lacks flexion, the thorax may flex too much and become chronically rounded to make up for the lack of flexion below it. Conversely, when the pelvis is chronically tucked, the lower back flattens and may also be restricted in extension.

WEIGHT SHIFTS AND LOCOMOTION

All mammals have evolved strong muscles in the lower body to propel them forward and to pounce on prey from a crouched posture. The crouch loads the joints of the lower limbs into flexion, building potential energy in the powerful flexors of the hips and legs in preparation for springing into extension. Since humans stand upright, our spring from a crouch has a more vertical thrust.

Although most people rarely crouch and spring as animals do, we do use a vertical thrust of the lower body to make transition from squatting to standing, and a forward thrust of the pelvis to walk or run. During any weight shift, the torso moves over the base of support, and the base of support usually widens in the direction of the shift. For example, a person tossing a horseshoe spreads his feet apart from front to back and rocks over his base of support to swing the horseshoe. The momentum of the throw is initiated by the swing of the arm and a shift from one foot to another.

Any time we make a movement that changes the body's base of support, we make a weight shift in some direction. Bartenieff identifies a **forward shift** or a **backward shift** of the pelvis, both weight shifts that propel the pelvis forward or back in the sagittal plane (Figure 10.49). We make a forward shift in the pelvis when we rise out of a chair or propel the pelvis forward in some kind of locomotion pattern. We make a backward shift when we lower the hips into a chair or into a squatting position.

Most weight shifts in the pelvis are some combination of a forward and lateral shift. A **lateral shift** involves a sideways movement of the pelvis in the frontal plane in such actions as getting into a car, sliding over on a bench to make room for someone else, and moving sideways during a tennis match (Figure 10.50). During a lateral shift, movement sequences from one hip to the other along the horizontal axis running through the *greater trochanters*. Lateral shifts

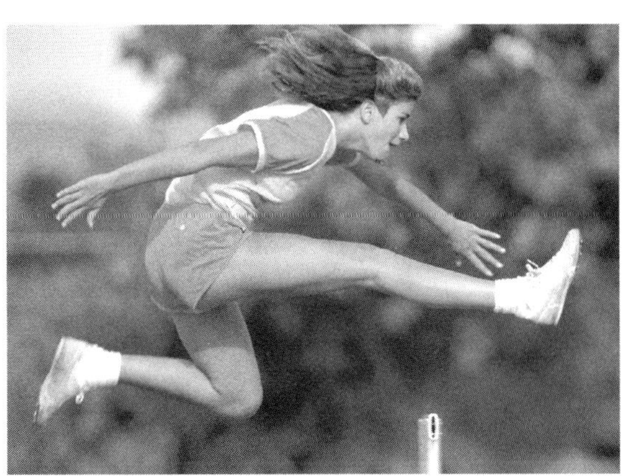

Figure 10.49 This athlete's jump is propelled by a forward pelvic shift.

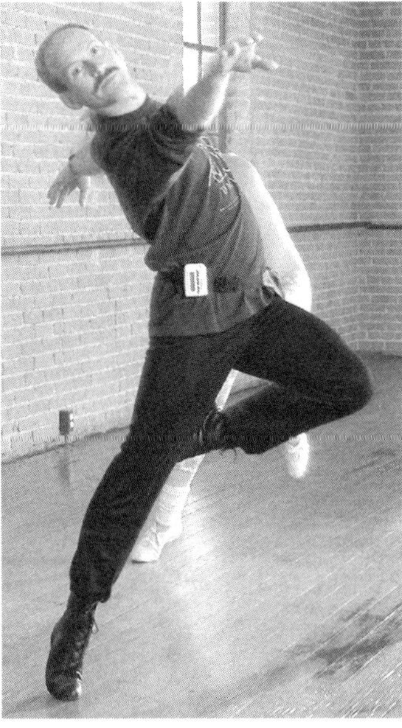

Figure 10.50 This dancer's movement involves a lateral weight shift.

also occur in the feet between the inner and the outer arches. There is slight lateral shift during walking, which is exaggerated when a person has a tendency to swing the hips. An efficient lateral shift moves through one hip to the other like a typewriter carriage sliding back and forth. Lateral flexion of the spine can be confused with a lateral weight shift, but a pure lateral shift lacks side-bending or hip hiking; it moves the pelvis directly sideways.

All pelvic shifts involve coordinated movements between the legs and trunk, and may even include the arms, such as rolling over to stand up (Figure 10.52a-b). These coordinations become apparent while practicing each action. Ideally, pelvic tilts and shifts begin in a neutral posture,

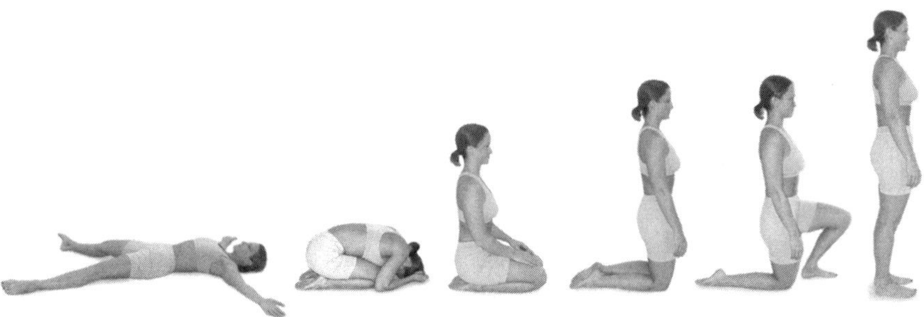

Figure 10.51a Sequence of a lateral weight shift from lying to kneeling to standing

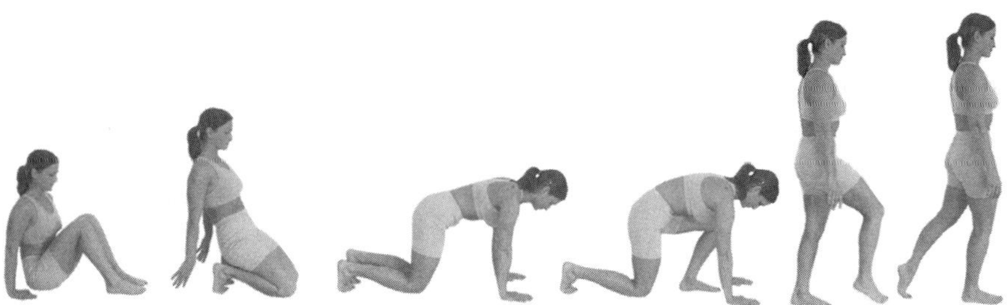

Figure 10.51b Sequence of a sagittal weight shift from sitting to standing

Patterning Exercise #111: Pelvic Shifts

1. Lie on your back with both knees bent, feet flat on the floor. Tilt your pelvis back by pressing your lower back against the floor.

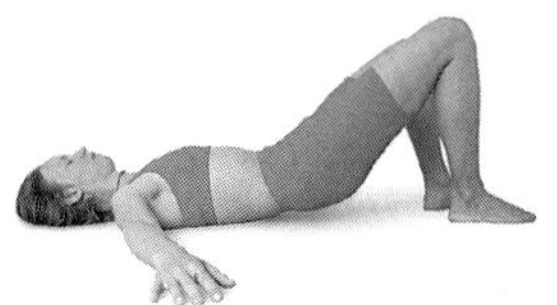

PE Fig. 111a

2. *Forward pelvic shift:* From this position, in one action, reach your tail and pelvis toward the back of your knees (PE Fig. 111a). This should shift your body weight slightly toward your knees and feet.
3. Then return your pelvis to your original position by pointing your tail toward your feet and reversing the movement. Your hips should land closer to your feet; move your feet away from your body to open the angle at the back of your knees and resume your starting position. Practice this several times in one smooth action.
4. *Forward and backward pelvic shift:* Sit on both knees. Reach your hand as you shift your pelvis forward, ending in the quadruped position (PE Fig. 111b-c). Then reach back with your tail in a backward pelvic shift to return to your original position. Practice going both ways several times, feeling the power of the pelvic shift propelling you forward and backward.

PE Fig. 111b

PE Fig. 111c

5. *Lateral pelvic shift:* Start in the quadruped position, on all fours. Avoid side-bending and hiking the hips during the lateral shift (PE Fig. 111d). Slowly shift your pelvis to one side, sensing the sequence through six bones:

   femur → hip bone → sacrum and pubic bone → hip bone → femur (PE Fig. 111e).

   Repeat this on the other side. Can you glide straight across these six bones? Take note of areas that are more difficult to move through and spend more time in these areas. Usually one side is easier that the other.

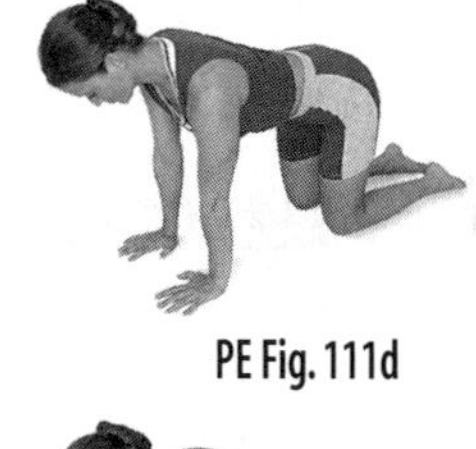

PE Fig. 111d

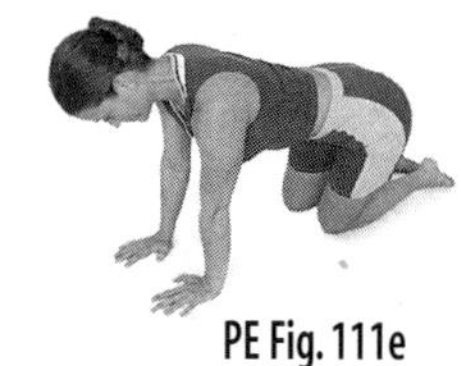

PE Fig. 111e

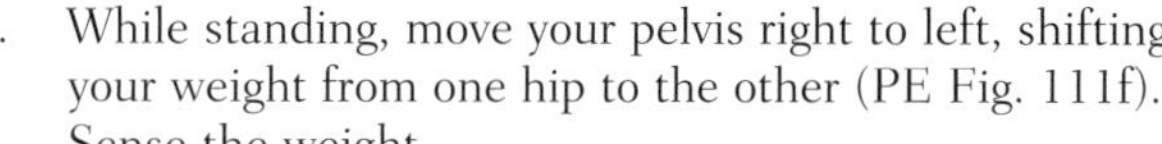

6. While standing, move your pelvis right to left, shifting your weight from one hip to the other (PE Fig. 111f). Sense the weight shift between the inner and outer arches on both feet. Move to one side, then to the other in an easy, smooth action (PE Fig. 111g). Avoid hiking up your hips (PE Fig. 111h).

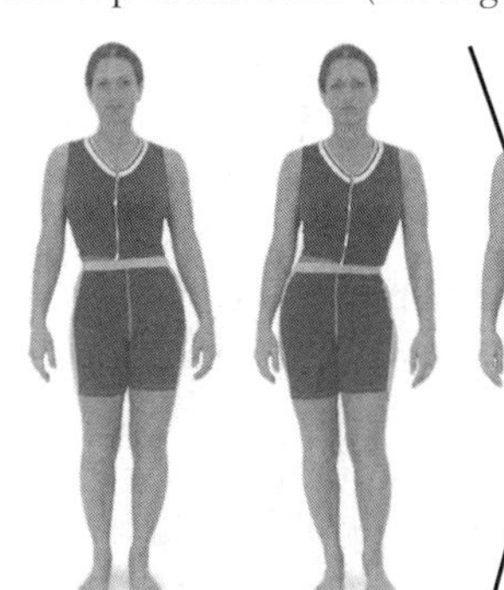

PE Fig. 111f **PE Fig. 111g**

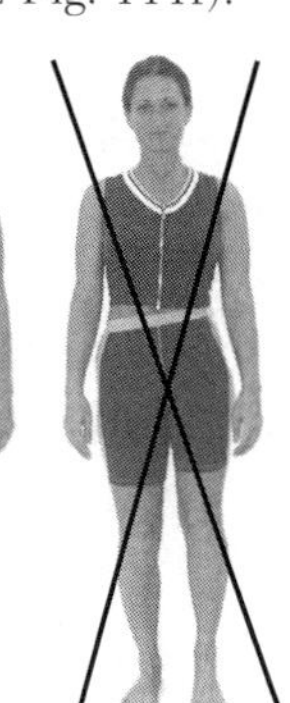

PE Fig. 111h

EMSPress.com

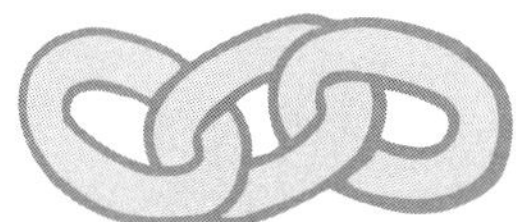

Links to Practical Applications

Observing Gait Patterns

An effective way to learn about efficient gait, other than feeling it, is to start watching other people walk. Sit in a park, airport, or mall and watch people pass by. Here are some things to look for:

- **Are the legs swinging under the body?**
- **Are the knees pointing forward?**
- **Does the front heel reach as the back toes push off?**
- **Does the person roll through five toes?**
- **Is there a spring in the arches or are the feet flat?**
- **Is the upper body over the pelvis?**
- **Or does the person lean back, walk on the outside of the feet, or lean forward and walk on the toes?**
- **Do the hips swing side to side? Does the pelvis swing back to front?**
- **Does the pelvis rise an inch or two as the pelvis shifts up and over the standing leg?**
- **Do the arms swing in opposition to each and in opposition to the legs?**
- **Are the head and neck responsive to each step, or are they rigid, thrust forward or held back?**

although if a person has a habit of chronically holding the pelvis in a tilt or standing with the weight shifted to one leg or hip, the action of the muscles working to maintain this position will be restricted during movement. Many people become habituated to standing on one leg with one hip thrust out to the side, which puts undue stress on the ligamentous capsule around the hip socket, or chronically tucking the pelvis under, which compresses the sacrum.

By practicing the range of motion in the pelvic tilts and shifts, a person can become aware of a neutral alignment in the pelvis and learn to move efficiently from this centered position. Also, practicing push and reach patterns in the legs and tail can help a person to become balanced and symmetrical in lower body movements, and therefore make more efficient pelvic tilts and shifts.

Walking

A person's gait can be as individualized as a written signature, although the mechanics of walking are generally the same for everybody. As mentioned in the last chapter, walking involves two primary phases in each leg—a *stance phase* and a *swing phase*. At any given point in the gait pattern, one leg supports weight while the other leg swings through. The stance phase begins when the heel strikes the ground and lasts as long as the foot is in contact with the ground. The swing phase begins at toe-off and lasts as long as the foot is off the ground. The stance phase is slightly longer than the swing phase so that one foot is always on the ground. A rhythmic alteration between the stance and swing phases continues throughout the gait.

Walking can be broken down into six primary movements of the lower body:

- pelvic rotation
- pelvic tilt
- lateral pelvic shift
- knee flexion and extension
- hip flexion and extension
- knee and ankle interaction

Each of these six movements contributes equally to an efficient gait pattern and has been discussed either directly or indirectly in previous text. By dissociating the individual components of movement, a person can determine which component to work with in patterning to improve the overall gait. Inefficiency of any one component, which usually occurs when one or more joints fail to go through their full range of motion, increases the effort and reduces the efficiency of the entire gait. For example, if the sacroiliac

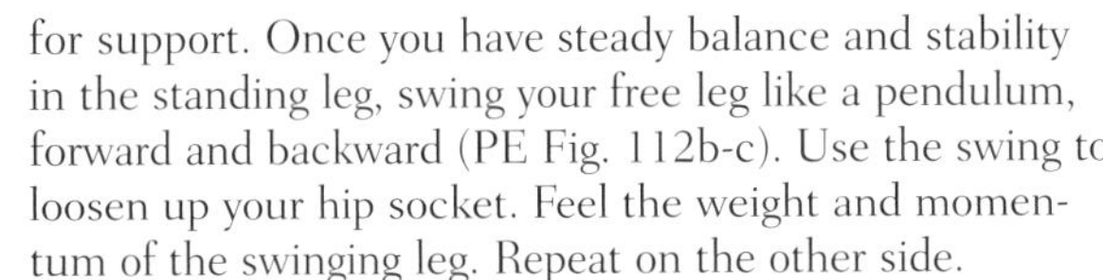

Patterning Exercise #112: Exploring the Stance and Swing Phase

1. *To explore balance and alignment in the stance phase*: Walk around, taking about five steps, then stop and balance on one leg (PE Fig. 112a). Continue to balance on that leg for several seconds. Then continue walking. Now stop and balance on the other leg. Continue to walk and stop, balancing on one leg, then the other.

Feedback: Do you step onto a straight, fully extended standing leg? If your gait is balanced, you should. People who walk with their knees bent, never reaching full extension, will have trouble stepping onto an extended stance leg.

PE Fig. 112a

2. *To explore the swing phase*: Start by standing comfortably. If you have trouble balancing on one leg, hold onto something stable (like a wall, doorknob, or table) for support. Once you have steady balance and stability in the standing leg, swing your free leg like a pendulum, forward and backward (PE Fig. 112b-c). Use the swing to loosen up your hip socket. Feel the weight and momentum of the swinging leg. Repeat on the other side.
3. When you are finished with both explorations, walk around and take note of any changes in your gait.

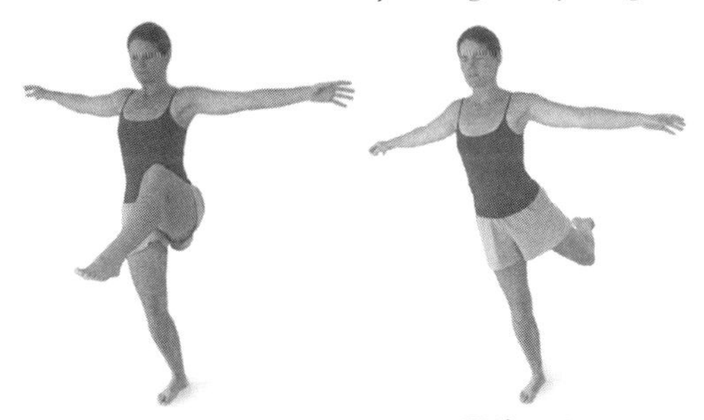

PE Fig. 112b **PE Fig. 112c**

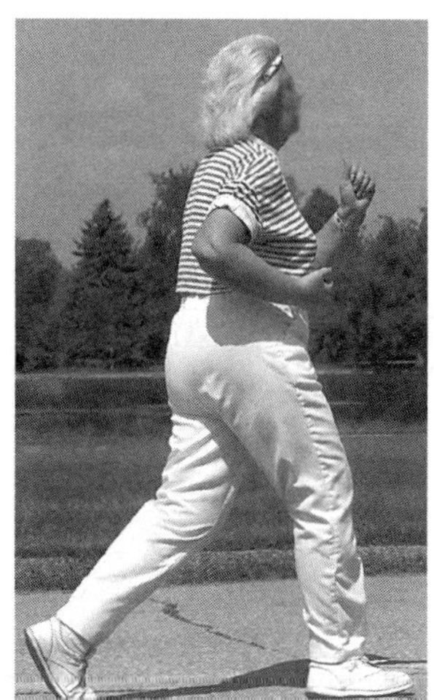

Figure 10.52 Is this woman walking or running?

joints around the sacrum are restricted, the hips cannot rotate forward and back. As a result, the pelvis will move in a rigid, block-like manner and rotational forces will translate to the next available joint. If the restriction is in the lumbar spine, the lower back might twist or tilt in an exaggerated manner.

What differentiates walking from running is that during walking the stance phase is longer than the swing phase because both feet are simultaneously on the ground for a period of time. During running the two phases are of more even duration because only one foot is weight-bearing at a time. There is a "float moment" when both feet come off the ground. Many amateur runners leave one foot on the ground at all times, which gives them a heavy, flat-footed gait pattern that prevents full flexion and extension cycles of the legs (Figure 10.52). This type of gait also lacks the push from the back foot and the spring action in the vault of the arches. People with this type of gait pattern would be better off taking brisk walks because a flat-footed run cannot adequately absorb the shock of impact on each stride and can easily lead to joint strain and damage.

Stepping through the Whole Foot

While walking, it is important to transfer weight through the whole foot, rolling from the heels to toes on each step. The back foot pushes off with the toes, flexing and bending all five *metatarsal joints* in a hinge-like action. The front foot reaches with the heel, which initiates the transfer of the body up and over the stance foot. Ideally, a push in the toes of the back foot is balanced with a reach in the heel of the front foot (Figure 10.53). The push-off needs to stretch all five toes evenly to fully extend the back leg and to transfer through the center of the ankle and leg.

Rolfers teach a simple exercise to encourage people to let the front of the ankle fall open at the end of pushing off with the toes. They have a client walk slowly, and as the client reaches the end of the toe-off movement, turn the ankle and drag the top of the toes a short distance on the floor (see PE Fig. 113f). This exercise exaggerates extension that a person gets in the ankle of the back leg by rolling completely through the toes and flexing the *metatarsophalangeal joints*. These joints must flex for a person to push off with the back

Patterning Exercise #113: Foot Reflexes and Walking

1. *Waking up reflexes in the feet:* Lie down on your back, and have a partner gently stimulate the soles of your feet to stimulate flexor withdrawal reflexes (PE Fig. 113a-b). Switch roles and repeat.
2. Sit comfortably and press the sole of your foot on a tennis ball several times. Repeat on the other foot.
3. Lightly bounce on a minitramp (PE Fig. 113c). Allow the force of the bounce to travel from your feet through the vertebral discs along the front of the spine. Sense the spring in your joints from your feet to your head.
4. Lightly jog on a minitramp to stimulate the spring in your feet and legs (PE Fig. 113d).
5. *Walking:* As you walk, reach with your front heel as you push off with your back foot and roll through all five toes (PE Fig. 113e). Allow each toe on your back foot to fully extend, particularly your big toe. Imagine lights on the bottom of each toe shining behind you as you roll through your toes.
6. Feel the front of your back ankle extend and open on each step. To exaggerate this, walk slowly and drag the toes on the foot behind you on each step (PE Fig. 113f). This will help you sense how the front of the ankle extends and opens.
7. Contrast this by walking with stiff toes. How does this change your gait?

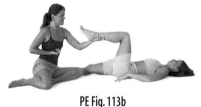

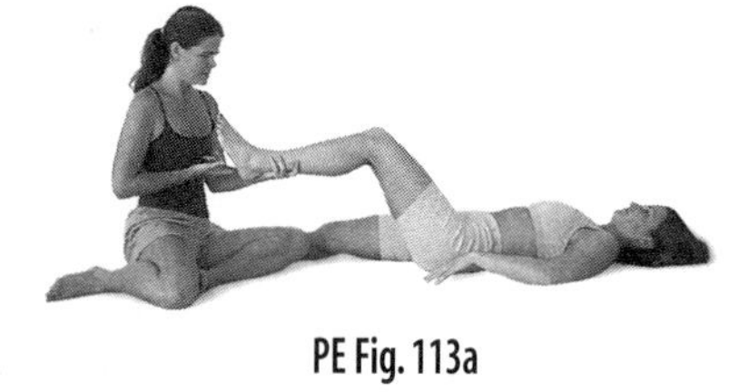

PE Fig. 113a

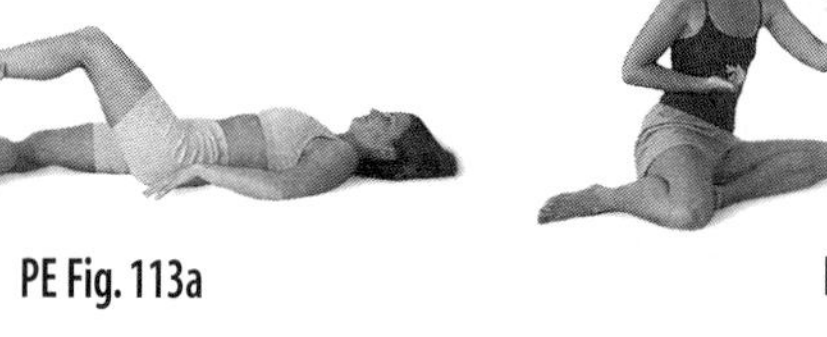

PE Fig. 113b

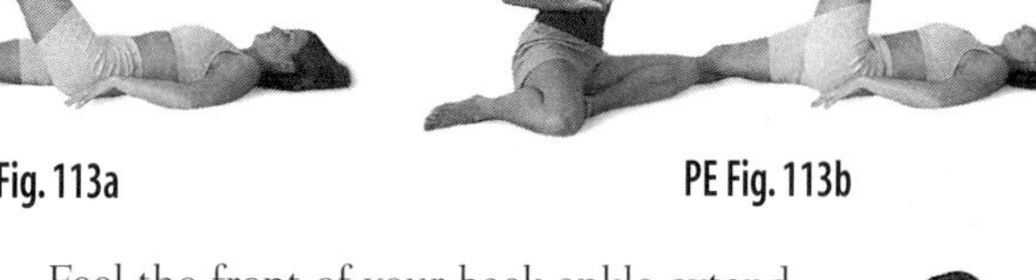

PE Fig. 113c

PE Fig. 113d

PE Fig. 113f

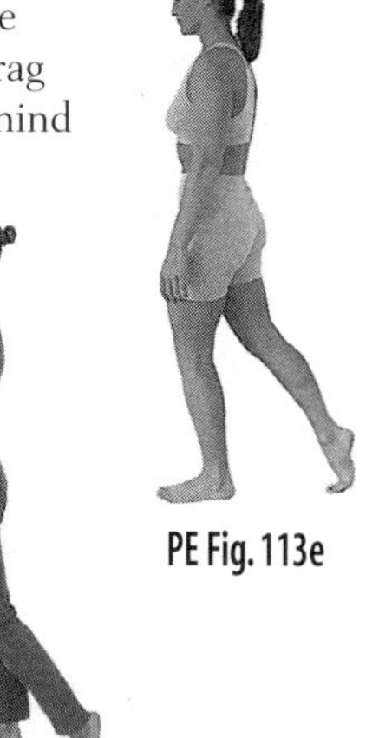

PE Fig. 113e

EMSPress.com

Patterning Exercise #114: Fall and Recovery Exploration

1. Stand on one foot (PE Fig. 114a). If you have good balance, close your eyes; if not, keep them open. Eventually you will lose your balance, and one leg will reflexively step out to catch you (PE Fig. 114b-c). Practice several times, then repeat on the other side.

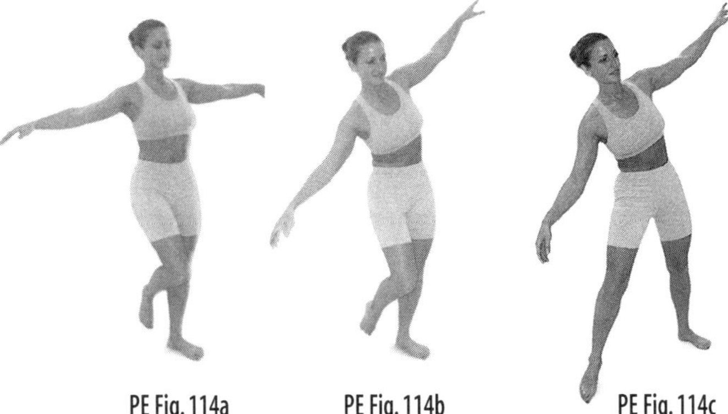

PE Fig. 114a PE Fig. 114b PE Fig. 114c

2. Stand about two or three feet from a stable table or counter. Put both hands on it to support you, then lean forward with your body vertically aligned, flexing only at the ankle joint (PE Fig. 114d).
3. Check yourself in a mirror if you can. Does your body break anywhere but at your ankles? If so, push yourself back up and lean again, isolating the flexion in the front of your ankles. You should be able to maintain your vertical alignment as you lean forward (the same way a person does during a push-up).
4. As you lean, let one knee drop forward so that the hip and knee bend (PE Fig. 114e). Then straighten it and let the other knee drop forward. Sense how each leg falls from the hip, the same dynamic that occurs in the legs while walking.

Caution: Read the entire instructions for the next step before you proceed. Attempt this exploration only if you are physically fit with no wrist problems, have good balance, and have good reflexes. This exercise is best done on a firm but flexible mat or well-padded carpet. If falling on the floor is too risky for you, explore falling into a couch or bed.

5. Stand in a relaxed, comfortable posture with both feet under you. Lean forward and fall, catching yourself with your arms (PE Fig. 114f). One leg and both arms should reflexively move to catch you. Your body should lean forward like a tipping column. Practice several times, catching yourself with the opposite leg each time.

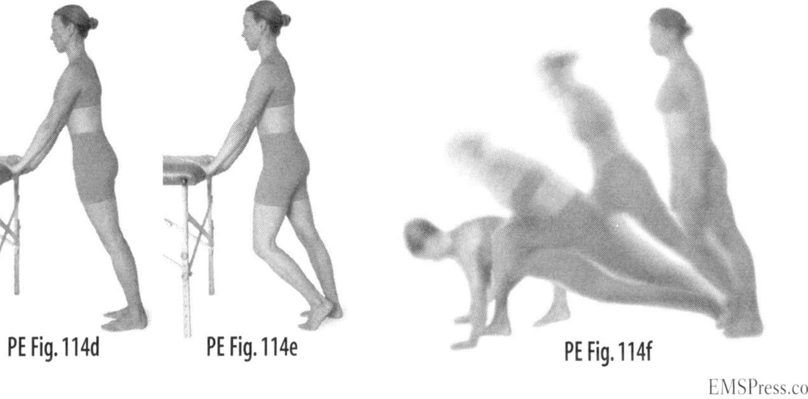

PE Fig. 114d PE Fig. 114e PE Fig. 114f

EMSPress.com

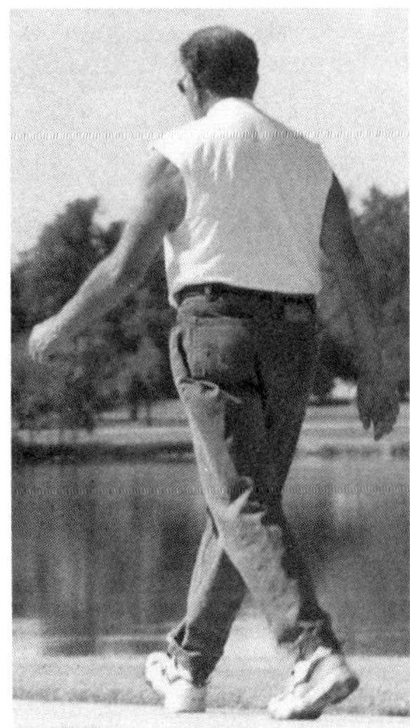

Figure 10.53 Walking involves a reach with the front foot and a push from the back foot.

leg, an action that propels a person forward.

Walking becomes lighter and easier when the spring action in the arches, which was described earlier, is active. Conversely, walking becomes heavier and cumbersome if the soles of the feet remain flat. Working with flexor withdrawal and extensor thrust reflexes in the feet can help restore articulation in the arches. Also, the arches can be strengthened with the "inchworm" exercise (see PE Fig. 108b-c) by jumping on a minitramp, or by rolling back and forth on a physioball and pushing off with the feet. A person can also have someone stimulate the reflexes in the feet and legs by stroking the soles of the feet in a manner that causes the person to withdraw the leg.

Walking is a constant cycle of **fall and recovery**, of losing one's balance and regaining it. Whenever a person falls forward, one leg naturally and reflexively extends to catch the body. For this action to be efficient, the entire body must maintain a stable yet responsive vertical alignment, and the joint action in the forward motion needs to occur mainly at the ankle joint. During walking, the ankle flexes and extends like a hinge between two distinct lever arms: the *foot*, which is oriented horizontally, and the *body*, which is oriented vertically. As we lean forward, the length of our feet determines how far we lean. For example, a clown can lean forward at a comic angle because his shoes are three feet long.

People tend to brace the body to prevent falling, particularly when the base of support is unstable. This bracing actually interferes with a person's ability to fall and recover without injury. Also, any break in the vertical integrity of skeletal alignment, which is secured by postural muscles, will interfere with the efficiency of the fall-and-recovery mechanism.

SUMMARY

This chapter is the last one in Part 2 on the practice of somatic patterning, which is a distillation of the actual movement mechanics of patterning. It provides an overview of the fundamental movement patterns that make up the myriad of activities we do every day. Although a thorough understanding of the biomechanics of kinesiology is an area generally left to experts, anyone can learn and practice the fundamental movement patterns of the human body.

By improving the efficiency of the fundamental patterns of flexion, extension, and rotation in the four limbs and spine, a person can begin to differentiate the elements that combine to make up more complex movement patterns. If any one fundamental pattern is faulty, isolating and working with that pattern can affect the economy of all movement patterns. Thus, by going through each fundamental pattern, a person will not only improve body awareness, control of parts, and overall coordination, but will also be able to identify what part of a faulty pattern reduces the economy of the overall motion.

The integrity and stability of a neutral posture in extension, particularly of the spine, provides a foundation for all of the fundamental movement patterns. Therefore, when exploring the fundamental movement patterns, it is important to be able to feel the neutral position of the skeleton in an extended, upright posture and to initiate movement from a neutral posture for economy of motion and optimal joint and muscle balance. To achieve this end, a person could first learn the isometric exercises for postural stabilization in Chapter 9, then use them to secure a stable posture while practicing the fundamental movement patterns. Practicing these exercises will not only improve economy of motion, but also will enhance comfort, may reduce pain, and will improve posture, which will ultimately improve performance in any activity.

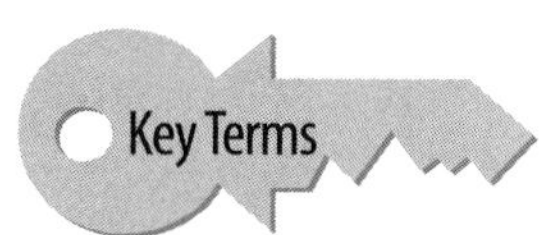

abduction
adduction
anterior tilt
arcing
backward rotation
backward shift
circumduction
depression
dorsiflexion
elevation
eversion
fall and recovery
forward rotation
forward shift
fundamental movement patterns
gradation with rotation
head righting reactions
inversion
inward rotation
kyphotic curve
lateral rotation
lateral shift
lordotic curve
lumbar-pelvic rhythm
outward rotation
plantar flexion
posterior tilt
pronation
protraction
retraction
scapulohumeral rhythm
supination

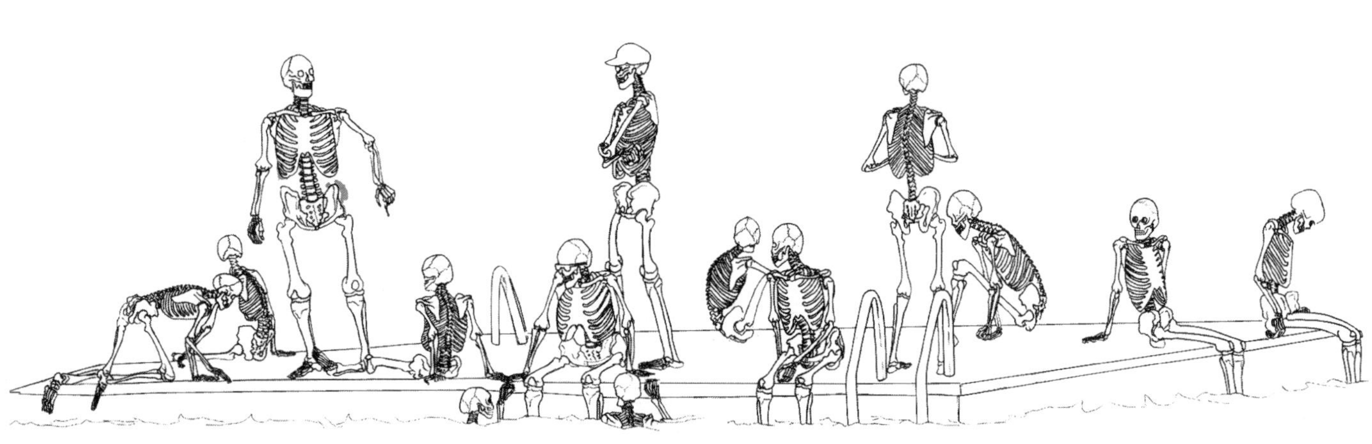

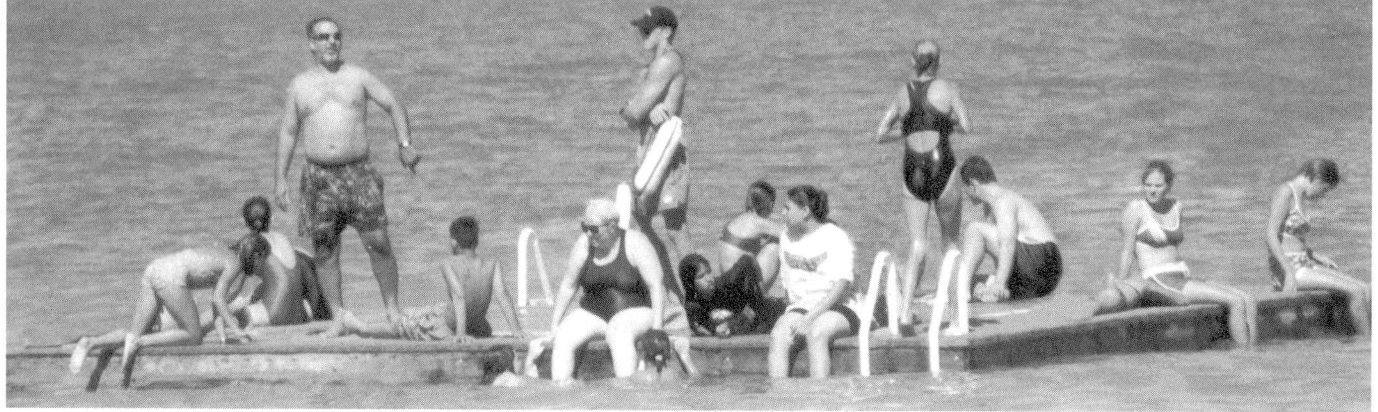

Part 3: History

Somatic therapies are being developed at a rapid pace. The proliferation of modalities and approaches in the general field of somatics can be confusing to the novice and practitioner alike. The chapters in Part 3 cover somatic principles underlying those modalities that work to change somatic patterns. These five chapters present an overview of diverse somatic approaches that work to change body-mind patterns of movement and psychophysiology. The overview is limited to what this author believes are the groundbreaking approaches in the respective areas. As a result, many useful and at times better-known second- and third-generation approaches that have grown out of these seminal works are not included here. Modalities and approaches are presented here in five categories, each a separate chapter of Part 3:

- Western movement therapies
- integrative manual therapies
- physiological patterning
- behavioral and cognitive patterning
- body-based psychotherapies

This history is not meant as a representation of how to practice any modality or system. Although such a history cannot help but reflect the views of the author, for the sake of accuracy, experts in each modality were given the opportunity to review the text on their respective system. Lastly, this history is presented as a background for the theory and practice found in Parts 1 and 2 of this book.

OVERVIEW OF CHAPTER 11

THE ALEXANDER TECHNIQUE
- Inhibition
- Verbal Directives and Light Touch
- Process Orientation and Philosophy
- The Johannesburg Trial

LABANALYSIS
- Movement Choirs and Pageants
- Effort Qualities and Personality Assessment
- Space Harmony

THE LABAN/BARTENIEFF INSTITUTE OF MOVEMENT STUDIES (LIMS)

FELDENKRAIS AND AWARENESS THROUGH MOVEMENT
- Roots of the Feldenkrais Method
- Functional Integration and Private Sessions
- Feldenkrais Concepts about Development and Movement

PSYCHOPHYSICAL MOVEMENT EDUCATION
- Ideokinetic Facilitation
- The Constructive Rest Position

SENSORY AWARENESS

BODY-MIND CENTERING
- Developmental Patterning: Reflexes, Reactions, and Responses
- Automatic Movement and Cellular Touch

CONTINUUM MOVEMENT

PILATES METHOD

CONTACT IMPROVISATION

11

Integrative Movement Modalities

> **In the esoteric schools of thought a Tibetan parable is told. According to the story, a man without awareness is like a carriage whose passengers are the desires, with the muscles for horses, while the carriage itself is the skeleton. Awareness is the sleeping coachman. As long as the coachman remains asleep the carriage will be dragged aimlessly here and there. Each passenger seeks a different destination and the horses pull different ways. But when the coachman is wide awake and holds the reins the horses will pull the carriage and bring every passenger to his proper destination.**
>
> ***—Moshe Feldenkrais***

The integrative movement modalities cover a broad range of approaches. This range reflects the fact that there are, of course, many qualifiers to movement. There is more movement or less movement, more ease or less ease, and greater flow or lesser flow. Some of the somatic pioneers who developed the systems reviewed in this chapter had strong ideas about what efficient movement should be like, while others worked in more organic styles, focusing on feeling and sensing the qualities of free-form movement explorations. But they all shared one precept: *when the mind becomes fixed on an idea, the body stops moving*. To elicit integrative movement—movement that is integrated into a person's ongoing thoughts and feelings—a method must promote fluid cognition (thinking); otherwise, a person assumes a rigid idea about the "right" or "wrong" ways to move, and this mental construct becomes fixated in the actual fibers of the posture.

Each modality presented in this section portrays a somewhat different perspective, yet as a group they share a similar premise. This premise is that the fluid and unencumbered movement of the body will dissolve the fixations of the mind. Each historical figure presented here felt that too narrow a system of movement education does not allow for individual differences, although their own unique differences influenced the nature of their work. And each of their modalities specializes in one or more aspects of a diverse yet holistic approach to somatic patterning.

Many of the integrated movement therapies developed out of their founders' personal needs. Some were looking for help with health problems that doctors said could not be remedied. Instead of passively accepting physical maladies deemed untreatable, they embarked on disciplined programs of self-study that led them to their discoveries. Rejecting the prevailing norms, many swam against the tide of popular culture to develop their work. Others came upon their discoveries by accident, and still others simply had the good fortune and right combination of circumstances for developing their approaches.

The history covered here is by no means complete. The presentation is more or less chronological and includes the somatic movement therapies that are most well known in the United States. A European, Asian, or South American writer might compile a completely different chronology. Rather than a strict chronological history, then, the purpose of this review is to provide an overview of the fundamental theories and applications of somatic patterning.

Many of the movement modalities presented here are slowly gaining recognition as specialties of *movement therapy,* apart from bodywork or traditional physical therapy. Certified graduates of a number of these schools qualify with the International Somatic Movement Education and Therapy Association (ISMETA) to become "registered movement therapists" (RMTs), a registry of the Department of Labor.[155] ISMETA has defined four principles that guide the practice of movement therapy:

1. to notice restrictive habit patterns that limit awareness;
2. to gain an increased awareness and control over body-mind habit patterns;
3. to learn how to use movement skills during daily tasks;
4. to use these skills to promote self-reliant health care.[156]

Keep in mind while reading this section that it was written to flesh out the basic principles of somatic patterning. Rather than focusing on a single system, it is useful to view the group as a whole body of work, with each system contributing an elemental part to the bigger picture.

THE ALEXANDER TECHNIQUE

Frederick Mathias Alexander (1869–1955), the creator of the **Alexander Technique**, was an Australian actor whose fledgling career was interrupted by a severe case of laryngitis, precipitated by hoarseness and gasping during his performances. In the 1890s, Alexander sought the advice of many well-intentioned doctors who prescribed long periods of rest and medications, only to have the hoarseness return when he went back to work reciting. Determined to solve his own problems, Alexander began to notice how he thrust his chest and chin forward just before beginning to speak. This fixed posture also arched his back and actually depressed his larynx, cutting off his breathing. After unsuccessfully working one by one with the parts of the pattern, he recognized the need to address the whole body pattern in order to solve his problem. Using a system of three-way mirrors to view his entire body from all directions, Alexander began to study his pattern of assuming a fixated posture before moving and speaking.

Inhibition

Alexander discovered that his senses, without help from the mirrors, were unreliable in providing the feedback he needed to change his pattern. When he relied on his senses alone, he merely created a new pattern on top of the old one. In essence, *what he habitually did in order to adjust his body created more tension.* Since habit did not usually yield the end results he sought, Alexander worked to gain conscious control over his habitual posture, to inhibit his faulty habits, and then direct his movement with more intelligent choices using conscious control.

His system of conscious control presented three choices of response to his postural dilemma:

- to respond in an old habitual way;
- to respond in a new manner;
- to not to respond at all.

This led Alexander to develop the concept of inhibition as a basis for his work. He inhibited the faulty head-neck muscle pattern that was squeezing off his throat and taught himself to initiate speech and motion with a subtle lift of the head. Over time, Alexander came to believe that inhibition improved not just physical health, but was the key to all human development, particularly in education, about which he stated, "Restoring inhibition so that it can perform its integrative function on a conscious level should be the primary aim of education."[157]

Verbal Directives and Light Touch

In the spring of 1904, Alexander moved to London with his younger brother, Albert Reden Alexander, and began promoting the Alexander Technique with letters to the press and articles describing his discoveries in the "use of the self." After practicing his method for a considerable time, the two brothers began teaching.

Recognizing how words can create specific neuromuscular responses, Alexander and his brother developed a precise system of carefully chosen verbal directives, or "orders," as Mathias Alexander called them. The directives are intended to help a student "aim and point" the muscles toward an intended movement. They are meant to help students inhibit chronic and habitual muscular effort and elicit the experience of light, effortless movement. One common directive Alexander used is: "Allow your head to lift forward and up."

This determined innovator also developed a system of light touch to guide a student's head forward and up while initiating movement (Figure 11.1). His tactile guidance was designed to evoke a set of reflexes that lengthened the entire spine. The effectiveness of the touch was in direct proportion to the lightness of the pressure applied—just enough to give the suggestion of where vertical is and to trigger a subtle reflex that brings the head over the body. This subtle yet intentional touch evoked a lift that many have described as a freeing and pleasurable sense of kinesthetic lightness.

During the same time that Alexander was developing his work, innovative physiologists such as Sir Charles Sherrington were identifying rudimentary reflexes in animals. It appears that the mechanism Alexander discovered and developed a technique to evoke involved head righting reactions. However, Alexander never identified the technique as head righting.

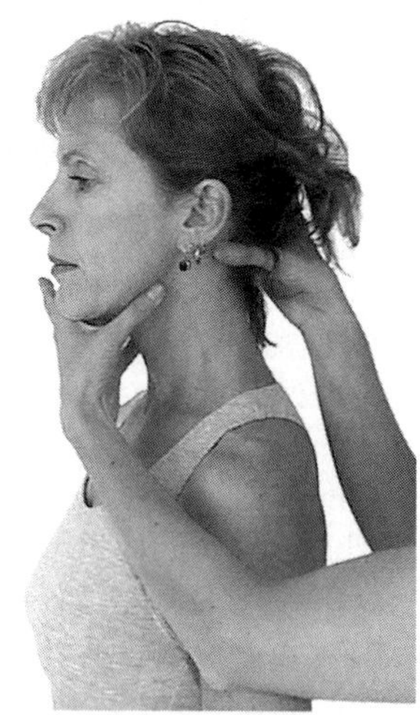

Figure 11.1 A practitioner helping a student find head righting

One of Alexander's advanced procedures, taught only after a student could adequately inhibit chronic tension and shortening in the neck muscles, is "the whispered ah," which demonstrates how inhibition affects speech and respiration. This experiential procedure is practiced in order to detect and inhibit extraneous effort involved in either speaking or breathing. It involves five steps, which are:

1. Relax the tongue by letting it rest with its tip touching the lower teeth.
2. Think of something funny, then smile without opening the mouth to relax the lips and the back of the mouth.
3. Open the mouth by sensing gravity's pull releasing the lower jaw forward and down, being careful not to tilt the head back.
4. Whisper the sound "ah." (Other sounds can be substituted, either whispered or spoken.)
5. Close the mouth and continue to whisper "ah" while keeping the air passages open in the back of the throat.[158]

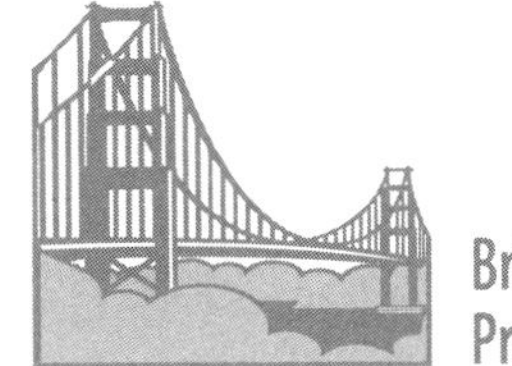

Bridge to Practice

Eliciting Head Righting Reactions

To elicit head righting in your client, stand at her side (she can be sitting or standing) and place your hand under her occiput, gently cradling the back of the skull while reaching your thumb and middle finger to the hollow place under her ear lobes. Make sure your touch is light so that you do not push your client off center or interfere with her balance. With your hands, give her a gentle nudge to lift the head up over the body, then release. The direction of the lift will depend upon where her head is resting in relation to her body. If it is back, lift it forward and up, then release. Although this lift may sound simple, it takes a lot of practice to be effective. Most practitioners use too much pressure and direction when first learning, which can elicit a guarding response.

Process Orientation and Philosophy

Alexander's work was a great success. Many prominent actors and physicians sought his services and referred students to him and his brother. In 1910, he published *Man's Supreme Inheritance,* at which point his work made a transition from a therapeutic approach to a philosophical approach. As Frank Jones explained in his well-known book *Body Awareness*, Alexander believed that "under the influence of civilization, man as a whole—as a human being—had degenerated, that he had reached a stage where his instincts were no longer reliable, and that if he were going to survive, his behavior had to be regenerated on a conscious level."[159]

In the 1940s, the prevailing systems of physical education were based on a military model in which a person was taught to tighten the body into a rigid posture. Alexander's work was in direct opposition to this model. It is unique in that it offers what he called a "means whereby" the student focuses on the process rather than a goal. The Alexander Technique was one of the first process-oriented systems of movement education, and it gained popularity because it was effective in improving posture and relieving pain.

What patterns of tension do you feel in your neck? Can you reach through the top of your head and elongate your neck in an effortless manner? If not, what prevents this motion?

The dropping of the atomic bomb in 1945 shook many people to the core, and Alexander was among them. He believed that the event would be considered a warning that reactive instincts rather than rational thinking guide human behavior. He felt that as a species, humans could either create our own destruction or harness the vast powers of inhibition to control human reactions, bridging conscious and unconscious actions. He wrote about this philosophy in *Knowing How to Stop,* published in 1946, in which he discussed the inhibition of subconscious reactions as a fundamental means of change for humanity as a whole.[160]

The Johannesburg Trial

Like the work of many pioneers with new ideas, Alexander's work was challenged when the enthusiastic students of Irene Tasker, an Alexander teacher in Johannesburg, started to introduce the technique into the schools of South Africa. They wanted to replace the orthodox system of militaristic physical education on the grounds that they were being forced to teach movement that was unrelated to how the children moved in school and in their daily lives.

This action started a controversy that was eventually taken to trial by two men named Dr. E. H. Cluver and Dr. Ernst Jokl, who sought to defend their relatively new but orthodox "science of physical education."

The trial began 16 February 1948, ran for three years, and was well publicized. Many witnesses and experts were called in on both sides to either defend or disclaim the Alexander Technique. In the end, the judge found no evidence to disprove the claims that Alexander's work actually did improve physical health and functioning. Yet while Alexander was awarded 1,000 pounds in damages after the trial, public schools in South Africa were still prohibited from using his technique.

Although this work was unable to gain a foothold in the public school systems, it did gain widespread recognition elsewhere. Like Alexander himself, many actors and performers continue to turn to this work to improve

Patterning Exercise #115: Head Righting Reactions

Use this exercise to elicit the reflex mechanism that brings the head from an off-center place to vertical, and to release neck tension.

1. Sit comfortably with your eyes closed. Slowly and subtly rock your head at the uppermost joints between the skull and first vertebra (PE Fig. 115a). Find the axis of these joints by placing your index fingers lightly in the hollow places under each ear lobe. Sense subtle weight changes through the skull and spine as you move. Feel when your head is off-center and when it comes back to vertical. How does this affect the rest of your spine?
2. Continue the movement until you can clearly feel the place where your head is centered effortlessly over your body. If you have a lot of neck tension, you may feel discomfort until the tension relaxes.
3. Now explore tipping your head off center, then moving it back to center in one simple action, using the least amount of effort possible (PE Fig. 115b-c). Explore it first with your eyes closed, then opened. When you feel that the movement of your head from an off-center position to an on-center position becomes automatic, the head righting reaction is working.

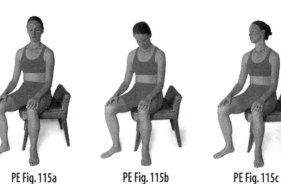

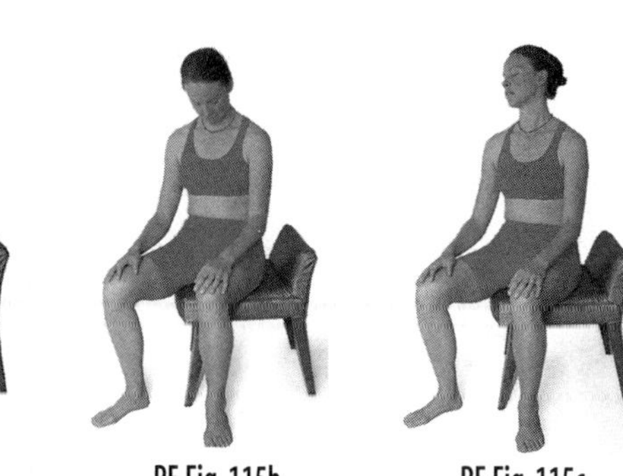
PE Fig. 115a PE Fig. 115b PE Fig. 115c

their speech, breath, and delivery. Numerous people with pain from injury or sustained misuse of the body also use the Alexander Technique to learn how to release tension patterns that form around the pain.

Alexander created what is now one of the oldest of the body-based therapies. He defined some fundamental patterning principles and techniques, specifically those that involve conscious control of body movement, the inhibition of faulty habits, the head righting mechanism, and the use of objective feedback rather than distorted kinesthetic feedback from the senses. Alexander also left a rich legacy of philosophical writings that delve into the relationships among the body, the mind, and the environment, particularly in regard to man's use of self and related ethical issues in the world at large.

During his lifetime, Alexander and his work had a great impact on many people and ushered in a new era of body-mind therapies. He had a number of influential students and supporters, including the American philosopher and educator John Dewey, the English author and critic Aldous Huxley, the Dutch ethnologist and Nobel Prize winner Nikolaas Tinbergen, and the well-known British playwright George Bernard Shaw. We could rightly call F. M. Alexander the "grandfather of somatic patterning."

LABANALYSIS

During the same period that Alexander was developing his work in London, Rudolph Laban (1879–1958) swam against the political tide in Eastern Europe and taught people how to express spiritual vision in the body through dance. Laban rejected the privilege, rank, and wealth of his father, a famous military governor in Hungary, and went out on his own to develop his artistic vision. Being a natural athlete, dancer, gymnast, and lover of nature who was also trained in painting and music, Laban chose poverty over a position of prestige and wealth in order to pursue what gave him the most pleasure in life—leading large groups of people through community dance celebrations.

To get a sense of Laban's work, imagine hundreds of Eastern Europeans tiring of shallow lifestyles, deciding to throw off the restraints of materialistic, spectator-based entertainment, and spending their leisure time exploring an unusual sport—large group dances designed to advance their collective spiritual growth. Now imagine numerous groups of 100 people each gathering over a number of years to rehearse for a community dance pageant. This is what happened in Nazi Germany when thousands of people paraded through the German streets in a collective dance concert. Our closest experience to Laban's pageants might be thousands of people gyrating together at a rock concert, yet they differed in motivation. The daring Laban ignited the gatherings with his longing to transcend the avarice and hate of the times with dances motivated by spiritual aspirations.

Other art forms flourished because there were ways to record them in songs or plays, but the restaging of dance depended on the memory of a proficient performer. This was another of Laban's many talents. In 1913, after exploring studies in art and music, Laban thoroughly devoted himself to improving the status of dance as an art form. He choreographed movement experiences designed to motivate people to dance in a way that inspired joy and gave people a sense of cooperative fulfillment. Like a loving father figure, Laban oversaw the physical and spiritual development of hundreds of thousands of dancers, perhaps a million in his lifetime.

Laban had a vision about the dynamics of movement that recast the way in which anyone who has studied his work views patterns. Out of his pursuit came **Labanalysis**, one of the most multifaceted systems of movement analysis ever created. Labanalysis moves a step beyond the traditional system of movement analysis found in biomechanics and kinesiology. It is a study of the qualities and personas of a movement phrase, a language for how psychology expresses in movement by exploring the intersections of *spatial*, *effort*, and *body* elements. Laban sought balance in the body by exploring the opposing tensions and efforts found in a full range of movement. He looked at *where we move*, *how we move*, *when we move*, and *what moves*.[161] Laban eventually codified movement into a system of written notation, later called **Labanotation**.

In what life situations do large groups of people move together in unison, and what effect does it have?

Laban passionately believed that dance is the great liberator of the heart and soul, and that only through a broad range of expressive movement experiences can one embody the full richness, joy, and inspiration that life has to offer. Exploring Labanalysis in movement improvisations can be quite therapeutic in every sense of the word. By doing so, individuals inevitably access unfamiliar styles of movement that expand the boundaries and limitations of each person's individualized range.

Movement Choirs and Pageants

Even more amazing than Laban's ideas was his ability to implement them. This charismatic man led large numbers of people through group dance performances in Germany, Switzerland, and Austria between 1913 and 1939. With innate skill as a body-based leader and his dynamic enthusiasm, Laban motivated hundreds of thousands of people to perform natural, joyous movement in "movement choirs." According to this innovative somatic pioneer, the sole purpose of these choirs was to "help people feel the joy of moving together, to strengthen their desire for community connections."[162]

The cultural and political events in Germany during the movement choirs underscored the power of the group mind. Laban's choirs illuminated the paradox that swept the German culture, juxtaposing the spiritually enlivening pageants of the trade workers with the foreboding marches of the Nazi legions. This paradox also brings up the universal dilemma: *how can a person remain a unique individual while still contributing to a sense of community?* Laban explored this question in his study of the individual motivations that people had to move. He carefully observed the natural movements of many different worker guilds (such as the rhythmic swings of the builders), and choreographed them into simple patterns for large groups to perform, bringing out the innate dancer within the working-class person. Thousands would gather on a hillside and move together in synchrony in a symphony of simple gestures and motions that Laban would orchestrate.

The movement choirs reached a zenith in 1929 when Laban was commissioned to produce a pageant procession of 10,000 laborers from many trades and guilds in Vienna. Laban's performers moved through the streets to choreography that was based on the natural rhythms and gestures of their working movements.[163] During preparation for another pageant to be performed at the 1936 Munich Olympics, Laban's work was cut short when the Nazis put him under house arrest and prohibited the use of his notation, the reading of his books, and even the mentioning of his name. Although the soul of the movement pageants was squashed out by the Nazi legions, Laban's work as well as Nazism give testimony to the enormous positive or negative power that can be generated in a crowd when people move together in synchrony.

Effort Qualities and Personality Assessment

Laban eventually fled from Germany to England, where he was hired by the British government to study the efficiency of movement in factory workers. During this time, he and Warren Lamb refined and compiled a system of movement analysis based on four **effort elements** that described the changing attitudes and contrasting qualities of movement. These elements—*free* or *bound* flow, *strong* or *light* weight, *direct* or *indirect* attention to space, and *quick* or *sustained* time—are what Laban at times referred to as the *how, what, where*, and *when* of movement (Figure 11.2).[164]

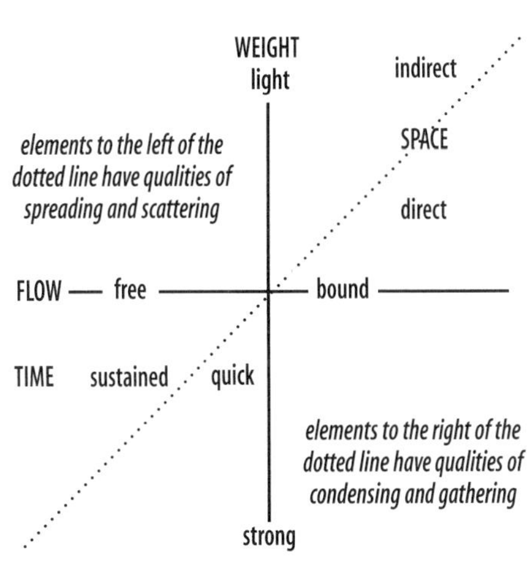

Figure 11.2 Laban's effort qualities

During his exile from Germany, Laban spent a considerable amount of time assessing the movement patterns of individuals in mental health institutions and concluded that repressed and undeveloped movement qualities reflected "shadow" aspects of the unconscious. He related the concepts of the inward and outward flow of motion to Carl Jung's introverted and extroverted

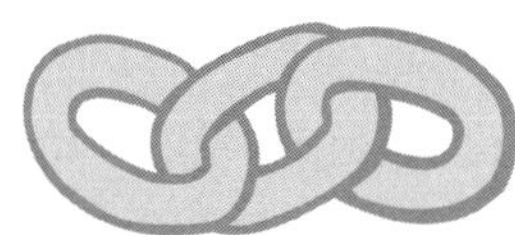

Links to Practical Applications

Letting Go of Control

When practicing any patterning exercise, explore doing the movement slowly, with a controlled, bound flow. Then contrast this by doing the same movement faster, with a free-flow quality, one that energizes circulation. For example, use a rocking or swinging motion. Using a free-flow quality will help you to let go of any tension you may have incurred doing a slow, controlled movement. It will also help you to pattern the movement to be more fluid and natural.

personality types, and correlated the four efforts—flow, weight, space, and time—with the four Jungian concepts of the mind: thinking, sensation, feeling, and intuition.

Laban believed from his studies that each person moves in and out of a personal repertoire of various effort qualities. These qualities communicate personality affinities and changing moods (or mood fixations) of a person. Hence, psychological issues can often be observed in the qualities with which a person moves. To be able to move with a broad range of effort qualities requires both psychological and physical fluidity and adaptability.

In terms of Labanalysts, flow can be free or bound. Free flow embodies a degree of ease, fluidity, and streaming abandonment, as seen in swinging or rocking motions. People who embody free flow qualities are often carefree and easygoing, able to flow through life without too many mishaps, and can bounce back from stress with minimal impact. Bound flow is just the opposite: restrained and controlled. It gives a person control over a movement because it requires the ability to stop at any point along a movement sequence, like the careful work of a surgeon's hands or of a tailor threading a needle.

Labanalysts also found that the dualities of flow modulate each other, crystallizing at different times in diverse activities and emotional states. As discussed in Chapter 6 under fluid qualities of movement, too bound a flow can result in rigidity, whereas too free a flow can result in the lack of direction or boundaries. "Shape flow" is an effort term used to describe the stream of changing shapes that flow through the body during movement, such as the expansion and deflation of respiration, or the undulating waves of a belly dancer.

Labanalysts describe the qualities of weight in terms of strength or lightness. Strong weight qualities are associated with having impact and power, being stable and grounded, or, on the less positive side, being compressed and immovable. Light qualities are associated with delicacy, precision, and levity, or with dreamy or flighty tendencies. In some patterns, one part of the body may move with a light quality while other areas move with strength.

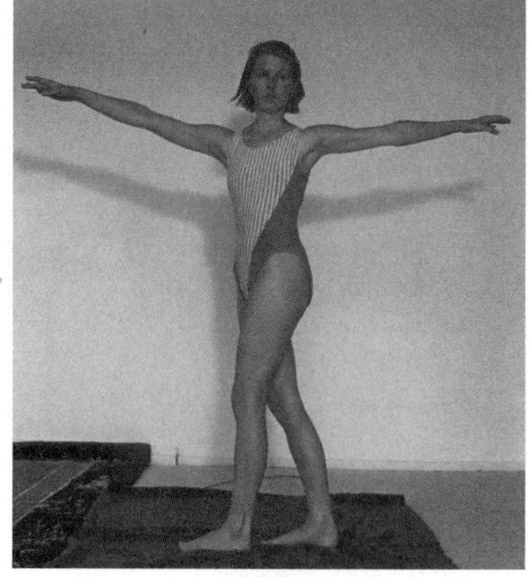

Figure 11.3 As this pose illustrates, two-dimensional movement is flat and unnatural.

Space can be attended to with either a direct or indirect attention. In a direct approach to space, a person zeroes in on a single focus. In an indirect approach, a person has an inclusive, encompassing focus and is able to attend to multiple directions at one time. Ideally, a person's movement repertoire encompasses both polarities, having the ability to focus concentration on one place while being flexible enough to focus more broadly.

In terms of the time frame that movement occurs within, Labanalysts note that time can be broken into small, quick impulses or can be drawn out and lingering, like the contrasting paces of the tortoise and the hare. Our contemporary difficulty with time is that it exists outside a person and is something over which we exert no control, yet each individual has innate, instinctual rhythms that express a quality of inner time completely separate from the influence of a clock. This creates a human dilemma: whether to attend to our natural rhythms or to follow the rhythms imposed on us. For example, do we eat when hungry, or always eat three times a day whether we are hungry or not?

Space Harmony

Laban not only mapped out effort qualities, he also mapped out shapes of movement—how the body forms itself in space—and spatial pathways of movement. His system used geometric forms to explore how a moving body passes through dimensions and planes, how pathways carve shapes in space, and how bodies move when free of the pull of gravity. A large misconception about range of movement comes from the linear movements presented in kinesiology. Although traditional kinesiological studies communicate valuable information for understanding joint and muscle function, typical movement rarely occurs in one direction or one plane (Figure 11.3). It is much more dynamic and flowing, literally sculpting tracers in space. Laban's spatial studies brought the dynamic nature of body movement to life.

His most eloquent explorations involved a study of the "transversals," which are curvilinear pathways that sequence from the corner of one plane to a corner of a second plane to the corner of the third. (Recall from Chapter 10 Bartenieff's simplified representation of the three planes as the "door, wheel, and table.") Since each plane has four corners, these twelve corners, when connected, make an icosahedron (Figure 11.4). Connecting three corners from three different planes makes up a "three-ring," a shape that we recognize in the pathways of planets in orbit. By exploring movement along transversal pathways, Laban Movement Analysts help their students to broaden and enliven their range of movement within all dimensions (Figure 11.5). This process not only expands a person's movement vocabulary, it can evoke movement through a previously unaccessed range, opening up new territory not only in the muscles and joints, but also in a person's psyche.

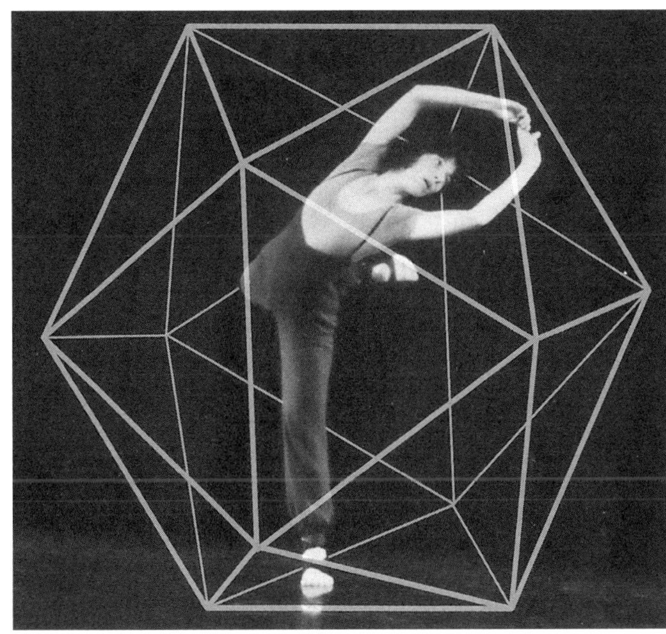

Figure 11.4 Dancer in an icosahedron (photos courtesy of M. Seereiter).

Laban's work is far too vast to do it justice in this short discussion. Also, his work, like many of the detailed somatic therapies, is like music: a written description cannot come close to expressing the experience of it. Still, other concepts of Labanalysis that should at least be noted here are the following:

- *Gestural* and *postural patterns*. Gestural patterns sequence through a single body part while postural patterns involve full-body movements that sequence through the entire body. These two terms were coined by Warren Lamb, Laban's associate.[165]
- *Emphasis*. Different elements can be emphasized in a movement sequence. The emphasis of a movement is the main statement the movement is making, the attitude of a motion. A person might habitually emphasize movement with a sustained pause, a sharp flick of the shoulder, or a tilt of the head. We can observe the artifacts that an emphasis leaves on structure, such as shoulder tension from a habit of repeatedly hiking, or pulling to one location in space, emphasizing that stress.

If a single effort quality were embodied fully in one person, what would this person's body type be? Personality?

- *Simultaneous* and *sequential movement*. Simultaneous movement occurs in the body all at once. Sequential movement progresses from one part of the body to another.
- *Central* or *peripheral initiation*. Central initiation of movement begins in the core of the body. Peripheral initiation begins at the ends of the limbs at the hands or feet.
- *Shaping* and *carving movements*. Those movements that sculpt spatial forms within or around the body, in either internal or external space. A symphony conductor carves forms in space; a baker shapes the frosting on a cake. Some shaping and carving terms that describe contrasting movements are: gathering/scattering, rising/sinking (up-down dimension), spreading/enclosing (side-to-side movement), and advancing/retreating (front-to-back movement).
- *Spokelike* or *arclike directional movement*. These movements create a boundary or bridge between a mover and an object (either space, a prop, or another person). A spokelike movement travels along a straight line, such as a fencer thrusting a sword, whereas an arclike movement creates a curvilinear pathway, such as swinging a baseball bat or swatting a fly.
- *Personal or shared kinesphere*. The area of space that surrounds a person, into which he or she can reach while still maintaining a stationary and stable base of support, or the space that we share with others. A shy, diminutive person might have a small kinesphere without much extension, whereas an aggressive person might have a large, overextended kinesphere; similarly, a noisy, aggressive group might have a large shared kinesphere.[166]

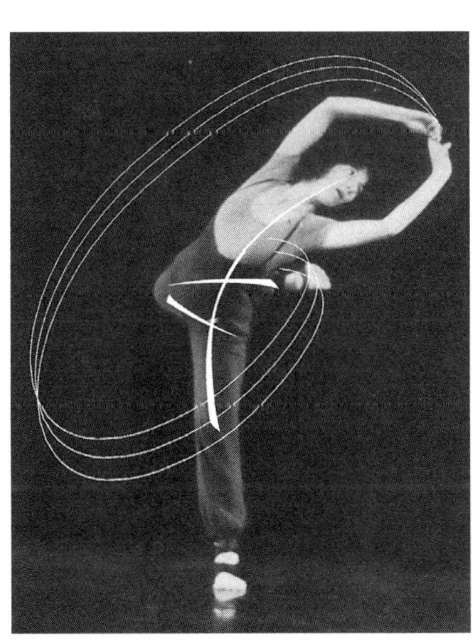

Figure 11.5 An illustration of the spatial pathways the dancer moves through and the spatial pulls within her body

Laban saw movement objectively through the eyes of both an artist and a mathematician. In his vision, he found that movement was the way to sculpt and shape the space around us, to extend our inner joy out to the external world. With his unusual perception, Laban created a language for describing movement that went

Patterning Exercise #116: Exploring Movement in the Three Planes

Movement is relative to the position of your body; therefore, you need to maintain a spatial relationship to feel dimensions with clarity as you move. To do so, keep the four corners of your body—two shoulders and two hips—facing directly forward as you move.

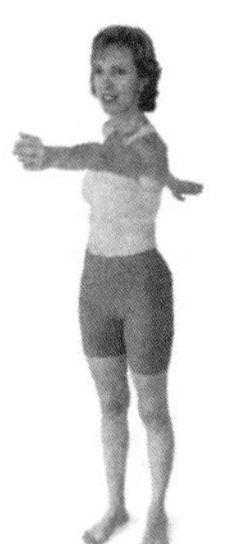

PE Fig. 116a

1. *To feel the axes:* Draw your hands up and down along the vertical axis of your body. Widen and narrow your hands across the horizontal axis of the body. Reach your hands directly forward and back along the front-back axis (chest or waist level) (PE Fig. 116a).
2. *To feel the frontal plane:* Stand as though you are in a wide door frame and touch your hands and feet to its four corners (PE Fig. 116b). Explore moving within this plane, which will involve lateral bending.
3. *To feel the horizontal plane:* Lie on your belly and reach your hands and feet out to the four corners of the room. Then, standing, tip your trunk parallel to the floor and reach both hands and one foot to three corners of the room (PE Fig. 116c). Change legs and repeat on the other leg. How far can you move in this plane?
4. *To feel the sagittal plane:* Imagine you are standing at the center of a large wheel, one that has been cut square. Keeping your hips and shoulders facing forward, reach your hands and feet to the corners of the floor planes. Then switch sides. Trace the corners of this plane with your hands.

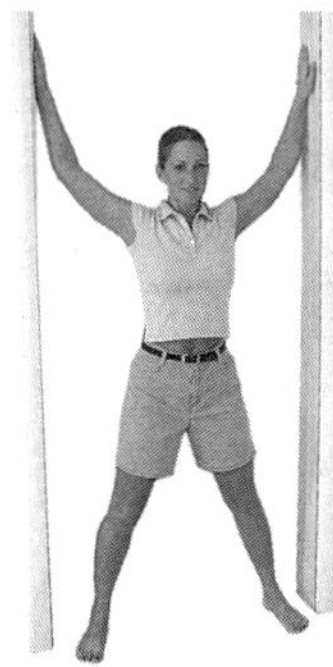

PE Fig. 116b

5. *To feel three-dimensional movement:* With one hand, draw the corners of each plane around your body. You should have 12 corner points in space around your body.
6. *To feel a three-ring:* Now, pick three corners, one from each plane, and draw an imaginary line with your hand to connect them. Notice how your arm naturally makes curvilinear movements. (There are 12 variations possible; 24 if you reverse them.) Next, begin to trace connections among three points, one from each plane, to draw a three-ring. Notice the three-dimensional shape of your movement. Then reverse the movement. What quality do you move with? Can you feel the swirling quality?

PE Fig. 116c

EMSPress.com

beyond body mechanics. He continued to lecture and teach until his death in 1958. Near the end of his life, he maintained his agility and, at age 70, could still perform outstanding aerial leaps.

Of all the movement therapies, Laban's work is probably the least understood by somatic practitioners. Labanalysis provides a system through which a person can access, embody, and unify the broad range of expression available in movement. Because it has been refined into such a precise analysis and notation, Labanalysis can seem mechanical and confined. The genius of this work is that it gives a person a detailed and precise movement-based language with which to explore and describe the psychological states inherent in specific effort qualities and geometric forms of movements.

How much of your kinesphere do you occupy, either physically or energetically? Stand in front of a full-length mirror to study how much of your body expands into your kinesphere.

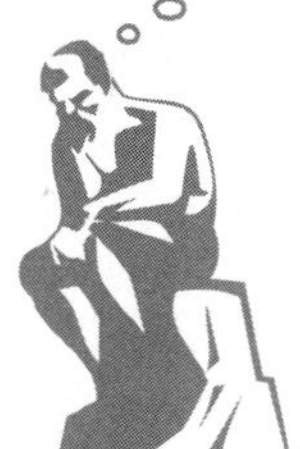

THE LABAN/BARTENIEFF INSTITUTE OF MOVEMENT STUDIES (LIMS)

One of Laban's students, a professional dancer named Irmgaard Bartenieff (1900–1980) fled from Germany to New York City with her Jewish husband in 1936 to escape the tyranny of the Nazis. She became a physical therapist and joined the Dance Notation Bureau, where she further developed Laban's material and, in 1978, founded the Laban/Bartenieff Institute of Movement Studies (LIMS).

Many of Laban's original concepts have been further developed by a second generation of Laban analysts such as Bartenieff. She pioneered a movement language that is used today by dance therapists as a framework to interpret the psychological motivations that underlie movement.

Other key Laban analysts who pursued the understanding of psychological drives through movement are Marion North, who did extensive research on combinations of effort qualities that crystallize in states and drives, which she wrote about in *Personality Assessment through Movement*, and Judith Kestenberg, who developed a system of personality profiling that is based on parent-child patterns of interaction and is also taught in many systems of dance therapy.[167]

Bartenieff's unique contribution to SP is her development of what she called the **Bartenieff Fundamentals**. They include a series of six basic patterns—the *thigh lift*, the *forward pelvic shift*, the *lateral shift*, the *diagonal knee drop*, the *body half*, and the *arm circle*—that Bartenieff delineated as a vehicle through which students of Labanalysis can explore and embody these concepts (Figure 11.6). They are also made up of a number of concepts and principles that include "dynamic alignment, breath support, core support, rotary factor, initiation and sequence, spatial intent, center of weight, weight transference, effort intent, and developmental patterning and its support for level change."[168] In her own words, Bartenieff explained the need for these fundamentals in movement education:

> We frequently observe in teaching choreutics that beginning students, who have been taught body movement mainly by imitation with emphasis on body parts and muscular tension, have difficulty with spatial exploration, that is, spatial intent. This is manifested, for instance, when they are given such tasks as reaching and exploring the areas around the body with the arms, particularly in the back. They may go into awkward contortions . . . exclaiming, "I cannot get there, I am stuck." Sometimes the teacher must manipulate the rotary element and direct the arm so the student can find a releasing action into the back area.[169]

Bartenieff began developing the Bartenieff Fundamentals while working as a physical therapist rehabilitating polio patients. Through her series of six basic movement patterns, Bartenieff integrated spatial concepts of movement with body mechanics to motivate her patients to move. As Bartenieff wrote: "The introduction of the spatial concepts required an awareness of intent on the part of the patient that activated his will and thus connected his independent participation to his own recovery."[170]

When a movement teacher guides a student's movement with clear spatial direction, to the amazement of the student, difficult movements are accomplished with surprising ease, efficiency, and increased range. During a class in the Bartenieff Fundamentals, the teacher gives students cues that elicit both effort qualities and spatial configurations to create dynamic, curvilinear movements that integrate the elements of body, space, and effort. During a thigh lift, for example, the teacher might suggest that students allow the shin to float effortlessly up toward the ceiling. During a diagonal knee drop, students might be asked to spiral the thighs while lowering both knees to the floor on one side. Or during a forward pelvic shift, students may imagine the coccyx and sacrum as a shovel that is scooping dirt forward and up.

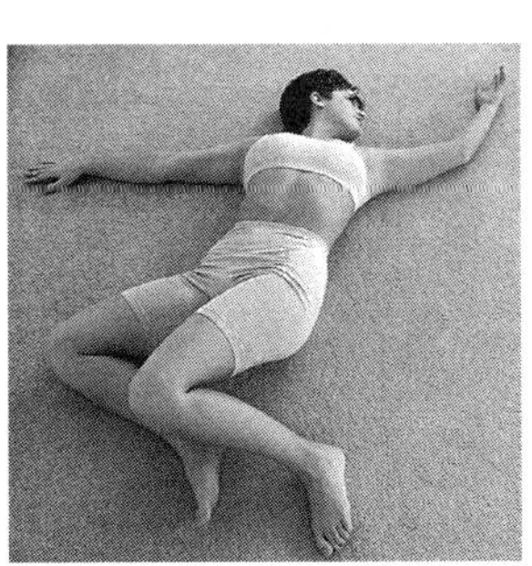

Figure 11.7 The diagonal connection between the upper and lower body

While training in the Bartenieff Fundamentals, students learn to initiate each action from the center, the core of the body. To prepare for a motion, students take a deep breath and exhale, allowing the weight of the abdominal organs to drop and sink into the lower back, "hollowing out" the lower abdomen. This allows movement to initiate in the contraction of the iliopsoas muscle, which begins

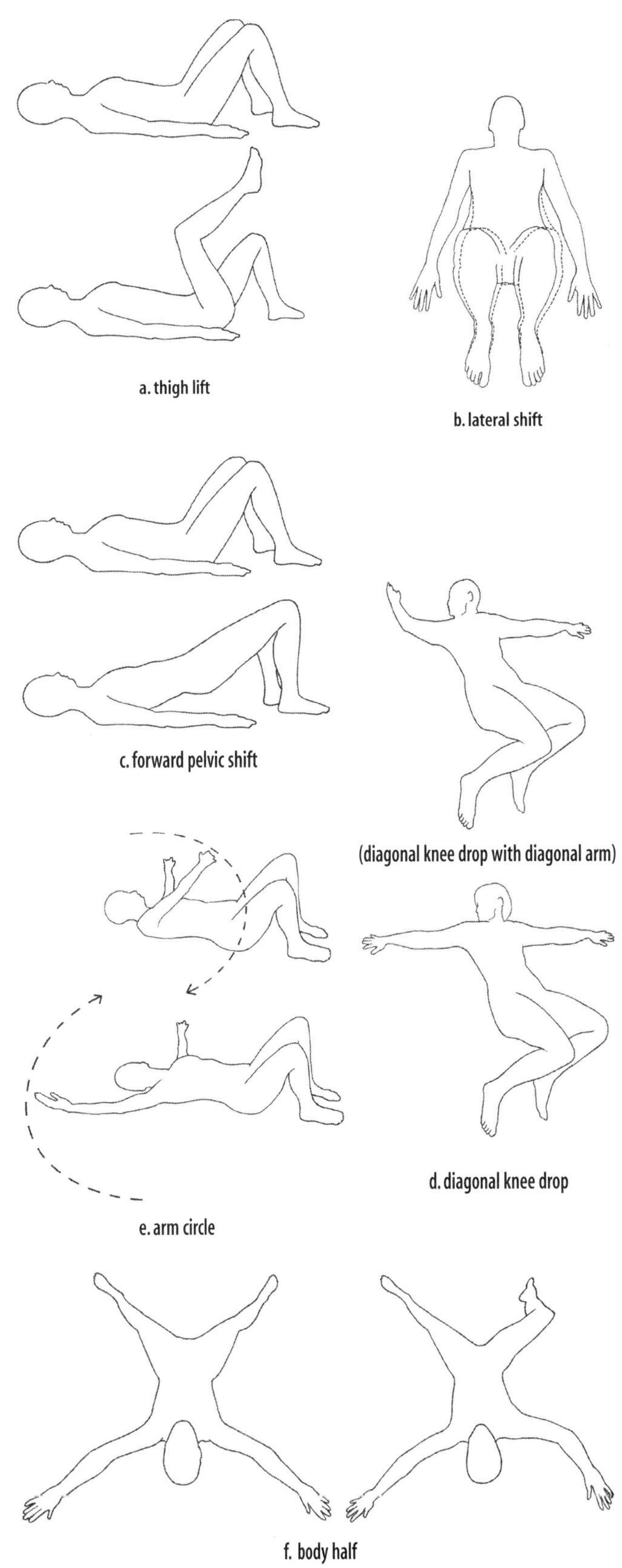

Figure 11.6a-f The Bartenieff Fundamentals

intrinsic flexion in the trunk and stabilizes the lumbar spine during each action. Students support movement along spatial pathways by internally shaping the body. To do this, they learn to shape the pelvis in either a concave or convex shape during the "in" and "out" phases of a movement—a flexion-extension cycle—and use this rounded shape to shift the lower body with ease.

All the Bartenieff Fundamentals stress a core connection between the upper and lower body (Figure 11.7). The movements of the arms are connected to the lower body through the center of the trunk and are explored along a full range of rotary pathways and diagonal arcs. Students also explore internal shaping by feeling the shapes of different tones, or sounds, within the body's cavities. For instance, the sound "aaah" makes a tall oval shape and reverberation in the throat and torso, whereas the sound "eeeh" makes a wide oval.

The Bartenieff Fundamentals are part of the primary curriculum taught in the LIMS program. LIMS students also study the elements of space and effort described in the previous section. LIMS teachers and certified practitioners have contributed widely to the fields of dance, and many of them are professional dancers. Bartenieff and her associates have also influenced the field of dance therapy with their rich psychological assessment of movement, which is often part of the core curriculum in dance therapy programs.

FELDENKRAIS AND AWARENESS THROUGH MOVEMENT

Moshe Feldenkrais (1904–1982) was a brilliant scientist and movement educator from eastern Europe. At the age of 14, he went to Palestine and fought in the Hanageh, a self-defense group of about 300 young men that protected Jewish people in the area from surrounding enemies in what is now the state of Israel. After seeing more than half of the Hanageh killed by Arab swordsmen, the young Feldenkrais analyzed the Hanageh's combat skills in Jujitsu to discover the source of their inadequacy in combat. Wanting to save lives, he then took three years to develop his own martial art, to teach it to the men in Hanageh, and then to write a small booklet about it. The booklet was published and distributed from Paris to protect Feldenkrais from capital punishment that the English were dispensing for such "crimes" at that time in their position as the protectorate of the Palestinian territory.

After his military work in Palestine, Feldenkrais went on to study mechanical and electrical engineering, as well as physics, and claims to have completely forgotten about the booklet.[171] To his surprise, in 1932 the Japanese Minister of Education and Japanese Ambassador to France contacted him. They had found in his booklet a technique they had never heard of that impressed them. Spurred by this discovery, they wanted to enlist him in their efforts to bring the Japanese martial art of judo to Europe. Feldenkrais trained with them, became the first European black belt, and began teaching judo while finishing his education.

After receiving a doctorate in physics from the Sorbonne, Feldenkrais worked with the famous French physicist Frédéric Joliot-Curie, and later returned to what had become Israel for employment in the Israeli Defense Forces.

Roots of the Feldenkrais Method

When in his forties, Feldenkrais was told by doctors that he had a 50-50 chance of recovering from a chronic knee injury sustained in soccer years before, and that he probably would never walk again. Determined to beat the odds, this avid athlete and scientist began researching anatomy, psychology, neurophysiology, and learning theories, upon which he based a self-directed process of rehabilitation. Out of this process, he not only healed his knee and taught himself how to walk again, but he developed a new method of reeducating habitual movements that evolved into the **Feldenkrais Method**.

Feldenkrais recognized that habitual movements involve a set number of motor pathways and that each habitual movement we repeat recreates the same limited

The Feldenkrais Experience

In a large classroom, 200 students lay on the floor while a Feldenkrais instructor gave Awareness Through Movement instructions over a broadcast system:

"Slowly, with awareness, move your right hand out to your right side . . . turn your head to the right and follow it with your eyes . . . reverse the movement, taking your head and hand to the left . . . again, slowly and with awareness, repeat that movement about ten times.

"Now take your right hand to the right as your head turns left, then reverse the motion . . . again, repeat that movement about ten times, being aware of each tiny increment your hand and nose pass through along an arc over your body.

"Next, move your head and hand to the right as your eyes go to the left, then reverse. Again, repeat ten times. Move the eyes slowly so that you do not strain them. Move only in a range that is comfortable."

As the teacher's directives went on, she kept adding new elements to the original movement, such as moving the right leg across the body, then opening it. By the time the exercise was complete, I had gone through every combination of moving the head, eyes, right hand, and right leg from side to side that was possible. Then the teacher had us rest and compare the two sides of our bodies.

My right side felt much more open and relaxed than my left, plus the range of movement there had increased considerably. Finally, the instructor talked us through the same sequence on the left side, only this time we only visualized the movement without actually doing it. Surprisingly, the results were the same—my left side changed just as much as my right side.

pattern of motion over and over again. He sought to restore motor balance in the nervous system by increasing a sensory awareness of a broad range of movements, thereby creating more neuromuscular pathways. To do this, Feldenkrais created hundreds of movement lessons. The sheer volume of his lessons made habit-forming repetitions of exercises within his method unlikely.

Feldenkrais believed that learning occurs only when it is brought to a conscious level of awareness and that movement is the basis of awareness. He also felt that movement is the basis of learning; therefore, a system of movement education that promotes self-awareness is essential to human development. In his work, there is no ideal body posture or way to move; the focus is on the learning process, the intention to move, and how movement in one part of the body affects another. Feldenkrais students are directed to find positions from which to move that are comfortable and easy, to move slowly with an awareness of the subtle sensations created by the motion, and to find pathways that feel the most natural for each individual. A hallmark of this work is a focused awareness of small increments of motion along spatial pathways.

Like Laban and Alexander, Moshe Feldenkrais was also a prolific author who wrote many detailed books about his theories and his philosophies. *Awareness Through Movement* is the most well-known of his books. It introduces Feldenkrais's theories and methods of his system of movement education, also called **Awareness Through Movement**, in a series of movement exercises.[172]

Functional Integration and Private Sessions

Using hands-on work, called **Functional Integration**, a Feldenkrais practitioner gently guides the client's body through new pathways of motion. People have said that Moshe Feldenkrais's touch created a communication between the brain and body that allows the central nervous system to take over and spontaneously reorganize. The new organization frees the neurological core of the body from its musculoskeletal container, resulting in easier and more effortless movement.

The Feldenkrais hands-on work and the Awareness Through Movement classes are done with clients or students lying down or sitting in relaxed positions. These positions promote relaxation and avoid habitual or conscious efforts that result in excessive muscular strain. Distinguishing features of the Feldenkrais Method include:

- taking long periods of rest between movements;
- sensing where one's body is in relation to the supporting surface before, during, and after the action;
- performing small movements within one's range to actually increase the range of motion;
- going through precise visualizations of movements;
- finding motion through the pathway of least resistance;
- moving one area to achieve flexibility in another.

Feldenkrais was adamant in his belief that movement teachers should never demonstrate patterns because doing so would create what he calls "idiots," which we infer to mean people who learn by imitating others. He felt that learning and movement typically initiate in response to random environmental influences rather than by conscious direction and choice. His work was designed to cultivate a conscious, intrinsic initiation of action.[173] Feldenkrais rarely spoke during private sessions to avoid imprinting the client with his notions.

Feldenkrais Concepts about Development and Movement

We know that humans are born with only a fraction of the instinctive movement abilities that other animals have at birth. We develop primarily through movement experiences, which are shaped by random events and the imitation of habits. Feldenkrais identified some fundamental concepts about the relationship of movement to human development. Consciousness, defined by Feldenkrais as "the quality of observing by the higher nervous centers what is happening in the lower ones," is a relatively recent human capability.[174] Consciousness exists in the forebrain and develops when a person becomes aware of motor actions; therefore, motor activity precedes awareness. Two primary aspects of consciousness—*spatial orientation*, the perception of our location in space, and *patterns of sequential thinking*—are unique to our state of human consciousness. They are not found in sleeping states, in which we are unaware of time and space.

Feldenkrais stressed that the transition from the state of consciousness to the state of awareness must involve the motor cortex. He believed that "human infants twist and taste for hours" in order to resolve the asymmetry found only in the forebrain, where neural connections are made more slowly than in other parts of the nervous system.[175] Hence, the essence of his technique is to slow down a movement to reconnect body consciousness with awareness to give the forebrain ample time to recognize and reorganize neuromuscular pathways. Therefore, all Feldenkrais exercises and hands-on techniques are explored slowly with deliberation to cultivate the core of the Feldenkrais method—the development of awareness through body movement.

PSYCHOPHYSICAL MOVEMENT EDUCATION

Mabel Todd was a physical education teacher well ahead of her time. A faculty member at Columbia University Teachers College in New York during the late 1920s and early 1930s, she introduced novel concepts of training in physical education and dance. At the time, traditional physical education was based on the notion that the body needed to conform to militaristic models of posture and form. Efficiency in movement was a new concept that was rejected by most physical education instructors. Todd's work, based on visualizations created from a sound understanding of body mechanics, was considered radical and was not easily embraced by mainstream instructors. Yet Todd endured. She meticulously outlined principles that underlie efficient and balanced movement. Her groundbreaking book, *The Thinking Body*, analyzes the mechanical and organic principles of movement that spring out of a study of anatomical relationships and developmental processes.[176]

Todd referred to her work as **psychophysical education** and describe the interplay between physical and emotional patterns in the following passage:

> Behavior is rarely rational; it is habitually emotional. We may speak wise words as a result of reasoning, but the entire being reacts to feelings. For every thought supported by feeling, there is a muscle change. Primary muscle patterns being the biological heritage of man, man's whole body records his emotional thinking.
>
> The explorer and pioneer stand up; the prisoner and the slave crouch; the saint leans forward, the overseer and the magnate lean back . . . Thus the stuff of ages goes into man's thinking, is interpreted and comes out in movement and posture again. Personality goes into structure—by denial or affirmation into person again. It is an aspect of life in evolution.[177]

The term "thinking body" stems from the intelligent use of mental processes to organize balanced posture and movement. Todd developed a number of images out of her vision of balanced anatomical structures and physiological processes. Some key concepts in Todd's work include:

- the importance of centering movement and weight through the core of the human structure;
- a balance between tensile pulls of the tissues and compressional forces of the joints and bones;
- the importance of using the mind to intelligently direct movement.

Ideokinetic Facilitation

Lulu Sweigard was a student and associate of Mabel Todd's and a research pioneer in the study of postural improvement. She coined the term **ideokinetic facilitation** (introduced in Chapter 8 under "Imagery and Ideokinesis") to identify Todd's method of changing movement through imagery. The premise of this work is that the image or idea of movement alone is enough to begin a movement sequence along its most efficient pathway.[178] Sweigard felt that by concentrating on the desired movement, our nervous system, with its remarkable ability to organize patterns subconsciously, would automatically organize the most efficient pathway for that movement. Initiating new patterns requires imagery coupled with stillness to first inhibit old patterns through conscious inaction. Put another way, the "workhorses" of muscular habit must be quieted if new pathways for motion are to be effectively organized.

In the process of ideokinetic facilitation, or *ideokinesis*, a person imagines a desired movement without exerting any muscular effort toward that movement. The new movement is performed only after a new neuromuscular pathway is clearly established in a mental picture, which often leads to a spontaneous impulse that initiates an effortless pattern. Students of ideokinesis describe the experience with comments such as, "My leg seemed to float up all by itself" and "My arm had a mind of its own as it lightly circled over my head."

In her book *The Human Movement Potential,* Sweigard describes three factors that are essential to changing movement through imagery:

1. The student needs to know the exact *location* of the desired movement.
2. The student needs to know the exact *direction* of the movement.
3. The student needs to have the *desire to move*.[179]

As first described in Chapter 8 under the section titled "Visualization and Ideokinesis," Sweigard measured her students before and after posture classes in ideokinesis and found that nine changes occurred in the same locations and directions in all subjects. These changes included an increase in height and a greater conformity to the principles of mechanical balance. Sweigard also found that each student's center of weight had shifted more closely toward the core and base of his or her body.

The Constructive Rest Position

Ideokinesis is often practiced while in the **constructive rest position (CRP)**. Todd and Sweigard both had their students assume the CRP for short periods of time, about 20 to 30 minutes, to practice relaxation, recuperation, and rejuvenation (Figure 11.8). By relaxing in this position and actively focusing on allowing each vertebra in the back,

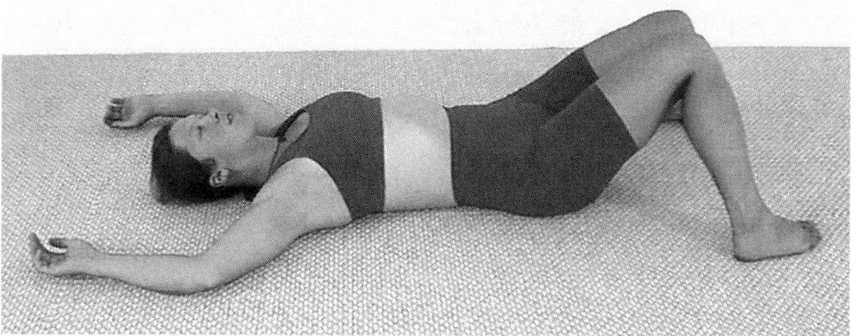

Figure 11.8 Variation on the constructive rest position, with arms overhead

particularly in the lower back and the area between the shoulder blades, to sink into the floor, a person can release chronic contractions in the spine and improve alignment. When the CRP is practiced regularly, people learn to consciously relax so that every time they return to it, the body remembers relaxation and rests a little more deeply than the time before. (The CRP or supine position with the knees up is also referred to as the **hooklying position**.)

Constructive rest underscores the fact that rest is an active process and that we need to practice it if we are to become adept at it. Todd stressed the importance of alternating periods of rest with every activity, even to the point of practicing some form of rest during continuous and rigorous activities, such as between strokes during swimming, or between steps while running. Constructive rest is now used so widely in dance training that it is not unusual to see dancers camped out on the floor in the CRP during breaks between rehearsals and classes.

One of Sweigard's favorite images using the CRP was to imagine the body as a wrinkled suit, then to visualize the wrinkles gradually flattening out. Another popular image, one that came out of Sweigard's posture laboratory, involves imagining the body as a peanut butter sandwich and visualizing the back slice of bread sliding down and the front slice lifting on each inhalation. Sweigard suggested that her students practice relaxing imagery in the CRP twice daily.

Todd's and Sweigard's anatomically sound images are widely used in dance training to pattern efficient movement. Although her classic text is out of print, Sweigard's images that grew out of her posture laboratory are still widely used in dance education and available in a book titled *Dynamic Alignment through Imagery*.[180]

SENSORY AWARENESS

At times it is easy to take our sensory apparatus for granted, overlooking the intricate processes in which information about the environment continually comes to us through our sense organs—the eyes, ears, nose, mouth, and skin. Most people receive sensory input unconsciously, yet in actuality, we selectively choose what comes into our awareness. We make choices every time we point our sense organs toward an object of perception. In short, perceiving is an active process.

Charlotte Selver (born in 1901) was a movement pioneer who refined the process of sensory reception into a process she called Sensory Awareness. **Sensory Awareness** is not a technique or a methodology: it involves no exercises or ideals. It is merely the process and practice of becoming more fully aware of sensory perceptions and refining this awareness.

Selver began developing Sensory Awareness in the United States in 1938, after which several prominent students popularized her work. Fritz Perls, the founder of Gestalt therapy (see Chapter 15) studied intensively with Selver in the 1940s. Perls used Sensory Awareness practices to develop Gestalt therapy, the first form of psychotherapy that incorporates body awareness into psychological process work. Alan Watts, the renowned philosopher, spiritual teacher, and writer, also studied with Selver. He described her work as "the living Zen" because he felt it truly was meditation in action.

In the practice of Sensory Awareness, a person focuses on expanding an awareness of his immediate experience, such as the sensations of the skin; the textures, colors, and smells of the environment; and the subtleties of sounds, temperature, and air currents. In a Sensory Awareness group, people often pair up and explore body awareness and touch, while the facilitator asks gentle questions that lead them into deeper levels of awareness and contact. She may ask students to notice the temperature of the skin, for example, as well as the quality of touch, responses to touch, and what happens when the area of contact shifts.

Each probe takes participants into deeper states of sensory awareness. This culminates in an altered perception and a more acute appreciation of the present experience. Participants begin to revel in the simple pleasures that are so easily overlooked, such as the smell of a flower or an appreciation of another person's smile or bright eyes. Selver's work quietly peels away the barriers that have built up through the habitual ways we have of interacting with people and the environment (Figure 11.9).

A Sensory Awareness workshop takes place in a simple, carpeted room without furniture, without distraction. Participants might start by sitting on the floor, then simply and slowly standing up while they are encouraged to observe the minute details of how they stand. They might be asked to stand with the eyes closed, in which case the participants become aware of how much they use vision for balance. As they locate where balance comes from with the eyes closed, their awareness of a standing balance changes. Or they might become aware of how the eyes are associated with thinking, and how closing the eyes affects thought patterns. Others may become aware of their eye lids resting over their eyes, or how the eyes flit incessantly when closed, still trying to look out behind closed lids.

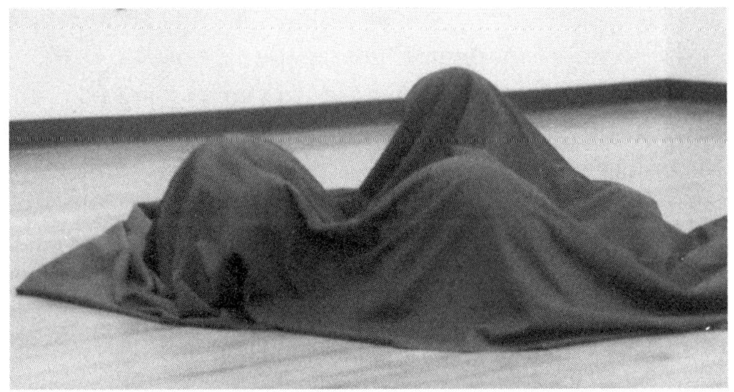

Figure 11.9 Play activities often involve sensory explorations, such as these children playing under the cloth (photo courtesy of K. Wasson).

Every Sensory Awareness experience is as unique as each person's individual mode of perception. Selver's husband, Charles Brooks, eloquently describes this process: "Attention to sensing quiets what is compulsive in our thought, so that the mind becomes free and available for its normal function of perception. The camper's lantern is blown out, and darkness fills with stars as the woods deepen and widen."[181]

Sensory Awareness builds upon the premise that intelligence is based on perception; therefore, expanding one's ability to perceive expands intelligence. This work effectively enlarges a person's present-moment awareness, allowing participants to appreciate the subtle and delicate nuances of the details of daily life.

Selver's work was groundbreaking when it began. She went on to teach it at Esalen in 1963. Today, Sensory Awareness as a practice is the foundation of many body-based therapies. Practitioners use its principles and improvisational form to track sensations in the body as they occur, to observe the nuances of the body's relationship to the environment, and to become more deeply aware of interactions between two people.

BODY-MIND CENTERING

Every summer near Amherst, Massachusetts, a large group of students gathers to participate in the study of **Body-Mind Centering (BMC).** The outside observer might have a hard time understanding what is going on in these unconventional classes in experiential anatomy and developmental movement, particularly if the group is submerged in an exploratory movement improvisation.

Unlike a typical dance or exercise class in which everyone is doing exactly the same movement, in BMC each person learns to follow her own intrinsic impulses. The outside observer would see only a jumble of twisting, swirling, slithering, and sliding bodies engrossed in a group improvisation. During this improvisation, the students are exploring the orchestra of physiological processes going on within their bodies, pulsing or floating, rocking and swaying to a sea of subconscious rhythms. Each movement reveals a hidden quality of the body's inner workings, creating impressions such as churning through the convoluted pathways of intestines, filtering across the walls of the capillaries, sliding down the filaments of the muscles, and rhythmically pumping out the arterial hoses.

As the students meander and twist in and around each other, their movement impulses permeate the group body, the group energy builds, the participants begin to play off each other's movements, and eventually move together as one group body. Movement themes ripple from one person to the next, transforming into new shapes and rhythms much as a crashing wave morphs into a new form at the shore. Many times these improvisations come to a spontaneous zenith and then settle, leaving the group in a resting huddle where each person basks in the afterglow of the exploration.

In a different type of BMC class, one focused on integrating cognition with experience, the observer might find the students strewn across the floor among scattered books and papers and drawings of the body, in pairs or small groups, practicing simple movements while cross-referencing anatomy texts. BMC seeks to integrate the body and mind by combining a cognitive study of the body with experiential study. To this end, BMC students explore anatomical details from textbooks, adding a subjective perspective by feeling the movement and touch qualities inherent in each tissue or movement pattern being explored.

Dancer and developmental movement specialist Bonnie Bainbridge Cohen created BMC. At the age of 16, Cohen began teaching dance to children with cerebral palsy and went on to become an occupational therapist and professional dancer. Cohen combined her many studies in martial arts, bodywork, yoga, voice, meditation, Laban Movement Analysis, and Kestenberg Movement Profiling to found the School for Body-Mind Centering in 1972. BMC students are a diverse group, often including dancers, bodyworkers, physical therapists, nurses, artists, psychotherapists, and many more. They are drawn together by a curiosity to study movement in a manner that balances cognitive processes with experiential learning.

The essence of BMC is to center one's conscious awareness in the experience of body, which is viewed as the physical expression of the mind. To do this, BMC students study anatomy and physiology by actually sensing and feeling the movements within themselves in the specific tissues *as they are occurring*. As one student described it, "I'm not only aware *of* my knee; I become aware *with* my knee." Each new awareness and movement leads to shifts in perception, which lead to new movement possibilities, which in turn create another new awareness. BMC students learn to volley their attention between a cognitive understanding of the body and the actual experience of the body, a body-mind process that has a calming and centering effect.

Cohen has created a myriad of experiential lessons in anatomy and developmental movement that include touch and repatterning exercises for each body system (organs, fluids, bones, muscles, nerves, and glands) and developmental movement patterns (see Chapter 7), as well as numerous movement and voice explorations. With each lesson, BMC practitioners experience how awareness can be centered in different tissues, which Cohen calls the "mind" of the movement: "The mind is like the wind and the body like sand; if you want to know which way the wind is blowing, you can look at the sand."[182] Like the wind, each tissue and body system expresses through the body in a specific rhythm, tone, and quality of motion. To access each aspect of a person, the mind of movement or the tone of touch must also vary. A BMC student uses these lessons to access every tiny part of his own anatomy through awareness, touch, and movement experiences, creating a continuity of sequence between sensing, feeling, and action.

BMC students also learn to access the parts of themselves that they are touching in another person during hands-on work. For instance, if one person is working with another person's heart, the first person tunes into the sensations of his own heart, and then touches with this awareness. During BMC touch and repatterning, BMC practitioners work to embody the consciousness and tone qualities of a specific tissue or movement pattern with which they are working with their clients or students, transferring information or eliciting body-mind experiences via a deepening level of somatic presence. In this sense, consciousness exists within each cell, tissue, or movement pathway, and it also exists non-locally in the transpersonal space between people.

Developmental Patterning: Reflexes, Reactions, and Responses

Cohen's unique contribution to the somatics field is her work with developmental movement patterning. BMC is one of the only systems of somatic education that extensively explores the role of developmental movement in neurological organization.

This system of developmental patterning is unique in three ways. First of all, developmental patterning is typically used to assess movement pathologies. Occupational therapists study early motor patterns at an arm's length; they learn to identify and teach the patterns yet do not actually practice them in their own bodies. Cohen created movement explorations for each of the developmental stages along with its underlying reflexes that a person goes through from birth to walking. Her developmental explorations liberated this valuable knowledge from the isolated world of occupational therapy and translated it into an accessible form that anyone can use to improve the overall coordination of movement.

Second, Cohen uses the educational vehicle she created—Body-Mind Centering—to explore these developmental patterns through experiential learning. BMC participants experience the benefits of developmental patterning processes on the overall organization of their bodies strengthening weak patterns and pathways while allowing overused pathways to rest. BMC participants also explore the psychological correlates, or "personality," of each developmental phase. For instance, push patterns support strength, separation, and the formation of boundaries, whereas reach pattern support a connection to others in relationship.

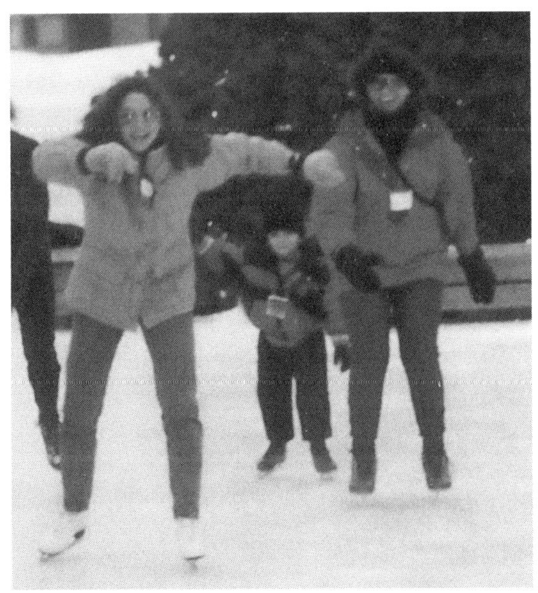

Figure 11.10 Notice the various strategies to maintain balance: lifting the shoulders and bracing, or holding the knees or ankles togethers (photo courtesy of L. Bright).

Third, Cohen has demystified the complex processes of neurological development by presenting them in a dynamic and easily understood continuum of primitive reflexes, righting reactions, and equilibrium responses.[183] She was motivated to do this by her frustration with the traditional view of the reflexes as "static, isolated reactions . . . [that were] too limiting when applied to integrated and efficient movements."[184]

The **primitive reflexes** are what Cohen calls the "alphabet of movement"—the earliest, simple reflexes such as the Babinski reflex, which causes the toes to fan when the top of the foot is lightly brushed. These simple reflexes eventually combine to form more complex movement patterns, akin to the way letters form words, phrases, and eventually full sentences. The spinal cord and brain stem control the primitive reflexes, which show up between birth and four months of age and disappear once they are integrated into the more complex patterns. Each primitive reflex has a modulating reflex; for example, the flexor withdrawal and extensor thrust reflexes counterbalance each other. Many movement problems develop as the result of a deficient reflex, one that has not developed or is not modulated by its counterbalancing reflex. By identifying the deficiency and developing a full range of reflexes, a person can fill gaps in motor development and build a harmonious movement vocabulary.

The **righting reactions** are the spontaneous, automatic patterns that bring the head and torso into alignment with each other along a vertical axis and bring the head to an upright position. They are coordinated at a midbrain level and include head righting, optical righting, neck righting on the body (NOB), and body righting on the body (BOB). Righting reactions help us maintain an upright orientation and also orient the eyes along the horizon. When a horse falls, head righting causes its head to pop up first. The righting reactions underlie movements that lift the body up against the pulls of gravity and are thus important for the coordination of tonic function and postural muscles.

The **equilibrium responses** are the most complex of the reflexive movement patterns, reestablishing balance in the body when the center of gravity or the base of support shifts

Patterning Exercise #117: Cellular Holding Exploration with a Partner

This is an excellent BMC exploration for parents to practice with young children, and for friends and lovers to practice with each other. It will increase tactile bonding and a positive touching connection, plus it can be very soothing and healing. Be aware, however, that it can also access deep places within a person, including strong emotions and memories, so make sure you and your partner have mutual trust. If, at any time during this exploration, any issues come up for either you or your partner, stop and discuss them with each other.

1. Find a partner and decide who is going to receive first. Begin by getting in a comfortable position and place your hands on a part of your partner's body that you are both comfortable with.
2. Focus your attention on touching the top layer of skin (whether you have direct contact with the skin or are touching through clothes). As you feel the contact between you and your partner, imagine the cell walls in each of you meeting at the place of contact.
3. Now shift your focus to the fluids inside the skin and cells. Feel or imagine the cellular fluids under your hands sensing the fluid bed under the skin in both you and your partner.
4. Have your partner also track your touch with his or her awareness.
5. Sense or imagine the cells as a conglomerate of millions of fluid-filled sacs resting in the cradle of your hands. Sense any fluid rhythms or subtle motions within them. Explore cellular touch for at least 10 minutes.
6. Discuss your experience with your partner afterwards. Then switch roles and repeat the exercise. Discuss the underlying quality of tone in tissues being held. Discuss if and when you felt you or your partner's tissues either relaxing into the contact or retracting away from it.

(Figure 11.10). They are coordinated at a forebrain level and show up as spontaneous movements that occur when a person loses balance, such as a protective step or spatial reach with arms, or a roll that follows a fall.

Automatic Movement and Cellular Touch

In Body-Mind Centering, there is no right or wrong way to move. Even movement patterns that we think of as problematic have an inherent purpose; they point us toward the missing link that we need to embody in order to achieve integration. All patterns are seen as "overlapping waves" of development. Each movement pattern has an intrinsic value as being the expression of some diverse part of a person, or in BMC language, as "the mind of the body." Cohen encourages students to discover *how* they learn and to honor the unique style and composition of each person's individual movement experience. From this approach, students develop the ability to stay with patterns that they find foreign and do not understand, rather than try to change or fix them. This creates a gentle, inclusive quality that encourages the acceptance of diversity.

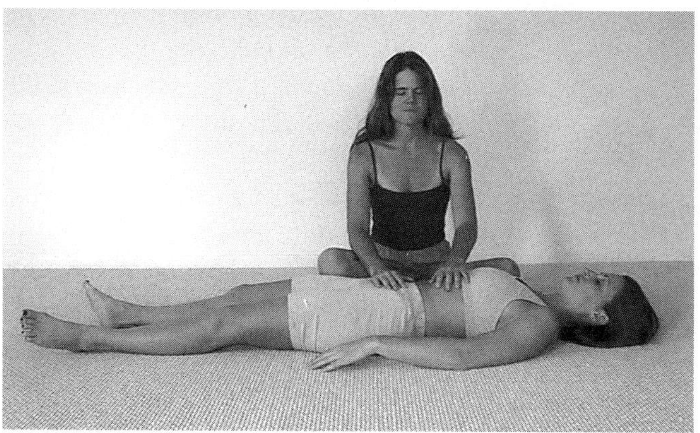

Figure 11.11 A practitioner and client exploring cellular holding

Approaching movement explorations with this open-minded curiosity cultivates the spontaneous, automatic impulses that arise for intrinsic body processes and allows them to evolve into full and expressive movement sequences. **Automatic movement** is Cohen's version of an improvisational movement practice she learned from Buddhist monks while living in Japan. This practice, called *katsugen undo*, or "Life-Force Movement," is practiced "to train the involuntary nervous system by awakening automatic movement."[185]

To practice automatic movement, a person lies, sits, or stands quietly and begins observing body sensations and organic impulses to move, allowing the smallest impulses to spontaneously unfold into a full movement sequence. This practice trains a participant to let go of the mind's control over the body's movement and cultivates fluidity in the body. From this fluid state, a deep somatic embodiment and healing can come forth.

Automatic movement begins in a quiet state of observation in which a participant becomes aware of a cellular fluid presence. Cohen associates the quiet rhythm of cellular fluid (fluid within the cells) with a state of presence. BMC touch and repatterning also begin with a quiet state of "cellular holding," a BMC skill in which a practitioner gently holds a client and focuses attention on cellular fluids (in self and other) with the intention of establishing contact and presence. Cellular holding serves as a neutral touch (without agenda) from which a practitioner begins to sense the automatic, organic movements happening within the client's body (Figure 11.11). This awareness initiates a

Tissue Surfacing

It is this author's experience that when a practitioner has the ability to move between body systems as described here, the client's body tends to be receptive on more levels, which can lead to interesting therapeutic encounters. An example from the author's practice illustrates this point:

In Body-Mind Centering training, we learned to track the physiological rhythms of each tissue and fluid through tactile and kinesthetic channels. We also practiced shifting our focus from one rhythm to another during hands-on explorations. By practicing this with clients, I have experienced a phenomenon many times that I began calling "tissue surfacing." This occurs when I rest my hands on a client in a receptive mode, and symptoms from one tissue layer, such as heat, pulsing, or even movement, become obvious. The tissue with symptoms seems to rise to the surface to meet my hands as though its symptoms were those of some kind of innate, self-healing intelligence that, when given the right conditions, bubbles to the surface to direct the healing process.

For example, I had my hand on the lower abdomen of a woman who came to me with hip pain. She had a long history of kidney problems. As I rested my hand on her belly, I began sensing the various tissue layers and rhythms. Something in her belly gurgled, her spine moved, and her bladder lifted up into my hand as though it knew my hands had the intelligence to adjust it. I lifted her bladder toward her head and gently pushed it back into her belly. Afterwards, the client commented on experiencing great relief. She said that she felt the area around her kidneys relax, felt a stretch from her kidneys to her belly (perhaps her uretors?), and also felt relief from the sensation she always has of needing to urinate. It was as though, since I was in a sensory mode, not knowing which system to work with, her body went into a motor mode and began moving toward more balance through self-correction.

touch and repatterning process that can unfold in a multitude of directions, into any tissue or movement pathway. The combination of automatic movement and cellular holding allows the movement initiated by a person's deep, intrinsic impulses to spontaneously emerge.

BMC students go through a broad and diverse exploration of movement qualities and pathways. Through this process, BMC students acquire a common language to describe diverse qualities of movement, and leave the four-year training with a developmental and anatomical understanding of the body as well as refined skills in touch and tracking movement through all the body's pathways and tissues.

CONTINUUM MOVEMENT

Emilie Conrad was born and raised in New York City, where she trained in both classical ballet and primitive dance. In 1955, she went to the West Indies to become the director and choreographer of a folklore dance company, steeping herself in the ancient, snakelike undulations of the Haitian rhythms for five years. After returning to New York, she had the unique body experience that she describes as falling into a "black hole":

> Your arms, legs, and torso begin to lighten and expand. You sense the spaces between cells and molecules and the smooth flow of fluids across membranes. Air ripples like liquid through your skin. You are floating now in a vast sea. Like an eel, you slither forward, then, formless as an amoeba, you spread out. You become a fish. You swim, rest, dissolve, merge with other creatures, then reform to swim again in an ocean of love.[186]

Conrad emerged transformed into what has been described as a fluid and organic being of pure liquid movement. She soon gave up imposing patterned movement on dance and began cultivating an awareness of the subtle sensations that occur while experiencing wave-like, organic movements. Through this process, she discovered that movement could dissolve body-mind boundaries and expand consciousness beyond the confines of the skin. Recognizing the strong effect culture has on movement patterns, she gave up a promising career as a professional dancer to develop her work in **Continuum Movement**.

In an effort to understand her Continuum experience, Conrad went to see Dr. Valerie Hunt, physiologist and internationally recognized researcher of human energy fields, at UCLA. Dr. Hunt was astounded by Conrad's physiological capabilities when Conrad participated as the movement expert in Dr. Hunt's research during 1974–1979. After 30 minutes of elegant, strenuous, technically proficient and complex yet extremely fluid movement, Conrad's heart rate had actually decreased, her blood pressure had dropped, her breathing was slower, and she had not even perspired. When Dr. Hunt asked her to describe how she had achieved these physiological feats, Conrad replied, "I create a field of energy and ride it." Hunt also measured a paralyzed polio victim's muscle loss before and after hands-on treatments with Conrad and found, to her amazement, that there was actually neuromuscular regeneration in the paralyzed tissues after the treatment. After a series of hands-on sessions with Conrad over four years, the woman, who had been paralyzed for 23 years, regained almost full function, confirmed by electromyographical (EMG) readings of neuromuscular regeneration.[187]

Conrad's work has challenged our beliefs about solid bodies. She feels that mental constructs and cultural conditioning create physical fixations that support and maintain rigid beliefs and ideas about who and what we really are. Once people have experienced the fluid state of Continuum, according to Continuum facilitators, they come away with an experience of the body merged with all life forms in a collective ocean of boundless fluidity.

Continuum Movement also challenges our notion of the central nervous system, which Conrad believes developed for the bipedal survival patterns of stalking prey and fleeing predators. Conrad feels that our centralized, hierarchical cultures are reflections of our notion that the body is commanded by a brain rather than by a deeper, biologically based intelligence that resides within each cell. She also equates fluid movement within the body with love—a power and energy that dissolves personal boundaries and opens the exchange of healing energies.

In a Continuum Movement class, participants explore wave-like movements combined with various sounds, such as "HU, AW, or SSS" to reawaken the mutable, fluid origins that humans share with aquatic life forms. The combination of sound and fluid movement seems to have an inexplicable effect on the body, dissolving the boundaries of the ego and reconnecting a person with the expansive ebb and flow of the collective biological pulsation of life. People who engage in this sensual, supple, organic form of movement often complete the Continuum Movement exploration feeling energized and reunited with some primordial essence forgotten long ago.

PILATES METHOD

Joe Pilates (1880–1967) had a sickly body but an iron will. Although his young body suffered the ravages of rickets, asthma, and rheumatic fever, he was determined to overcome his physical frailties and, as a child in Germany, embarked on a self-disciplined regimen of gymnastics, dance, sports, yoga, and body-building. Out of this, Pilates built both an outstanding physique and a steely determination.

At age 32 Pilates moved to England. When WWI began, he was interned as a German "enemy alien" in a British camp. During this confinement, Pilates created exercise programs for himself and his fellow internees. He also invented crude exercise devices for the disabled prisoners to use for rehabilitation, such as cords hooked into walls to pull on for resistance. This was the birth of the **Pilates Method**.

Pilates continued to develop new exercises and machines for his method after the war. He immigrated to New York in 1926, where he and his wife (a nurse he met on the transatlantic ship) opened their first studio. Together they taught this innovative form of conditioning. Within a short time, many famous dancers—Ruth St. Denis, Ted Shawn, and Martha Graham among them—flocked to Pilates to condition with him. They found his philosophy of "lengthening while you strengthen" congruent with the subtle articulations and refined gestures of their dance choreography.

Joe Pilates originally called his method "contrology" because each exercise is done slowly with concentration and focus on proper form. Using precise control, an individual contracts the deep postural muscles first, then maintains an aligned posture with core support in the trunk while exercising. This aspect of Pilates makes it an unusual form of exercise: it may be the only program that integrates postural stabilization with conditioning.

As a student practices Pilates, a teacher helps the student change habitual patterns by coaching him to focus on several important elements:

1. pulling the abdominal wall back into a hollow shape to stabilize each movement with a core contraction;
2. lengthening the spine and limbs to elicit stabilizing contractions along the waist;
3. coordinating the movement with breathing to expand the ribs and improve respiration;
4. engaging an entire chain of muscles, from the head to feet, hands to tail, during pushing or pulling movements, to achieve full-body integration.

The Pilates Method provides a person with a postural education typically absent in regular conditioning programs. It teaches a person to work out in a manner that engages and strengthens core muscles. Pilates exercises require an intense concentration on form and efficiency, which in itself improves the body-mind connection. Since eccentric contractions elicited by lengthening employ less motor units than concentric contractions, these fewer motor units work harder to move the same load. Thus Pilates can work the muscles hard. And each Pilates exercise is done with an awareness of the entire body, integrating postural muscles with working muscles, and coordinating a sequence of contractions along a chain of muscles rather than in a single group.

Although Pilates was used almost solely by dancers until the 1960s, it has been spreading through the fitness world like wildfire in recent years. There seem to be several reasons for its growing popularity. First, Pilates has gained a reputation for building lithe, lean, streamlined bodies. Pilates also focuses on "core movement" that initiates in the iliopsoas muscles—an approach also advocated in the Bartenieff Fundamentals and in Rolfing Movement. And since core movement, particularly in the pelvis, is effective in improving alignment and releasing the holding patterns caused by pain from injury and poor posture, Pilates is rapidly becoming a widely used system for rehabilitation. Physicians are recommending Pilates to patients recovering from injuries, surgeries, or chronic pain conditions; many physical therapists are training in Pilates; and some insurance companies are now willing to pay for it, all of which make Pilates as popular for rehabilitation as for general fitness.

CONTACT IMPROVISATION

Whether or not Contact Improvisation should be included in this survey of the integrative movement therapies is debatable because it is an improvisational dance form. What is unique about it, and the reason it is included, is

Patterning Exercise #118: Following and Leading

This exercise is designed to help you become aware of when you're following your partner's movement with touch, and when you are leading your partner's movement.

1. Sit or stand beside your partner, and turn to face him or her. Without compressing your partner's body or moving him or her off balance, place one hand on the front of your partner's body and the other on the back (PE Fig 118a).
2. Have your partner slowly begin to move with organic, intrinsic movements. Follow the movements with your hands (PE Fig. 118b).

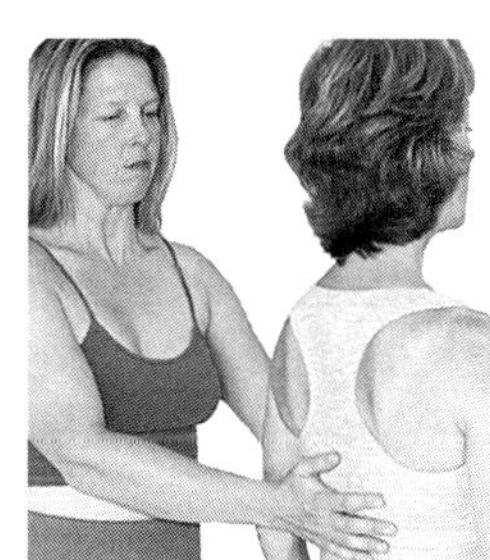

PE Fig. 118a

3. Then switch to leading or directing the movement with your touch. Alternate between the two. Ask your partner to become aware of when he or she is following or leading.

Feedback: Give each other feedback about each role that each person is in at any time during the exercise. What did you discover? Was it always clear who was following and who was leading? Discuss the exploration after you have finished and are no longer touching.

4. Switch roles, and repeat the exercise.

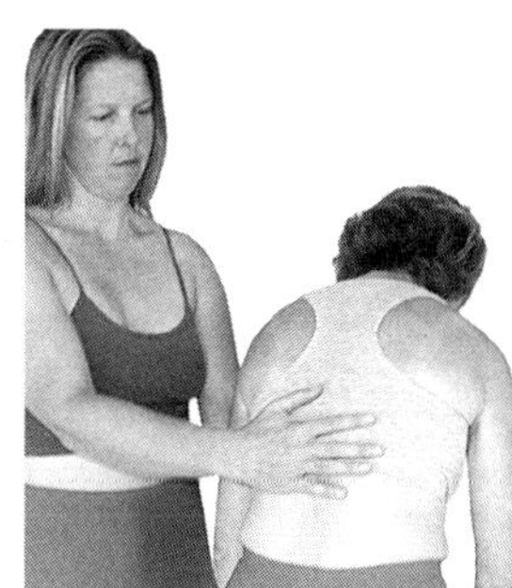

PE Fig. 118b

EMSPress.com

that **Contact Improvisation** is based on the spontaneous responses between two people when they come into physical contact with each other. The many somatic practitioners who practice Contact Improvisation have found that it not only expands their movement abilities, but it also creates a sensitivity to body contact unlike any other.

Body contact is not new to dance or sports. It occurs in partner dancing and the random meetings of players in contact sports such as football. When two bodies unexpectedly meet, the responses of each person span a wide range, from impact and crashing to the cooperative execution of a roll or lift done with grace and ease. Graceful contact involves timing, focus, and the ability to trust releasing one's physical weight into the support of another person's body.

In the 1960s an innovative dancer named Steve Paxton had been experimenting with dance forms that involved body contact between dancers, an improvisation that crystallized into organic and fluid falls, throws, rolls, and lifts (Figure 11.12). After more than a decade of playing with this form, Paxton and others named it Contact Improvisation, which precisely describes what it is.[188]

Although Contact Improvisation does not include a hands-on modality, it has helped many movement therapists learn how to follow spontaneous movement in themselves and others. The off-center positions dancers move through during Contact Improvisation require a tolerance to disorientation from the usual vertical posture. Contact Improvisation participants learn how to yield into body weight and into present-moment sensations and experiences, letting go of tendencies to determine movement, allowing spontaneous reflexes to take over. As one person's body tips off-center into another person's body and into gravity, new and dynamic reflexes and responses are automatically patterned into a participant's movement vocabulary.

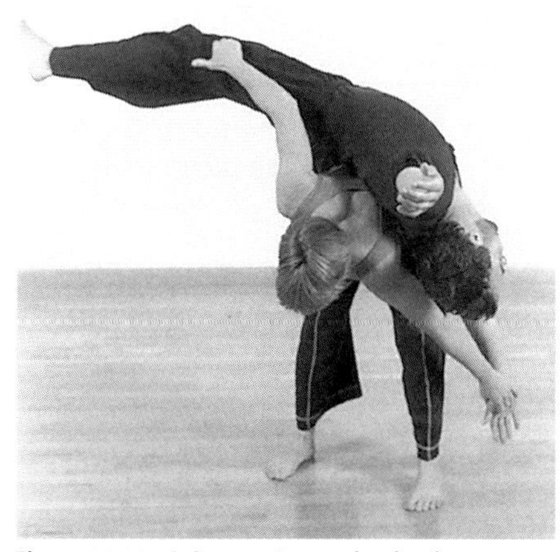

Figure 11.12 A Contact Improvisation jam (photo courtesy of Annie Brook, from *Contact Improvisation and Body-Mind Centering: A Manual for Teaching and Learning Movement* [2000]).

Initially, Contact Improvisation can be difficult because it requires letting go into unknown and unfamiliar spheres of motion. It takes time to learn to release the body's weight into unusual positions. The beginner might be hesitant and stop the flow of the improvisation to think about how to move, or get stuck in a pattern that might have formed around the fear of falling. But soon this cortical planning falls away to the pure sensation of allowing the body to move with another person in spontaneous, interactive, and mutually supporting dance. Contact Improvisation is akin to problem solving in action; it forces people to think—through their bodies—on their feet. Solutions to shifting weight, balance, and position arise out of spontaneous responses to sensation and fluid transitions of one body in relation to another.

Contact participants progress through stages of developing sensitivity to body contact and trust in each other's responses. Unless Contact dancers already are adept movers with high degrees of agility and strength, they can get hurt throwing the body into a contact jam. Sensitive teachers introduce Contact with stress on safety and on trusting the body's instinctive movement. Teachers have students start contact with slow improvisations that help students learn to relax and loosen up. As the participants become familiar with making body contact, they develop more trust in their instinctual movement responses. Teachers help build trust by having students practice movements that will cushion a fall, such as bearing weight on their hands or rolling when they fall. The more confident participants become in their innate responses to contact, the more fluid, daring, and enjoyable their improvisation becomes.

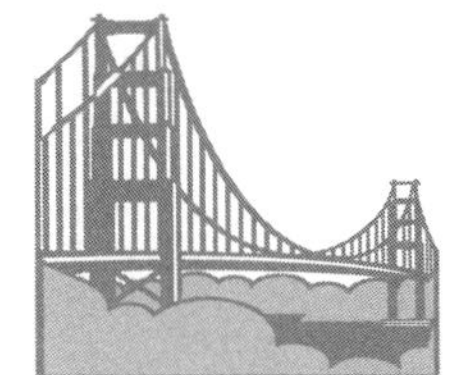

Bridge to Practice

Improvising with Contact during Touch

A dialogue between two responsive bodies during movement and interactive touch is an essential patterning skill. The more you can feel, follow, and shape the flow of intrinsic and subtle movements within your own body and within your client's body, the deeper your somatic awareness of intrinsic and organic movement will become. During a patterning process, the internal spontaneous responses of the body can guide the flow of the process in the same manner that body contact plus the forces of falling weight, momentum, and inertia determine the dance that arises out of Contact Improvisation.

SUMMARY

The initial idea and research for this text were based on a survey of only the somatic patterning methods that focus on movement education, specifically, those described in this chapter. Once the research began, it became clear that the movement modalities draw extensively from many other somatic fields that also address somatic patterns; therefore, the text was expanded to cover the broad range of methods described in the subsequent chapters.

Still, the movement modalities in Chapter 11 could be thought of as the core of somatic patterning because they work the most directly with actual body movement. Each modality in this chapter contributes a specific element to a comprehensive picture of movement education within somatic patterning. The Alexander Technique works with head righting reflexes, the Feldenkrais Method with tonic function, Ideokinesis with anatomically based imagery, Sensory Awareness with present-moment awareness, Body-Mind Centering with experiential anatomy and developmental movement, and Continuum with fluid and organic movement practices. Pilates stands alone as one of the only exercise programs that focuses on developing core stability in the body.

All of these modalities share the recognition that body movement is an ongoing expression of a person's psyche. Movement is also a vital integrating link between the body and mind. Ultimately, every expression we make, every activity we are involved in, and every somatic study we undertake involves the movement of the body, so the integrative movement therapies are essential to a comprehensive somatic patterning process.

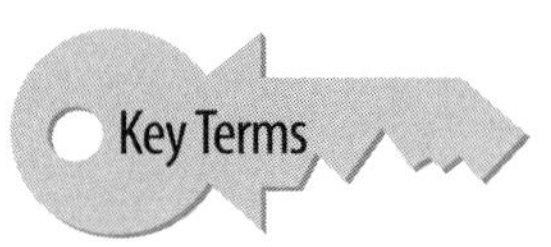

Alexander Technique
automatic movement
Awareness Through Movement
Bartenieff Fundamentals
Body-Mind Centering (BMC)
constructive rest position (CRP)
Contact Improvisation
Continuum Movement
effort elements
equilibrium responses
Feldenkrais Method
Functional Integration
hooklying position
ideokinetic facilitation
Labanalysis
Labanotation
Pilates Method
primitive reflexes
psychophysical education
righting reactions
Sensory Awareness

OVERVIEW OF CHAPTER 12

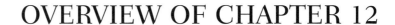

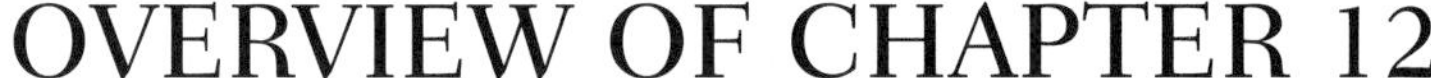

12

Integrative Manual Therapies

As a person develops there are at least three major factors that influence adult posture: heredity, disease, and acquired habit. Of the three, the last is the least well-understood. However, it is the factor that can be influenced most by treatment.

—Rene Cailliet

In the last chapter, the movement therapies that grew out of alternative somatic practices were reviewed. Most of the movement therapies use hands-on methods as an adjunct to movement education. Conversely, this chapter covers the bodywork modalities that grew out of some form of manual therapy (therapy delivered through hands-on techniques) and use movement education as an adjunct to hands-on work. Most people are familiar with massage, which is a hands-on manipulation of the tissues via rubbing and kneading strokes used for its general therapeutic benefits. Bodywork and manual therapy have more defined goals than massage, using specific techniques of releasing myofascial and joint restrictions with the goal of restoring structural balance to a person's posture and movement.

Massage and bodywork sprang from similar roots. From the turn of the century until the 1960s, movement was a standard part of massage therapy. By 1930, the Charter Society of Massage and Medical Gymnastiks had more than 12,000 members throughout the United Kingdom and its dominions.[189] These early practitioners, called "gymnasts," used Swedish massage plus a system of both passive and active stretches and exercises to restore flexibility and circulation to the physical body. This unique combination is returning today. Many bodywork pioneers have recognized the integrative benefits of combining movement education with manual therapy. This chapter covers these integrative methods. Each modality reviewed here uses hands-on techniques to release myofascial tensions, balance posture, and restore economy of motion; and uses movement education to change structure and improve function.

The various schools and techniques of integrative bodywork are too extensive to present in a book this size; the methods included here are ones that were the first to establish or popularize a particular innovation in the field. Most of the methods in this chapter were developed within the field of orthopedics, osteopathy, and physical therapy, such as cranialsacral therapy, proprioceptive neuromuscular rehabilitation, and stability training. Although there are numerous other mainstream methods of manual therapy, the methods included here are widely used or emulated among somatic practitioners and educators, as well as bodyworkers and massage therapists. We now begin with a groundbreaking method of structural realignment called Rolfing.

ROLFING: STRUCTURAL INTEGRATION

Ida Rolf (1896–1979), a biochemist and physiologist trained at Columbia University, promoted the importance of what she called structural integration, which is, basically, good posture. An avid yoga practitioner, Rolf felt that many health problems deemed untreatable by doctors were actually tissue restrictions in the body that developed as postural responses to the stress of gravity's constant pull. These stresses distort the three-dimensional balance of the body and shorten it with chronic rotations. To get a picture of this, imagine twisting a pliable hollow tube; it loses both length and volume. As a result of the off-center posture, myofascial adhesions—fibrous buildup in the muscles and their associated fascias (introduced in Chapter 2)—develop to shore up the body and maintain some semblance of vertical balance. Ironically, the adhesions that develop to solve one problem create another. They literally twist and glue body parts together, which restricts motion and creates postural distortions that affect mechanical, physiological, and even psychological imbalances.

The **fascial network** is so pervasive that one could hypothetically remove all the other tissues and bones and still be able to see the shape of the body in the fascia. Rolf calls the fascial network the "organ of support" because it connects every part to the whole, wrapping and binding every organ, bone, muscle fiber, gland, joint, and structure in the body together.[190] Rolf developed her bodywork, originally named "structural integration" but later known as **Rolfing**, to release fascial restrictions that distort body posture and movement. Over the course of some 50 years of research, Rolf developed a 10-session series to systematically release myofascial restrictions and, in the mid-1960s, held the first certification program in Structural Integration at the Esalen Institute in California.

Basic Principles of Rolfing

Rolf considered structural integration a system of education because it teaches people how to balance their bodies within the field of gravity. Using deep and sustained pressure with the hands and elbows to stretch myofascia, she helped people reorganize their body structures by releasing and realigning fascial planes, allowing muscles to once again slide over bones and movement to occur between parts. Although other myofascial release systems have since been developed, Rolf's work is unique because she was the first bodyworker to focus on relationships among body parts to create an overall integration of the structure.

Recall from Chapter 6 that fascia is thixotropic: it loosens and stretches under sustained pressure. A Rolfer applies sustained compression and stretch to myofascia in a systematic fashion, beginning with the ribcage to expand respiration, then releasing superficial fascia, and proceeding with a focus on relationships among body parts. In this way, a practitioner will stretch superficial fascia evenly throughout the top layer, creating a continuity of release in the "top skin of the onion" before delving into deeper layers.

Rolfers have a saying, "gravity is the therapist." This sums up their belief that releasing fascial restrictions in the extrinsic musculature facilitates support from the intrinsic muscles, which creates the lift that people often describe feeling after a Rolfing session. Rolfers call this experience "being on your Rolf line," referring to the vertical line of gravity around which a balanced body is organized. Their theory is that when we let down into the pull of gravity we come on our line and get a lift that is a result of relaxing the superficial tensions that shorten the body.

Rolfing does seem to lengthen the body and affect intrinsic muscles, yet how it does so is not completely understood. Generally, if the intrinsic muscles are inhibited, a person must actively contract them to turn them on. In a widely used Rolfing technique, the practitioner puts the client in an aligned position, then puts pressure on a particular body part and asks the client to move. Perhaps the movement cues a Rolfer gives a client elicit the contractions of intrinsic muscles. Or the deep pressure a Rolfer applies restricts the contraction of the extrinsic muscles and limits the size of the movement, which forces a client to do small, internal movements that engage the intrinsic postural muscles.

Examining Myths

Myth: After having myofascial restrictions released to align the posture, the body spontaneously assumes an upright posture.

Although many proponents of structural integration work from this premise, upright posture is learned. If it were an instinctive behavior, like sucking or swallowing, a newborn would be able to stand up at birth. Therefore, releasing restrictions is a preliminary step to developing upright posture, but a person also needs to learn to recognize what the sensation of upright posture feels like, and then to use this recognition to move from a faulty position to an aligned posture. Most importantly, a person needs to have the desire, willingness, and commitment to learn how to improve posture to make it more upright.

The Body as a Tensile Structure

Ida Rolf envisioned the myofascial network as a **tensegrity structure**—a three-dimensional grid supported by its tensional forces (Figure 12.1). Tensegrity structures were first developed in architecture by Buckminster Fuller in the 1930s. Fuller designed the geodesic dome, an efficient structure based on his guiding premise of "doing more with less." Fuller originally got the idea that led to the innovative dome from one of his architecture students, who presented Fuller with a three-dimensional structure made of wooden dowels and rubber bands. This led Fuller to develop the sturdy dome built out of self-bracing triangles.

Rolf applied Fuller's tensegrity concept to the connective tissue network within the body, viewing it as a three-dimensional grid of guylines, each aligned along a path of geometric tensions that support the body's shape and volume (Figure 12.2). Rolf compared fascial adhesions to snags in a sweater that pull on the fibers of the connective tissue fabric, translating pulls from one fascial plane to another, thereby distorting the dimensional integrity of the structure.

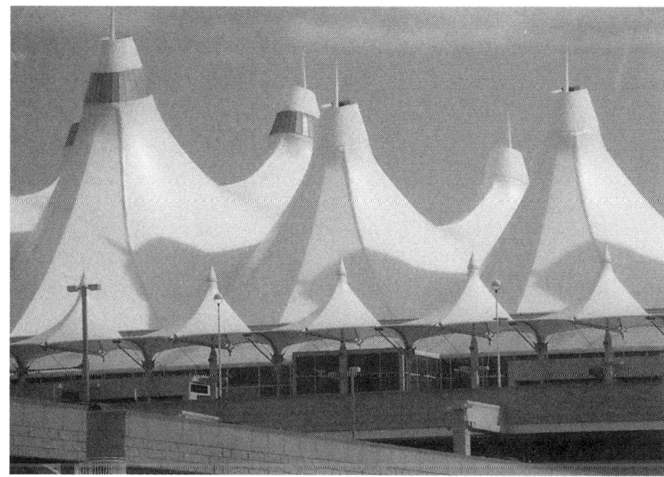

Figure 12.1 A tensegrity structure in which tensional forces provide support

Recall from Chapter 2 that fascia binds one muscle to another across joints, wrapping them in bundles around bones and translating motion from one part of the body to another. In fact, what many people feel elongating when they stretch are actually fascial sheaths stretching. As fascial sheaths become more supple and pliable, they create more space for the muscles that they wrap to move within, thereby increasing one's range of motion. Conversely, fascial adhesions restrict the space that muscles have to work within. Adhesions also transfer forces, meaning that adhesions in one area of the body can create movement restrictions in other areas.

A tensegrity network of connective tissue fibers extends throughout the body even on a cellular level. Every single cell is supported by and connected to other cells through a continuous network of microscopic fibers, or cellular tubules. This network gives each cell shape and dimension similar to the way fascia shapes the entire body. Connective tissue fibers, sheaths, and tubes function as slings and straps for all cells, organs, and tissues, stringing together body parts within a tensional network.

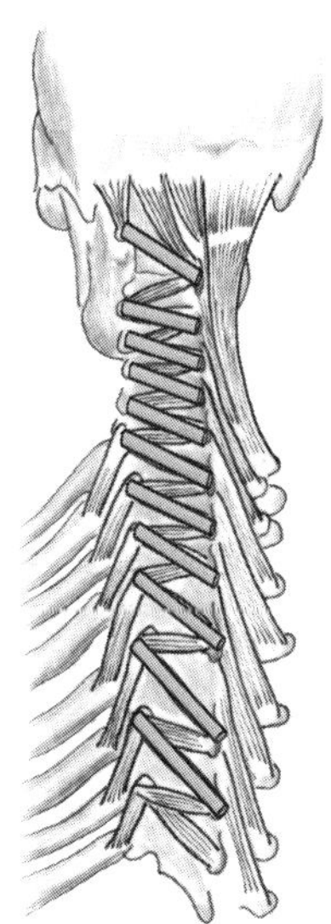

Figure 12.2 Tensegrity pulls along the spine

Rolfing theorists offer insight into the role of connective tissue in immune function, pointing out fascia's conduction properties as a semi-liquid crystal. The connective tissue network not only passes mechanical tensions, such as the impact of a heel strike in walking, through the body; it may also serve as a conduit for electromagnetic and vibrational frequencies to pass through the body, which are thought to affect autonomic tone and strengthen immune function. James Oschman, a biologist and researcher who has written extensively about the scientific basis of bodywork, has hypothesized about the *piezoelectric effect* within connective tissues: when fascial areas are compressed, an electrical field spreads through the entire fascial network, softening and increasing conduction properties throughout the body.[191] In his book *Energy Medicine,* Oschman discusses a hypothetical role of connective tissue tubules in the body:

> Electrical engineers know that an antenna works best if its length corresponds to the wave length of the signal being transmitted or received. When a person moves, tensions set up within the body change the lengths of the molecular antennas of the myofascial system, and therefore change their resonant frequencies.[192]

The Confusion between Myofascial Release and Rolfing

Since its inception, Rolfing has spawned second-and-third generation schools of manual therapy, such as Postural Integration and Hellerwork. In fact, Rolfing has become so integrally associated with deep tissue massage and myofascial release that the word "rolf" is often used as a verb to connote this meaning. In addition, numerous myofascial release techniques have developed over the last twenty years, many used by Rolfers, yet myofascial release and Rolfing differ because Rolfing is a process rather than a single technique. Unless a bodyworker has been trained to use the structural integration recipe, she or he is not practicing what is officially defined as Rolfing.

The 10-session series works logically from the outside in and the bottom up. It begins with the manual stretching of the superficial fascia in order to release overall extrinsic tension and open up respiration. Then a practitioner works to establish the feet as the base of support. Next, bilateral right-left balance is established by separating tissues on the

Ida Rolf and Moshe Feldenkrais

Ida Rolf and Moshe Feldenkrais were contemporaries. They knew each other and were said to have behaved in the European tradition—showing respect by contradicting each other. They often criticized each other's work in public, yet many felt that they were two geniuses who actually respected, challenged, and influenced each other.

Feldenkrais believed that function determined structure, and Rolf believed that structure determined function. It is said that when Feldenkrais met Rolf in the 1940s, he decided she was doing a fine job developing the structural work, so he focused on functional work based on movement. Rolf took Moshe Feldenkrais through her 10-session series, but she would not allow him to try his methods on her in turn. When asked why, she declared: "I am afraid my body would lose its [Rolf] line."[193]

front of the body from those on the back by working with the client in a side-lying position. This is followed by work on the inner line of the legs to establish a core connection up the lower limbs. The series continues up into the pelvis and along the front of the spine to integrate the lower limbs with the trunk. Now the client is ready for bodywork in the upper body, to balance the thorax over the lower body, integrate the arms into the spine, and release fascial tensions in the head and neck to integrate the head with the body. Finally, the series culminates with several sessions that focus primarily on integrating the entire body and working with structural considerations unique to that individual.

Several techniques that Rolf used and taught differ significantly from typical myofascial release work. Instead of releasing a trigger point in the muscle, then having the client stretch afterward, Rolf would glide over a number of sore points within a muscle. She would also have clients actively move as she put pressure on the restricted tissues. Using movement, the clients literally pull their bodies out of the restriction and, at the same time, establish new neuromuscular pathways. The client's active movement during session allows Rolfing to make the leap from a structural approach to a functional, neurological approach.

Rolfing Movement

In 1970, Rolf decided that there needed to be an organized system of movement instruction that Rolfers could use to direct their clients during each session, which led to the development of an adjunct system. **Rolfing Movement Education** is a body of exercises and body awarenesses that teach a person to focus on the sensation of weight in the body, particularly in the core, to achieve effortless posture and movement. This sensation of weight helps a person to relax excessive muscular effort and holding, particularly in the extrinsic muscles, and to feel intrinsic muscles contract in the initiation of any motion.

In a typical Rolfing Movement session, clients first become aware of how they move in relationship to their vertical alignment and to gravity. To do this, teachers help clients feel how the head is aligned over the thorax, the thorax over the pelvis, and the pelvis over the legs and feet. Then clients lie down to reduce the downward pull of gravity on the body, and the teacher guides them through a series of exercises that are intended to realign the body and increase a person's perception of weight.

In Rolfing Movement exercises such as "arm drops" and "leg drops," clients lie supine and lift their arms or legs toward the ceiling, moving the limb until it feels heavy, then passively drop it to release the limb into gravity's pull. Other exercises to align other parts of the body, such as the pelvic tilt, are taught to release low-back tension and activate the intrinsic muscles. Falling from the front of the ankle is taught to help people feel the effects of the pull of gravity on their bodies while walking. Although a person used to be able to get certified as a Rolfing Movement teacher without doing the basic Rolfing training, certification in this adjunct system is now limited to Rolfers, who use it as an educational tool to enhance their bodywork.

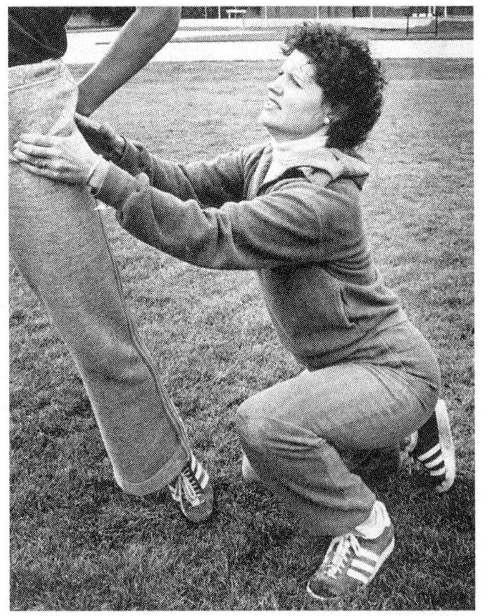

Figure 12.3 Judith Aston working with a client (photo courtesy of J. Aston).

ASTON PATTERNING

Some of us learn through sympathy, relating to what another person feels and thinks; others learn through opposition, rebelling against the status quo to develop new ideas. The latter was the path Judith Aston took to make a discovery that led to her development of **Aston Patterning** (Figure 12.3).

In 1963, Aston began teaching dance at Long Beach City College in California. Her work was interrupted in 1966 and again in 1967 by car accidents that left her with severe whiplash and sciatic pain, requiring her to wear a back brace. Told that she would never dance again, Aston went to Ida Rolf for treatment at Esalen, where she not only got Rolfed, but also began her training as a Rolfer. After the training, Rolf asked Aston to develop movement exercises that Rolfers could teach their clients to help them move with symmetry and balance after getting Rolfed. In response to Rolf's request, Aston and several others (Rachel Harris and Dorothy Nolte among them) developed movement exercises that they began teaching to Rolfers in 1971.

Initially, Ida Rolf insisted that Rolfers work with straight hands and move in straight lines. But while using pillows to prop up a five-year-old boy paralyzed from a swimming accident, Aston discovered that if she supported the shape of the stress pattern, she could effect deep change. She formed her hands to the shape of the boy's body and spiraled into his tissue pattern to get release, much as one pushes a knotted rope together to loosen it. Excited about her discovery, Aston soon began to teach Rolfers her principles of matching tissue with corresponding hand shaping and of moving in spirals.[194] She encouraged bodywork practitioners to use spiral shaped strokes and hand movements to match the shape of clients' asymmetrical bodies and .

Eventually, Aston recognized that her theories of spiral movement and bodywork were at odds with Rolf's notions of linear core alignment and linear pathways of movement. In 1977, she split off to form her own school of Aston Patterning, built on the premise that all the tissues, joints, and muscles are three-dimensional and curvilinear in form so that the imposition of straight lines creates stress within the body.

Aston Patterning has evolved into a number of forms. They include several forms of *Aston bodywork* such as *myokinetics*—in which each stroke follows the grain of the tissue in and out of three-dimensional patterns, and *arthrokinetics*—in which a practitioner gently spirals tissues along the bones in and out of the joint patterns. *Aston Movement Education, Aston Fitness,* and *Ergonomics* are forms of movement education designed to help people follow asymmetrical movement patterns during common activities such as sitting, walking, or exercising.

Central to Aston's work is an exercise called arcing, in which a person collapses the spine into flexion during exhalation and extends the spine during inhalation, then finds the place in between where the body weight can rest into a neutral position (introduced in Chapter 10).[195] To use Aston's words, "A person's neutral position can become an excellent point of departure for any action."[196] From neutral, the body flows, sways, and is fluid; it is responsive to weight shifts in any direction. Using this understanding as a basis of her thought, Aston developed techniques in direct opposition to Rolf's rigid notion that the body should be organized in a straight line. She took traditional Rolfing and made it more fluid. In traditional Rolfing Movement exercises, such as toes-up, toes-down, arm drops, and knee drops, a person moves a limb while sensing support in the core. Aston's work, in contrast, centers more around the dynamic movement in the core, so that the core is thought of as organized around fluid, spiral-shaped motion rather than a positional line.

CRANIALSACRAL (CS) THERAPY

Traditionally part of osteopathic medicine, **cranialsacral (CS) therapy** began being used in bodywork when several osteopaths determined that it was too valuable a therapy to remain in the confines of their field. In the early 1900s, William Sutherland was the first osteopath to study the movement of the cranial bones—still a debatable subject among many medical doctors who believe that the sutures are fused and immovable. Sutherland felt that the interdigitated and beveled sutures between the cranial bones suggested that they were capable of subtle motion, so he began experimenting with wearing elaborate helmets lined with screws that lightly jabbed into his skull during subtle cranial motion. The helmet provided Sutherland with proprioceptive feedback from which to study cranial motion. Out of his research came a model of inherent motion throughout the cranial system, fueled by the circulation of *cerebrospinal fluid* (CSF) produced in the ventricles (spaces) of the brain and filling the subdural spaces around brain and spinal cord. Sutherland described the movement of fluid in the CS system as a rhythm that he called the "breath of life."[197] He felt the breath of life was a more primary rhythm than diaphragmatic breathing because of its supposed healing and integrating effects on the nervous system.

Although cranialsacral (CS) therapy does not involve an active system of movement education, it has been shown to effect deep changes in somatic patterns. The primary tool in this work is touch. Practitioners use hands-on techniques to access the physiological rhythms of the fluid that circulates around the brain and spinal cord. CS therapists believe that this rhythm, called the *cranialsacral (CS) rhythm*, spreads through the fascial network of the entire body and can be palpated anywhere on the body. Restrictions in the rhythm indicate areas where the tissues are dysfunctional, lacking normal physiological motion. These movement restrictions result from fascial restrictions that form around holding patterns from emotional traumas or the sites of previous injuries.

There are forms of cranial manipulation that use cross-fiber friction on the sutures to move the bones, or use direct, firm pressure to loosen tissues attached to the cranial bones to mobilize them and bring the cranial bones into symmetrical rhythms. Numerous other approaches to cranialsacral therapy work with fluid rhythms. The only one that will be discussed here, the Upledger method, is widely used among bodyworkers and employs passive motion to unravel myofascial tensions and release autonomic tension. Upledger's first text on cranialsacral therapy, written in collaboration with an architect, emphasizes how the architectural features of the cranial bones (such as the beveled edge of the temporal bone) reflect the nature of their constant physiological motion. In his text, Upledger clearly explains a simple 10-step protocol

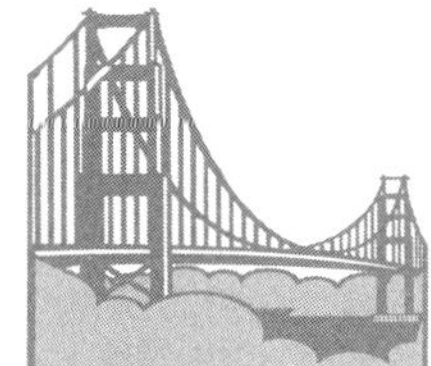

Bridge to Practice

Unwinding

As practitioners familiar with unwinding know, it is important that a client continues to relax on a deeper and deeper level during a session in order for him to sink into a deeper parasympathetic state. If he is truly relaxing, the unwinding usually becomes slower and slower. If it speeds up, the faster movement can literally wind your client into a deeper tension pattern. It is easy to mistake winding-up for unwinding. Winding-up cycles in repetitive loops that seem to go on without resolution. Its movement creates a rubbery quality in the tissues. To avoid this, encourage your client to slow the unwinding down and relax. Also, suggest that he sense a deeper level of his body than the layer that is unwinding, and then keep his attention focused on this deeper place.

for using the cranial bones as anchors on the dura and myofascial membranes, then lightly pulling the bones in specific directions to traction the membranes and increase normal physiological motion.

The Upledger Institute

In CS therapy, mobility is restored to the body by following the rhythm and flow of CSF into areas blocked by fascial adhesions and tension. Dr. John Upledger, an osteopath who has popularized CS therapy among bodyworkers, hypothesizes that the pumping action of cerebrospinal fluid (CSF) intermittently filling the ventricles located in the brain acts like a semi-closed hydraulic system on a pressurestat model: as fluid pressure changes, it provides feedback that in turn regulates the pump.[198]

The cranialsacral rhythm creates changing tensions in the tissues around the brain and spinal cord, which are continuous with the body's fascial network. Restrictions in the CS system, including fascial restrictions throughout the body, create changes in amplitude, symmetry, and rate of the CS rhythm; therefore, cranialsacral palpation can be used as a diagnostic tool.

Cranialsacral therapy has provided many practitioners with valuable tactile and sensory skills in tracking physiological rhythms. CS practitioners learn to follow the subtle CS rhythm in and out of oscillating cycles of action and rest. They also learn how to manipulate the CS rhythm by following the CS pattern into the direction of restriction—an **indirect technique** that follows a person into the pattern and holds it there until the system spontaneously rebalances; or pulling the restriction open—a **direct technique** in which an outside force is applied to pull the tissues out of the pattern (Figure 12.4).

When flexion and extension cycles are imbalanced, a self-correcting mechanism called a **stillpoint** rebalances the system. To induce a stillpoint, (a direct technique), a CS practitioner makes his hands immovable against the cranial rhythm so that pressure builds in the CS system. This increased pressure opens fascial restrictions; when the pump starts again, it normalizes the rhythm. On a mechanical level, inducing a stillpoint is like compressing a spring to build up pressure that expands upon release, or like pushing a stuck door in order to pull it open. Compression on the CSF pump forces fluid into areas of restriction, which opens them.

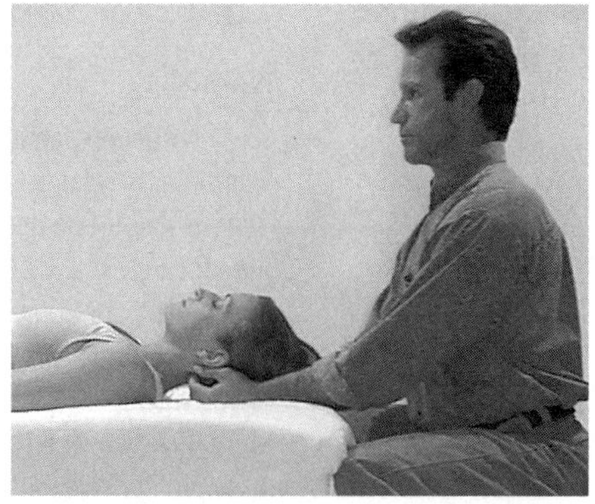

Figure 12.4 The occipital release this practitioner demonstrates is basic to cranialsacral therapy.

Unwinding and Somato-Emotional Therapy

When cerebrospinal fluid (CSF) begins to flow into areas that were once restricted, the release spreads out into the fascia, gently unraveling tension throughout the entire body. This unraveling occurs in nonlinear pathways that follow the natural spirals found in the structure of both connective tissues and muscular tissues. Upledger developed a technique called **unwinding**, in which the therapist gently follows the spiral-shaped movement activated by cranialsacral (CS) rhythm to help the client unravel fascial adhesions throughout the body. During unwinding, a CS practitioner tracks the CS rhythm and uses it as a guide to lead a client through subtle, passive movement. The movement unwinds tension in the CS system, which in turn releases restrictions and restores balance in the autonomic nervous system. This finely focused work teaches practitioners to sense the subtle intrinsic and organic movements within a client's body.

Unwinding is used within the context of another therapy Upledger developed, called "somato-emotional release," which clears the body and mind of the physical and psychological residues accumulated from past traumas and negative experiences. Upledger believes that when people have unresolved trauma, whether physical or emotional, as the result of a blow that impacts the body, they have a subconscious, adaptive response that isolates the injured area. This occurs when the trauma condenses into an "energy cyst," which forms an energetic wall around the injured area. Upledger describes an energy cyst as "a localized area of increased particle activity [that] is synonymous with increased entropy. By this we mean that the ions and molecules are moving in a disorganized and chaotic way so that they are not performing usual work and serving the whole body efficiently."[199] In short, the body literally adapts to trauma by compressing and encapsulating it.

During somato-emotional release, the practitioner "holds the intention" of pulling the energy cyst out the point of entry in reverse while feeding what Upledger describes as healing energy into a place on the opposite side of the client's body. The client is then gently guided by the practitioner's touch through unwinding movements, often moving into the original position of trauma and reenacting the original injury, which may be physically and emotionally uncomfortable until the trauma releases. Exactly how somato-emotional release works is unknown, but it seems that moving into the position of a trauma could trigger a state-dependent memory of that trauma, bringing up the original charge and making an old wound available to new healing possibilities.

Somato-emotional work is a gentle synthesis of movement, touch, and emotional discharge that can provide practitioners with useful skills in following subtle, full-body patterns of physiological motion into release. CS therapy has increased the touch sensitivity of many practitioners, and, in turn, deepened clients' body awareness of subtle patterns of stress and relaxation. Many people, particularly those with high levels of stress in their bodies, have found enormous relief from chronic pain, nervous tension, and headaches after receiving CS therapy.[200]

PROPRIOCEPTIVE NEUROMUSCULAR FACILITATION (PNF)

Proprioceptive neuromuscular facilitation (PNF), first discussed in Chapter 3, is a longstanding physical therapy approach that is rapidly becoming a popular modality among bodyworkers. So many different versions of PNF are springing up in the somatic field that they tend to obscure what PNF actually is. In its most basic sense, PNF is as broad and fundamental a term as the word "stretching." (Stretching is used as a method of PNF.) PNF includes all methods that stimulate body awareness (proprioception) through assisted (facilitated) movement (neuromuscular function). Its biological definition is "any method used to activate neuromuscular mechanisms by stimulating proprioception." PNF describes any method of increasing movement range and coordination through awareness. Even massage could be considered a PNF technique if the massage practitioner is engaging the client's active participation in contraction, relaxation, or stretching techniques.

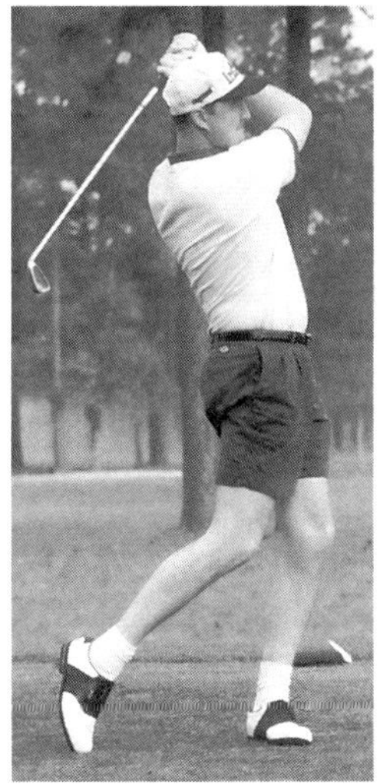

Figure 12.5 PNF rotations in sports activities (photo courtesy of L. Foster).

The PNF techniques, PNF patterns, and PNF stretching are actually three separate yet related aspects of PNF that can be used together or separately. Two widely used PNF approaches involve *facilitated stretching* (see Chapter 8) and *moving against resistance*. Both are used in therapeutic settings to increase, or facilitate, body awareness. The outcome of increased awareness, or proprioception, is the reorganization of the neuromuscular pathways. This reorganization can result in improved relaxation and contraction of individual muscles and groups of muscles, enhanced coordination among muscle groups, injury prevention due to increased movement efficiency, and rehabilitation from both structural and neurological injury. PNF creates neurological changes affecting how the nervous system organizes motion by increasing an awareness of motion. The goal of PNF is not so much to facilitate a muscle (to get it to contract), but to be able to feel when a muscle or group of muscles is working (contracting), and to sense the optimal sequencing of a chain of muscles during movement.

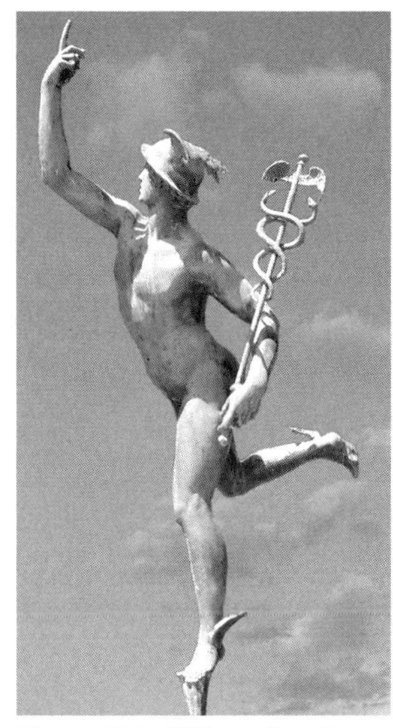

Figure 12.6 PNF rotations in classical sculpture

The PNF patterns are patterns of natural rotation that allow people to move in the familiar twisting and turning actions that they normally use during common daily activities and in sports (Figure 12.5). These rotations are commonly depicted in art and sculpture (Figure 12.6). PNF patterns affect the maximal number of neuromuscular (NM) structures in a movement sequence because they take all the joints in a kinematic chain through their full range of rotation. More stationary movements that lack rotations in the limbs, such as the homologous movement of pushing a wheelbarrow, involve only a part of the arc of a PNF pattern; the rotational relationships are still present in some of the joints, but they do not sequence through the entire body.

PNF Patterns

A systematic method of PNF therapy using rotational PNF patterns was first developed in the 1950s by a neurophysiologist named Herman Kabat, who created this unique system of diagonal movement patterns and facilitation techniques to treat polio patients.[201] Kabat's method of PNF has since been used by physical therapists to treat numerous musculoskeletal and neurological disorders, as well as orthopedic problems.

Patterning Exercise #119: Feeling Natural Rotations

Explore the following movements to feel how natural rotational patterns are for our bodies. You will not need any equipment to do this exploration; simply imagine the soccer ball you are kicking or the discus you are throwing as you go through the motion. Notice the shape of the rotations in the spine and the four limbs as you perform each action.

1. Kicking a soccer ball.
2. Hitting a tennis ball.
3. Throwing a bowling ball.
4. Throwing a discus.
5. Throwing a baseball.
6. Cross-country skiing.
7. Walking a tightrope.

The original elements of Kabat's method are:

- maximal resistance through a range of motion;
- movement that combines rotation with either flexion or extension;
- specific positions;
- the stimulation of primitive movement patterns, postural reflexes, and righting reflexes;
- progressive motion from the strongest part of the range to the weakest;
- stretch applied to synergist muscles for greater proprioceptive stimulation;
- repeated muscular contractions to gain range and endurance.[202]

In 1949 Kabat added several important elements to refine PNF techniques. He would have a patient isometrically contract the agonist muscles against his resistance, then contract the antagonist, in a technique he called "rhythmic stabilization." He also discovered the importance of using an **isotonic contraction** to facilitate motion. In this type of contraction, the muscle tension is even throughout the movement. All isotonic contractions are either concentric or eccentric, during which the agonist has a facilitating effect on its antagonist, causing inactive antagonist muscles to contract. In Kabat's technique called "slow reversal," a practitioner provides slow resistance for a patient to push a moving limb against.

Then Kabat realized that a spiral, diagonal shape of a PNF pattern caused the maximal elongation of muscles. In 1951, he defined four diagonal patterns (D1 and D2 in both the arms and the legs) designed to take a person through a full range of rotary patterns (Figure 12.7a-b). Each pattern follows the three-dimensional topographical alignment of the muscles and takes all the joints in the moving limb through a complete range of three-dimensional motion by combining three movements: *internal or external rotation, flexion or extension,* and *movement toward or away from the midline of the body.* The PNF stretches take the three components of the diagonal pattern to their full range of motion, getting the person to move to her limit of range so she can maximize the benefit of the PNF patterns.

Kabat's system utilizes a combination of both PNF patterns and techniques. For instance, if a person has a chronic posterior tilt in the pelvis, the hamstrings are too tight, which restricts the movement pattern. Therefore, a PNF stretch technique is applied while a client moves through a PNF pattern not only to increase the range of motion that elongates the hamstrings, but also to improve coordination by changing neuromuscular pathways. While PNF naturally enhances flexibility, flexibility is not its primary goal because this system works to improve neurological function, of which flexibility is simply one component.

The PNF patterns are designed to:

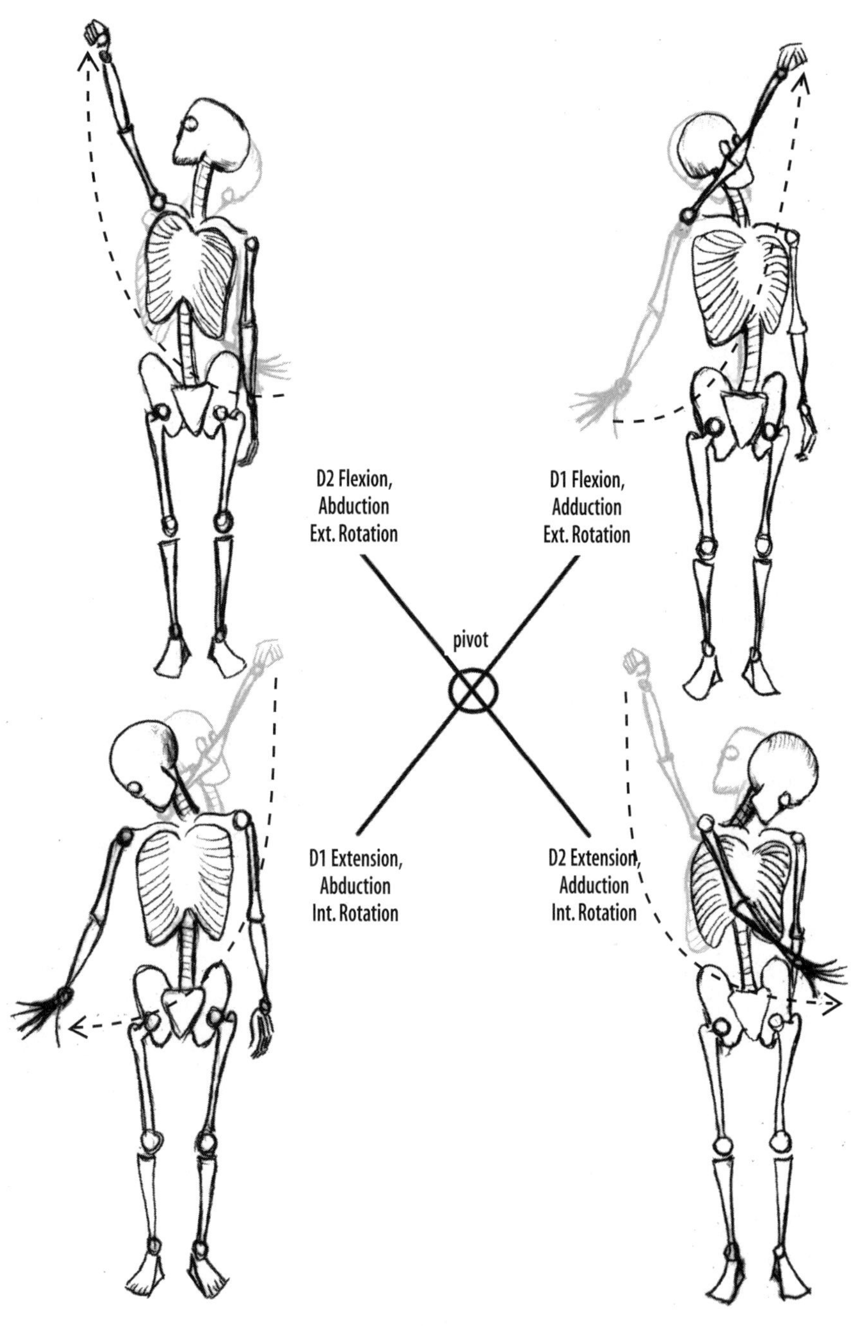

Figure 12.7a The PNF patterns of the upper extremities

- create rotational, diagonal movements that increase proprioceptive stimulation;
- improve coordination;
- balance tone between agonist and antagonist muscle;
- organize a chain of motion that sequences through two or more joints;
- increase joint flexibility;
- improve overall coordination and neuromuscular function.

The basic PNF patterns, D1 and D2, each has a flexion and extension phase so that the end of one pattern is the start of another. D1 flexion in the upper extremity approximates the movement of wrapping a cape around the neck, or wrapping an arm around the face to scratch the back of the head. D1 extension of the upper extremity resembles a backstroke in tennis or the arm gesture a baseball umpire makes to indicate a player is safe. D2 patterns of flexion and extension in the upper extremity are often called "drawing a sword" and "sheathing a sword," respectively, because they resemble these actions. D2 extension is also similar to pull-starting a lawnmower.

Once a person has become proficient at D1 and D2 flexion and extension, he or she can practice them together, doing D1 patterns in one arm and D2 patterns in the other, moving in simultaneous flexion and extension patterns or in opposing patterns. At the beginning level of the patterns, the knees and elbows are extended during the entire movement. At advanced levels, the elbows and knees are flexed and extended in different variations. The patterns seem complex at first because they cover precise spatial pathways and require precise movements. Still, they clarify the normal rotational patterns that are coordinated between the limbs and trunk during most activities, particularly sports.

D1 flexion of the lower extremity resembles kicking a soccer ball forward and across the body with the inside edge of the foot. D1 extension is a reversal of this action. It resembles reaching a foot behind the body to kick a door closed. D2 flexion resembles kicking a soccer ball forward with the outside edge of the foot. A bowler uses a D2 extension pattern to counterbalance his body with his back leg while throwing the bowling ball forward.

By going through every possible combination of PNF patterns in both the arms and the legs, we can move our joints through their full rotational range, which will expand our range of neuromuscular pathways. This improves not only the range of motion in the body, but also muscular coordination as well as the coordination of movement between the limbs and the trunk.

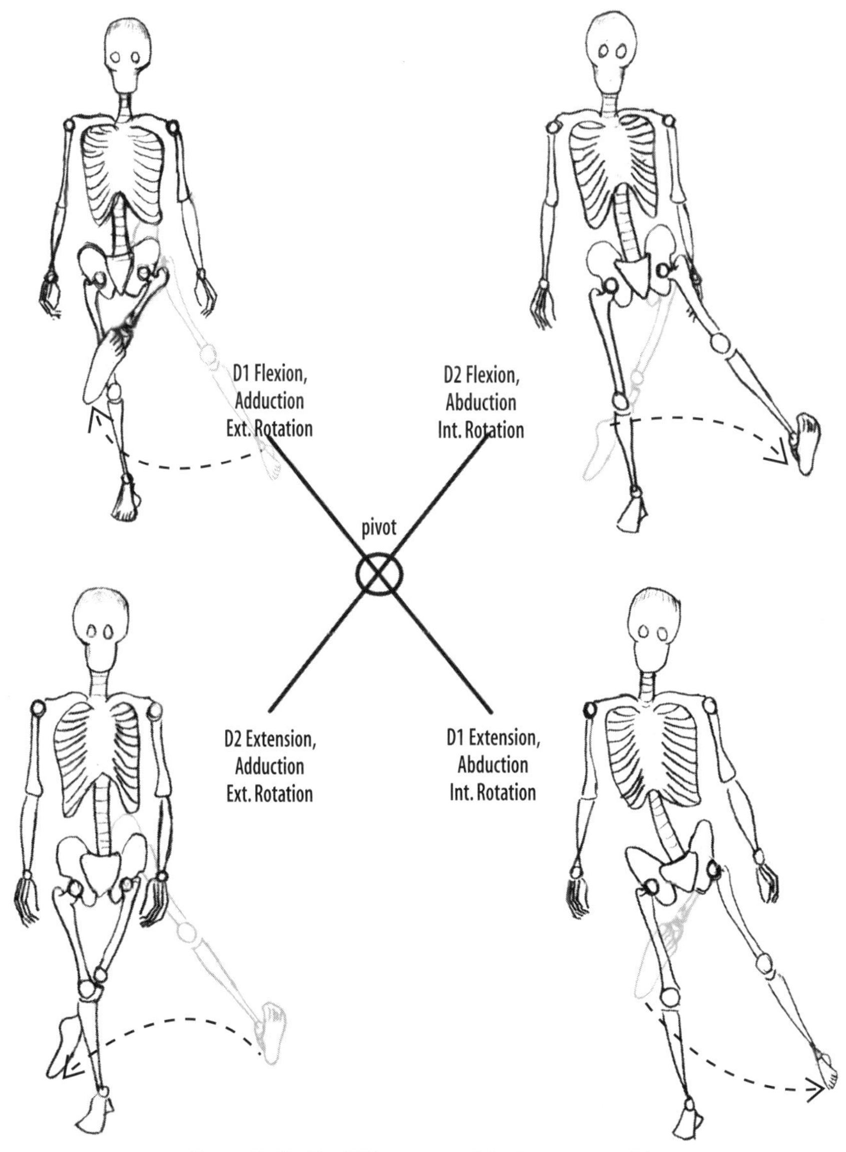

Figure 12.7b The PNF patterns of the lower extremities

PNF Techniques

As mentioned earlier, PNF is a neurological technique. Its neurological effects are broader than just awareness because PNF accesses and patterns the reflexive neuromuscular structures in the muscles. During the practice of PNF techniques, the brain receives input from the *muscle spindles,* which are sensory and motor fibers in the muscles that respond to changes in length. The brain also receives input for the *golgi tendon organs* (GTOs), which are sensory fibers in the tendons that respond to changes in tension.

Both the muscle spindles and GTOs serve a protective function in a muscle and its tendon to prevent overstretching

Patterning Exercise #120: D1 Patterns of the Upper Extremity

Explore these movement patterns with a focused awareness of what your arm is doing, taking each component of motion—flexion or extension, internal or external rotation, and adduction or abduction—into full range.

1. Begin in a standing position with both arms hanging at your sides, palms facing forward.
2. *D1 flexion:* Simultaneously make a fist with your right hand and flex your right wrist. The DI flexion pattern begins here.
3. Bring your right arm forward, up, and across the front of your body while externally rotating your right *humerus* at the shoulder joint. Your right humerus should be in front of your face, your fingers and wrist all flexed, your right fist pointing toward you (PE Fig. 120a). This is the end of D1 flexion.

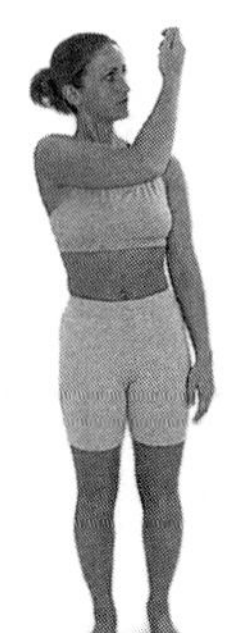

PE Fig. 120a

4. *D1 extension:* To begin D1 extension, open your right hand, turning the thumb first toward your face, then toward the floor. Keep turning your right thumb away from you as your forearm rotates.
5. Internally rotate your right upper arm in the same direction as your thumb and forearm while you move your arm across your body (in internal rotation, abduction, and extension). Move until you feel a stretch and your extended palm is facing backward (PE Fig. 120b). The D1 extension pattern ends here. (D1 flexion begins here with step 2, which starts the D1 flexion and extension cycle over.) Repeat D1 flexion and extension several times with the right arm.
6. Switch arms and repeat steps 1–6 .
7. *Both arms in synchrony:* Simultaneously practice the same pattern with both arms, beginning with both arms extended, hanging at your sides.
8. *Both arms in opposition:* Simultaneously practice opposite patterns with both arms—doing D1 flexion with the right arm while doing D1 extension with the left arm, and vice-versa.

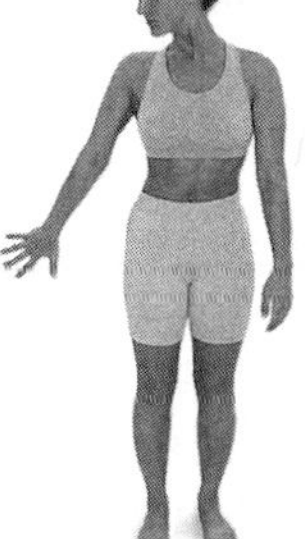

PE Fig. 120b

Note: This exercise can be practiced with an extended or flexed elbow.

EMSPress.com

which could cause injury. The muscle spindles and GTOs have the opposite effect on the same muscle. For instance, say a man's arm muscles are starting to overstretch during a game of tug of war. The muscle spindles will trigger reflexes that contract the arm muscles so he can pull harder to protect his arms from overstretching. Conversely, the GTOs trigger reflexes that relax his arm muscles so that he can release the rope to prevent muscle or tendon pulls and strains. In each

Patterning Exercise #121: D2 Patterns of the Upper Extremity

Move with an awareness of what your arm is doing, taking each component of motion—flexion or extension, internal or external rotation, and adduction or abduction—into full range.

1. Begin in a standing position with your right arm crossed in front of your body, your right hand and fist flexed at about the level of your left hip bone (at the *anterior superior iliac spine*) (PE Fig. 121a). The D2 flexion pattern begins here, at the end of the D1 extension.
2. *D2 flexion:* To begin D2 flexion, flex your wrist and make a fist as though you were closing your hand around a sword. Then externally rotate your arm and raise it across your body and up to your right side. This is the end of D1 flexion.

PE Fig. 121a **PE Fig. 121b**

3. *D2 extension:* To begin D2 extension, open your fist and extend your fingers and wrist (PE Fig. 121b). Then internally rotate your right arm, and, leading with your thumb, take your hand and arm across you body and down to your left hip. This is the end of the D2 extension. (D1 flexion begins by flexing the wrist and making a fist.)
4. Repeat D2 flexion and extension several times with your right arm.
5. *Left arm:* Switch arms and repeat steps 1–4 on the other side.
6. *Both arms in synchrony:* Simultaneously practice the same pattern with both arms, beginning with both arms extended, hanging at your sides (PE Fig. 121c-d).

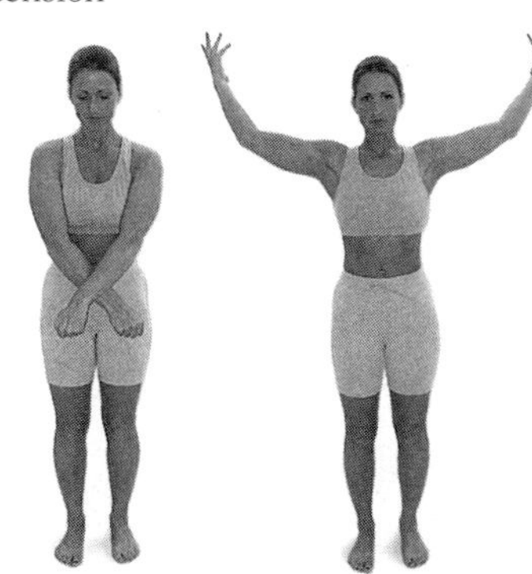

PE Fig. 121c **PE Fig. 121d**

7. *Both arms in opposition:* Simultaneously practice opposite patterns with both arms—doing D2 flexion with the right arm while doing D2 extension with the left arm, and vice-versa.

Note: Any of these patterns can be practiced with either an extended or flexed elbow.

EMSPress.com

Patterning Exercise #122: D1 and D2 Patterns of the Lower Extremity

1. *D1 patterns:* Begin in a standing position with your right leg crossed in front of your body, knee extended, foot flexed, and hip internally rotated (PE Fig. 122a). This is the end of the D1 flexion pattern.
2. *D1 extension:* To begin D1 extension, simultaneously point your right toes and externally rotate your right hip (PE Fig. 122b). Then take your leg in a sweeping motion to your side and behind you, ending with your toes on the floor (PE Fig. 122c).

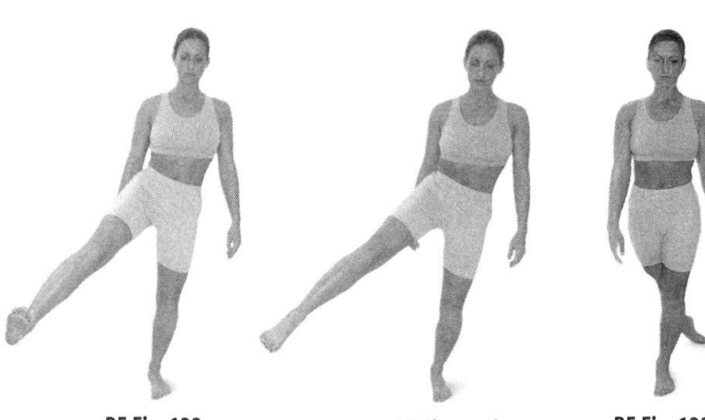

PE Fig. 122a PE Fig. 122b PE Fig. 122c

3. *D1 flexion:* To begin D1 flexion, flex your ankle, then internally rotate your leg and sweep it forward, up and across your body, ending in the starting position described in step 1.
4. Repeat steps 2 and 3 several times until you can make smooth transitions between the two movements.
5. Repeat steps 1–4 on the left leg.
6. *D2 patterns:* Begin in a standing position with your right leg extended in front of your body slightly out to the right side, foot flexed, and hip internally rotated (PE Fig. 122d). This is the end of the D2 flexion pattern.
7. *D2 extension:* To begin D2 extension, simultaneously point the toes of your right foot and externally rotate your right leg by turning your heel (PE Fig. 122e). Then sweep your leg back, across, and down to the floor, ending with your leg behind you (PE Fig. 122f).
8. *D2 flexion:* To begin D2 flexion, flex your right ankle and internally rotate your right hip as you sweep your leg forward and up, ending in the starting position described in step 6.
9. Repeat steps 6–8 several times until you can make smooth transitions between the two movements.

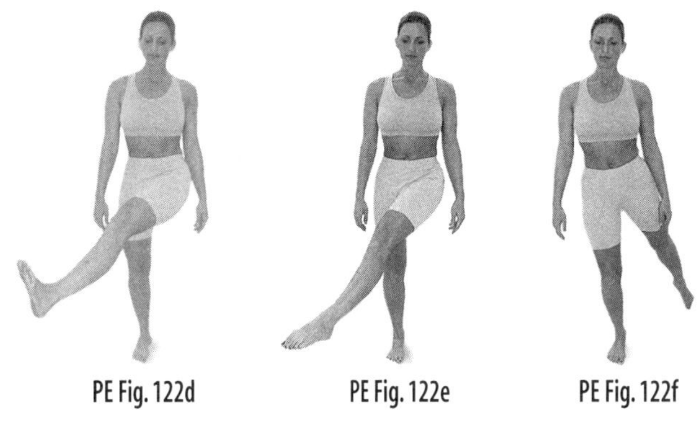

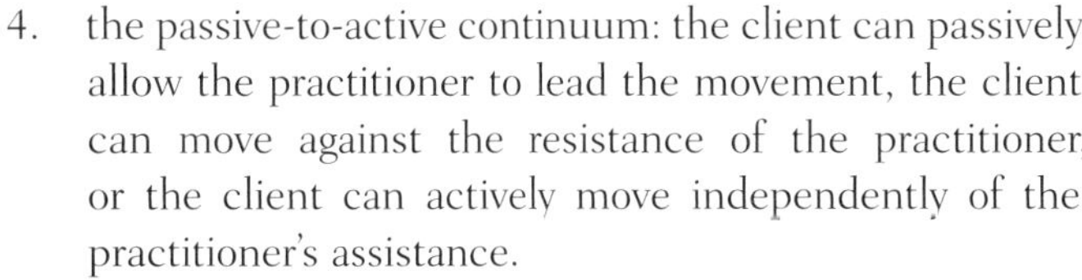

PE Fig. 122d PE Fig. 122e PE Fig. 122f

10. Then repeat steps 6–8 on your left leg.

Note: The lower extremity patterns can also be practiced while sitting in a chair with one variation: the knee should be flexed whenever the leg goes behind the body.

EMSPress.com

case, the proprioceptive awareness of the extreme pull on the muscles triggers protective reflexes to prevent injury.

Proprioception has to do with an awareness of what happens within a muscle cell. However, a practitioner can facilitate a client's muscles without the client's conscious awareness of muscle reflexes. A PNF practitioner uses many different techniques while guiding a client through the PNF patterns.[203] These basic techniques are used in conjunction with other variable elements:

1. the client's push against the practitioner's resistance or the practitioner's push against the client's resistance;
2. the speed of contraction, of relaxation, and of movement reversal;
3. the position in the range that the contraction, relaxation, or stretch takes place;
4. the passive-to-active continuum: the client can passively allow the practitioner to lead the movement, the client can move against the resistance of the practitioner, or the client can actively move independently of the practitioner's assistance.

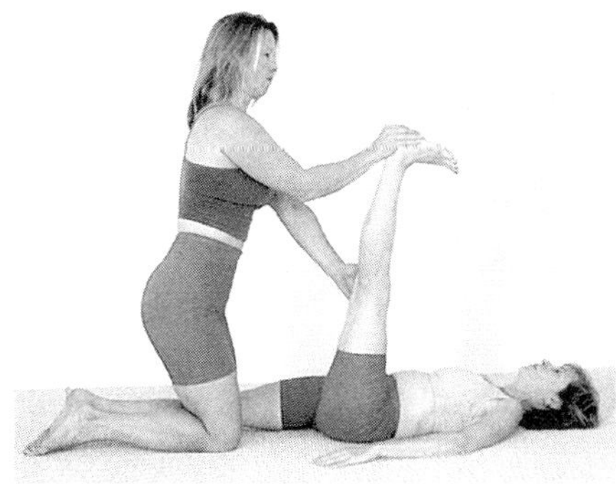

Figure 12.8 A practitioner providing resistance for the client to push against

PNF patterns can be practiced in a number of ways. People can explore the patterns on their own or can be guided through the patterns by practitioners who provide them resistance when needed (Figure 12.8). Resistance can enhance proprioception and increase the strength of a contraction or the range of a stretch. People can also practice the patterns on their own while moving against the resistance of something like a towel, theraband, or rubber bungee. Resistance may be applied with steady pressure or with rhythmic pulsation. However, when resistance is used, it is always applied against the medial or lateral side of the hand or foot to increase tone there during the initiation of the PNF pattern. Resistance has the advantage of strengthening the limb and reorganizing the chain of muscular actions.

The eight basic PNF patterns (D1 and D2 flexion and extension in the upper and lower extremities) can be done in 120 different combinations to create 120 patterns. Each of the different PNF techniques can be used with each pattern. Given this complexity of the PNF system, it is likely that any of the popular bodywork modalities claiming to use PNF methods are using only a small part of the complete system. Regardless, PNF techniques and stretches can be highly effective in reorganizing neuromuscular functions even within a limited application.

STABILITY REHABILITATION

Traditionally, spinal instability is defined as excessive joint play due to abnormal range at the end range of motion. But the orthopedist Manohar Panjabi's model of the stabilizing system of the spine challenges this definition. Panjabi points out that spinal joint stability comes from an interdependent relationship among joint structure, muscle function, and the control a person has over neuromuscular mechanisms (Figure 12.9). In 1989 he defined the concept of a *neutral zone* in the spine (introduced in Chapter 2) as "the displacement between the neutral position and the initiation point of spinal resistance to physiological motion."[204] This concept describes the amount of play there is in a spinal joint before there is any effective resistance offered from the spinal muscles to stabilize it. When a joint is stable, the neutral zone is relatively small, but as a joint becomes less stable, shear forces increase the size of the neutral zone.

Although Panjabi's concept of the neutral zone stems from a study of passive joint and ligamentous structures, his definition of stability—the ability to control the entire range of motion of a joint—has laid the groundwork for a new approach to stability rehabilitation. Stability rehabilitation exercises are used by physical therapists to treat chronic pain caused by a *stability dysfunction* (introduced in Chapter 2), a condition is which joint play has become so excessive that light movements actually damage the joint. Traditional rehabilitation exercises involve strengthening muscles around the damaged area. In this new approach, a person learns to control specific intrinsic muscles around the injured joint using light isometric contractions that stiffen the joint.

Exactly which specific muscles control joint stability, especially in the spine, has become a topic of much research. For example, a group of Australian researchers observed that in stability dysfunctions in knees, although the specific muscle that supports and controls joint position was inhibited, typical stability exercises given in rehabilitation weren't specific to that muscle. In progressive rehabilitation programs, a patient learns control over the *vastus lateralis oblique muscle* (a small, intrinsic muscle going from the knee to the distal third of the inner thigh) in order to control joint position and thereby stabilize the knee.

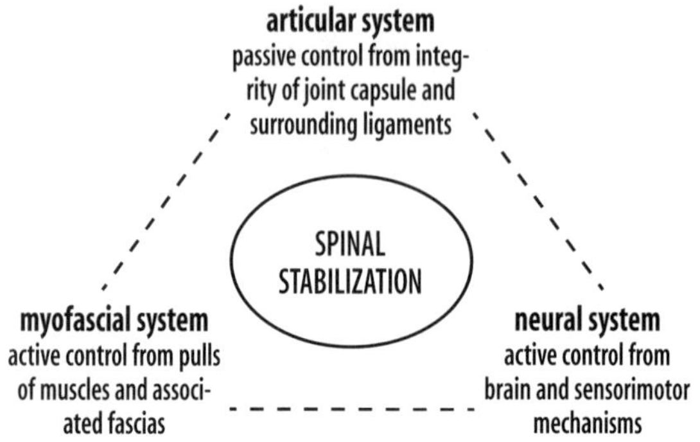

Figure 12.9 Panjabi's model of spinal stabilization

Using the same logic, a group of researchers hypothesized that by identifying exactly which muscles control segmental stiffness in the spine, they could teach a person to control these muscles to alleviate low back pain caused by a stability dysfunction from the lack of segmental stiffness.[205] They began to develop specific tests to target the stabilization function of specific muscles, and found evidence indicating that their hypothesis was valid with results indicating, for example, that the *multifidus* and *transversus abdominis muscles* were consistently weak in people with chronic low back pain (see Chapter 9). In one study, only 10 percent of the subjects with chronic low back pain could control the transversus abdominis muscles compared to 82 percent of those without chronic pain.[206] They then hypothesized that low back pain could be alleviated by learning to control the transversus abdominis and other muscles that control segmental stiffness in the lumbar spine. Learning to control stabilizers became the basis of this innovative approach to stability training.

Another enterprising Australian physical therapist named Mark Comerford combined and expanded the stabilization rehabilitation concepts and methods into a comprehensive training program for physical therapists called **Kinetic Control**. Comerford took the approach to lumbar stabilization of learning to control stabilizing muscles in the pelvis and expanded the application by applying the same type of treatment to problematic joints in the entire spine. Protocol is based on awareness and timing rather than muscle strengthening. A person learns how to control the dysfunctional muscle—dysfunction meaning that it is either not firing or firing too late—contracting it at the right time in the appropriate sequence.

This innovative program offers a progressive training that begins with learning to control the **local stabilizers**, then the **global stabilizers**, and then the *mobilizers* (the concept of stabilizer and mobilizer muscles was introduced in Chapter 2).[207] To review, the muscles are classified as local or global based on their mechanical roles. The local muscles of the spine are usually intrinsic and control the segmental stiffness of a specific joint. The larger muscles of the spine are usually extrinsic, span two or more joints, and are involved in moving the spine as well as transferring load from the upper to the lower body.[208] The local stabilizers of the spine work independently of motion both in a stationary posture and while the whole body is moving. They control segmental stiffness of the spine independent of the direction or range in which the spine is moving. The global stabilizers come into play to control range during movement. For example, the diagonal fibers of oblique muscles wrapping the waist control the degree of rotation in the waist during twisting motions.

The type of training for each stabilizer (see Chapter 9 for information on specific muscles) depends on its function and on the person's baseline skill level. The first step in stability training is learning to control the neutral range of a joint. During this stage, the emphasis is on learning isolated contractions of the local stabilizers in a nonmoving position. It is crucial that a person be able to contract and control the stabilizers without contracting the mobilizers. By doing this, a person learns to control the sequence in which the muscles fire so that the stabilizers fire before the mobilizers.

Making sure the right muscle is contracting is an important aspect of this approach. Usually, this takes accurate feedback from a trained professional such as a physical therapist who has been trained in Kinetic Control. Repetition is also key: it takes a long time to control and tone a tonic muscle whose slow motor units have evolved to sustain a continuous contraction. Turning a stabilizer on and keeping it on can take anywhere from 30 to 90 days of conscious, methodical repetition. Although this seems excessive, the payoff makes it worthwhile. When a person suffering chronic pain from a stability dysfunction is able to isolate, activate, and control the muscle that stiffens that unstable joint, the relief can be almost instantaneous. Stabilizing muscles should be doing their job whenever we are awake; therefore, learning to control them makes repetition of training critical.

The second phase of training for the local stabilizers is learning to produce the isolated contractions in different positions. After this, a person learns to simultaneously contract, or co-contract, two or more local stabilizers. Once proficient at controlling the local stabilizing muscles, in isolation and as a unified group, the person is ready to add the next phase of the training.

The third phase entails learning to use the global stabilizers, without losing the underlying support of the local stabilizers, to *stabilize movement through range* (Figure 12.10). People with instability problems usually lack control in both the local stabilizers. To stabilize movement through a range, a person practices activating the local stabilizers while in a neutral posture, then progresses to the eccentric control of slow movements. For example, when lifting or lowering the knees one side from a hooklying position—lying on the back with both knees bent, feet flat and parallel—the oblique muscles on the opposite side work eccentrically to elongate the waist and control the lowering of the knees. Eccentric control works similarly to an elastic line being let out a bit at a time to keep a descending weight from dropping too fast. During forward bending, the gluteus maximus works eccentrically to the rate at which the trunk descends.

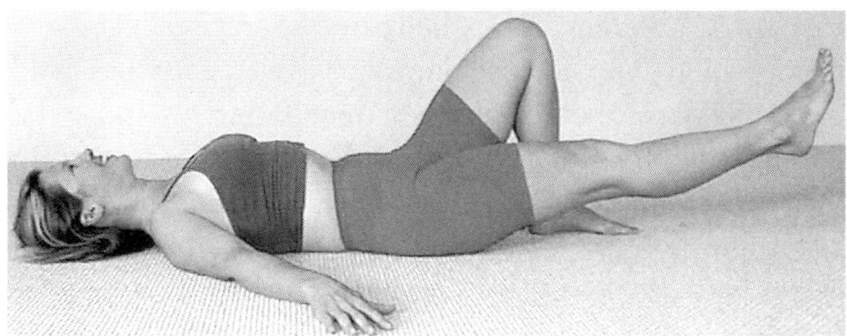

Figure 12.10 Lifting the leg while keeping the pelvis stable

When the mobilizers lose their extensibility, changes occur in the tissues. Connective tissue that builds up in the myofascia can make the muscles too taut to stretch or contract effectively. In the most advanced stage of stability training, a person practices "mobilizer extensibility." During this stage, a person practices precise movements that stretch and lengthen the mobilizers, particularly chronically contracted mobilizers that restrict range of motion.

Stabilization is integrated into daily activities in a number of ways. A person can practice any of the stability isometrics during any activity. The red dot technique is also suggested—red dot stickers are put around areas of common use—over the mirror in the bathroom, for example, or above the kitchen sink or on the telephone. Anytime a person sees a red dot, he or she practices a stabilization exercise.

SUMMARY

This chapter is a mix of traditional and alternative approaches to neuromuscular education and manual therapy. This mix is included for several reasons. First of all, the traditional approaches presented here are widely used by somatic practitioners and bodyworkers. Also, both the alternative and traditional therapies that use neuromuscular education to change faulty body-use habits that lead to pain are working toward the same goal in regard to patterning intrinsic musculature for postural support.

Although there are many different approaches to myofascial release, Rolfing is unique in that it is an educational process, a 10-step protocol in which myofascial tension is unlayered in an organized and logical manner. Aston Patterning is similar, only more organic, viewing the core of the body as a dynamic spiral around which we can move in and out of tension patterns in a fluid manner.

Many Rolfers and bodyworkers specializing in myofascial release are also drawing on the techniques used in cranialsacral therapy and proprioceptive neuromuscular facilitation (PNF). Cranialsacral therapy has provided an invaluable education to many somatic practitioners in becoming able to sense the movement of physiological rhythms in the body. By allowing these rhythms to be present during patterning exercises, a person can both release autonomic tension and integrate intrinsic organic processes with mechanical neuromuscular patterning. PNF provides a comprehensive system to work with neuromuscular reflexes and rotational patterns in order to improve coordination and expand range.

It is interesting to note that many orthopedic doctors and physical therapists are currently investigating *exactly* which intrinsic muscles function as postural stabilizers, and are applying this work to stability rehabilitation with a precision generally absent in the alternative methods of developing postural muscles such as Pilates and Rolfing Movement. Their research findings and therapeutic methods will definitely be helpful to somatic practitioners using neuromuscular patterning to improve posture. Conversely, somatic therapies such as Rolfing contribute an integrative model of structural integration to give myofascial release holistic direction, and cranialsacral therapy provides bodyworkers and physical therapists alike with refined skills to sense the subtle fluid rhythms that are restricted by myofascial tensions. Although the alternative and traditional practitioners come from opposite ends of the healthcare system, they seem to be headed toward similar conclusions about what constitutes healthy neuromuscular function and optimal postural support.

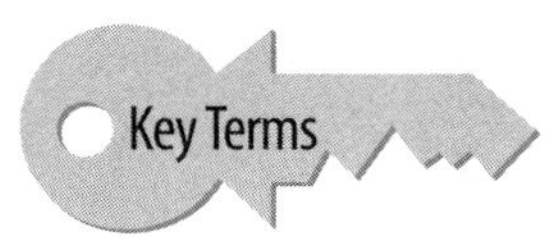

Aston Patterning
cranialsacral (CS) therapy
direct technique
fascial network
global stabilizers
indirect technique
isotonic contraction
Kinetic Control
local stabilizers
Rolfing
Rolfing Movement Education
stillpoint
tensegrity structure
unwinding

OVERVIEW OF CHAPTER 13

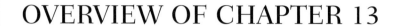

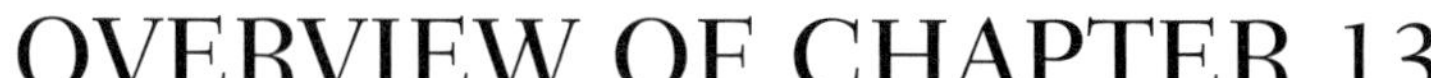

13

Physiological Patterning

Evidence that the mind and body influence each other abounds. And suggests something much stranger: That awareness isn't confined to the brain: it operates 'nonlocally,' beyond the biochemical lines between brain and, say, immune system. This consciousness revolution is rattling the very foundation of Western medicine.

—M. Barasch

Since the early 1900s, paradigms in Western medicine have been shifting in terms of our understanding of the causes of pathologies. By about 1960, the primary causes of death in the United States were no longer microbial in nature.[209] Stress had replaced infection as the number one cause of illness and disease, and it continues to hold that role today. At the same time that many of the movement and bodywork therapies were developing, a number of progressive physiologists and physicians had begun to recognize that body and mind are integrally connected and that many stress-related problems have psychosomatic roots. Researchers were beginning to uncover the physiological basis of stress and metabolic balance. Scientists began searching for new treatment modalities that were based on gaining conscious control over unconscious body functions. Their research revealed that thoughts and emotions not only create stress and affect physiology, but that thought may also affect nonlocal conditions, as evidenced in research findings validating the healing power of prayer.[210]

In 1932, physiologist Walter Cannon coined the terms *fight-or-flight* and *homeostasis* to describe physical states of alarm and balance, respectively. About this time, psychiatrist Edmund Jacobson found through extensive research that muscle activity accompanies all mental processes. In the 1950s, John Basmajian began studying muscle activity with electromyography and found that it is possible for a person to gain conscious control over a single motor unit. And in the 1960s, Elmer and Alyce Green began studying the effects of self-regulation on physiology and on treating various health problems. Out of all this work came biofeedback therapy, a relatively new modality developed to teach people how to regulate physiological patterns of stress and tension through mental control using physiological feedback.

This chapter covers the history and methods of biofeedback and psychoneuroimmunology. Biofeedback research is proving that the mind *does* affect the body and that we can effect changes in physiology through thought. Research in psychoneuroimmunology takes this knowledge one giant step further; it is beginning to uncover the biochemical relationships between thought and emotion, revealing *how* the mind actually affects the body.

STRESS

Although most people now understand the effects of stress on their health in a general way, our understanding of the impact of stress is relatively recent. It began when the Viennese physician Hans Selye took the word "stress" from the realm of physics and gave it a biological definition in the 1950s. Selye defined stress as "the body's non-specific response to any demands placed upon it, whether that demand is pleasurable or not."[211] Although initially tempted to

PARASYMPATHETIC	SYMPATHETIC
Heart rate slows down	Heart rate speeds up
Breathing slows down	Breathing speeds up
Vegetative functions are dominant (e.g., digestion, regeneration)	Blood is sent to the muscles to prepare for action
Blood is primarily in abdominal organs	Capillaries vasoconstrict
Capillaries vasodilate	Perspiration (electro-dermal response) increases
The body relaxes	Pituitary stimulates adrenals to release adrenaline and epinephrine
Feelings of peace, security, and safety arise	All senses are heightened, fear may arise
Tissues regenerate	Eyes dilate to focus more specifically

Figure 13.1 Autonomic Responses

define stress as wear and tear on the body, Selye chose to emphasize more accurately that stress is not the actual wear, but the symptoms caused by the wear.

Selye's definition of stress explained the many maladaptive, vague symptoms such as headaches, fatigue, joint pain, and indigestion that occur prior to the onset of stress-related conditions, such as arteriosclerosis, arthritis, and late-onset diabetes. His revolutionary concept of stress opened up an era of new approaches in medical treatment, approaches based on lifestyle choices.

The first step in treating a stress-related problem is to understand what stress does psychologically and physiologically. Cannon, who influenced our thinking about how emotional excitement relates to changes in physiology, used the phrase **fight-or-flight response** to describe organisms' behavioral responses to stress, which occur when a person is frightened or threatened. Whenever the hair trigger of a defense mechanism is set off, stress ensues and the person experiences a broad range of physiological reactions marked by anxiety. A fight-or-flight response triggers an increase of sympathetic tone in the autonomic nervous system, creating physiological responses that are in opposition to the parasympathetic tone that naturally exists in a relaxed state.

Keep in mind that our bodies are always shifting between sympathetic and parasympathetic states as we move in and out of action mode; therefore, sympathetic tone is not synonymous with being stressed (Figure 13.1). Stress occurs when we become stuck in a sympathetic state and are unable to recover from it.

The flight-or-flight response also involves a preliminary stage called the **freeze response**. Neuroscientist Joseph LeDoux points out that the freeze response is automatic and always occurs before a fight or a flight.[212] In fact, freezing when faced with danger, particularly a predator, creates a playing-dead bluff that increases the odds of the potential prey surviving longer. Most physiological damage actually occurs when the fight-or-flight mechanism is mobilized but the organism repeatedly locks down into a state of immobilization. Trauma specialist Peter Levine describes this response as a *tonic immobility*, a natural pattern he observed in wild animals who play dead by actually entering a suspended state that slows down physiological processes after a chase to avoid being killed. Tonic immobility becomes problematic for people when its physiological state remains long after an attack or trauma has ended, a condition often found in people with post-traumatic stress.[213]

To understand what happens during a freeze response, imagine what occurs in a person's body when he slams on the brakes to avoid a collision: adrenaline floods into the bloodstream, the heart races, a sweat breaks out, the stomach lurches up through the throat, and thoughts of death race through the mind. These reactions race inside of the driver's body while he sits frozen, immobilized, usually with white knuckles clutching the steering wheel. Internally the physiological engine is revved up, while externally the body remains locked in a freeze.

How many times are you able to carry your defense reactions into action and resolve them with actual body movement?

As first mentioned in Chapter 1, the aroused and unresolved physiological state that occurs in a freeze response could be compared to flooring the gas while the car is in park. When a person freezes, the body has made a physiological preparation for survival, for a defensive fight or flight, and this burst of energy has nowhere to go. The incomplete movement sequence puts stress on the physiological engine. Stress occurs whenever a person is unable to recover from a stress response, such as a fight-or-flight reaction not carried into action, a common occurrence in most modern lifestyles. Dr. Charles Stroebel, author of *QR: The Quieting Reflex*, estimates that most people experience more than 50 stress-causing situations every day.[214] According to his figures, the average person has fight-or-flight responses two or three times per hour.

The General Adaptation Model

We cannot avoid stress in our lives. In fact, we need stress to become stronger. Healthy stress, or **eustress**, builds resistance. Seyle describes eustress as the type of stress that results in a healthy adaptive response, that builds strength in the body and mind, and that fortifies the system.[215] People who lack the normal stress of an active life in both the body and mind may suffer from soft bodies (lacking muscle tone) and low levels of motivation.

We all respond to stress with some type of adaptive behavior. To identify the adaptive approaches we use to handle stress, Selye researched the cumulative degeneration that occurs during prolonged exposure to a **stressor**, the factor that induces a stress responses. Prolonged exposure to stressors creates a cumulative degeneration that can lead to what Selye calls **diseases of adaptation**. These include metabolic disorders or diseases such as obesity, diabetes, and hyperthyroidism; liver disease, gout, heart diseases, cancer, ulcers, and immune dysfunction; and inflammatory diseases such as arthritis and rheumatism. Selye speculated that physiological wear and tear builds up after each episode of stress until the body is no longer able to return to normal. He developed a **general adaptation syndrome** (GAS) model to describe the cumulative stages involved in stress responses:

1. *Alarm reaction*: This is the body's "call to arms" of its defenses. The initial reaction, if extreme, can lead to death or shock; when mild, the adrenal cortex secretes hormones and glandular stores are depleted.
2. *Resistance stage*: Continued exposure to stressors creates resistance, and the symptoms involved in the alarm reaction disappear. Glandular stores are replenished and the organism is strengthened.
3. *Exhaustion*: After long, continuous exposure to stressors, the adaptation response is exhausted, alarm reactions reappear, physiological changes are irreversible, and the organism usually dies. [216]

Stressors can range from thinking self-deprecating thoughts to living in a violent family or war zone. Most people go through the first two GAS stages many times, yet Selye feels that many activities can take us through all three stages. As he describes it: "First we have to get in the swing of things, then we get pretty good at them, but finally we tire of them."[217] By recognizing the stages involved in recovering from stressful states before reaching exhaustion, we can learn to manage stress responses and actually use them to increase our resistance levels to stressors.

Autonomic Flexibility

Autonomic flexibility (introduced in Chapter 4) is a term coined in biofeedback therapy to describe the ability of a person to move from a stress reaction into a relaxed state, from sympathetic tone to parasympathetic tone. The degree of autonomic flexibility is gauged by the amount of time it takes a person to recover from a stress response. The key to developing autonomic flexibility is not in becoming relaxed and remaining so, but in having the ability to move from a state of high arousal to a state of relaxation.

The degree of autonomic flexibility a person has is an indicator of that person's stress-coping abilities, similar to a barometer or a thermostat. A high degree of flexibility indicates that a person can recover from stress in a manner that discharges the negative effects without incurring the damaging side effects. A person without a healthy level of autonomic flexibility tends to function from a baseline of high sympathetic tone and thus is deeply aroused by even minor stressors.

Links to Practical Applications

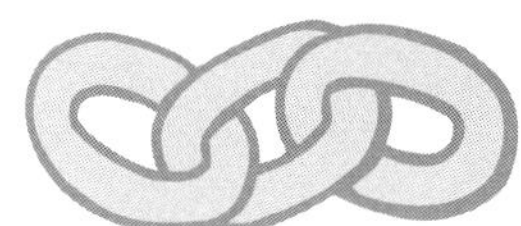

Dealing with Stress

Notice during the course of a day how many times your fight-or-flight responses are triggered. You might sense them while flinching to avoid a swerving car or while thinking about a stressful life situation. When you feel them, take a moment to recover: breathe slowly, relax your body, and tell yourself everything is okay. With practice, you will become more adept at taking a moment for recovery and will develop control over your ability to relax after the stress response has been triggered.

Relaxation skills are taught in biofeedback training (to be discussed shortly) with the goal of improving autonomic flexibility. There are numerous types of relaxation skills, autogenics being one of the oldest modern methods.

Autogenics

Before the concept of physiological stress was clarified by Dr. Selye, Johannes Schultz, a German physiologist and neurologist, created a technique called **autogenics** to teach people how to reduce physiological and psychological tension. In 1910 Schultz began teaching his patients this technique of putting oneself into a mild state of self-induced hypnosis that is incompatible with states of tension.[218] During autogenic training, a person gets into a quiet place and assumes a relaxed position. Then she repeats a series of phrases for a 20-minute period, such as: "My arms and legs are getting heavy and warm . . . I feel warmth flowing into my limbs . . . my heartbeat is calm and regular . . . my body breathes itself."[219]

The autogenic phrases are designed to elicit specific physiological responses. The term "heavy" is equated with relaxation, and "warmth" with vasodilation. By focusing on heaviness and warmth in the limbs, a person learns how to control vasodilation by relaxing capillaries in the periphery of the body so that warmth rushes into the limbs. Schultz developed this series of verbal formulas with a focus on the relaxation of skeletal muscles, the vascular system, the heart, and breathing; on warming the abdominal area; and on cooling the forehead.

Autogenics has proved effective in the treatment of hypertension, stuttering, bed-wetting, insomnia, headaches, chronic constipation, bronchial asthma, and phobias. It has also been used in the treatment of Raynaud's disease, a condition in which a person has poor circulation in the hands and feet, causing the extremities to always be cold.

A significant therapeutic aspect of autogenics is its focus on helping a client to take active control over his own condition. Studies by many researchers have found that one of the most stress-producing agents in any life situation is lack of control or the perception of lack of control. Holmes and Rahe researched several occupations in which control was severely limited by job status or environment. They found in a study of secretarial workers that their work is one of the most stress-inducing jobs because secretaries have huge amounts of responsibility with little or no control over their jobs. In an evaluation of how men living on a navy ship adjusted to the new lifestyle, the researchers found three main factors to indicate healthy adjustment:

- having the ability to accept change as a challenge;
- having a sense of control over their lives;
- having a sense of commitment, which gives life purpose.[220]

Many people "try" so hard to do things the "correct" way that their efforts block change. Healthcare practitioners, if your client is caught in this dilemma, how can you help her enter into a state of passive volition?

Autogenics was designed to counter the negative effects on health of modern tensions by helping people to gain control over their body states. A hallmark of autogenics training is an attitude of *passive volition* (introduced in Chapter 4), which creates a state of "allowing" rather than active "doing." Passive volition enables relaxation to passively spread throughout the body without a person contributing any conscious effort to the process. It also allows an individual to direct a healing or learning process without creating stress from working too hard through too much conscious involvement in the process. Skills in passive volition and relaxation have been integrated into many somatic therapies.

BIOFEEDBACK THERAPY

Robert Stern and William Ray, the authors of a primer on biofeedback, describe the powers of biofeedback in the treatment of psychosomatic conditions:

> Let's use a hypothetical example of a person who complains of frightening attacks of heart palpitations: that is, his heart seems to pound rapidly in his chest. When Mr. R. first comes to see us, he reports that he is not aware of his heart beating except when he has an attack. We have Mr. R. take off his shirt so we can tape a small microphone to his chest. We then amplify the sound of his heart beating and permit Mr. R. to hear it over a speaker. He is now encouraged to relax and let his heart rate decrease. After a few minutes we tell him to think arousing thoughts, and in so doing cause an increase in heart rate. We do this for 30–40 minutes twice a week for 6 weeks. By now Mr. R. can make his heart rate go up and down at will. The next time Mr. R. starts to have an argument with his wife over a trivial matter, he will listen to his heart, accepting the warning as he senses that it is speeding up, and back off from the situation in time to avert an attack.[221]

Biofeedback (BF) therapy is a multidisciplinary approach to treating health problems, particularly those caused or complicated by stress. Although this discussion falls under the category of physiological patterning because of the results it yields, BF is primarily a cognitive process because it uses a person's awareness and mental influence to slow down physiological processes. Somatics is based on the fact that the body and mind are not separate, and BF therapy takes advantage of their integral connection. BF

Patterning Exercise #123: Autogenics—Warmth and Heaviness

First read this script into a tape recorder, taking a three-second pause after each statement. Next sit or lie in a relaxed and comfortable position, in a warm and quiet setting. Then play the tape and repeat each phrase during the pause.

1. My arms feel heavy and warm; warmth is flowing into my arms.
2. My hands feel heavy and warm; warmth is flowing into my hands.
3. My shoulders feel heavy and warm; warmth is flowing into my shoulders.
4. My hips feel heavy and warm; warmth is flowing into my hips.
5. My legs feel heavy and warm; warmth is flowing into my legs.
6. My feet feel heavy and warm; warmth is flowing into my feet.
7. My stomach feels heavy and warm; warmth is flowing into my stomach.
8. My heart feels calm and regular; my heart feels calm and regular.

therapy combines behavioral and cognitive therapies with stress management techniques and physiological feedback to teach people how to self-regulate the maladaptive stress reactions that precipitate many health problems. As a therapeutic modality, BF is used in a number of settings, from schools to hospitals, with a variety of conditions, combining several modalities. For example, the fictitious Mr. R. learned how to control his heart rate using BF instrumentation, which was only the beginning of his treatment. For the therapy to be effective, Mr. R. also needs to modify his stress-inducing behaviors, to practice these skills at home, and then, most importantly, to put these skills into action when he is in a stress-inducing situation.

The view of BF as a single treatment using machines such as electromyographs, which amplify muscle activity, is inaccurate. A typical biofeedback session usually includes two or more of many modalities, combining self-awareness and relaxation techniques with imagery, behavorial therapies (see Chapter 14), and self-regulation skills.[222] There are several types of machines for learning self-regulation, each providing a different kind of physiological feedback.

- *Thermal feedback* provides feedback of peripheral blood flow, monitored as skin temperature. This is the easiest method to monitor overall relaxation because thermistors (small apparatuses that monitor skin temperature) for fingers are cheap and easy to use.
- *Electrodermal resistance (EDR)* provides feedback of sweat gland activity, measured from fingers. EDR is used to build self-regulation skills in autonomic nervous system control.
- An *electromyograph (EMG)* provides feedback about muscular activity. EMGs are widely used to help people learn muscle relaxation skills and to reduce pain caused by chronically contracted or dysfunctional muscles.
- The *electroencephalograph (EEG)* provides feedback of brainwave activity, measured in different locations on the scalp. The EEG is used to help a person learn relaxation skills that occur during altered states of consciousness and to control such conditions as epilepsy and migraines.
- A *perinometer* provides feedback of contraction in the sphincter and pelvic floor muscles. It is used for incontinence and bladder control.

Biofeedback training using instrumentation addresses both physiological imbalances and muscular imbalances. A person is hooked up to a machine that measures physiological responses such as heart rate, skin temperature, skin resistance or sweating (the type of feedback used in lie detector tests), electrical activity in muscles, or brain wave activity. Feedback is delivered through either auditory or visual channels, by listening to an intermittent beep or watching a blinking light. The feedback acts like a mirror, reflecting the internal state of the body, providing a person with immediate information that he or she can use to regulate involuntary functions. In the example of the hypothetical patient Mr. R., he learned to control his heart by listening to the sound of its beat then slowing the beat down at will.

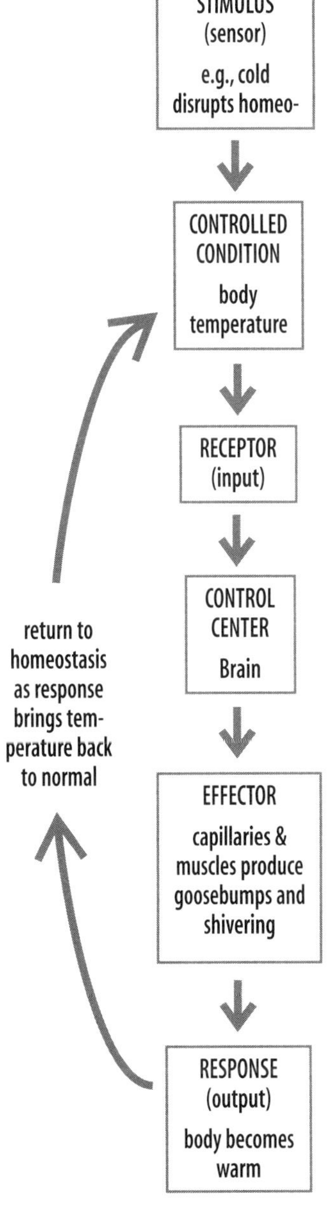

Figure 13.2 Homeostasis of body temperature in a negative feedback loop

The body has many internal feedback loops that function automatically and regulate physiological balance, or homeostasis, among body systems.[223] **Homeostasis** is the normal state of physiological equilibrium in which all of the body systems work together. Excessive amounts of stress upset homeostatic balance. Internal feedback systems regulating homeostasis steer the interacting body systems toward equilibrium after a stress response, returning the body to its normal equilibrium.

The feedback loops controlling homeostatic systems tend to be negative. This means that the feedback decreases or shuts off as the physiological changes move toward and reach homeostatic balance. BF employs a negative feedback loop. For instance, the blinking light on a BF machine slows down as muscle relaxation increases. Negative feedback loops control homeostatic systems that need to be maintained at a steady level or narrow range (Figure 13.2) Thus, everything remains quiet in the body until something needs to change; then signals such as pain or hunger become louder.

Positive feedback loops are just the opposite: they control episodic, infrequent events. For example, a positive feedback loop regulates the birthing process. Hormones pour into the system to escalate events toward delivery. The hormones provide a laboring mother's body with the rapidly changing physiological feedback needed to increase contractions and deliver a baby. Positive feedback systems can easily spin out of control. The initial feedback may appear positive, but the underlying adjustment is negative. For example, a person who feels pain may want the painful area to be deeply massaged by a practitioner, yet before this person knows it, what initially feels like relief from the massage can escalate into increased pain and a protective spasm. The surface feedback of changed sensation from the massage can mask the underlying spasm and increase pain.

Biofeedback therapy is based on using accurate feedback about physiological process to make changes to counter the ill effects of stress on homeostasis. With BF, people get immediate, ongoing information about their internal biological processes. The Greens, a husband and wife team who were early pioneers in BF research, compared it to Pavlov's classical conditioning exercise with dogs, only with the added element of human awareness. BF therapy is based on sound biological principles because external feedback from machines mimics internal feedback loops in the body. As the Greens explain: "In order to develop voluntary control of behavior, it is necessary to become conscious of (or focus consciousness on) the present behavior and at the same time visualize (imagine) the desired behavior. The difference between the two, between the fact and visualization, [guides the learning process]."[224]

BF researchers and educators Judith Green and Robert Shellenberger stress in *Essentials of Complementary and Alternative Medicine* that biofeedback is based on **biopsychosocial medicine**. The term biopsychosocial was coined by George Engel "to reflect the importance of understanding the multifactorial interactions of biological, psychological, and social influences in a patient's presentation."[225] The biopsychosocial approach focuses on illnesses whose origins are clearly behavioral.[226]

Shellenberger and Green also caution about the "ghost in the box" syndrome that can easily occur when using biofeedback instruments as tools for learning.[227] A person might feel that the machine is the healing agent, not realizing that the machine is merely an empty box without power, a mirror reflecting that person's state. The healing comes with what a person does with the information provided in the reflection. In this sense, BF is a self-motivated therapy, only as effective as the commitment and focus a person brings to it. It requires that people take full responsibility for changing their patterns. Therefore, it empowers people to take charge of their psychosomatic processes and thus their approach to life once they become aware of the patterns through BF.

The benefit of using BF machines to effect change is that physiological feedback is completely accurate. For instance, if a person has stress responses about a particular situation caused by unresolved emotions, the machines will accurately reflect the stress response. In a psychotherapy session, the client might feel justified in projecting the responsibility for a reaction on the therapist, yet would clearly see how foolish it is to project responsibility on a machine.

Physiological Feats

Controlling physiological responses may be relatively new in Western culture's biofeedback therapies, but it has long been cultivated in Eastern spiritual practices as a way to prepare the adept's body for spiritual enlightenment. Take the case, for example, of a group of monks in India with unusual abilities to control their physiology. Researchers wired the monks to devices that measured changes in body temperature. The monks sat in below-freezing temperatures surrounded by snow with their naked bodies wrapped only in wet sheets. To the amazement of the researchers, the sheets began to steam and dry as the monks' body temperatures rose as much as 17 degrees above normal. Within 45 minutes the sheets were completely dried.[228]

Brain Wave Feedback

The brain emits small oscillating voltages or waves that can be detected by electroencephalogram (EEG) machines. Researchers have identified four different types of brain wave patterns—beta, alpha, theta, and delta, which are measured in the number of brain wave cycles per second. Each type of brain wave is associated with a specific state of consciousness (Figure 13.3). Beta waves are most prominent during concentrated mental tasks, occurring at 14 to 30 cycles per seconds and even faster in people suffering from schizophrenia and other forms of mental illness.

Alpha waves run at 8 to 13 cycles per second and are associated with a detached yet alert and diffuse state of awareness, one cultivated in many forms of Eastern meditation and considered to be a bridge between the conscious and subconscious mind. Alpha waves generally appear when the eyes are closed or when a person is internally focused. When the attention of a person engaged in conversation drifts inside into a memory or interior process, the eyes may glaze over, which can indicate alpha waves are present.

Theta waves occur at 4 to 7 cycles per second, are active when a person is drowsy or dreaming, are associated with a creative state, and are present during moments of creative insight. The slowest, delta waves, occur at ½ to 3½ cycles per second and are prominent during nondreaming sleep and during waking psychic and healing experiences.

BETA WAVES ⟶ 14–30 cycles per second
ALPHA WAVES ⟶ 8–13 cycles per second
THETA WAVES ⟶ 4–7 cycles per second
DELTA WAVES ⟶ .5–3.5 cycles per second

Figure 13.3 Brain wave rates

When a person crosses the threshold from alpha to theta, he reaches a state of **reverie** in which **hypnagogic images** tend to bubble to the surface of consciousness. These images can be surprising and even startling because they seem to pop out of nowhere. They are thought to be a projection of impulses from the unconscious mind and have been found beneficial in the process of psychoanalysis. A number of biofeedback researchers feel that if a person could stay in reverie, he could access levels of creative thinking and imagery not available in normal waking states. In order to recall the images that bubble up, a person needs to have a minimal level of muscular activity because total muscle relaxation tends to induce sleep. To stay in reverie, psychologist Charles Tart recommends a person lie down to rest, but keep the forearms vertically balanced on the elbows. When the person begins to fall asleep, the arms will drop and wake him up, creating a moment conducive to recalling hypnagogic images.[229] Upon waking, the person can write down the images much as a person would do in the morning to analyze his dreams, then later process the meaning of the images.

Massage clients often frequently experience the twilight state of reverie and may comment on having a parade of images pass through their minds. Perhaps the stimulus of the practitioner's hands is just enough to keep the massage client from falling completely asleep. Likewise, meditators tend to access the consciousness between sleeping and waking states, being prevented from falling asleep by the muscular activity and/or discomfort needed to maintain a meditative posture. When people practicing a meditative discipline linger at the alpha-theta threshold, they have access to subconscious processes because they are able to bridge the unconscious and conscious mind, a process that is invaluable to successful psychotherapy. Also, if alpha and theta waves are prominent during states of alert relaxation and creativity respectively, then learning how to assume a state that hovers around the alpha-theta threshold would give a person some reprieve from the stressful demands of prolonged mental concentration. This hypothesis has spurred a number of brain wave researchers to explore various states of consciousness.

In 1958, research psychologist Joe Kamiya found that people were able to control alpha brain waves with feedback from EEG equipment that he designed. His research subjects, mostly college students, were also able to learn to distinguish alpha states from beta states, and to control brain wave activity in a very short time. It is important to understand that we cannot feel brain wave patterns because the brain itself lacks sensory nerves. Changes in brain wave patterns can only be detected by shifts in states of consciousness with accompanying changes in muscle tone, in heart rate or respiration, and in body temperature. The point of Kamiya's studies was not to teach people how to produce particular brain waves, but to produce the states of consciousness that accompany them. Kamiya felt that learning to produce the detached calm associated with alpha waves provided people with a natural alternative to taking sedatives for the alleviation of hypertension, a benefit long realized by meditators and yogis. He proposed the possibility of developing a psychophysiology of consciousness through the study of brain wave patterns.[230]

In the late 1950s, researchers B. K. Bagchi and A. Wenger studied the physiological changes of experienced Zen meditators in India.[231] They found that the meditators consistently demonstrated a rise in skin resistance that is associated with relaxation, a decreased breath rate, and a high amplitude of alpha brain waves during meditation (Figure 13.4). Kasmata and Hirai, who studied the brain wave patterns of master Zen monks in the early 1960s, found that they initially produced alpha waves as they turned the monks attention inward, then began to produce theta waves as they entered the meditative consciousness that they described as a state of "knowing" rather than "thinking."[232] These findings are consistent with those made by Anand, Chhina, and Singh shortly before. They found that people who practice yoga-based meditation are able to enter a profound state of relaxed yet detached consciousness in which they produce theta waves and are completely undisturbed by noxious stimuli such as loud gongs and flashing lights.[233]

These findings suggest a beneficial state of consciousness when the brain waves reside near the alpha-theta threshold. This state produces deep relaxation, bridges the conscious mind with the unconscious mind, creates a state of detached awareness that can improve emotional well-being, accesses creative and healing images and thoughts, and may even be a key to deep psychophysiological healing.

Still, the brain is far too complex to assume that only one or two rhythms are present at any given time. It is more likely that a combination of waves occurs within a group configuration, some being more dominant than others in different parts of the brain at different times. This was the focus of C. Maxwell Cade in the 1980s, a biophysicist and yogi who studied the brain wave patterns of thousands of yogis, healers, Zen masters, and clairvoyants in an effort to see if they exhibited a unique brain wave pattern that could be the signature of the enlightened mind. Cade invented a novel feedback machine that he called the "Mind Mirror," which provides an overall picture of brain wave activity by measuring all four types of wave patterns simultaneously in both hemispheres.[234] Cade

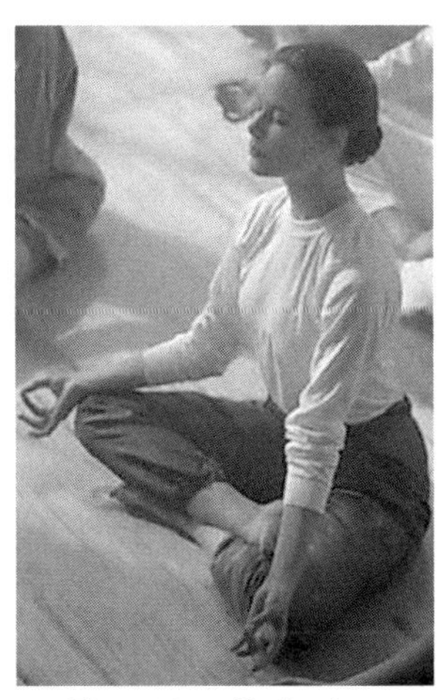

Figure 13.4 Meditation

found a pattern that seems to function as a bridge between the unconscious and conscious mind, in which alpha waves produced in a meditative state carry over into waking states. This pattern, which he called the "Awakened Mind" pattern, differs from the relaxed alpha state that Kamiya described. It is bilaterally symmetrical, embodying both the creative, abstract qualities of the right hemisphere and the linear, logical qualities of the left hemisphere, and is accompanied by feelings of creativity, bliss, and illumination. Cade describes in his book *The Awakened Mind* many different exercises and visualizations to balance right and left hemispheres and evoke integrated brain wave patterns.[235]

Ultimately, each person needs to find the process that works best for him or her to enter a desired state of consciousness. For instance, a person can visualize a peaceful or blissful setting, such as sitting by a bubbling brook in the middle of a lush, green forest. The more senses used in the visualization, the deeper a person is likely to go into a specific state. A person can imagine breathing fresh and invigorating air; walking on soft moss as a gentle wind brushes the cheek; tasting clean, refreshing water from a nearby brook; hearing the gentle sounds of leaves rustling and birds chirping; or feeling sensations of peace and ease while out in nature. Images of climbing down a tunnel or walking into a cave seem to help a person drop from beta through alpha to theta waves; likewise, the hypnotist often has a person count backward and imagine getting sleepier to induce changes in consciousness.

Progressive Muscle Relaxation and Electromyography

Other early BF researchers linked muscle tension with emotional stress. In the 1930s, Edmund Jacobson, a psychiatrist who was a pioneer in the study of muscle activity in sedentary patients, discovered a relationship between muscle tension and states of anxiety.[236] He was also one of the first researchers to use a simple form of electromyography (EMG), employing a crude device designed to pick up electrical signals in the motor units of muscle fibers to determine levels of muscle contraction. This EMG machine did not, however, provide feedback to the patients and was used solely for research, so technically it was not a biofeedback machine.

Jacobson felt that one of the aims of therapy was to reduce or make less severe the tensions found in the "welfare response," a term he coined to describe the responses that all organisms need for survival and reproduction.[237] Much of his extensive research over 35 years tracked the correlation between emotional states and increased sympathetic tone, recorded by EMG measurements of increased firing in the skeletal muscles.

Initially surprised to find muscle tension in bedridden patients who were supposed to be resting and recovering, Jacobson found that the muscle activity was related to mental stress arising from worry over recovery, which actually interfered in the recovery of his bedridden patients. He concluded that mere thought is enough to trigger muscular contractions, that "minuscule neuromuscular contraction patterns [from voluntary, striated muscle fibers] . . . are in part the physiological basis of what in the past has generally been called mental."[238]

Jacobson coined the term **muscle bracing** to describe this phenomenon and developed the technique of *progressive relaxation* to treat it. Progressive relaxation (PR) emphasizes the conscious release of tension in skeletal muscles which can be controlled voluntarily. People practice PR by systematically contracting and releasing each muscle group, one by one, until they are able to relax the entire body. PR is a widely used method

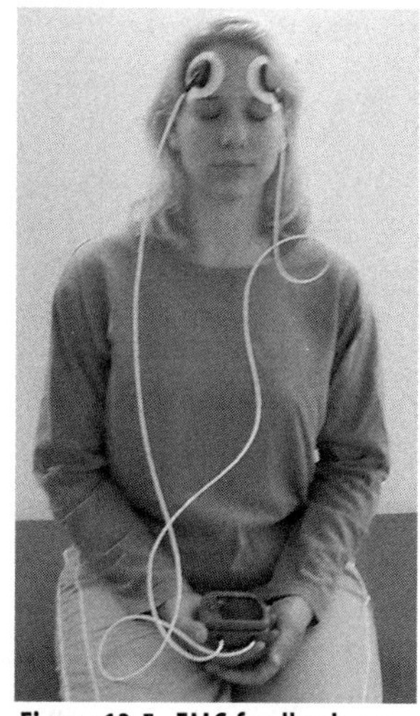

Figure 13.5 EMG feedback on the frontalis muscle

Patterning Exercise #124: Progressive Relaxation

1. Sit or lie in a comfortable position (PE Fig. 124).
2. Focus on one area of your body at a time. Slowly and gradually contract the muscles in that area. Notice the tightening sensation the contraction creates. (Note: Only contract to a level that is manageable; avoid cramping, especially in the neck and legs.)
3. As you exhale, quickly release the contraction. Notice the sensation the release creates. Compare it to the previous sensation of contraction.
4. Progressively contract and relax each of the following areas: Scalp, eyes, nose, mouth, neck, shoulders, arms, hands, between the shoulders, abdomen, lower back, buttocks, thighs, lower legs, and feet.
5. Take several relaxed breaths, letting muscular tension go on each exhalation.
6. Now scan your body from head to feet. If there are any areas that still feel tight, contract them slowly, then relax them as you exhale.

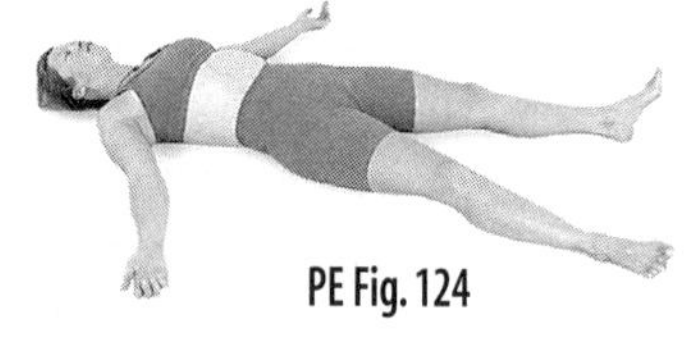

PE Fig. 124

Patterning Exercise #125: Progressive Relaxation Imagery

First read this script into a tape recorder, taking long pauses after each statement. Repeat each statement three times before moving on to the next. Next, lie down and relax in a quiet, comfortable position. Play the tape and sense each area of your body as you listen to it.

1. My forehead is smooth and unwrinkled.
2. My eyelids settle like ripples on a pond coming to rest.
3. The bridge of my nose widens and opens.
4. My jaw loosens and falls slack.
5. My ears widen and open.
6. My head sinks and widens.
7. My neck relaxes and loosens.
8. My shoulders widen and fall open.
9. My breath rises and falls.
10. My arms become heavier with each exhalation.
11. My legs become heavier with each exhalation.
12. My knees sink as I relax.
13. My ribs are round and weighted.
14. My back muscles lengthen and relax.
15. My hips sink with each exhalation.
16. My belly settles and sinks into my spine.
17. My body drifts down through the floor with each exhalation.
18. I am loose and relaxed.

EMSPress.com

of relaxation because it is easy to do, can be practiced anywhere, and cultivates muscular proprioception.

In the same vein, Basmajian performed numerous studies using EMG readings on the muscular control of flaccid tissues. Basmajian discovered during his research in the 1950s that it is possible to gain conscious control of a single motor unit. When using EMG with biofeedback, the clinician places electrodes directly on muscles to pick up electrical signals at neuromuscular junctions (Figure 13.5). Adjustable auditory signals feed back information about the degree of contraction in the muscle. Basmajian demonstrated that a person can use this information either to gain conscious control of flaccid muscle groups or to relax overactive groups.[239] Later research by Budzynski, Stoyva, and Adler found that relaxation in the *frontalis muscle* (located on the forehead) resulted in full body relaxation. They also found that patients who received feedback about muscle tone learned to relax faster than patients who did not receive such feedback.[240]

Today, EMG feedback is used in the treatment of tension headaches, partial paralysis, incontinence (lack of bladder or bowel control), temporomandibular dysfunction (TMD), stuttering, and bruxism (teeth grinding), among other conditions. It is also widely used to promote general relaxation. The value of EMG feedback is that it helps people regain proprioceptive awareness that they have lost over muscle groups. EMG feedback is also used in postural education, for neuromuscular reeducation, and for improving physical performance. Biofeedback training with EMG machines is often used with beginners in a treatment protocol because it teaches people to regulate tension in the skeletal muscles of the somatic nervous system, which is voluntary and therefore more easily controlled than functions of the autonomic nervous system like heart rate and skin temperature.

Unusual Pain-Control Abilities

We read about people who can pass sharp objects through their bodies without pain or bleeding, or yogis who can bury themselves alive for more than a month and survive. If these stories are true, how are these feats accomplished? And what is the value of such unusual abilities? Many early BF researchers had these same questions, which led them to study people with these unusual abilities. Researchers discovered that these seemingly exceptional people demonstrate profound healing powers that all people have the potential to develop.

Elmer and Alyce Green studied the physiological responses of a man with exceptional abilities named Jack Schwarz. This unusual man can stop pain in both himself and others, can read other people's thoughts and their pasts accurately, and can heal himself from severe injuries. To demonstrate these abilities, Schwarz passes large needles through his muscles and puts his hands into fire without pain or injury. He sleeps an average of a mere two and one-half hours per day. When asked how he is able to do these extraordinary acts, Mr. Schwarz replied that he simply asks his body to do what he wants, and then waits patiently for the response. Schwarz emphasized the importance of asking and not commanding. Elmer Green describes a time when Schwarz pulled a large needle out of himself and began to bleed: "Much to my surprise, the hole in the skin seemed to close as if drawn by purse strings."[243]

The Greens' Biofeedback Research

By the 1970s, more than 400 books and journal articles had been published in Europe on autogenics, compared to only four in the United States. At this time, American researchers were just beginning to recognize the role of stress in many nonspecific illnesses and were beginning to study yogis and meditators who could perform unusual physiological feats. Elmer and Alyce Green, two of the most prominent BF researchers, went to work at the Menninger Clinic in Kansas to study the physiological changes that occur during autogenics training. They understood that people who are adept at autogenics have produced physiological changes similar to those found in advanced meditators, and they hoped to discover the relationship between the effects of autogenics and meditation.[241]

In one famous study, the Greens recorded the physiological changes made by a yogi who could control a number of autonomic functions at will, including his heart rate. They found that a slowing of the heart rate was accompanied by an increase in capillary vasodilation, specifically an increase in blood flow to the limbs. They also found that alpha brain waves were consistently present during the altered states people would enter to control pain, stop bleeding, raise body temperature, and slow heart rates.[242]

The Greens experimented with different types of biofeedback training to teach thermal control to their research subjects, mostly housewives and students. By chance, one woman found she could relieve her migraine headache by warming her hands. This led to the development of temperature training and limb-warming skills for the treatment of migraines and tension headaches. The Greens developed machines to measure galvanic skin responses (GSR), electrical changes in muscle tone (EMG), and changes in brain wave patterns via electroencephalogram (EEG). Their many discoveries laid the foundation for important protocols in BF therapy.

The clinical results of the Greens' work were remarkable. Through the use of a number of BF modalities, their patients were able to stabilize a variety of mental and physical disorders, and improve respiratory, cardiovascular, vasomotor, gastrointestinal, and endocrine functions. The Greens demonstrated a 60 to 90 percent success rate in treating people with long-standing disturbances such as insomnia, headaches, asthma, chronic constipation, anxiety, phobias, stuttering, and bed-wetting.[244] All their patients were given exercises to do at home so that the patients were gradually weaned from dependence on the BF equipment. With homework, patients learned to integrate their new skills with physiological self-regulation into their daily lives.

Biofeedback and Feldenkrais

The pioneering biofeedback researchers Elmer and Alyce Green felt teaching a person to control the single-motor-unit firing in a particular muscle bundle might help treat spastic behavior, such as that found in epilepsy and cerebral palsy (CP). While looking into this, the Greens discovered Moshe Feldenkrais, whom they felt was doing some of the most exciting body-mind work at the time.

The Greens met with Feldenkrais in London in 1974 and shared information about working with CP patients. Feldenkrais demonstrated his work with a severely disabled patient. He explained to the Greens that the man's problem stemmed from the fact that as a child he was told to expect the out-of-control movement that Feldenkrais felt special training could help alleviate, and yet the man never received that training. The lack of training broke the feedback loop he needed for normal development under circumstances of CP. Feldenkrais put his hands on the client's foot and explored moving it in a variety of ways. After a series of repetitive slaps to the foot and occasional pauses, Feldenkrais stopped moving the foot and began talking to his client, pointing out that he had found the muscle group that was out of control. At first the patient felt nothing but soon began to feel trembling in his calf. Then the spasms in the man's foot stopped.

As Feldenkrais explained, he had provided his client with the feedback he needed from the striated muscles to restore the loop between the muscles and the central nervous system.[245] During spasticity, the feedback loop between the muscles and brain breaks. Feldenkrais's touch and movement provided the feedback necessary to reconnect the broken loop, and once the spasm stopped, Feldenkrais did not need to keep working with the man's foot. Similarly, as people learn voluntary control in BF training, they gradually lose their dependence on the equipment and learn to use body awareness for feedback.

The Relaxation Response

During the 1960s, R. K. Wallace studied the physiological changes that occur in people who practice transcendental meditation (TM).[246] He measured their oxygen consumption, cardiac output, respiration rate, arterial blood pressure, EEG measures, and carbon dioxide elimination, and found that their physiological patterns correlated with the quieting of the nervous system.

Another physician named Herbert Benson felt that these physiological skills were not unique to TM meditators. Benson developed a system to evoke the states TM meditators enter which he called the *relaxation response* (introduced in Chapter 4).[247]

Benson also found in his research that numerous people had routines that they made up themselves to help them relax when they felt stressed. Many times, these routines were integrally connected to their belief systems or spiritual practices. One research subject, for example, who became upset when her doctors insisted that she would need surgery and bypassed her requests to explore spiritual healing first, repeated a prayer over and over again, like a mantra, a prayer she had practiced for years when faced with adversity. This short prayer had a calming effect on her body and mind, eliciting a sense of peace from her belief system.[248]

Benson found that any phrase, whether it reflects a person's values or spiritual beliefs, or is just chosen to help a person learn how to become calm, has the same physiological effect: as the mind quiets, the body relaxes. The word or phrase need only be repeated like a mantra for several minutes to elicit the calming effect. For example, Benson discovered that a runner, by rhythmically counting his steps during a jog, will actually reach the relaxed state called "runner's high" four times as fast as the average runner. The primary steps to elicit the relaxation response are:

1. to repeat a word, sound, prayer, phrase, or muscular activity. A person could also focus on a repetitive process, such as the cycles of the breath.
2. to passively disregard thoughts that come to mind and return the mental focus to the object of repetition.[249]

When a person begins to practice the relaxation response, it is helpful to be in a quiet environment, without interference such as phones or doorbells, and to assume a position of comfort. Benson recommends practicing it twice daily, with the eyes closed, 10 to 20 minutes in each practice period. Afterward, it is important to sit for a minute with the eyes open before standing.

Naturally, relaxed breathing is an important part of inducing a relaxation response. Relaxed breathing is different from deep breathing because in the latter, a person focuses on taking full inhalations to expand the lungs and draw in as much air as possible. Deep breathing can actually raise autonomic tone and rev up sympathetic responses, helpful to do when a person wishes to become alert. To have a calming, relaxing effect, breathing should be natural and even, and the exhalation should be longer than the inhalation.

Biofeedback and Imagery

The use of imagery in evoking the relaxation response is not necessarily direct in affecting physiology because the brain has to interpret the image. Autogenics does not involve imagery; the phrases used are designed to evoke a direct physiological experience free from the directing influence of an image. In biofeedback, physiological feedback is direct from either a machine or from body sensations such as warmth spreading in the limbs. Biofeedback bypasses the need for cognitive interpretation and creates a direct physical experience in the form of a blinking light or sound, which provides enough information about the physiological processes for a person to influence them.

The BF mechanism of change is similar to Sweigard's process of ideokinesis (see Chapters 4 and 11), in which the results are attributed to the innate intelligence of the nervous system to organize the most efficient and effortless patterns when given the chance. The images Sweigard created to guide neuromuscular pathways work well because they reflect accurate anatomical architecture. Likewise, images to evoke physiological change are effective when they reflect the desired physiological response, such as becoming warmer, heavier, or slowing down.

People can evoke physiological change by imagining a favorite place they go to for rest and relaxation (Figure 13.6). Imagery does have its drawbacks because images that work are highly personal. For instance, a person could visualize holding his arms and legs near a warm fire to get warm from increased circulation in the limbs. Although the image of fire might produce a warming effect for one

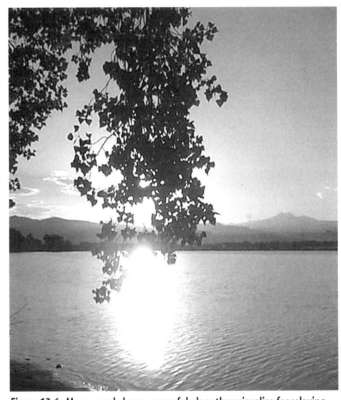

Figure 13.6 Many people have a peaceful place they visualize for relaxing.

Patterning Exercise #126: Breathing for Relaxation

Take about 5 or 10 minutes for this exercise.

1. Sit or lie in a comfortable position, in a quiet, warm place. Breathe easily, allowing the exhalations to be longer than the inhalations.
2. Breathe in for two counts, out for four counts. Or, as you breathe, repeat the following phrase, "inhale, one, two, exhale, three, four, five, six."
3. As you exhale, sense or imagine your body drifting and sinking down through the ground.
4. Visualize breathing *in* relaxation, breathing *out* stress.

Feedback: Afterward, do you feel more relaxed? What are the sensations of relaxation? Practice this simple exercise for about one minute during the day whenever you feel stress.

EMSPress.com

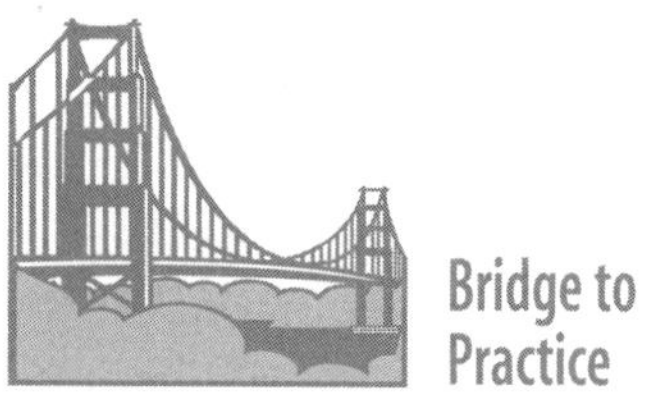

Helping Clients to Quiet Stress-Inducing Thoughts

Help your clients become aware of the thought patterns they have that maintain chronically high levels of muscular tension. To do this, ask your clients to identify what thoughts they have when they feel muscular tension and what thoughts they have when they feel a relaxation response. Tell your clients that they do not need to share their thoughts, but simply to notice the effects these thoughts have on body states of tension or relaxation.

person, it could produce a startle response in another who has had a bad experience with fire.

HOW THE MIND LIVES IN THE BODY

Most people understand that the times when they are under extreme psychological or work-related stress are the times when they are most susceptible to becoming sick. It seems just simple common sense that prolonged stress lowers the body's abilities to fight off minor illnesses such as a cold, flu, or chronic infections. If this is true, then it follows that the opposite would be true, that positive emotions could boost immune function. This is the premise of the relatively new field in medicine called psychoneuroimmunology (PNI).

Research in PNI is beginning to shed light on the actual biochemical processes that link the body with the mind and produce these effects. The negative effects of emotions on the body have been widely documented. For instance, stress coupled with depression has been associated with lower immune responses.[250] Increased levels of stress prior to surgery have been associated with slower recovery after surgery.[251] And the vulnerability to physical illness and death increase during the first two years after a spouse loses a mate.[252] Even common, marital conflict can considerably raise blood pressure and increase the numbers of natural killer cells in a person with an already cynical and hostile affect.[253]

Stress and the Brain

Stress alters brain chemistry. During a stress response, the adrenal glands release a surge of adrenaline to boost the body's energy in preparation for fight or flight. The adrenals function along a complex neuro-physiological circuit that begins in the brain. When a person becomes aware of a threat, whether real or imagined, the *cortical-pituitary-limbic-adrenal axis* is activated. In layman's terms, this means that the perceived threat stimulates cortical activity, or thinking, which triggers the *pituitary gland*. At the center of the pituitary lies the *hypothalamus gland*, also called the "master gland" because it regulates many others glands and creates a vital link between the endocrine, immune, and nervous systems.

Recall from Chapter 4 that the hypothalamus and limbic system, located in the midbrain near the limbic system, regulate our emotional responses. When we become aware of a threat or a stressor, this awareness (a forebrain function) triggers a lightning chain that sequences through the brain between a perception, an emotional response, a physical reaction, and a defensive response. The type of defense reaction depends upon a person's coping skills. Some people react before thinking, others freeze, and others think before acting and wait until the emotional charge has settled before responding. Generally, most people find that emotions cloud thinking, so it is difficult to make an intelligent response when the response is charged with emotions.

The process happens so fast that rarely do we realize how perception ignites the process. Yet without awareness of a stressor, there is no stress. Take, for example, a search team of frantic parents looking for a lost child. These adults will probably undergo tremendous stress from their catastrophic thoughts about what may have happened to the child, only to find the child innocently and curiously playing in a remote area, totally oblivious to her parents' stress and herself without any stress responses. The stress of parents is caused by their projected fears about what may have happened to their child, rather than any actual physical danger or injury to the child. Until they know the child is safe, their brain chemistry keeps the reactive loop ignited. In short, the perception of stress is in itself a powerful stressor.

The notion that positive emotions can reduce and even reverse the symptoms of stress and boost immune function breaks down the long-held view that the functions of the central nervous system are separate from the functions of the immune and endocrine systems, and builds a case for the biological basis of psychosomatic conditions. Psychosomatic causes have long been considered a valid diagnosis for unexplained health problems. Although biofeedback researchers have proven that we can change the homeostasis of our bodies through awareness and intention, they have not been able to explain how these changes occur. Now neuroscientists and immunologists are actually beginning to uncover the physiological mechanisms that explain how thought can alter physiology. These groundbreaking discoveries illuminate the biochemical basis for how the mind lives in the body.

Neuropeptides: The Chemical Communicators

During the late 1970s and early 1980s, neuroscientist Candace Pert, at the National Institute of Mental Health, researched opiates and their receptor sites in the brain.

Opiates are a class of drugs, or chemical messengers, that reduce the perception of pain. Shaped in unique three-dimensional configurations, they function like keys that lock into very specific receptor sites, or "keyholes." When an opiate binds to its receptor site in the brain, it acts like a biochemical trigger, starting a cascade of physiological responses that the user perceives as feelings of euphoria similar to what is sometimes called a runner's high. What astounded Pert and her colleagues was the discovery of receptor sites not only in the brain, but throughout the entire body, which implied that the brain can actually produce opiates to affect the body. Further investigation revealed that tissues in the body other than nerve cells actually produce chemical messengers like opiates.[254]

Pert's findings revealed a complex biochemical network of messengers that relays information among the nervous system, the immune system, and the endocrine system, creating mood alterations and shifts in immune function. Her surprising discoveries, as well as those of other researchers, are now shaking the pharmacological foundation of Western medicine, whose drug treatments are based on the belief that the immune system and nervous system function independently of each other.

Until discoveries like Pert's, communication within the nervous system was thought to occur primarily between nerve cell synapses (junctions) in a linear fashion through the release of molecules called neurotransmitters. **Neurotransmitters** (which include neuropetides, hormones, and lymphokines) are chemicals produced by nerve cells that communicate messages to other nerve cells to stimulate a response. **Neuropeptides** are a type of neurotransmitter produced in the brain as well as in various places throughout the body. Since neuropeptides have receptor sites all over the body, Pert refers to them as a vast, nonlinear network of intercellular communicators wherein the mind "chatters" with the body and the body "chatters" back. In essence, communication via neuropeptides diffuses through the fluids circulating in all the body's tissues rather than being limited to the linear "telegraph lines" of the nervous system.[255]

The discoveries of Pert and her colleagues shook up the notions held dear by many scientists about the separation between mental and physical processes. This work has been controversial and has been scoffed at by scientists who hold the body-mind split dear to their technologies. We are reminded of how scientists initially rejected Louis Pasteur's discoveries of foreign germs that invade the body and cause disease, yet his work later became the foundation for modern allopathic medicine.

Pert and her colleagues also found that *monocytes*, large white blood cells involved in the immune response, not only produce neuropeptides but also have receptor sites, revealing another important piece of this biochemical puzzle. A fundamental property of immune system cells is their ability to move throughout the body. This finding expanded the territory and influence of the unfolding communication network between the brain and the immune system, implying that biochemicals affecting emotional states also control the migration and routing of the immune system cells. This implies a strong biochemical link between emotions and immune functioning, a finding congruent with what BF researchers have long since realized. In other words, emotional responses regulate both behavior and survival functions. Because neurotransmitters are thought to both create and regulate many different emotional states, Pert calls them the *biochemical mediators of emotions.*[256]

Psychoneuroimmunology

In essence, Pert's research points to the fact that chemicals not only run our brain and our body, but they also run our emotions.[257] In fact, communications among the body, mind, and emotions could be much more interconnected than modern neuroscientists can yet imagine. We now know, for example, that neuropeptides and their receptor sites even line the digestive track, from the esophagus to the large intestine. "Gut feelings" do have a biochemical basis.

These findings have birthed a whole new field in Western medicine called **psychoneuroimmunology** (**PNI**). This term was coined by psychologist Robert Ader, who, in 1974, discovered that rats could be conditioned to depress immune system function through mere mental associations.[258] Ader fed the rats water sweetened and mixed with a medicine called Cytoxan, which causes nausea and suppresses immune responses. The rats learned to associate sweetened water with nausea, and when fed only sweetened water with no Cytoxan, first developed nausea, then began dying of infectious diseases.[259] In short, the rats had actually learned to suppress their own immune responses. These groundbreaking research findings supported the premise that the central nervous system and thought can alter immune system functions, findings which launched PNI as a viable field.

Another important link between the immune system and the nervous system was discovered in 1987 by the husband-and-

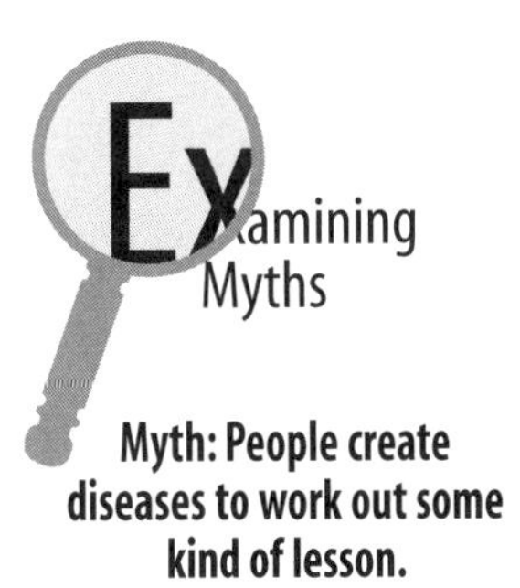

Myth: People create diseases to work out some kind of lesson.

Although it is well-documented that chronic depression, anger, and negative emotions elevate physiological stress and make a person more susceptible to illness, disease processes are complex and often beyond our control. It would be detrimental for people to believe that they are solely to blame for their illnesses. In fact, this belief could lead to a downward spiral of self-blame that might interfere with healing.

Healing Cancer with Imagery

Norman Cousins, in his famous book *Anatomy of an Illness*, describes one of the most popular cases of healing using the powers of PNI. After contracting a form of fatal cancer, Cousins holed up in his hotel room for several months with a VCR and numerous tapes by comedians such as the Marx brothers. Combining megadoses of vitamin C with positive thinking, he watched the tapes and literally laughed himself to wellness.

Also, a woman with a bulging cancerous tumor on her breast was referred to Norman Cousins after she refused surgery. Cousins began by addressing her most basic sense of physical comfort. Upon discovering that cold hands and feet bothered her, Cousins taught her a simple visualization to bring warmth to her limbs. Once she learned and practiced the visualization, the temperature in her hands shot up 14 degrees. After two weeks of practicing, she returned to see Cousins. To his amazement, her tumor had completely disappeared.[263]

wife team of researchers, neuroscientists David Felton and Suzanne Felton. While studying spleen cells (the spleen is an important lymph system organ that recycles old red blood cells), the Feltons found nerve fibers running throughout these cells. This flew in the face of traditional medical dogma that claimed the nervous system and immune system lack any connection and function separately. The Feltons undertook pioneering work tracing nerve fibers from the central nervous system to the spleen and thymus, and eventually to every organ of the immune system. They found that cutting the nerve fibers between the CNS and the spleen or lymph nodes stopped immune responses cold, demonstrating that these nerves are involved in immune function by enabling the brain to influence the immune system.[260]

Healing and PNI

Research in PNI still remains in its infancy, although since Pert's initial discoveries, more than 80 neurotransmitters have been discovered. Perhaps the most widespread application of these discoveries in the medical establishment has been an increase of psychiatric drugs in both range and use. Many physicians are warning people to use PNI as a supplement to traditional medicine rather than a replacement until more is known about its effectiveness. Still, many sensitive physicians now recognize how important a patient's attitude, perception, and especially participation are to a successful healing process.

In short, psychoneuroimmunology is based on the premise that emotions and thoughts affect the immune system. The precise mechanisms of *how* PNI works remain largely a mystery; yet, rather than wait for definitive answers, numerous doctors are testing this premise in the treatment of stress-related disease. For example, Dr. Bernie Siegel, author of *Love, Medicine, and Miracles,* studied the effects of group therapy on cancer patients to assess the claim that the right mental attitude could help conquer cancer. He took two groups of cancer patients and treated one with traditional care—radiation, chemotherapy, and drugs. The second group received exactly the same treatment, but with the addition of weekly group therapy sessions. Siegal found that the second group's members reported less depression, anxiety, and pain, and that they actually lived an average of 18 months longer than those in the first group.[261]

Along the same lines, Dr. Carl Simonton investigated the personality profiles of people who recover from cancer and those who do not and found attitude to be the key difference between the two groups. Simonton developed healing visualizations for people with cancer to practice, such as imagining the lymphocytes as cellular "Pac men" ingesting cancerous cells. Simonton's techniques of cancer treatment using visualizations and positive thinking led to higher rates of remission among cancer patients at his healing center.[262]

SUMMARY

Biofeedback therapy developed as a remedial therapy for the multitude of stress-related problems and illnesses that are prevalent in our modern society. Biofeedback provides us with the physiological feedback we need to start regulating the homeostatic mechanisms within our bodies. In this sense, biofeedback training is "physiological patterning."

Initially, a person in BF training depends on feedback from machines to control physiological responses. Yet after minimal training, people can use sensory feedback coming from their own bodies, such as heart or breath rate, temperature changes, or even vague sensations of ease, to guide the process of relaxation. A person can even use BF to learn how to cultivate the brain wave patterns that accompany relaxation and healing. The primary skill learned in BF training is to use thought and physical awareness to actively induce a relaxation response. Since stress is a natural part of life and we need it to make us hardy, it would be folly to assume that it is possible to always be relaxed. More important is the ability to move from an agitated to a calm state, which cultivates autonomic flexibility.

BF researchers are not sure how the physiological changes occur when we direct internal body processes with physiological feedback. But what they do know is that it is possible to learn how to control these physiological responses. Although BF research has proved that thought patterns can change physiology, *how* the mind actually changes the chemistry of the body has begun to be illuminated by researchers in the field of psychoneuroimmunology. PNI is based on the knowledge that a person's psychology, neurology, and immune responses are integrally connected. These connections were first revealed by research that mapped opiate receptors in the brain, which led to the discovery of receptors all through the body.

The findings of PNI researchers imply that the elements that trigger illness are not just bacterias and viruses, but are also driven by our own thoughts and feelings. This revolutionary concept has a flip side: if thought and imagery can trigger disease, then perhaps they can also boost immune function, improve general health and well-being, and trigger healing processes. Although the evidence is largely anecdotal with research still in its infancy, case after case of people "curing themselves" from cancers and other potentially fatal diseases using the power of visualization, positive thinking, prayer, and laughter have been reported.

In the combined application of BF and PNI, visualizations are used not just to induce relaxation, but also to induce healing processes, tapping the powerful abilities of the mind to heal the body by boosting immune response. If we compare these findings to what we knew of body-mind patterns 50 years ago, we can only wonder what the next 50 years will reveal. All these studies and theories point us to the incredible healing potential that may lie latent in our own patterns of thought, emotion, physiology, and movement.

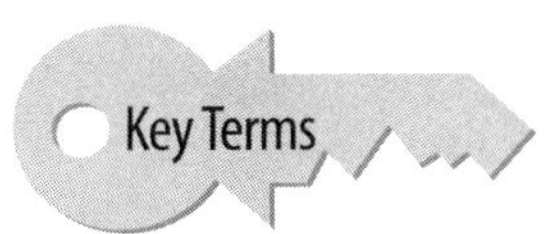

autogentics
biofeedback (BF) therapy
biopsychosocial medicine
diseases of adaptation
eustress
fight-or-flight response
freeze response
general adaptation syndrome (GAS)
homeostasis
hypnagogic images
muscle bracing
neuropeptides
neurotransmitters
psychoneuroimmunology (PNI)
reverie
stressor

OVERVIEW OF CHAPTER 14

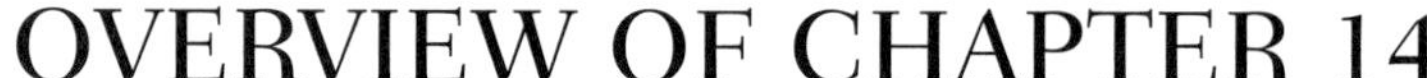

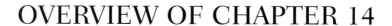

14

Behavioral and Cognitive Patterning

> **Reality is perception; perception is reality. To change one's reality, one must change one's perception.**
>
> —*G. F. Buens*

As we learned in the last chapter, biofeedback and psychoneuroimmunology offer practical methods with which we can use thought and awareness to reduce stress, to influence physiological processes, and to boost the strength of our immune system. In essence, these fields have helped us tap the innate power that our thoughts and emotions have in promoting wellness, and have reunited us with our intrinsic abilities to heal ourselves.

In this chapter, we will look at the behaviors that can lead to illness and holding patterns, and at the behavioral and cognitive therapies that restructure maladaptive thought patterns that underlie psychological problems and destructive behaviors. Although behavioral and cognitive therapies are usually employed to help a person work through psychological issues, many of the somatic modalities also use these methods to help change the mental patterns that sustain problematic somatic patterns. In order to understand the relationship between psychological theories and somatic patterning, we begin with a brief history.

Initially, behaviorism was built on the premise that human behavior is conditioned by positive and negative reinforcement. A transition in modern psychology from behaviorism to behavioral therapy began when researchers started exploring how behavior is shaped more by the habitual patterns of internal dialogue than by conditioned responses to external environmental influences. Then the power of using thought patterns to change behavior was tapped as a therapeutic tool by psychotherapists. In the 1960s, cognitive psychologists began to uncover the thought processes that underlie maladaptive behaviors; their research findings about learned helplessness rendered obsolete the operant conditioning theories of behaviorists that dominated modern psychology until then.

Later, in the early 1970s, Richard Bandler and John Grinder began to experiment with nonverbal communication in psychotherapy, modeling the body language and linguistic habits of effective psychotherapists. By viewing hours of taped and live psychotherapy sessions (through two-way mirrors), they observed the nonverbal behaviors of both successful and unsuccessful psychotherapists. From this research they developed neurolinguistic programming (NLP), a system of linguistics and communication based on the conscious use of body postures and language, as well as the three representational channels: visual, auditory, and kinesthetic. The premise of their work is that thoughts are like mental "software," that we can change our reality by reprogramming our thoughts. Thus, NLP identifies the structure of successful communication without getting lost in content.

The bulk of this chapter focuses on NLP because many of the practical elements found in the behavioral therapies were outlined by the NLP founders in a format that is easily understood. Bandler and Grinder felt that by extracting the dynamics of successful communication, they could teach these elements to therapists and professional communicators, bypassing the years of trial and error that psychologists often go through to develop these skills. As a result, many of these elements have been absorbed into a number of schools of psychotherapy, as well as numerous somatic therapies.

The elements of behavioral therapy naturally show up in somatic patterning because posture is not only physical, it is also behavioral. Recall from Chapter 1 that posture is an attitude as well as a body position; it is an emotional and mental stance that we act out through our behaviors and in our body's stance. Habitual behaviors tend to solidify into observable holding patterns. Understanding the fundamentals of behavioral therapies can help us work effectively to change somatic patterns because, in short, a relaxed mind is the key to a relaxed body.

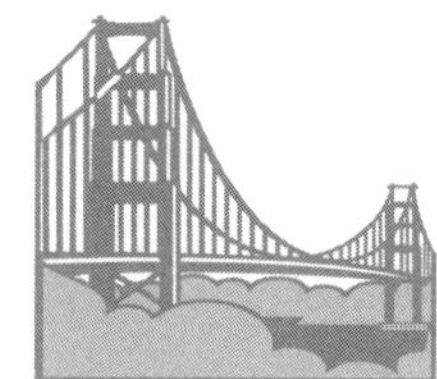

Bridge to Practice

Behaviorism in Bodywork

Bodyworkers, you can use simple forms of positive and negative reinforcement to support a therapeutic focus. For instance, if your client is talkative and talking tightens his body, stop and remove your hands until he stops talking, then put your hands back on him and go back to work.

BEHAVIORISM AND BEHAVIORAL AND COGNITIVE THERAPY

Behaviorism is a school of psychology that developed during the first half of the twentieth century and is based on the influence that environmental factors such as reward and punishment have on behaviors. Behavior in this sense is strictly the observable action of people, the manner in which people conduct themselves.

Most people are familiar with behaviorism in the famous case of "Pavlov's dogs." Ivan Pavlov, a Russian physiologist (1849–1936), experimented with operant conditioning on dogs by using variable levels of positive or negative reinforcement to condition them to salivate at the sound of a bell. A psychologist named John Watson (1878–1958), generally considered the founder of behaviorism, took Pavlov's work a step further. He applied principles of animal behavior taken from objective observation of conditioned responses to human behavior, while excluding the possibilities of the subjective experiences of human thought and reasoning. One of Watson's students, the research psychologist named B. F. Skinner (1904–1990), applied behavioral principles to human learning and transferred Pavlov's methods to the study of humans. Skinner envisioned a utopian society based on behavioral principles in his novel *Walden Two*.[264]

Watson was eventually hired as a consultant to the advertising industry, where conditioned responses are widely used today to entice consumers into buying more merchandise. In a conditioned response, two seemingly disparate elements become associated in a phenomenon called **coupling** (Figure 14.1). For instance, a man may have fond memories of fishing with his father; therefore, every time he smells fishy odors, which other people might find foul, he is overcome with pleasant feelings. Advertisers couple products with common experiences. For example, this fish-fond fellow is likely to buy a certain brand of beer that is advertised in a photo of two men happily fishing because our fellow is influenced on a subliminal level.

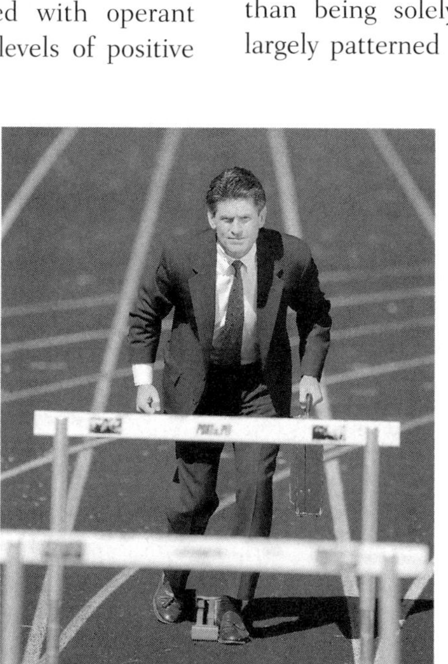

Figure 14.1 Advertising is such a pervasive part of our lives that the message behind coupling disparate elements, such as this businessman about to jump hurdles, is easily interpreted.

Although behaviorism was the approach most taught in academic settings from the 1920s through the 1960s, today most psychologists are uncomfortable with it. The reason is that researchers have found that behavior, rather than being solely shaped by environmental factors, is largely patterned by individual styles of cognition, which include a person's thoughts, attitudes, beliefs, expectations, and perceptions. Still, vestiges of the conditioning principles of behaviorism remain in many psychological paradigms because it is only natural for a person to associate certain experiences with the thoughts, feelings, beliefs, and assumptions that were present during the first few times that experience took place. Likewise, a widely held hypothesis in this field is that every health problem that a person contracts has associated thoughts, feelings, and beliefs, which either aid healing or exacerbate illness.

Typically, conventional medical practices have focused on the objective causes of disease, which has left unexplained the illnesses with no particular etiology, such as rheumatoid arthritis, asthma, and ulcerative colitis. In an effort to understand the causes of such diseases, behavioral researchers began looking at the subjective aspects of illness, such as a person's behaviors, beliefs, and thoughts. They found that thoughts are powerful because they pattern behavior. For instance, in his research, the psychiatrist Aaron Beck decided to investigate the thoughts that depressed clients were thinking rather than focus on theories about the causes of depression. Beck found that depressed people think negative thoughts repeatedly, almost like a personal mantra. Their thoughts were short, automatic, impulsive, critically negative, and irrational. Beck concluded that depression is the sum of its symptoms and is caused by negative thought patterns. He then treated depressed people with **cognitive therapy**, a form of **cognitive restructuring** in which a person learns to listen to subconscious thoughts and change them from negative ones to positive ones (Figure 14.2).[265] Cognitive therapy has become one of the primary methods used in behavorial or, more succinctly, biopsychosocial medicine.

Behavioral medicine is a multidisciplinary approach based on the theory that there is an intimate relationship between mental and physical processes. This approach to healing has origins in psychiatry, specifically within the study of psychosomatic illnesses like Beck's research with depressed clients' thought patterns. Behavioral therapists, as opposed to behavioralists, examine both the objective and subjective aspects of a client's illness, distinguishing between an illness and the subjective experience a person has of this condition, particularly the personal meaning and social context that health problems have for each person. By doing so, a therapist helps a patient understand how negative thoughts, poor lifestyles choices, and daily stresses are the precursors of many health problems, and then encourages the patient to take a more active role in recovery and prevention. Although behavioral medicine is not typically taught in medical schools, it has had a widespread application in the treatment of conditions caused or exacerbated by smoking and obesity, and is also widely used in the field of biofeedback.

Cognitive Therapy

The response a person has to any life event can be either adaptive—moving a person toward homeostasis and growth, or maladaptive—creating stress and perpetuating illness. In the last chapter, we discussed how thoughts create muscular and physiological responses. For instance, excessive worry over a situation can drive the average person into a panicked sweat, whether or not the worry is realistic and justified. An acrophobe may break out in an alarm reaction at the mere thought of standing on the edge of a cliff, regardless of the fact that this person has total control over whether or not she ever has to step into this threatening position.

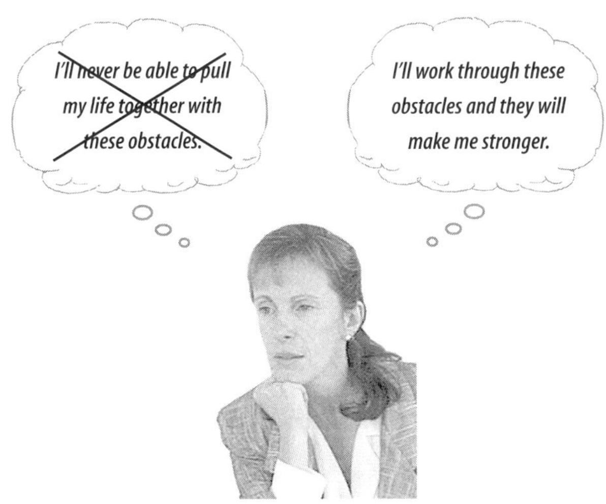
I'll never be able to pull my life together with these obstacles.
I'll work through these obstacles and they will make me stronger.

Figure 14.2 Cognitive restructuring

Patterning Exercise #127: Transform Negative Thoughts into Positive Ones

1. Begin to observe your automatic thoughts. Identify any dysfunctional thoughts or maladaptive assumptions that you habitually make, such as "I'll never amount to anything."
2. Write your maladaptive thoughts down, including what time of the day you tend to have them.
3. Begin to dispute maladaptive thoughts. Recognize and question your assumptions. Counter them with reality checks. For example, is it really true that you will never amount to anything? To counter this assumption, you might ask yourself, "What have I accomplished? How did I accomplish this? What do others see as my accomplishments?" Don't allow yourself to answer with your negative automatic thoughts. Instead, make yourself stop and think of honest answers to these questions.
4. Make a written list of your answers. Then use them to counter maladaptive thoughts whenever you have them.
5. Change your explanatory style. Make it more general if it involves an absolute, which is a mode of black-and-white thinking such as "I'll never . . ." In this case you might say to yourself "I wasn't successful with that situation, but I have been successful in others," or "I can learn the elements of success."
6. Do homework. Take notes. Chart your progress. Add up your successes. And most importantly, make sure to counter an automatic thought each time it comes up. In the last example, you could say, "I was successful in certain situations, and will be again," and "I can do this."
7. If depressing or ruminating thoughts keep popping up and you are unable to counter them, distract yourself from them. Get busy doing something else, writing, gardening, cleaning your house. You might even keep on hand a list of chores you need to get done to remind yourself about activities that will distract you.

EMSPress.com

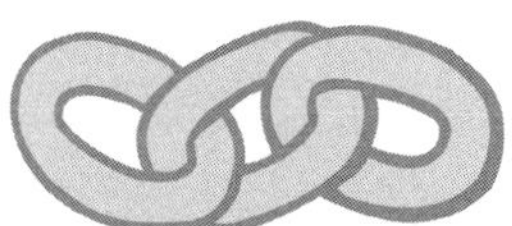

Combining Patterning and Psychotherapy

The more deeply entwined your physical problems are with your psychological problems, the more you will benefit from combining psychotherapy with somatic patterning. By sensing the body postures you go into when in the midst of psychological turmoil, you can feel the effect of the problem in both your body and mind, and work on it through both channels. Clients often only recognize this connection after starting SP and are then able to find an appropriate psychotherapist to work with in conjunction with SP.

Cognitive therapy requires an objective appraisal of a person's fears, specifically of the thoughts that create stress, to determine what is real and what is imagined. Through this appraisal, the acrophobe may come to realize that there is no pending threat of having to stand on a cliff, and that the threat may have come from a recurring and subconscious memory of having tripped near the edge of a steep precipice as a child. Once the appraisal has been taken, a person can then begin to identify resources and options. In doing so, the acrophobe may realize that she is in complete control of whether or not she goes to a location of great height. And if she ever does have to stand or walk along the edge of a threatening height, she can stand back far enough to block or minimize her view of the drop.

There are many techniques of cognitive therapy, or restructuring, which include *stress inoculation* (practicing coping skills in an imagined or real situation of stress), *visualization* (picturing the desired outcome), *values clarification* (identifying the subconscious rules of one's behavior), *systematic desensitization* (training for coping with threatening situations or pain), and *learned optimism*.[266]

The psychologist Martin Seligman developed the method of **learned optimism** after realizing that the difference between how a pessimist and an optimist view the same situation determines the failure or success of the outcome. Seligman also participated in research that uncovered the phenomenon of **learned helplessness**, in which people learn to give up trying when their actions prove futile.[267] Since people with severe illness or injuries are susceptible to slipping into a state of helplessness, it is imperative that they find some way to have control over their situation. Generally, control entails being actively involved in their own therapy, making decisions about the kinds of treatment they undergo, and learning self-regulation skills.

The discovery of learned helplessness more or less pulled the conceptual rug out from under behaviorists, who had believed that behaviors were learned solely as responses conditioned by external reward or punishment without the influences of internal self-talk. If helplessness can be learned, so can hopefulness; likewise, pessimists can learn to change their explanatory style of self-talk and begin to think like optimists. A pessimist imagines the worst will happen in any situation, believes the situation will last a long time, and is more likely to suffer from depression, listlessness, and health problems. Conversely, an optimist perceives a problem as a temporary and surmountable learning experience, is able to overcomes challenges easily, tends to be successful in school and work, and usually has excellent health. After 25 years of research, Seligman found consistent evidence that maladaptive thoughts, images, and beliefs can be replaced with adaptive ones, a concept now widely used in behavioral medicine. In short, pessimists can learn to become optimists by restructuring their habits of thought.[268]

Transcending the "Story"

Internal dialogue not only patterns thinking, it also evokes muscular responses. For example, it is common for people to read only as fast as they can talk because each word is silently spoken as it is read. Notice how people move while they talk to themselves, "acting out" their thoughts. An attentive practitioner can notice when a client who is lying on the massage table with his eyes closed trying to relax has thoughts racing through his mind because the eyes will dart under the eyelids and the muscles of his throat will

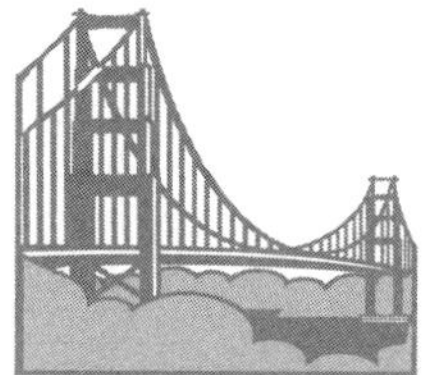

Bridge to Practice

Releasing Tension in the Throat without Talking

Many clients talk excessively during a session. Talking can be very helpful in opening the throat and discharging nervous tension although it can create a double bind. This is because the content of the words tends to keep the mind busy, which often gets in the way of the client relaxing.

If your client talks excessively in an effort to discharge nervous tension, but actually becomes tenser in the process, you might suggest that the client quietly sense this pattern. Then suggest that your client sense the muscles inside the mouth and throat; this awareness alone may help her to relax any muscle tension in this area.

Also, you might suggest that humming, sighing, or doing some kind of abstract vocalizing may be a more direct way to open the vocal channels and release muscular tension around the throat while relaxing the brain. Even opening and closing the mouth and moving it in a way that stretches the muscles around the lips, jaw, and tongue can release nervous tension through the throat.

There are other clients who lack overall body strength yet are good at making biting, sharp comments. In this case, you'll notice that the throat and mouth have high tone while the rest of the body has low tone. Encourage these clients to express their busy thoughts through movement in the arms, legs, and pelvis to bring the tone up in these areas while allowing the throat channel to relax.

move as if he were speaking. To learn how to speed-read, a person has to learn how to inhibit muscular responses in the face, throat, and neck.

A holistic approach to patterning includes monitoring thoughts and emotions that accompany postures and movement patterns, and working to change them accordingly. The challenge of somatic patterning is to be able to work with the effects of psychology on the body and behavior without getting lost in the content, or "story," behind the physical pattern. A relaxed mind is a prerequisite for a relaxed body. The contents of the client's thoughts are not as important as the client's ability to let them go and quiet the mind. Addressing content remains in the scope of psychotherapy, although psychotherapy may be needed in conjunction with somatic patterning when a body pattern is rooted in a persistent psychological issue.

When thought patterns become habitual and limiting, corresponding body patterns also become habitual and negative. Many people who have been traumatized will recall the traumatic incident over and over again, actually recreating the same stress responses that occurred in the body during the original trauma. When this happens, the "story" becomes the negative thought, and each recounting of it deepens the effects of the trauma on the body. The story also becomes habitual, or automatic. Automatic thoughts create muscular and other physiological responses that realize the commands of the thoughts. These physiological responses are well documented by stress researchers. Negative thoughts may also trigger endocrine responses that accompany emotional states, which is a basic premise of psychoneuroimmunology.

NEUROLINGUISTIC PROGRAMMING

As discussed at the beginning of this chapter, one popular method used to reorganize cognitive patterns as they manifest in speech and body patterns is called **neurolinguistic programming** (**NLP**). NLP grew out of a research project set up to answer the question: What are the behavioral elements of successful psychotherapy?

NLP began when, in the early 1970s, two enterprising men with unusual perspectives named Bandler and Grinder started to work on developing a method of changing behavior by reprogramming thought patterns. Richard Bandler, originally a student of mathematics and computer sciences, switched his track to pursue studies in psychology. He found that by modeling the behavior of several well-known therapists, he was able to achieve successes similar to theirs. John Grinder, a professor of linguistics, found that by assuming cultural behaviors and accents, he was able to assimilate into foreign cultures and discover the hidden grammar within their thoughts and actions.[269]

Bandler and Grinder teamed up and used their combined backgrounds in computer technology, linguistics, and psychology, as well as their similar skills in modeling nonverbal behavior, and together started to explore the dynamics of personal and relational change. They began by copying the mannerisms and professional techniques of Fritz Perls, the founder of Gestalt therapy. They went on to study the nonverbal mannerisms of many other psychotherapists, including famed family psychotherapist Virginia Satir, foremost hypnotist Milton Erickson, and systems thinker Gregory Bateson. From their observations, Bandler and Grinder made a fundamental discovery: "How people think about something makes a crucial difference in how they will experience it."[270] For instance, they found that people who are chronically depressed often spend most of their time thinking depressing thoughts. They developed the main premise of NLP out of this research, which is that all thoughts are like "software" for the "computer" of the mind: they make up the mental program a person uses to operate and maintain any psychological or physical state.

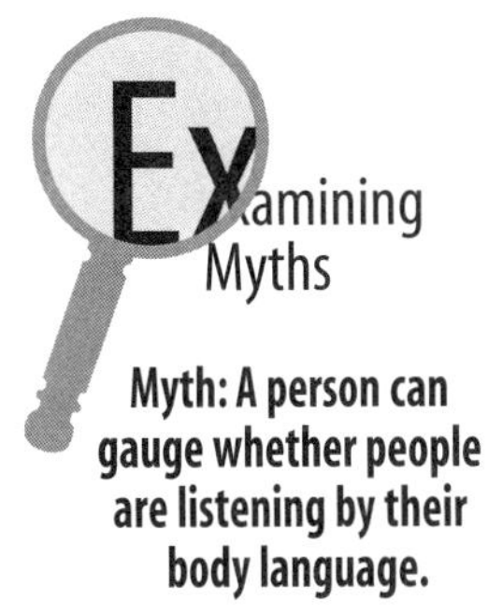

Myth: A person can gauge whether people are listening by their body language.

This is not necessarily true. For example, a man might believe that a woman is not listening to him because she does not look at him as he speaks, or crosses her arms across her chest in response. However, this may be a projection on the man's part because the woman may be an auditory type, hearing better when the visual field is turned down. Or she may simply be crossing her arms because of back pain. When in doubt, a person should always ask the other person what is going on rather than make assumptions. Each person communicates with a different style, and what a person finds upon inquiry may be a surprise.

Studies in psychology have traditionally focused on all the things that go wrong with the human mind. Bandler and Grinder studied what works, how people are successful, and what thought patterns support success and achievement. They systematized this information into neurolinguistic programming, first calling it Modeling Human Excellence. Through NLP techniques, people learn how to rearrange patterns of thought in order to release limiting behaviors and achieve their goals. Since NLP stems from a study of the mechanics of successful communication, many of its working premises are likely to be familiar to the already successful communicator.

Tracking Responses

NLP is based on some basic principles that can serve as guidelines for facilitating change in a person's thoughts and behaviors. One of the most fundamental premises is: "The meaning of your communication is the response you get."[271] A person assesses whether a communication has been received by noticing body cues in the recipient, such

Rearranging Reality with NLP

Richard Bandler, the cofounder of neurolinguistic programming, describes an approach to psychosis that he finds most useful in this excerpt from his text Using Your Brain—For a Change:

Enter the psychotic's reality and then spoil it for him. There are a lot of ways you can do this, and some of them aren't obvious. For instance, I had one guy who heard voices coming out of electrical outlets, and the voices forced him to do things. I figured if I made his hallucinations real, he wouldn't be schizophrenic any more. So I hid a speaker in an outlet in my waiting room. When he came into the room, the outlet said "Hello." The guy turned around and looked at it and said, "You don't sound the same."

"I'm a new voice. Did you think there was only one?"

"Where did you come from?"

"Mind your own business."

That got him going. Since he had to obey the voice, I used that new voice to give him instructions that he needed to change what he was doing. Most people get a handle on reality and respond to it. When I get a handle on reality, I *twist* it! I don't believe people are broken. They have just learned to do whatever they do. A lot of what people have learned to do is pretty amazing, and frankly I see more of that outside of mental hospitals than inside.[272]

as breathing patterns, verbal responses, gestural or postural shifts, and spontaneous movements.

The two most basic responses are acceptance or rejection, a yes or a no, which are observed in the client's body responses. Generally, the body does not lie: it either opens or closes it either retracts or expands. An astute person can see, feel, or hear acceptance in another's eyes and voice, through open or closed gestures and postures, but most accurately through shifts in autonomic tone.

Recall from Chapter 1 that somatic retraction is usually a defensive response regulated by the autonomic nervous system. It affects the physiological tone of the body in a systemic response that runs deeper than a gesture or posture. Although a gesture or posture can reflect whether a person is opening or closing to an experience, it can also habitually cover up what is occurring within a person on a much deeper level. Therefore, to accurately track somatic responses, a practitioner needs to by able to pick up cues about shifts in autonomic tone, such as changes in breathing, skin color, temperature, or even vibrational shifts (usually obvious in nervousness or in changes in the tone of voice).

Likewise, to accurately track the effectiveness of communication, a practitioner can also pick up clues about whether or not a client is internally accessing or processing information. When people are processing internal information, they become quiet and internally focused, and may even furrow their brow. Also, they might assume a far away or searching look in the eyes as they sink into thought.

Whenever people go inside themselves to access information and process it, either by thinking about it or feeling it, they can no longer take in more outside information. During this time, it is important for practitioners to wait for a response.

Representational Systems

Ask three people to describe the same event and one person might paint an elaborate picture of the experience, another might describe the sounds and tempos of the speakers at the event, and the third might describe how he or she felt during this event. Each person recalls the event through a different **representational system**: the first is

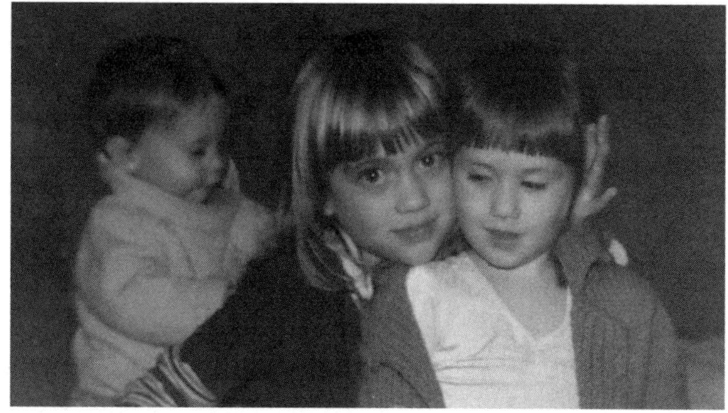

Figure 14.3 Each child is focused in a different channel; one is touching, one is looking, and one is listening.

Patterning Exercise #128: Exploration with Representational Systems

1. For five minutes, listen to your partner describing the details of what he or she had for breakfast this morning. Take notes, jotting down words that reveal which representational channels your partner uses. The verbs used in the description indicates the channel, such as "I saw," "I listened," "I felt", etc.
2. Switch roles and repeat step 1.
3. Now give each other feedback about the channels you heard, naming the words that were auditory, kinesthetic, or visual.
4. Change gears and have a discussion with each other for five minutes. Notice how your two representational systems interact. Are they in synchrony?
5. End this exploration by discussing your findings with your partner. Give examples of what was discovered. Discuss what occurs when the channels you and your partner use do not match. Lastly, discuss how you can build bridges across these communication gaps.

EMSPress.com

Links to Practical Applications

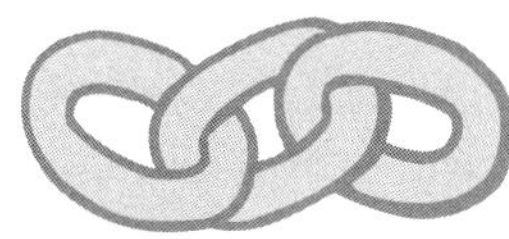

Communication Channels

Listen to the verbs and adjectives you use during the course of a day to determine which channels you communicate in: visual, auditory, or kinesthetic. Listen to the descriptive language of someone you are close to and compare them with yours. Do you communicate through the same channels? Now listen to the verbs of someone you have conflict with and compare your channels.

visual, the second auditory, and the third kinesthetic (Figure 14.3).

After reviewing many, many psychotherapy sessions, both taped and live, the developers of NLP found that communication problems often occur when two people cannot find common representational systems. For instance, a client might describe how he *sees* a situation, elaborating on his perspective, while the therapist continues to interpret the *feelings* the client had. The client gets frustrated because the therapist does not *see* his perspective. The therapist becomes annoyed because she feels that the client is not willing to *feel* his feelings, and she labels him as "resistant." In this example, the client is operating in a visual system and the therapist is operating in a kinesthetic one; the two will only meet if one person switches over to the other's system.

Having an awareness of the different representational systems can expand how we structure experience and how we communicate with others. Representational systems can be tracked through eye movements and gestures, or cues from language, such as "I see," "I hear," "I feel." Since each person usually learns through a predominant channel, ability to discern which representational system is being used is helpful for therapists, teachers, or anyone working as an agent of change with others. Here are some general cues for discerning which representational system is being used:

- People in the auditory system appear to be listening to silent voices.
- People in the visual system often look to certain locations in space while accessing information.
- People in the kinesthetic system make gestures that simulate sensory experiences and often involve touch or movement.

Some people may learn through a primary representational system, yet most people move among systems in habitual patterns. Representational systems are like channels that we can tune into or switch between. Also, the representational components tend to occur in sequences. An example of a visual-kinesthetic-auditory sequence follows: "Every time I think about how *bad she looked* I get a *gut feeling* that I needed to *listen more closely* to find out what was really wrong." A person with a kinesthetic-auditory-visual sequence might say, "I *felt unnerved* by how depressed she was but didn't *feel comfortable* commenting about how *worn out she looked*." Still another says, "I *can see* that she *never talks* about her feelings because she's *hurting inside*."

A representational sequence shows how a person internally structures thoughts and perceptions. If someone is having an experience that he or she does not want to be having, the sequence of *how* the experience occurs can be interrupted. The previous body story titled "Rearranging Reality with NLP" is an account of a man experiencing auditory hallucinations. Bandler interrupted the order of this man's hallucinations by introducing a new voice, which disarmed the man's inner voice.

Matching and Rapport

Matching behavior creates a common ground on which relationships between people can be based. When this naturally occurs we refer to it as "making a connection" with another person, or "being in sync." Couples who have good **rapport** in their relationships often begin to look alike, walk and talk alike, and match each other's rhythms and mannerisms on very subtle levels. NLP practitioners describe many successful sessions in couples therapy where clashes in communication channels have been identified and rectified by helping couples communicate in matching modes. For instance, a husband might compli-

Rapport with a Hospice Patient

A massage therapist describes how she developed a rapport with a dying woman who had lost her ability to speak:

Mary, a client dying of a long-term illness, was brought to me by her family to receive massage therapy as a way to help relieve swelling and pain. This woman had lost over 50 percent of her speech and memory functions and got incredibly frustrated when she could not finish a sentence, which contributed to her tension and pain.

We began our sessions with a relaxation exercise that involved slowing the breath rate down into long, rhythmic cycles. Initially, I counted the cycles in a soft, hypnotic voice, saying, "breathe in . . . breathe out . . . breathe in . . . breathe out." Once this rhythm was established, I matched the rhythm of my massage strokes with the movement of her breath. When the client was able to synchronize her breath with this rhythm, she began to relax and let go of her frustration. Over time, we got to the point where, when she got tense, I would begin to breathe in the long audible rhythms, then she would breathe in synchrony with me, and we both would enter deep states of relaxation.

Shortly before Mary passed away, I went to see her. By this time she had lost all her speech functions, so communication was nonverbal and primarily tactile. That day I was particularly tense because of pressing deadlines. Mary saw this and reached for my hands. She held them and began breathing slowly, bringing me into a cadence with her rhythm and reminding me to relax. Several hours later, she closed her eyes and died gracefully and peacefully.

Matching Desire and Action

Robert, a physical therapist, was helping John, a clerk, with an ergonomic problem at his workstation. John explained that his back and neck always hurt, and that he was suffering from severe headaches. He felt it was related to something he was doing on the job and wanted Robert to help identify this.

Robert asked John to show him his work posture. John leaned back his swivel chair, turned sideways to the desk, and stretched his feet out, then twisted his keyboard around so he could reach it.

To correct the ergonomics, the physical therapist swiveled John's chair so that he faced his desk. John sat there for a few minutes, looking quite uncomfortable. Eventually he exclaimed, "Good grief! This is the first time I have ever looked at my work straight on. What a shock! I just realized that I hate this job. No wonder I'm in such pain. I'm coming and going at the same time. My body is turning away while my mind forces me to stay." Shortly after this session, John decided it was time to listen to his body and find work that was enjoyable to him. He quit his job and began a landscaping business.

ment his wife by telling her she looks great. The wife, who is a kinesthetic person, feels he is just saying this because she really does not look very good, and wonders why her husband doesn't hug her to show approval. Once the husband understands these dynamics, he can learn to offer a compliment with a hug to bridge the communication gap of his visual channel with his wife's kinesthetic channel.

From their research, Bandler and Grinder found that successful therapists were highly skilled in matching and building rapport with clients, and unsuccessful therapists were not. They also found that what therapists typically call "resistance" is most commonly a communication problem, the result of the client and therapist communicating with different representational systems. There are many ways a therapist can change the situation. An astute therapist can match the client's representational system with his own to develop rapport, or can link the client's predominant system with ones the client does not use to expand the client's channels of awareness and communication. For instance, if the client is visual and the therapist is primarily auditory, the therapist could practice visualization techniques to communicate effectively in the client's channel. Or the therapist could help the client enter an auditory channel by asking the client what sounds his or her internal pictures have.

Matching is a widely used skill in both SP and in bodywork, although it is practiced primarily in the realm of movement and tissue quality. SP practitioners use matching not only to build rapport, but for a number of other reasons as well. A practitioner might try to sense a client's body pattern by taking it on, giving a client feedback about a holding pattern by modeling it. Also, in one widely used technique, a practitioner actually moves the client's body into a tension pattern so that the client cannot only feel the pattern, but can gradually release it by letting the practitioner take over the effort required to hold the tension. This method is known as *indirect technique,* a classical hands-on technique akin to pushing a stuck door into the frame to open it rather than trying to pull it open. In SP, this method of matching the client's pattern is often referred to as "taking the client into the pattern" or "taking over the pattern."

Reframing

Destructive behaviors at the very least tend to confuse us, and frequently cause us and others harm. All actions and behaviors, beyond their primary purpose, have a *secondary gain,* or payoff, or people would not do them. For example, a beautiful woman gains 100 pounds to protect herself subconsciously from relationships with men, or a man habitually complains because he learned, at some point in his life, that complaining gains him sympathy and support from family members. In both of these cases, the negative behavior became fused, or coupled, with the gain.

Reframing is an NLP technique used to separate the behavior itself from the gain or intention of the behavior.[273] We reframe a situation when we see it from a new perspective (Figure 14.4). For instance, a client must reframe her view by seeing what she once thought of as a problem as an opportunity to change and grow.

To get a sense of the reframing process, let's consider a fictitious man named Mike who had a tendency to whine. When Mike was a child, he actually learned that whining was an effective behavior to elicit sympathy. Because he had cancer as a child, he was in and out of hospitals and learned how to manipulate his caretakers by whining. Mike's parents gave him a lot of sympathy, especially when other children teased him. Therefore, whining and getting support became linked or coupled. Now Mike decides his behavior is driving friends away, so he goes to an NLP practitioner to learn how to change it. The reframing process consists of the following steps:

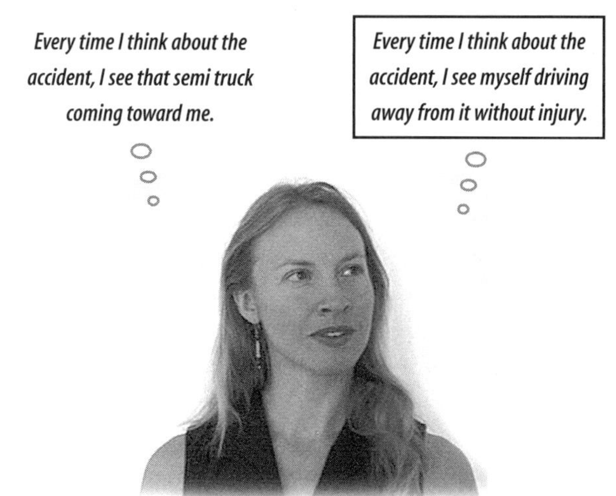

Every time I think about the accident, I see that semi truck coming toward me.
Every time I think about the accident, I see myself driving away from it without injury.

Figure 14.4 Reframing involves seeing a difficult situation from another perspective. It can be used to take the charge out of a traumatic memory.

1. *Identifying the undesirable behavior and the person's attitude toward the behavior*. In our example, Mike is embarrassed because he feels that whining is a weakness, yet it persists because it has been programmed into his unconscious mind. The part of him that views the behavior as weak is the part of him that rejects this aspect of his unconscious self. In other words, his conscious actions and unconscious beliefs are not congruent.
2. *Establishing communication and rapport with the unconscious part of the pattern*—in this case, the weak self. The practitioner suggests that all behaviors serve a function and perhaps whining was a great way to get something at one time. Upon hearing this, Mike realizes that he initially got an enormous amount of sympathy and support, which he truly needed at the time, by complaining in a whiny voice. Now that the payoff is identified, Mike has gained access to an unconscious part of himself and quits rejecting it by labeling it as weak.
3. *Separating the behavior from the intention of the behavior*—in this case, separating whining from the need for support.
4. *Identifying alternative behaviors.* The practitioner asks Mike to imagine or feel some other ways that he can get support from people. Once Mike has come up with a number of different choices, he begins to visualize himself in a variety of life situations using some of his newly imagined behaviors.
5. *Sensing whether the body is relaxing or tightening, indicating whether the unconscious mind is accepting or rejecting the new behaviors.* Acceptance or rejection responses may occur in any representational system, depending upon the person. A kinesthetic person might have a pleasurable feeling of expansion or a feeling of contraction. An auditory person might hear a yes or a no. A visual person might see himself shaking his head yes of no. For unwanted behaviors to be dissected from the function they serve, the unconscious mind must accept the exchange of these behaviors for new ones. Only then can new behaviors be consciously chosen to replace the old.

In this example, Mike learns to recognize congruency between the conscious process and the unconscious mind by asking yes and no questions, learning to feel when something is being accepted or rejected. Once new options are in place, he can begin creating future scenarios where he uses the new options he dreamed up to get the support he needs. Although lifelong behavioral habits like Mike's usually take time and diligent effort to change, once the dynamics of the behavior are clearly illuminated, the change can be immediate. In fact, people who have spent years in psychotherapy to change negative behaviors often comment that NLP cuts through the emotional webbing directly to the structural dynamics of faulty relationship, providing simple, concrete tools that can be implemented in an instant.

Psychological patterns that become habitual, such a Mike's behavioral pattern of whining, usually have a corresponding posture. When a person reframes a situation to move past behavioral fixations, it is helpful to also feel the corresponding postures for the old and new behaviors, and to change the postures accordingly. In fact, by becoming aware of an old postural habit setting in again, a person gets helpful feedback that he or she may be unconsciously or habitually acting out an old behavioral pattern, and can then make changes accordingly.

NLP Applications

A retail merchant recounts the following story about applying NLP skills and patterning principles in a tense situation:

I was driving to an important business meeting and could feel the tension within me mounting. It was the final meeting in a series of negotiations that were not going well, whose outcome would make or break my business. As I thought about the guy I would be negotiating with, the back of my neck tightened, my knuckles slowly bore down on the wheel, and my body became increasingly more tense.

"Think," I told myself. "You know how to work with patterns; you can move through this. Think. What is the first step?

"Feel. Yes, awareness. I feel my body shrinking.

"What does the meeting look like from this perspective? The man I am about to negotiate with is looking very big.

"Think. What is this pattern teaching me? Tension. No! That's a polarity—being set against the enemy. Find the common ground to create a win-win basis for the meeting. If we close this deal, it will help both of us succeed.

"What is my perspective now? I am sitting next to the man on mutual ground and he is the same size as me.

"Feel. I'm starting to relax but am still a little short of breath. I feel kind of claustrophobic, like sitting next to him is too close. But I know that I do have a choice, I can move.

"Think. I can see us sitting at a distance from each other. I feel far enough away from the situation to relax now. I feel more objective, less emotional, and my body has relaxed. I'm now ready for the meeting."

The negotiations went great. I was relaxed, somewhat detached, and very clear. Even the other guy seemed more relaxed. It was our smoothest meeting to date, and we closed the deal.

The whole experience felt like a crystallization of all NLP and patterning work I had learned. In less than 10 minutes I was able to use patterning principles to move through an old place of tension and help to create a successful experience for all the parties involved. I never cease to be amazed at how I can apply these principles to so many aspects of my life.

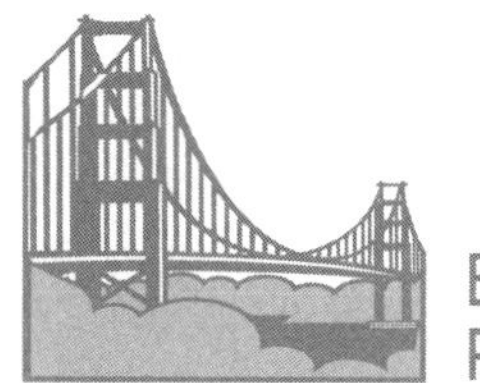

Bridge to Practice

Touch Transference with Bodywork Clients

If you are doing hands-on work with a client, watch and sense how each client responds to your touch. Does your client relax or draw away? If she draws away, stop what you are doing and verbally acknowledge the retraction. Your client may not even realize that her body is retracting, so by mentioning it, you provide an opportunity for her to increase her awareness of how she does or does not like to be touched.

Many times, clients ask for deeper pressure yet at the same time pull away from the pressure. If this happens, point out the incongruency between what they are asking for and how their body is responding. This will bring your clients' patterns to a conscious level, which gives them an opportunity to understand certain patterns.

Also, before putting your hands on a client, get a commitment from the client to speak up if she or he finds your touch uncomfortable for any reason. Even with a commitment, unconscious transference can still occur. Still, your client's verbal commitment to speak up establishes an important boundary in the therapeutic relationship for several reasons: the client is taking responsibility for what occurs, the client is learning to trust her responses, the client is learning how to track and break negative associations, and you are both developing rapport.

A simple way for a client to communicate discomfort is through a hand signal that bypasses the mental and verbal channels and is much more immediate. Ask your client to pat the table or raise a finger if she or he feels uncomfortable with your touch.

Association, Dissociation, and Transference

One of the early NLP discoveries was that people who are stuck in phobias recreate the memories of phobias with associations. A person associates with memories when he goes back and relives them through his own thoughts. For example, someone with a fear of snakes may habitually visualize himself sweating and gasping every time he thinks of a snake. Bandler and Grinder found that people who got over phobias saw themselves as if they were watching someone else in a film, dissociating themselves from the phobia with an objective distance.

In **dissociation**, people view the memory from any point of view other than their own eyes. In NLP, conscious dissociation is used as a personal resource to create distance from an unpleasant experience. Although most somatic therapies encourage developing an increased awareness of body sensation, there are times when tracking sensation is not therapeutic. On a physical level, dissociation can help a client desensitize, or detach, from an uncomfortable sensation, such as chronic pain.

Association can be used positively, as well, to build connections to pleasant and successful experiences. People often associate gestures, verbal inflections and tones, postures, or expressions with people from the past. In psychotherapy this is called **transference**. Most people can walk into a crowded room, look around, and find at least one person who reminds them of someone else. If that someone else was pleasant, the association will be pleasant. If that someone else was unpleasant, the association will be unpleasant as well. For example, a woman's father could have shaken his finger whenever he yelled at her. Now, every time this woman encounters someone shaking a finger, she has the same uncomfortable feeling she had with her father because she unconsciously transfers her negative responses to her father onto the person shaking the finger. Another woman might have a pleasant association of her childhood vacations in the country every time she sees or smells lavender. So if someone is wearing lavender scent, this woman unconsciously transfers her pleasant association onto that person.

Changing Associations

NLP includes several techniques for changing associations. The first step is to become aware of associations and determine if they are happening in first or second person. For instance, a person might be plagued by a childhood memory of punishment in which he sees the legs of the punisher standing before him in a clear, colorful image, and then feels the terror of the memory shudder through his body (Figure 14.5a). To shift the memory to second person, he can visualize himself watching himself looking at the legs from a distance. To change the memory in his mind, he might shrink the person with the legs and enlarge himself, then shrink the whole scene and look at it from an objective distance (Figure 14.5b). He could also turn the picture, fuzz the picture, take the color out, and then place it in a boat and allow it to float away down a river. The more he distorts the picture, the less association there might be.

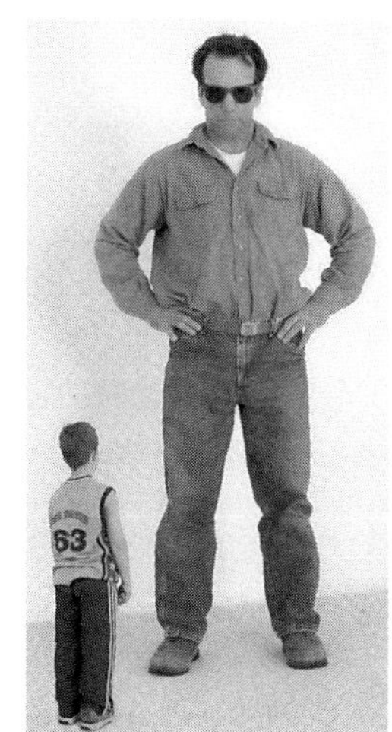

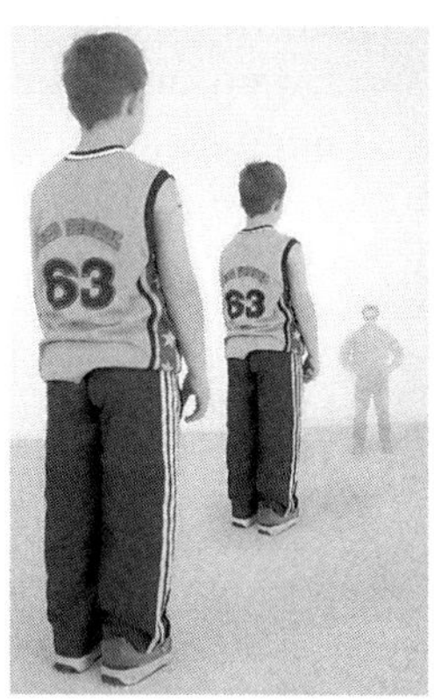

Figure 14.5a-b An NLP technique to change a negative memory or association by altering the image that it evokes

One beauty of NLP is that the practitioner can help a person go through the process of changing an association without even learning the content of a person's problem. A practitioner might ask the client to describe *how* he sees the picture without actually disclosing what the picture is. In this way, the content of a somatic or psychological process is secondary to the structure of memory or the structure of experience. We can identify the structure of a person's experience by the elements of behavior that are being discussed, particularly in a person's style of interacting and communicating with other people.

As mentioned earlier, behavioral patterns usually have corresponding postures. When a person experiences a negative association, for example, she usually contracts and cringes on some level. By noticing these postural habits, a person can become aware of when a negative association is playing out and dissociate from the pattern by not only changing the association on a cognitive level, but also on a physical level. For example, for the fictitious person above to deal with the memory of his abuser, this man could also plant both his feet on the ground, take an aggressive stance, and shrink the memory with the strength of his posture.

Transference through Touch

Associations with certain qualities of touch run incredibly deep because tactile interactions are one of our most primitive channels of communication. The way in which an infant or child was touched by caregivers and others imprints how he or she likes to be touched as an adult. Whereas one person might love having her feet or neck massaged, another person might recoil at any touch in these areas because of negative associations.

Associations develop in an instant and often last a lifetime, particularly negative associations. We tend to transfer negative tactile associations from one relationship to another. Touch transference explains why one person might enjoy a specific type of massage or bodywork on a specific area while another person will recoil at massage of the same quality or on a specific body part. One massage therapist noticed that every time she was working near a certain client's fingers, that client would wince. It turned out the client's last massage therapist had a habit of painfully snapping the woman's fingers, which she silently endured in an effort to be cooperative. Her association showed up in wincing, which she was unaware of, an example of transference through touch. The client transferred her unconscious response to the previous massage therapist onto the new one.

Touch transference comes up with people all the time. It is particularly common in people who have been physically or sexually abused. During abuse, a person is often helpless to set boundaries and stop the abuse; therefore, people with this history often silently endure receiving touch that they find disturbing. Fortunately, more parents and therapists are teaching their children and clients how to set boundaries about how and where they are touched, and to recognize inappropriate touching. Still, if a person has a strong reaction to an acceptable form of touch, chances are that there is a negative association to the touch for that person.

Timeline

A **timeline** is an NLP concept developed to teach people how to recognize their relationship to time, and how to link or bridge the past, present, and future in healthy ways.[274] Notice how each of the following sentences creates a different feeling:

- If we listen carefully to the speaker, we can track the timeline he is in.
- If we had listened carefully to the speaker, we would have heard the timeline he spoke in.
- If we can listen carefully to the speaker, we will begin to hear what timeline he is in.

The verb tenses of each sentence indicate the location in time of the action being discussed. The first is in present tense, the second past tense, and the third future tense. Many times, clients who are stuck in limiting body postures are also stuck on some part of a past-present-future continuum. The use of appropriate verb tenses is a powerful therapeutic tool. It helps us recognize how we relate to time so that we can build appropriate bridges between the past, present, and future. On the other hand, the unconscious use of inappropriate verb tenses can signal that a person is stuck on the time continuum and can also program negative events in the future. For example, an NLP teacher describes a situation in which a client kept saying to her therapist, "Every time he yells, I get angry." This statement sets a powerful program for the future of this relationship by using a verb tense that describes the action as ongoing. To put the behavior in the past, the therapist

Patterning Exercise #129: Exploring Timeline

(This exercise is adapted from Bandler.) To explore timelines, think of positive changes you want in your life, then reflect on them as you read each of the following sentences.

1. What will it be like when you have made these changes? How will your body feel different?
2. How will your future improve? How will your posture change?
3. Look back and reflect on what you sensed your life was like before you thought of making these changes. How was it different?
4. What is your view of your life situation now, as you sit in this room and think about the changes? Did your posture change?

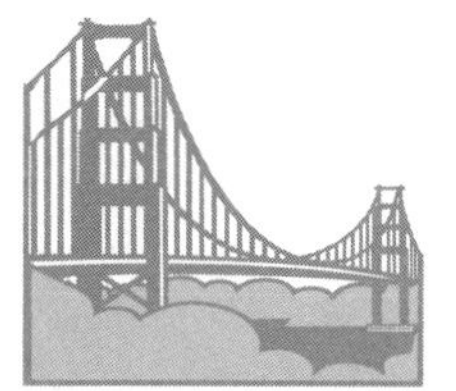

Using Timelines for Integration

The present and future can be linked together at the end of a session to help a client integrate the changes that he made during this session into his life. To do this, ask your client, "How do you want to take these changes into your life?" or "How will ____________ (*fill in the blank with something about your somatic patterns*) be different from this new perspective?" "How will your body feel different?" "How will your posture and movement change?" You can also ask your client to visualize an upcoming situation in which he could apply and embody the shifts he just went through.

By reviewing the change, you will get a clearer picture of what really occurred during the session rather than what you may think has occurred (the difference can be surprising!). The client also gets an opportunity to review what has just passed, how it passed, and how he wants it to affect his future. More importantly, by reviewing the process that he went through to make changes, the client leaves the session with a clear method for invoking the same kind of change in other situations.

rephrased it, asking, "Are you saying you got angry every time he yelled at you?"

People project the present into a negative future when they tell their children to "be careful not to get hit by a car." Bandler and Grinder feel that the unconscious mind does not hear positive or negative qualifiers. The child hears "get hit by a car" and is imprinted with some experiential representation of this, in an image, a feeling, or even a sound. To more effectively program the behavior they want, parents would be better off saying to their children, "You will be safer if you cross the street when all the cars are stopped."

The components of time are of immense value when working with body patterns. After all, the body exists only in the present moment. When people focus on physical sensations as they occur, they cannot help but connect with their present time reality and make direct contact with their bodies. Only the mind can effectively project into the past or the future, yet this ability carries with it the possibility of programming activities for the body that could either enhance or diminish the quality of a person's life, depending on how and what the mind projects. From Bandler's perspective, "about 90 percent of what goes on in [effective] therapy is changing kinesthetic responses that people have to auditory and visual stimuli."[275]

SUMMARY

The premise of the behavioral therapies and cognitive reorganization is that it is not so much the internal or external stressors that lead to problems in our lives, but *how* we view these stressors and respond to them. If negative thoughts cause stress and maladaptive behaviors, by changing the way that we think, we can reduce stress and learn positive, adaptive behaviors. The original behaviorists were Watson and Skinner, who trained rats to respond through classical conditioning with positive reinforcement for the desired behaviors and punishment for undesired behaviors.

Behaviorism has come a long way since the early days. It has evolved into cognitive therapy skills practiced by behavioral therapists, who work with people's subjective views of their situations, helping them to identify and change the thoughts, beliefs, and assumptions that underlie maladaptive behaviors. Like biofeedback, cognitive therapy is only as effective as the efforts that a person puts into it and the choices he or she makes. Most cognitive therapies use some form of cognitive restructuring, a method in which maladaptive thoughts are reorganized, such as replacing habitually negative thoughts with positive thoughts, or changing self-defeating internal dialogue into supportive phrases.

NLP is a distillation of the behavioral skills that underlie effective psychotherapy. These skills are body-based. They involve being aware of what is happening in the present moment by tracking the client's body postures and language patterns (specifically visual, auditory, or kinesthetic representational systems); by matching the client's channels of communication, breath, and posture to build rapport; and by helping a client see a situation from a different perspective by reframing a situation, changing associations to it, or looking at it from a different timeline.

NLP skills have been integrated into many somatic therapies because they are so effective in changing maladaptive behaviors. In a sense NLP is "behavioral patterning" without the content. It drops content out of the process of change, allowing people to reprogram the structure of their experience without getting lost in the story line of their problems.

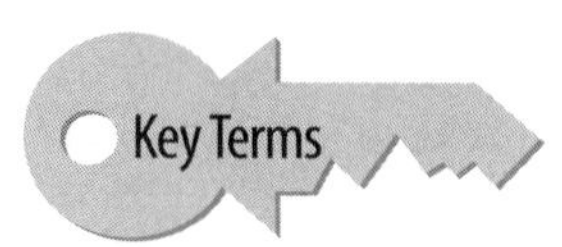

association
behaviorism
cognitive restructuring
cognitive therapy
coupling
dissociation
learned helplessness
learned optimism
matching
neurolinguistic programming (NLP)
rapport
reframing
representational system
timelines
transference

OVERVIEW OF CHAPTER 15

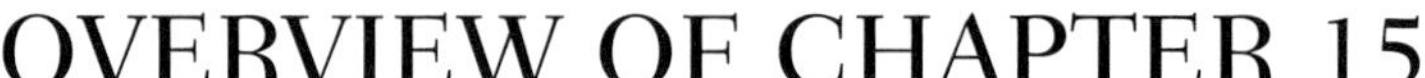

15

Body-Based Psychotherapy

> The life of the body is the life of the individual. [All too often], the body becomes an instrument of the will in the service of self-image.
>
> —*Alexander Lowen*

Modern psychology developed during the twentieth century as a science of behavior. Traditionally, this field has separated the study of the mind from the study of the physical body, a general approach that has remained dominant. Yet in the last few decades, body-based approaches to psychotherapy have begun to grow almost as a remedial system to reintegrate the body and the mind. Body-based approaches to psychotherapy arise from the premise that all psychological processes occur within the body and thus all psychological patterns have physical components. In terms of body-based psychology, psychological problems are believed to manifest in body fixations or maladaptive somatic patterns, making our bodies the most tangible evidence we have of our psychological states. While this chapter is about body-based psychotherapy, somatic patterning (SP) draws on this knowledge to deepen an understanding of body-mind patterns. The SP focus is on changing body patterns rather than processing emotional or psychological issues

An understanding of the body's role in psychological processes actually began with the psychoanalytical work of the Austrian neurologist Sigmund Freud (1856–1939). Freud had his patients recline on a couch to minimize distractions from external stimuli, thereby supporting the emergence of unconscious associations. The therapist sat behind the couch so that the patient would not be distracted by any visible responses on the part of the therapist. The couch served to isolate the patient somewhat in order to encourage him to tune into himself and his intrapsychic processes.

Most psychological therapies are based on the relationship between cognitive and emotional disorders. Early body-based or somatic psychologists also took this focus, but the field is more recently starting to identify and focus on the body components of psychological health. The original recognition of psychosomatic connections in psychiatry began with a condition Freud identified as hysteria. Freud began to correlate body symptoms with the repression of psychological problems, and his basic theory of repression became a major element in many psychotherapy schools. In Freud's view, psychological problems, especially painful memories and feelings, get repressed into unconscious parts of the psyche, literally fragmenting the psyche. Freud's work developed on the premise that breaking open the barriers to the unconscious mind heals this fragmentation and reunites the person with aspects of self that have been split off from the conscious self.

Freud's work seeded the idea that the unconscious is synonymous with the body, resulting in several generations of body-based psychiatrists. Among those influenced by Freud was his first lab assistant, Wilhelm Reich, who began a new field of psychoanalysis based on innovative theories of muscular armor and character structure. Like many body psychotherapists who followed him, Reich sought ways to improve the efficiency and effectiveness of psychoanalysis, which in the Freudian tradition took many years, perhaps even a lifetime. Reich noticed that change did not occur in the body through free association, but it did when insight was coupled with emotional response. He began body psychotherapy during the 1930s with a famous case in which he first touched a client, massaging the client's jaw, after which the client experienced a release of deeply suppressed rage.[276]

Reich's work influenced many body psychotherapists and became a major influence in European psychoanalysis. In his time, Reich was the only psychotherapist in Norway; today 40 percent of all psychotherapists in Norway specialize in body psychotherapy. Reich's work not only seeded the field of body psychology, but it influenced systems of bodywork as well. In fact, Reich's work has probably been more influential that anyone else's in the development of various types of body-based therapies.

Many second and third-generation psychotherapists influenced by Reich have also made notable contributions to the field. Prominent among the first generation of body psychotherapists were Reich's students Alexander Lowen and John Pierrakos, who developed *bioenergetics* in the 1950s. Reich believed that the circulation of energy in the body was based on sexual energy. Lowen and Pierrakos challenged this belief with their recognition that any feeling, not just sexual, can affect the circulation of energy in the body. Stanley Keleman, whose work followed on the heels of bioenergetics, introduced the principle of vibratory pulsations in the body as the basis for the cycles of human experience. Keleman's work—a unique blend of cognitive and biological principles—addresses the sequences of change the body goes through during mental and emotional processes.

Dance therapy developed when psychotherapists who were also dancers began using expressive movement for therapy in both psychiatric wards and private practice. In the 1950s, the dance therapist Mary Whitehouse developed a therapeutic process of "movement in depth" that has evolved into what is now called *authentic movement*. In this unique therapeutic process, the therapist acts as a witness, observing a client while she explores an expressive, improvisational movement as a type of free association by the body.

About the same time, psychiatrist Fritz Perls made another major contribution to the field by introducing the use of the client's own body awareness as a basic tool in psychotherapy. Perls incorporated an awareness of one's immediate experience advocated by Zen practices and Sensory Awareness (see Chapter 11) into his work, developing what is known as *Gestalt therapy*. The influence of Perls's work extended in many directions, including into the body psychotherapy community, the bodywork community (Perls and Rolf were teaching at Esalen during the same period), and neurolinguistic programming (NLP). The founders of NLP studied videotapes of Perls to observe and understand his techniques of keeping clients in a present-moment body-based experience (see Chapter 14).

The psychiatrist Eugene Gendlin also made an enormous contribution to the field of body psychology and somatics with his work in the technique of *focusing*. During his research in the 1970s, Gendlin found that, without fail, people who undergo successful psychotherapy have a profound body experience and shift during the course of the process. He coined the term *felt sense* to describe the body sensations, emotions, and thoughts that psychotherapy clients experience during effective psychotherapy, and developed a process called focusing that accesses somatic sensations to reach the core of a psychological issue.

The material in this chapter outlines some of the main elements of body-based psychotherapy that are widely used in somatic patterning. Many of the principles and techniques presented here are based on sound biological principles that many therapists and teachers come to on their own and through work with and observation of clients. Yet it is important to note that many of these principles and techniques have also been verified by research such as that done in biofeedback and psychoneuroimmunology.

REICHIAN THERAPY

> People who are brought up with a negative attitude toward life and sex acquire a pleasure anxiety, which is physiologically anchored in chronic muscular spasms.
>
> — Dr. Wilhelm Reich

Wilhelm Reich (1897–1957) has been referred to as the "father of somatic psychology" because his enormous body of work describes the patterns of character traits in which energy flows through the body of healthy individuals but becomes blocked in neurotic and psychotic individuals. An Austrian-born psychoanalyst, Reich was Freud's first clinical assistant. He had many ideas and activities that were considered radical at the time, including involvement with Marxism and the belief that all neurosis is based on a lack of sexual satisfaction. Reich promoted sex education, the distribution of condoms, and the availability of abortion, a few of the radical ideas that later led to his exile from Europe.

Reich's interest in body patterns began in the early 1930s when he was in a relationship with a dancer named Elsa Linderberg. Linderberg studied with the movement educator Rudolph Laban, who analyzed the emotional components of gestures (see Chapter 11). Linderberg also studied with Elsa Gindler, the founder of Gymnastiks and the teacher of Charlotte Selver (also see Chapter 11). Although it is difficult to know how much influence Linderberg had on Reich, after their relationship ended, Reich's work became focused solely on the flow of energy through the body and the psychological fixations that block this flow.

When Reich refused to terminate his political activities, he was expelled from the German Psychoanalytic Association. (Keep in mind that this was also the time when Margaret Sanger was imprisoned for advocating contraception in the United States.) After a series of professional and personal conflicts, Reich left Europe in 1939 for the New School of Social Research in New York. There he eventually founded the Orgone Institute and continued his research both on sexuality and the flow of biological energy.

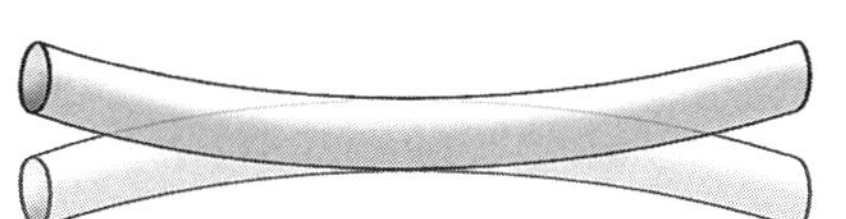

Figure 15.1 Schematic of alternating flexion and extension in what Reich called the orgasm reflex

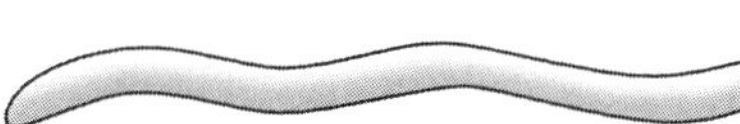

Figure 15.2 Schematic of the wavy, plasmatic movement that runs along the spine

Reich was the first psychoanalyst who recognized that in order for deep change to occur, people must link their mental, emotional, and physical processes. Unlike Freud, Reich sat patients where he could see them and have direct contact with them. This enabled him to observe **muscular armor**, a concept he developed to describe the chronic muscular patterns of tension. According to Reich, muscular armor blocks the flow of energy from the core of the body to the periphery, thereby repressing unmanageable and uncomfortable emotions, particularly those that cause anxiety. It creates a protective muscular rigidity, a psychological defense mechanism Reich called **character structure**. Reich's goal with psychoanalysis was to help patients surrender to involuntary movements and spontaneous impulses, thereby releasing the muscular armor that maintains character structure and restoring a normal flow of energy in the body.

Inspired by Freud, Reich searched for the biological basis of energy underlying Freud's concept of *libido,* which Reich called *"orgone energy."* He based his theories about the flow of biological energy on the idea of polarities of pleasure and anxiety. In his terms, *pleasure* is the natural expansion of an organism toward the periphery of the body and into the world, while *anxiety* is the retraction of an organism away from the world toward the center of the body. Armor forms around anxiety. As Reich stated, "In the armored human organism, the orgone energy is bound up in the chronic muscular spasms . . . [When armor releases,] the organism [often] reacts to these first streamings [of the release of orgone energy in wave-like pulsations] . . . with renewed armoring . . . [which] clearly shows the struggle going on between streaming impulse and armor block."[277]

To release muscular armor, Reich integrated psychoanalysis, deep-breathing exercises, and deep-tissue massage. His goal was to induce what he called the *orgasm reflex*, which is not a sexual orgasm, but a pulsation or streaming of energy and movement along the longitudinal axis of the body, reflected in strong pulsating cycles of spinal flexion and extension (Figure 15.1). The release of these "plasmatic streamings" and "emotional excitations," and the restoration of the orgasm reflex were essential parts of Reichian therapy: "When a plasmatic current cannot run along the body because the transverse blocks make it impossible, a transverse movement develops which secondarily means *no*. . . . It is not by accident that *no* is expressed by sidewise movement of the head and *yes* by nodding [along the longitudinal axis] (Figure 15.2)."[278]

Bands of Armor

According to Reich, bands of muscular armor develop in horizontal rings around the trunk in relation to the issues and energies they repress. The following list outlines Reich's seven segments, or bands, of chronically fixed muscles, their corresponding attitudes, and his suggested remedies to loosen or free them (Figure 15.3):

1. The *ocular segment* around the eyes relates to issues about the metaphorical inability to see. Rolling the eyes and encouraging free movement of the eyes in the head can help dissolve ocular armor.
2. The *oral segment* around the mouth and throat corresponds to issues about nourishment and verbal expression. Sucking, biting, moving the lips, and making sounds can help dissolve oral armor.
3. The *neck segment* around the deep muscles of the neck and the tongue carries issues of repressed verbal expression and the "swallowing of emotion." Screaming, yelling, and gagging can help dissolve neck armor.
4. The *chest segment* around the heart, lungs, chest, and arms holds issues of longing or desire, and holds back emotions

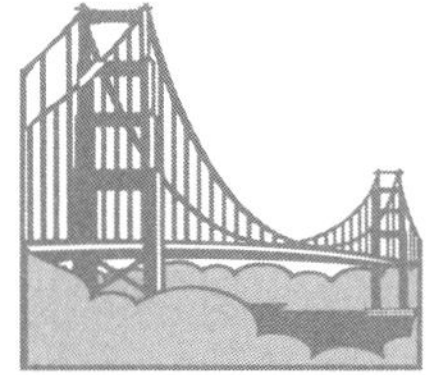

Allowing Emotions to Sequence

If your client has an emotional release during a patterning or bodywork session, remind the client that he has a choice—either to tighten his body to guard against feeling emotions or to open the body to allow the emotions to sequence and release. Allowing emotional responses to sequence might be more difficult than it sounds for someone who habitually blocks them, but with practice and a clear intention, most people quickly learn that they do have a choice. If the issues that trigger your client's emotional responses tend to surface again and again, suggest your client see a psychotherapist.

of anger, sadness, and grief. Deep breathing, plus expressive movements in the arms such as hitting, punching, and reaching out can help to dissolve chest armor.

5. The *diaphragmatic segment* around the solar plexus and diaphragm tends to show up in a pattern of excessive lordosis, a forward sway of the lumbar spine. Because people hold their breath to stifle overwhelming emotions, particularly anxiety and rage, releasing diaphragmatic armor can be difficult. Deep breathing, eliciting the gag reflex, and, in extreme cases, vomiting can help dissolve armor in this area.
6. The *abdominal segment* manifests as a contraction in the middle of the abdomen and relates to issues of fear and digestion. Abdominal armor is easier to release than all other segments and can be dissolved through belly breathing and abdominal massage.
7. The *pelvic segment* consists of all the muscles around the pelvis, the reproductive organs, bladder, and adductor muscles of the inner thighs. It holds issues of rage, sexuality, the inhibition of pleasure, and being out of touch with reality, or "ungrounded." Pelvic armor can be dissolved by mobilizing the pelvis and legs in expressive actions, such as kicking.

Releasing Character Fixations

Reich not only elaborated on Freud's concept of character, but he was the first psychoanalyst to actually help patients release the physical restrictions created by muscular armor. Reich observed his patients' posture, breathing, and movement habits, moving from an objective intellectual analysis to actually working with the body patterns that corresponded to psychological issues. He mapped out character structure by noting the physical areas of the body that tighten and armor during various stages of psychological development. For instance, if the child undergoes emotional injury during the oral stage of development, when mouthing and rooting patterns are prominent, the character fixation centers on issues of nourishment, resulting in muscular armor around the mouth. If the child undergoes emotional injury during the genital stage of development, the character fixation centers on issues of sexuality, resulting in muscular armor around the pelvis.

From his years of research and practice, Reich concluded that physical armor and psychological armor were two manifestations of the same pattern. Reich helped his patients become aware of character fixations by asking them to go deeper into their patterns, to further tighten their chronically contracted muscles. He also used touch. He was one of the first psychotherapists who actually touched his patients, applying deep pressure on areas like the jaw or lower back to release muscular armor, which often evoked cathartic screaming and streaming of repressed energy. He considered his patients free of their character fixations when they could enjoy the full orgasm reflex and the natural flow of orgone energy throughout the body.

Even though a conservative society and its psychoanalysts disdained him, Reich continued to promote his theories. In the 1950s, he developed large boxes called "orgone energy accumulators." His patients would sit inside these specially equipped boxes to expose themselves to concentrated orgone. In 1954, the U.S. Food and Drug Administration (FDA) obtained an injunction to prohibit him from selling orgone accumulators. Reich violated the injunction with continued research and sales, and in 1956 was found in contempt of court and sentenced to prison. In 1957, he died of heart disease while still in prison. Many felt that Reich was a man ahead of his time and that he actually died of a broken heart. Since his death, there has been no known research about his theory of orgone energy.

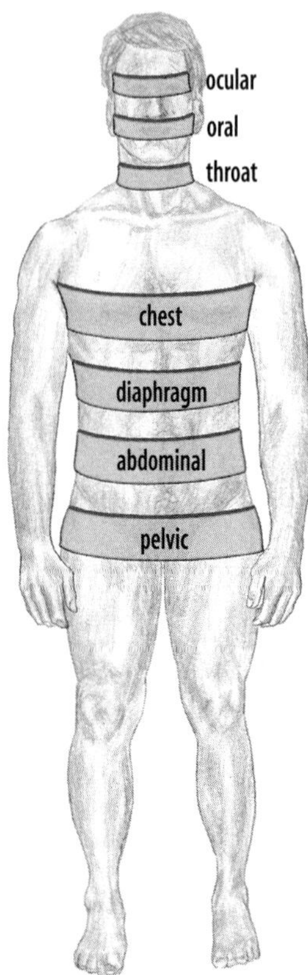

Figure 15.3 A schematic of Reichian bands of armor

Touch and Psychotherapy

As mentioned earlier, Reich initiated the use of touch in psychotherapy. His pointed touch has been described as being free of emotion, almost medical. Malcolm Brown, a student of Lowen's and the founder of *organismic psychotherapy*, also incorporated touch into psychotherapy with the help of his wife, Katherine Brown, a massage therapist. Together they practiced long periods of gentle, supportive touch that enabled clients to release emerging feelings. The Browns found that touch could never be neutral because it reflected not only the client's issues and patterns, but also those of the therapist, and the relationship between the two. Subsequently, the use of touch in psychotherapy opened the door to many possibilities, although it is still considered controversial by most traditional schools because of the ethical issues it raises.

Neo-Reichian massage is based on Reichian theories of how energy flows within a healthy individual. The main goal of this method is to help massage clients during a massage session release trapped energy, both emotional and physical, from the core of the body out the limbs. Neo-Reichian techniques consist primarily of long strokes that gently move and milk trapped energy away from the center of the trunk, down and out the arms and legs, and of connecting strokes shaped as figure eights that integrate one part of the body with another. Because this form of massage often triggers emotional releases, practitioners of the form learn how to support their clients in releasing pent-up emotions.

BIOENERGETICS

Alexander Lowen and John Pierrakos, both students of Reich's, felt that Reich was overly focused on the role of repressed sexual energy as the underlying component of blocked energy in the body, particularly along the spine. They felt that any emotion that creates anxiety in a person, not just sexual excitement, tends to be suppressed by chronic muscular tension that inhibits the flow of spontaneous movement. Together they evolved the Reichian approach by expanding it to address all blocked emotions rather than just repressed sexuality. They also added the circulation of energy in the limbs and developed the concept of grounding, one of their primary contributions to body-based psychotherapy.

Grounding is a simple process in which a person centers himself and gets in touch with reality by making a physical and energetic connection down the body through the feet and into the ground (Figure 15.4). To induce grounding, they would have their clients stand in stressful positions, such as arching the back, which made it possible to circulate energy between the body and the ground via the pelvis and legs. (Malcolm Brown later introduced the concept of "horizontal grounding," in which the client grounds energy through the supporting surface of the body while lying down.)

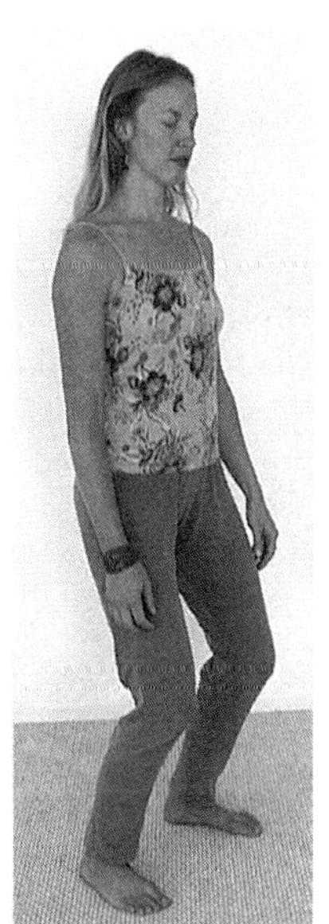
Figure 15.4 A grounding exercise: sensing weight in the feet

Lowen and Pierrakos generalized Reichian theories into a form of therapy call **bioenergetics**. In 1956, they began the Institute for Bioenergetic Analysis, where they taught other therapists principles of psychotherapy based on the language of the body.[279] Like Reichian therapy, bioenergetics is designed to help people release body fixations through psychoanalysis coupled with breathing exercises, grounding exercises, and self-expression through movement.

Lowen and Pierrakos elaborated on Reich's concept of character structure, particularly exploring how energy circulated in each character type. They were concerned with the source of a person's energy and with a person's ability to go through complete cycles of energetic charge and discharge in the body. **Charge** refers to the buildup of energy in the body, **discharge** to the release of energy. Certain character types become fixated on building energy without releasing it, thereby swelling the body and blocking the normal cycles of give and take inherent in healthy relationships. Conversely, other character types become fixated on the discharge of energy within a relationship, continually depleting their supplies without replenishing them, ultimately collapsing the body.

Character Types

The five basic **character types** described by Reich and further developed in bioenergetics are the *schizoid, oral, psychopathic, masochistic*, and *rigid*. (Note that the schizoid and psychopathic are in this case personality traits and *not* mental illnesses, such as schizophrenia and psychopathy.) The schizoid is the earliest of the character types to form so that a person with schizoid tendencies usually has psychological injuries that occurred early in life, probably during infancy. Other character types form during subsequent stages of the developmental process, and each type has energetic, physical, and psychological patterns:

1. *Schizoid:* Energy is withheld from the periphery of the body and gets frozen in the core. The schizoid-type body is thin and contracted, the face masklike, and the personality paranoid. Many describe the schizoid body as a group of spare parts that have been pieced together. Because of the amount of internal compression needed by the schizoid to contain the energetic charge, the schizoid type often experiences a sensation that the body could explode. Also, thinking is split from feeling. A weak ego boundary (sense of self) corresponds to a lack of energy in the periphery of the body. The schizoid energy pattern forms during early neglect or rejection of an infant by its caregivers.

   The challenge of a person with schizoid issues is to gain an ability to yield and bond, especially through touch, and in cases involving an overactive neocortex, to relax and reduce the exaggerated sense of vigilance.

2. *Oral:* Energy flows out of the periphery of the body, weakening the structure. The oral body type is often linear and collapsed with long spindly limbs, locked knees, a tendency toward shallow breathing, and an emphasis on reaching and longing through the throat and mouth. The oral body compresses the organs, making this type appear malnourished. The oral personality has a tendency to cling to others for support and nourishment. This character type also experiences feelings of emptiness, probably from early deprivation and lack of emotional nourishment.

   The challenge of a person with oral issues is to take in psychological nourishment, integrating a sequence of movements in mouthing patterns that brings fullness to the organs.

3. *Psychopathic:* In an effort to rise above others, this character type pulls the body up, inflating the upper body and blocking the energy flow through the spine, pelvis, and legs. Inflated and overcharged in the chest and head, the psychopathic type has a split between the upper and lower body. The psychopath has a tendency to constrict the diaphragm, which squeezes the body in the middle, so that the upper half appears larger than the lower half. This type can also be seductive with a snake-like body, a hyperflexible back, and an overcharged pelvis. Personality characteristics include a distrust of others, a need to control, and a denial of needs, all of which develop from a relationship with a seductive and/or competitive caregiver.

   A primary challenge of a person with psychopathic issues is to gain a sense of power and control from self-mastery rather than mastery over others. Push patterns, particularly the spinal push, can aid in developing an internal sense of core support and in integrating an upper/lower body split.

4. *Masochistic:* Although fully charged energetically, the masochistic type holds the charge in, compressing and collapsing the body, digging the heels in, and tucking the tail under, which makes the thighs and hips appear unusually heavy and thick. Impulses to act are choked off by chronic muscular tension at the neck and waist, creating internal anxiety. Attitudes of submission and of wanting to please others cover a deeper attitude of spite and hostility. The masochistic personality forms when caregivers are loving yet put a lot of pressure on the child, such as in forced toilet training. The child feels stuck in the middle, simultaneously loving and hating the parents, and learns to stubbornly bear down.

   The challenge of a person with masochistic issues is to allow pleasurable impulses to flow through the body and spine. This may involve movements that lengthen the spine, such as undulations or reach patterns.

5. *Rigid:* The rigid type tends to hold a strong energetic charge back in the periphery of the body, especially in the head and tail, actually bowing the back into a rigid posture. The posture of this character type may look balanced and integrated, but is actually rigid and lacking in fluidity, coordination, and vitality. The rigid body type has chronic spasms in both the flexor and extensor muscles of the spine. Personality characteristics include a fear of submission or collapse. Rigid character types are often overachievers with a high degree of control over their behavior. They are also ambitious and competitive. The classic rigid posture is seen in the military posture.

   The challenge of a person with rigid character issues is to let go of ideas or beliefs about how a person "should" move and simply explore movement without an agenda.

How can you experience a cathartic release without being hurt in the process or spinning into an overly stressful fight-or-flight response?

Examining Myths

Myth: Venting negative emotions by kicking and screaming is therapeutic.

Perhaps these actions can be therapeutic under certain circumstances, but not necessarily. We all appreciate it when an overly angry person can keep the rage under control, lest there be a violent explosion. The notion of venting anger by screaming, kicking, and punching was once popular in some expressive psychotherapies, but many people actually damaged their vocal cords in primal screams and pulled muscles beating pillows. Although it is certainly not healthy to suppress negative feelings, venting negative emotions with loud, expressive words and movements can damage tissues and create more stress. Therefore, if a person needs to vent negative or volatile emotions, it should be done with some kind of protective containment.

Lowen reminds us that therapists do not treat character types; they treat people. He encourages psychotherapists to always keep the character structure in the background and place the client in the foreground.[280] Also, it should be noted that there are diverse opinions about character types: some therapists believe that they are fixed, others believe that they can change over time, and still others believe that parts of various character types are pieced together to make up unique personalities.

Critics of both Reichian and bioenergetic therapies feel that the techniques are overly dramatic and cathartic, with too narrow a focus on moving pent-up emotions through and out of the body. For example, the "ventilationist" technique, in which the client kicks and hits and screams, can actually increase hostile and aggressive tendencies and risks becoming a reenactment of physically and emotionally injurious events (Figure 15.5). Since Reich's time, many body-based psychotherapists have taken a gentler approach. Ron Kurtz, who created a gentle style of the body-centered therapy called Hakomi in the early 1980s, felt the character types developed out of intelligent strategies

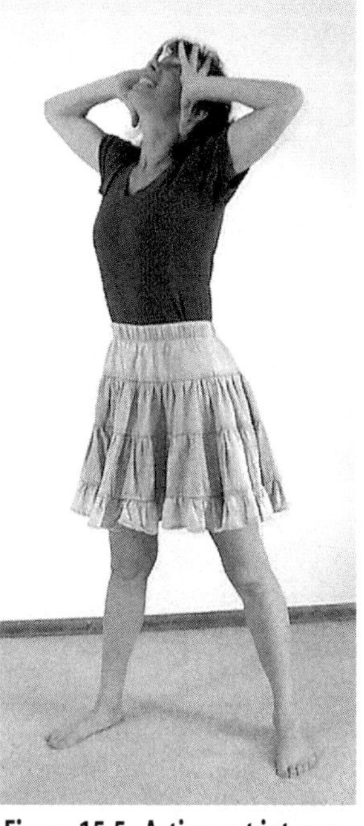
Figure 15.5 Acting out intense negative emotions can be self-damaging.

to survive deep emotional angst. He created new names for the types to more accurately reflect their behavioral strategies rather than their negative fixations: the schizoid is "sensitive-withdrawn," the oral "dependent-endearing," the psychopath either "tough-generous" or "charming-manipulative," the masochist "burdened-enduring," and the rigid "industrious-over-focused."[281]

Energetic Studies

Up until now, we have been discussing how we *have* psychological processes. Stanley Keleman's work seems to shift this paradigm and suggest that we continually *form and reform* ourselves through ongoing waves of body experience. Keleman, a psychologist who trained in several disciplines before he studied with Lowen, went on to develop a unique and dynamic perspective on how energetic processes occur. His **formative principle** is based on the notion that our bodies are constantly shaping and reshaping, a process that constitutes our psychology.

> To form is to grow. A crystal expands itself in an additive way; a tree, in a geometric extendedness. We humans grow by increasing our motility and coordination and by inventing new behavior, new shapes and feelings and responses. The intricate connectedness of developing shape and responsiveness that we usually call growing, I call forming.[282]

In short, we are in flux. We live our lives in a **formative process**, a continual reforming of shape and energetic flow around feelings and actions. This process occurs within the complex and interconnected series of sacs, tubes, and pumps that make up the fabric of every cell, organ, and tissue within our bodies.[283] Keleman brings his theory to life in detailed descriptions of how he hypothesizes the formative process sequences. The following excerpt is from *Your Body Speaks Its Mind*:

> I have a film that very clearly shows how protoplasm is capable of forming structure from itself. The protoplasm is pulsating, streaming. One layer of the streamings thickens and creates a membrane which acts as a channel for the main flow, giving it more form. This containing creates an individuation of velocity and rhythm. The different rate of excitement and the asymmetry of vibrating and resonating qualities result in a body. The protoplasm has been bodied.[284]

The Formative Process

According to Keleman, the formative process has three phases: expansion, containment, and expression.[285] In the *expansion phase,* energy and excitement from experiences build, expanding the body and charging the tissues with a vibratory aliveness. If the expansion continues without bounds, the energy dissipates.

Balance occurs with the next phase, the *containment phase*, in which the charge of emotional excitement is contained, driving the pulsation deeper into the tissues, allowing a person to collect herself, incubating and digesting her experience. During containment, boundaries begin to form. The internal expansion of feeling actually creates pressure on the walls of the body, fortifying and strengthening containment. Boundaries then become not just the psychological ability to distinguish between self and other, but an actual pressure, a physical strengthening and bounding of the tissues in the body. The development of boundaries leads to an increase in proprioception, which in turn builds body awareness and a greater sense of self.

The *expression phase* begins as excitement is expressed and charge dissipates. During this phase, we interact with the world and with other people, sharing the energetic fullness that has accumulated during the containment phase. With expression, the formative process has completed a full cycle, which naturally leads us to the beginning of the next cycle.

In Keleman's view, every life situation generates either the whole cycle or some part of it, creating new feelings and relationships that continually sequence through formative processes. These cycles can occur in situations as short as five minutes or as long as several months. Discord occurs when the natural cycles are incomplete, frozen, or amplified. Keleman explains how insults and injuries that occur in our lives create fixations in the formative process.[286] This causes an inhibition or distortion of continual formation, and the self becomes frozen in a personality role.

Keleman describes how fixations during the formative process create four psychophysical structures: *rigid, dense, swollen*, and *collapsed*.[287] When a person becomes *stuck in the containment phase*, the personality fixates around gathering and building energy, and the tissues swell. When a person becomes *stuck in*

Links to Practical Applications

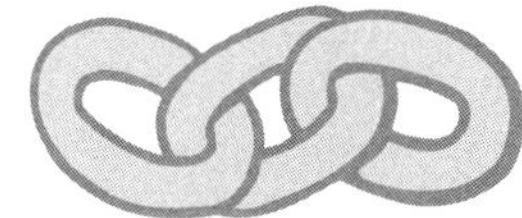

Breathing during Emotional Processes

Many people tighten the body and hold their breath when they have uncomfortable feelings or intense emotions. Whatever manner you breathe in during an emotional process patterns a relationship between your feelings and your respiration. Therefore, it's a good idea to practice deep, slow, and easy breathing during strong emotional states, particularly when you feel overwhelmed.

Also, whenever you go through emotional processing, your body needs more oxygen. At these times, breathe gently, taking in oxygen to circulate or "ventilate" your feelings. Inhale into your mouth to take in oxygen through a larger orifice. To avoid hyperventilation, breathe slowly. To relax, take slow, easy exhalations, pausing at the end of each breath.

the expression phase, the formative charge never gets a chance to adequately build; physical energy as well as psychic energy becomes depleted, and the body collapses. When a person becomes *fixated in time*, he or she inhibits the natural rhythms of the emotional process and becomes rigid, never changing body shapes or feelings. Finally, when a person's *impulses are crushed or betrayed* his or her tissue become compressed and dense.

Keleman believes that many tissue types can layer within one body based on the person's experience, creating many different combinations. For example, a person can be swollen in the periphery of the body while being dense at the core, or can be externally collapsed around a rigid core. Therefore, working with the formative process requires addressing patterns as they arise within tissue qualities and energetic layers. People with collapsed or swollen structures need a psychophysical restructuring and reorganization, while people with rigid and dense structures need to deconstruct and disorganize psychophysical fixations. In other words, the former need to build a new structure while the latter need to break down their fixed structure.

The Accordion Practice and Embodying Process

Keleman suggests that many emotional problems occur because we do not know how to organize or disorganize emotional patterns in our bodies around our psychological experiences. The function of an *organizing process* is to maintain pulsatory rhythm in response to whatever form is building and unfolding in a person's body. The function of a *disorganizing process* is to disassemble somatic patterns that lead to fixation.[288]

To embody process is to allow the energetic flow of a psychological process to move and evolve within the tissues. Keleman created a system for embodying experience in order to reestablish the pulsatory flow or continuum that occurs during the formative process. Since the formative process is ongoing and affects the psychology of our daily lives, Keleman's process of embodying experience provides us with practical self-help tools for self-management. He uses the analogy of the accordion (to be explained shortly) to demonstrate the organizing principle in action during the formative cycle. The natural pumping actions of our bodies support or inhibit pulsating cycles, tightening and expanding, shortening and lengthening the cycles. As Keleman explains, "The changing shape of cells creates pressure: that increasing and decreasing pressure is central to the somatic process."[289]

To help people reestablish formative cycles, Keleman encourages them to alternately organize and disorganize their somatic-muscular holding patterns with the accordion process. This process builds pressure through alternating compression and decompression; compression brings tissue surfaces together, connecting and integrating parts, while decompression dissolves patterns and rigid forms.

At the Center for Energetic Studies, which Keleman founded in 1976, he offers somatic education programs that enable people to embody their experiences and live more fully in their bodies. His describes the process of disassembling outdated behaviors and reorganizing them into new ones in *Embodying Experience: Forming a Personal Life*. In the first step in his five-step process, a person asks himself, "What is my image of myself in my present situation?" The answer arises while waiting and developing an experience of the present moment both by listening to inner dialogue and feeling the current body shape. In the second step, a person asks, "How do I muscularly create this image and perpetuate it?" Awareness of this psychosomatic state is illuminated by compressing into the physical pattern similar to how one would push in on an accordion. Then a person explores a way to end the pattern and disorganize the muscular shape by coming out of the pattern, or "pulling the accordion open." This leads to the fourth step of the embodiment process, that of dealing with what happens once the limiting pattern has been taken apart. This step involves taking a long pause to begin an incubation state and wait for a new form to organically occur. The process culminates by using what has been learned to reorganize a new form that more truly expresses a deeper aspect of one's current self.[290]

Some questions that Keleman has people ask themselves to illuminate the formative process are: How am I doing such and such? How is an event taken in, circulated, and responded to? How do I shape my response? Is my conflict internal or external? What roles or characters have I taken on? Have they rigidified? Are they fluid? [291] Keleman's process-oriented work encourages psychological processes to fully sequence in the body, on a moment-to-moment basis, by directing the ongoing flow of biological processes that enliven the tissues and continually reshape the mutable form of an embodied life.

DANCE MOVEMENT THERAPY

> It was an important day when I discovered that I do not teach Dance, I teach People.
>
> — Mary Whitehouse

A dynamic form of body-based psychotherapy, **dance movement therapy**, was developed in the 1940s by two pioneering psychotherapists who also happened to be dancers. They both began using expressive movement in their work with psychiatric patients and private clients. Marion Chace, in Washington, D.C., and Mary Whitehouse, in San Francisco, both experimented with ways to help the client move through psychological processes while engaging in improvisational and expressive dance movement.

Marion Chace observed how mental patients communicated predominantly through movement, generally avoiding movements that brought them into more contact with people and the world. She assumed that their movement fixations reflected areas within them where growth was inhibited due to trauma and injury. Chace would connect with her patients on an energetic level, then interact with them and follow these interactions into a transformational movement experience.

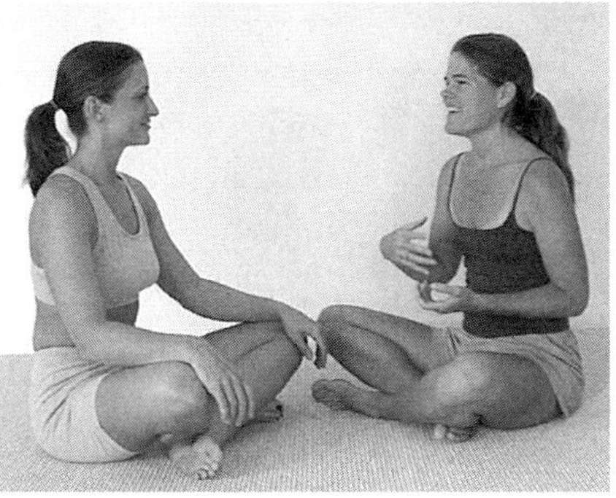

Figure 15.6 Being seen, heard, and acknowledged by another person is an important part of the therapeutic process.

Mary Whitehouse, both a dancer and a Jungian analyst, developed an approach to movement therapy called **authentic movement**. Authentic movement is a form of experiential psychotherapy usually done within a group process. In this form, a therapist observes a group of people while they explore improvisational movement. To begin, all participants sit, stand, or lie with their eyes closed and begin to sense their inner body-mind processes, allowing these processes to sequence through a spontaneous, expressive movement exploration. The movement exploration has several functions. It allows participants to explore psychological processes as they move through the body in the same manner that a verbal free-association helps participants explore psychological processes as they pass through the mind. Participants also use movement as a vehicle for working out psychological issues.

In Whitehouse's approach, the therapist serves as a **witness**, passively observing the members of the group as they move with their eyes closed. The role of the witness is to observe the individual processes of members of the group while holding the "container," the boundaries of the therapeutic process within which healing can occur. The witness has a healing presence in the role of a loving observer, like a parent, who observes the painful emotional processes until the client is able to develop his or her own inner witness (Figure 15.6).

Witnessing is a fundamental skill used by dance therapists to cultivate a therapeutic presence. The witness stays attentive to what is occurring in the client's process as it expresses through the body, without interfering or superimposing anything that would interrupt the client's organic process. Witnessing skills develop as a therapist learns to oscillate her attention between self and other, whether the therapist is working with an individual or with a group. This oscillating, roving awareness allows the witness to continually scan her own sensations, thoughts, feelings, and spontaneous movements in order to stay grounded within herself during the therapeutic process while still tending to the client or group process.

Authentic movement is practiced in groups and in private sessions. The improvisational movement of the authentic mover serves as a personal expression of the unconscious mind. The movement becomes authentic when the participants allow the unconscious to move them rather than consciously initiating movement. Dance therapist Joan Chodorow describes this in her book *Dance Therapy and Depth Psychology*: "Perhaps Mary's [Whitehouse] greatest contribution . . . was her ability to differentiate between the experience of *letting it happen* in contrast to *doing it*. . . . Mary helped her students understand the difference between movement that is directed by the ego and movement that comes from the unconscious. She emphasized the ability to develop *both* ways."[292]

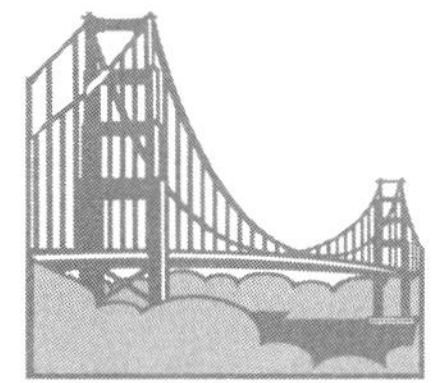

Bridge to Practice

Witnessing and Reflecting Your Clients

Many people are not used to tracking changes in their bodies and view their physical selves as stationary, solid objects. By tracking posture and movement in the body, a client can learn to monitor change (movement is change from moment to moment).

To help your client learn how to track body responses, call attention to changes the client has made in her posture, breathing, and movement over the course of several sessions. Compare objective data that you recorded on your intake form in the first session—information about posture and movement, self-image and awareness—to her body state now. Point out changes that you see on a periodic basis. Use comparisons such as: "When you first came in, you were complaining of low back pain and a swayback. Now your lower back looks more relaxed and straighter, and you no longer mention the pain."

Make sure your feedback is objective, the type that two people could easily see, hear, and agree upon. Better yet, take photographs or videotapes of your client in the first session and compare these to current pictures of your client. Objective data will disarm any skeptic. Help your client periodically reflect on the changes that she has made so that she learns to witness her own growth and to make changes on her own.

PRENATAL AND PARANATAL PSYCHOLOGY

Another form of body-based psychotherapy, **prenatal and paranatal psychology**, delves into the most primitive experiences thought to shape the psyche of an individual. This recent branch of somatic psychology has grown out of the belief that the experience a person has in the womb, during birth, and immediately after birth assembles a template for all psychosomatic patterns (Figure 15.7). According to this theory, the psychosomatic patterns that develop as a result of early traumas, particularly birth

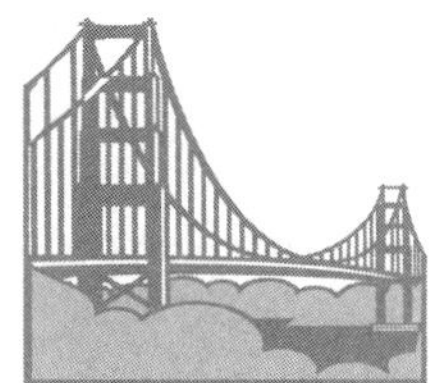

Helping Self-Critical Clients

Many clients are critical of themselves, especially their bodies. They feel that they are too fat or too thin, too tall or too short, too dark or too light. Sound familiar? This self-critical behavior is prevalent in a narcissistic culture that bombards us with advertising images of beautiful and slim actors and actresses with "perfect" bodies. Most people know what they want to get rid of rather than what they want to build or gain. If your client is self-critical, point this out. Defend your client against her inner "critic" until she learns to stop picking on herself. Gradually your client will learn, with your help, to see the parts of her body that she likes, and she'll *build* upon these rather than trying to get *rid* of some aspect she does not like.

traumas, are carried in a person's cellular memory, and these patterns repeat themselves until they are resolved. For instance, a person whose birth was interrupted by anesthesia might get foggy every time unconscious issues start to surface, or recapitulate her interrupted birth sequence by not being able to carry tasks through to completion. The theory holds that when prenatal and paranatal patterns surface in psychotherapy, they provide an opportunity for working out deep psychosomatic issues.

Otto Rank was one of the first psychoanalysts to work from the premise that birth trauma was the source of neurosis, writing one of the first books on the subject in 1993.[293] According to Rank, prenatal and paranatal trauma occurs when the organic, spontaneous rhythms of the fetus and newborn are interrupted and disturbed by an outside influence. For example, the toxins of a drug-addicted mother, the chaotic environment of a screaming and angry set of parents, or the forceful grip of forceps compressing and twisting the newborn's skull all interrupt the normal prenatal development and birth. Rank believes the preborn literally marinates in the mother's drug ingestion or loud, angry affect, and by birth, has an addictive or raging predisposition.

Psychologists in this relatively new field suggest there is mounting anecdotal evidence that prenatal and paranatal experiences may stamp us with behavioral imprints that we carry with us through our entire lives.[294] Dance therapist and teacher Christine Caldwell discusses how the toxic environments that many people endure during prenatal development create patterns of ingesting toxic substances, either physical substances such as drugs and alcohol, or toxic emotions such as rage, hate, and depression.[295] Caldwell believes that an early intake of toxicity gets confused with the intake of nourishment, setting up the template for addictive behaviors to develop later in life.

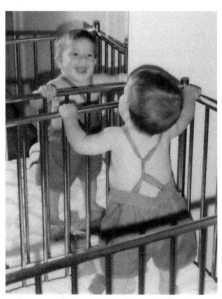

Figure 15.7 At what age do we really see who we truly are? (Photo courtesy of L. Bright.)

FRITZ PERLS AND GESTALT THERAPY

The Gestalt Prayer

I do my thing, and you do your thing.
I am not in this world to live up to your expectations,
and you are not in this world to live up to mine.
You are you and I am I,
And if by chance we find each other, it's beautiful.
If not, it can't be helped.

—Fritz Perls

This prayer, first popularized in the personal growth movement of the 1960s, is a guiding maxim written by Fritz Perls (1894–1970), the founder of **Gestalt therapy**. Perls was a strong, outspoken man who captured the hearts and minds of many people fascinated with his bold, honest, and effective approach to human development.

In his psychotherapeutic work, Perls incorporated Charlotte Selver's practice of Sensory Awareness (see Chapter 11), making him the first to integrate the client's body awareness into psychotherapy. By sensing the body, a person in Gestalt therapy learns to stay with an awareness of the present moment (since the body only exists in present time) rather than ruminating on the past or worrying about the future. In Perls's worldview, anxiety is the gap between the past and the present, and it creates "holes" in a person's personality. His therapy is based on the existential truth that all we have is our present-moment experience, and that living in the past or in artificial social roles punches holes in our **gestalt**—the totality of our experience.[296] A gestalt is a pattern so integrated as a functional unit that it has properties that far exceed the sum of its parts.

Perls wrote: "Once you have character, you have a rigid system. Your behavior becomes petrified, predictable, and you lose the ability to cope freely with the world and with all your resources. You are predetermined to cope in just one way, namely, as your character prescribes it."[297] In Gestalt therapy, the "end-gain," or outcome, is differentiated from the "means-whereby," or process of living. The client learns to make choices about the means whereby he or she lives in the present moment, to release the controlling nature of an end-gain, or goal orientation, and develop a realistic perspective and sensitivity to his or her own life situation.

During sessions, Perls would often completely ignore what his clients were saying, focusing instead on their gestures, postures, intonation, and repetitive habits. Then Perls would reflect back to them an accurate picture of what they were doing in the present moment, pointing out their body language or nuances in the tone of their voice, their breathing patterns or posture. Perls would continue his reflection of behavior until a gestalt surfaced, and the client could reunite with the totality of his or her experience. According to Perls, "This type of organismic self-regulation is very important in therapy because the emergent, unfinished situations will come to the surface. We don't have to dig in. It's all there . . . the organism knows all and we know little."[298]

The aim of Gestalt therapy is to help the client discover that she can do many things, usually many more than she thinks she can. Perls was so adamant about allowing the sessions to unfold from within the client's experience that there were times when he actually told the client to wake him if something happened, then proceeded to doze off. Perls would also intentionally frustrate his clients to the point where they would quit depending on an outside person for support and figure out how to support themselves.

Perls felt that any intention toward change actually achieves the opposite and becomes just another attempt to control or be controlled. This dual theme of the controller and the controlled is a fundamental aspect of the Gestalt view, where the "topdog" and the "underdog" battle for supremacy within a person. Perls believed that the only element that controls anything is the situation. The well-adjusted person chooses his behavior according to the present moment situation, remaining conscious of the center of his world, recognizing the two poles of every event, and not being limited by the conflicting personality roles of the topdog and underdog. Perls often had a client playact a conversation between roles until a negotiation between parts began to resolve conflict and the polarities merged into one whole.

In terms of body awareness, Perls tracked clients' movement and gestures that accompanied conflicting issues, first as a way to reflect to them what they were doing in the present moment, and also to help them connect these gestures and integrate them into a gestalt. An NLP technique that arose out of Gestalt therapy involves symbolically placing the images of conflicting polarities in each hand, then bringing the hands together to merge the polarities back into a unified whole along the midline of the body.

Gestalt therapy was one of the first psychotherapies to focus totally on what was happening in the present moment experience. As mentioned earlier, it was also the first work to truly integrate body awareness into psychotherapy. The effectiveness of Gestalt therapy shows us that cultivating an awareness of all the intersecting aspects of a present-moment experience is, in itself, curative.

FOCUSING

During the 1970s, at about the same time that the NLP founders were conducting similar research, University of Chicago psychologist Eugene Gendlin did extensive research on the question: What makes therapy successful? By watching videotapes of psychotherapy sessions and interviewing clients, Gendlin started to identify the elements of successful therapy. He got to the point where he could spot whether therapy was going to succeed or fail within the first few minutes of watching a session. Through his research, Gendlin made a profound discovery: therapy does not heal people; rather, people heal themselves, and *the outcome of therapy depends only on what people do inside themselves*.

Gendlin went on to identify the internal processes that a psychotherapy client goes through in effective therapy. He found that the client accesses a vague state of body-mind thinking and awareness that Gendlin refers to as "thinking with the body." This level of body-mind awareness, which Gendlin calls a **felt sense**, is like a hunch or "gut feeling," a holistic sensing that is more inclusive than an emotion or a feeling; it is a body awareness of a situation, person, or event. Gendlin describes the body as a "biological computer" that has an innate "sense of what is wrong . . . with [in] it, . . . [and also has] a sense of the direction toward what is right."[299] In short, Gendlin found that the solution to a problem is inherent in the felt sense. Since a felt sense includes physical, emotional, and mental aspects, it has a naturally integrating function that people feel as a deep yet relaxing body and emotional shift from previously conflicting states.

Gendlin began teaching his students how to access the felt sense of a particular psychological issue that each was experiencing, and out of this he developed a therapy called **focusing**. The six steps of focusing are:

1. "Clearing a space for yourself." Staying quiet and listening.
2. Getting a felt sense of the problem. Feeling the whole problem at once, with a soft focus.
3. Finding a "handle," a word or image that accesses the essence of the felt sense. A person knows when the handle accurately fits the felt sense because a deep body shift occurs.
4. Checking the handle against the felt sense, to see if the two resonate. If they resonate, there will be a deep body shift, or change of state, such as relaxing. If they do not resonate, go on to step 5.

5. Asking the felt sense what it is. The premise here is that the body never lies.
6. Receiving and accepting whatever information comes from the body without judging it.[300]

Like many of the concepts presented in this chapter, such as muscular armor or streaming, Gendlin's concept of felt sense has been incorporated into many schools of body-based psychotherapy. Felt sense is also widely used in the field of somatics as a primary tool for deepening a body awareness of a psychological issue. Since the advent of somatic therapies, many people recognize that body patterns, particularly holding patterns maintained by chronic muscular contractions, often have psychological components that perpetuate them. By accessing a felt sense of the holding pattern, people can both access the body patterns that maintain psychological issues, and access the psychological issues that underlie holding patterns and pain.

SUMMARY

Generally, body-based psychotherapies are based on the premise that the body cannot lie and that we can trust in the innate wisdom of the body. All the therapies presented in this chapter work extensively with monitoring the relationships among body sensations, emotions, and thoughts. Therapists observe whether their clients' bodies are advancing or retreating, whether the clients' tissues are expanding or compressing, and where there is movement or fixation in any part of the body, then use this information to guide the clients' processes. Likewise, they teach their clients to gain the same awareness of their own bodies. Body-based psychotherapy clients learn how to use body awareness to track the physical sensations that accompany their psychological processes and to process psychological issues within the ground of body sensation, movements, and energetic patterns. This is similar to biofeedback, only without the precise physiological feedback and with more focus on psychological issues.

A general theme shared by many of the body-based psychotherapies is the reintegration of the body and mind through a balancing of polarities. Many of these therapies work from the premise that a part of the personality can become isolated in a specific character role and exclude everything that it is not. When the personality or the belief system polarizes, the polarity itself ultimately reveals what is missing and what can be brought to consciousness to balance the split. For instance, a person may become rigid in the shoulders and arms in an effort to repress the expression of vulnerability when this very expression would release rigidity and heal the psychic wound. By revealing the counterbalancing forces of any polarity, the two extremes merge, creating new possibilities and moving a person toward integration and wholeness.

In some modalities, the therapist leads the client in tracking body sensations. In a way, techniques that guide a client through a body awareness exploration don't necessarily empower the client, although they can help a person lacking skills in somatic awareness develop them. Some models integrate body-centered awareness with client-initiated processes. Other models allow an organic unfolding of the client's processes, assuming that all psychological material is present in a client's gestures and postures, and will reveal itself to the client at the appropriate time.

Body-based psychotherapists tend to use their own body awareness, sensations, and feelings as therapeutic tools. They model for their clients what it is like to live in their bodies. Also, when therapists track their physical responses during psychotherapy, they model a healthy integration of body and mind, subconsciously teaching clients how to track their own responses.

As a whole, body-based psychotherapies seem to be moving toward more cellular and neurological models of processing and away from Reichian models that focus on muscular holding patterns. The field also seems to be moving toward more client autonomy in which a therapist does less leading of the client through body processes and more allowing of the client's organic processes to naturally unfold and lead the direction of the process. Similarly, many somatic patterning practitioners are recognizing that movement problems usually have a psychological component and are integrating more organic, client-based processes to allow the body level of psychological issues to be addressed and resolved within the somatic patterning process.

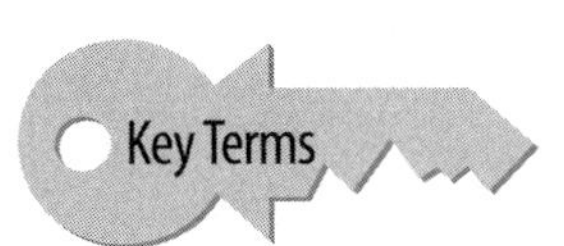

authentic movement
bioenergetics
character structure
character types
charge
dance movement therapy
discharge
felt sense
focusing
formative principle
formative process
gestalt
Gestalt therapy
grounding
muscular armor
prenatal and paranatal psychology
witness

ENDNOTES

Chapter 1

1. The term "somatic" is also used in medical terminology to distinguish autonomic nervous system function from the somatic functions of the muscles and joints, which are controlled by the skeletal nervous system.
2. T. Hanna, *Somatics: Rediscovering the Mind's Control of Movement, Flexibility, and Health* (Reading, Mass.: Addison, Wesley, 1988).
3. Many of these physicians are contributors to *Alternative Therapies in Health and Medicine*. Larry Dossey, the author of the books *Healing Words, Prayer Is Good Medicine,* and *Reinventing Medicine,* is the executive editor of this peer-reviewed journal. For information call 1–800–899–1712, or check out the website at www.alternative-therapies.com.
4. National Center for Complementary and Alternative Medicine Home Page (May 2002): <http://nccam.nih.gov/an/general>.
5. See both W. Jonas and J. Levin, eds., *Essentials of Complimentary Alternative Medicine* (Baltimore: Lippincott, Williams, and Wilkins, 2000) and J. Spencer and J. Jacobs, eds., *Complimentary Alternative Medicine: An Evidence-Based Approach* (St. Louis.: Mosby, 1999).
6. Jonas and Levin, *Essentials*, 582.
7. E. Dacher, *Psychoneuroimmunology: The New Mind/Body Healing Program* (New York: Paragon House, 1991).
8. D. M. Eisenberg et al., "Trends in Alternative Medicine Use in the United States, 1990–1997: Results of a Follow-Up National Survey." *Journal of the American Medical Association* 280, no.18 (1998): 1569–75.
9. From the mission statement of *Alternative Therapies in Health and Medicine* (1998).
10. F. M. Luskin et al., "A Review of Mind-Body Therapies in the Treatment of Cardiovascular Disease," *Alternative Therapies in Health and Medicine* 4, no. 3 (May 1998): 46–61.
11. U.S. Department of Health and Human Services, *Healthy People 2010: Understanding and Improving Health* (Washington, D.C.: Government Printing Office, January 2000).
12. C. Darwin, *The Descent of Man* (1871; reprint, Norfolk, Conn: Easton Press, 1979).
13. In a discussion of the health-threatening condition of escalating childhood obesity in the 3 July 2000 *Newsweek* article titled "Generation XXL," Geoffrey Cowley reports that "fewer than half the nation's schools offer PE [physical education classes]," and "the proportion of high-school kids in daily gym classes fell from 42 percent to 29 percent during the 90's" (44).
14. J. Basmajian and C. DeLuca, *Muscles Alive: Their Functions Revealed by Electromyography*, 5th edition (Baltimore: Williams and Wilkins, 1985).
15. H. Maier, *Theories of Child Development* (New York: Harper & Row, 1969).
16. In *The Case of Nora: Body-Awareness as Healing Therapy,* a volume in the

series Adventures in the Jungle of the Brain (New York: Harper & Row, 1977), the author, Moshe Feldenkrais, stresses how important it is to first address brain functions that occurred earlier in evolution, i.e., movement and touch, in order to rehabilitate higher neurological centers. Feldenkrais assisted Nora, a stroke patient, in relearning reading skills by drawing lines on her body and by moving her fingers under the words (after which she was able to draw lines under sentences which led to gradually relearning how to read).

17. J. Ayres, *Sensory Integration and the Child* (Los Angeles: Western Psychological Services, 1972).
18. B. Cohen, *Sensing, Feeling, and Action* (Northampton, Mass.: Contact Editions, 1993).
19. M. Gazzaniga, *The Mind's Past* (Berkeley: University of California Press, 1998).
20. B. Cohen, "Practitioner Training," class notes, Northampton, Mass., 1992.
21. K. Lorenz, *King Solomon's Ring* (New York: Cromwell, 1952).
22. M. Feldenkrais, *Awareness Through Movement* (New York: Harper & Row, 1972), 10.
23. S. Greenspan, *The Growth of the Mind: The Endangered Origins of Intelligence* (Reading, Mass.: Addison-Wesley, 1997).
24. M. Feldenkrais, *Awareness Through Movement.*
25. M. Feldenkrais, *The Case of Nora.*
26. Neuroscientist John LeDoux states in his text *The Synaptic Self: How Our Brains Become Who We Are* (New York: Viking, 2002) that the freeze response always occurs first, even if only for a millisecond, before the fight or flight responses kick in.
27. E. Jacobson, *The Biology of Emotions* (Springfield, Ill.: Charles C. Thomas, 1967).
28. D. Dusenbery, *Life at a Small Scale: The Behavior of Microbes* (New York: Scientific American Library, 1966).
29. *Taber's Cyclopedic Medical Dictionary*, 17th ed., s.v."startle reflex."
30. P. Levine, "Hakomi Bodywork Training," class notes, Boulder, Colo., 1992.
31. T. Hanna, *Somatics.*
32. C. Sherrington, *The Integrative Action of the Nervous System* (London: Cambridge University Press, 1952).
33. K. Luttgens, H. Deutsch, and N. Hamilton, *Kinesiology: The Scientific Basis of Human Motion,* 8th ed. (Dubuque, Iowa: William C. Brown Communications, 1992).
34. U.S. Department of Health and Human Service, *Healthy People 2010.*

Chapter 2

35. W. Diamong and S. Coniam, *The Management of Chronic Pain* (Oxford: Oxford University Press, 1997).
36. University of Kentucky, "Statistics on Chronic Pain," University of Kentucky Healthcare Website, 1998 (4 June 1998):<http://www.ukhealthcare.uky.edu>.
37. E. Marieb, *Human Anatomy and Physiology,* 4th ed. (Redwood City, Calif.: Benjamin/Cummings, 1989).
38. G. Tortora and S. Grabowski, *Principles of Anatomy and Physiology,* 8th ed. (Menlo Park, Calif.: Addison Wesley Longman Co., 1996).
39. R. Cailliet, *Soft Tissue Pain and Disability,* 3rd ed. (Philadelphia: F. A. Davis, 1996).
40. Mark Comerford states in his course tutor "Movement Dysfunction: Dynamic Stability Rehab of the Local and Global Muscle Systems in Sacro-Iliac Dysfunction" (Harrow, U.K.: Self-published, 2000) that the model of stabilizer and mobilizer muscles was initially classified by Rood and later developed by Janda and S. A. Sahrmann.
41. It is erroneous to call a specific muscle "tonic" or "phasic" because a muscle can work with both tonic function in an isometric, sustained contraction that does not generate movement and with phasic function in a strong, concentric contraction that generates movement.
42. M. Panjabi, *Clinical Biomechanics of the Spine* (Philadelphia: J.B. Lippincott Co, 1990).
43. S. Sahrmann, *Diagnosis and Treatment of Movement Impairment Syndromes* (St. Louis: Mosby, 2002); C. Richardson et al, *Therapeutic Exercises for Spinal Segmental Stabilization: Scientific Basis and Practical Techniques* (London: Churchill Livingstone, 1999).
44. J. Pearce, *Evolution's End: Claiming the Potential of Our Intelligence* (San Francisco: Harper & Row, 1992).
45. E. Wilson and C. Schneider, *Human Activity: A Primer in Psychobiology* (Boulder, Colo.: Self–published, 1988).
46. Ibid.
47. H. A. Kein, author of *Clinical Symposia: Scoliosis* (vol. 30, no. 1, Summit, N. J.: CIBA, 1978) identifies several types of scoliosis, primarily structural scoliosis, which is usually straightened using a combination of braces and corrective exercises, and the more severe idiopathic scoliosis, which is thought to have a genetic cause and is usually treated surgically to fuse the spine.
48. B. Cohen, *Sensing, Feeling, and Action.*
49. J. Pearce, *Evolution's End.*
50. A. Montagu, *Touching: The Human Significance of Skin,* 3rd ed. (New York: Harper & Row, 1986).
51. E. Wilson and C. Schneider, *The Challenge of Chronic Muscle Pain* (Boulder, Colo.: Self-published, 1988).
52. M. Siegfried and D. Simons, *Muscle Pain: Understanding Its Nature, Diagnosis, and Treatment* (Baltimore: Lippincott Williams & Wilkins, 2001).

53. R. Cailliett, *Pain: Mechanisms and Management* (Philadelphia: F. A. Davis, 1993).
54. M. Schacklock, "The Chronic Back: An Evidence-Based Approach to Prevention and Treatment of Persistent Back Pain" class handout, self-published, 2002.
55. J. Travell and D. G. Simons, *Myofascial Pain and Dysfunction: The Trigger Point Manual,* vol. 1 (Baltimore: Williams and Wilkins, 1983).
56. Ibid.
57. T. Melzack and P. Wall, *The Challenge of Pain* (New York: Basic Books, 1982).

Chapter 3

58. Dr. Thomas Milani, a German biomechanical researcher and visiting faculty member at the University of Colorado at Boulder, gave this definition during a presentation on proprioceptive neuromuscular facilitation (PNF) in Longmont, Colorado, in March 1999.
59. D. Voss, M. Ionta, and B. Myers, *Proprioceptive Neuromuscular Facilitation: Patterns and Techniques*, 3rd ed. (New York: Harper & Row, 1985).
60. From the mission statement of the journal titled *Alternative Therapies in Health and Medicine*. This peer-reviewed journal "is a forum for the development and sharing of information concerning the practical use of alternative therapies in preventing and treating disease, healing illness, and promoting health. . . . This journal encourages the integration of alternative therapies with conventional medical practices in a way that provides for a rational, individualized, and comprehensive approach to healthcare."
61. *An Outline of Chinese Acupuncture: The Academy of Traditional Chinese Medicine* (Peking: Foreign Language Press, 1975), 33.
62. See U. Laumer et al., "Therapeutic Effects of the Feldenkrais Method of Awareness Through Movement in Patients with Eating Disorders," *Psychotherapy Psychosomatic Medical Psychology Journal* 47, no. 5 (May 1997): 70–80. See also C. Stallibrass, "An Evaluation of the Alexander Technique for the Management of Disability in Parkinson's Disease: A Preliminary Study," *Clinical Rehabilitation* 11, no. 1 (February 1997): 8–12; and R. J. Dennis, "Functional Reach Improvement in Normal Older Women after Alexander Instruction," *Journal of Gerontology and Biological Medical Sciences* 54, no. 1 (January 1999): M8–11.
63. N. Moore, "A Review of Alternative Medicine Courses Taught at U.S. Medical Schools," *Alternative Therapies in Health and Medicine* 4, no. 3 (May 1998): 90–101.
64. M. Wetzel, D. Eisenberg, and T. Kaptchuk, "Courses Involving Complementary and Alternative Medicine at U.S. Medical Schools," *Journal of the American Medical Association* 280, no. 9 (September 1998): 784–87.
65. F. Luskin et al. "A Review of Mind-Body Therapies in the Treatment of Cardiovascular Disease," *Alternative Therapies in Health and Medicine* 4, no. 3 (May 1998): 46–61.
66. It is difficult to decide whether to call the Western movement modalities "practices" or "therapies" because a number of the movement modalities presented in Chapter 9, while therapeutic, are not considered therapy methods. Therefore, I have chosen to interchange the two terms "practices" and "modalities" throughout the book.
67. A number of professional somatic therapists, innovators, and teachers who call themselves the "Somatic Study Group" have been meeting periodically throughout the 1990s to discuss and refine their modalities and determine directions for growth and research. The group consists of representatives from Feldenkrais, Continuum, Aston Patterning, Rolfing, Body-Mind Centering, Sensory Awareness, Lomi, and somatic psychology. It also includes scientific consultants and medical advisers who provide feedback on the direction of somatic research.
68. Psychologist Daniel Stern discusses the core self as the body ego that first develops when an infant is between two and six months old. In his book *The Interpersonal World of the Infant* (New York: Basic Books, 1985), he defines the core self as a "separate, cohesive, bounded, physical unit, having a sense of their own agency, affectivity, and continuity in time" (7).
69. A. Lowen, *Narcissism: Denial of the True Self* (New York: Collier Books, Macmillan Publishing Co., 1985).
70. W. Reich, *Character Analysis,* 3rd ed. (New York: Noonday Press, 1949).
71. Healing Touch, a form of energy work developed by Dolores Krieger, author of *Accepting Your Power to Heal: The Personal Practice of Therapeutic Touch* (Bear and Company, 1993), is widely practiced by nurses and was originally called "Therapeutic Touch." In most Healing Touch sessions, the theory holds that a practitioner channels healing energy by holding the hands over the client's body and manipulating the client's electromagnetic field.
72. C. Andrade and P. Clifford, *Outcome-Based Massage* (Philadelphia: Lippincott Williams and Wilkins, 2001).
73. E. Green et al., "Anomalous Electrostatic Phenomena in Exceptional Subjects," *Subtle Energies* 2, no. 3 (1991): 69–97.
74. E. Green, *The Ozawkie Book of the Dead: Alzheimer's Isn't What You Think It Is* (Los Angeles: Philosophical Research Society, 2001).
75. R. Gerber, *Vibrational Medicine: New Choices for Healing Ourselves* (Sante Fe: Bear and Company, 1996).

76. M. L. Schulz, *Awakening Intuition: Using Your Mind-Body Network for Insight and Healing* (New York: Three Rivers Press, 1998).
77. H. Pagels, *Cosmic Code* (New York: Bantam, 1982).

Chapter 4

78. M. Seligman, *Learned Optimism* (New York: Knopf, 1991).
79. C. Simonton, *Getting Well Again* (Los Angeles: Tarcher, 1978). Also see L. E. Sweigard, *Human Movement Potential: Its Ideokinetic Facilitation* (New York: Harper and Row, 1974).
80. P. A. Levine, *Waking the Tiger: Healing Trauma* (Berkeley, Calif.: North Atlantic Books, 1997).
81. D. Goleman, *Emotional Intelligence* (New York: Bantam, 1995).
82. J. LeDoux, *The Emotional Brain: The Mysterious Underpinnings of Emotional Life* (Simon and Schuster, New York, 1996).
83. E. Greene and B. Goodrich, *The Psychology of the Body* (Baltimore: Lippincott, Williams, and Wilkins, 2004).
84. H. Benson, *The Relaxation Response* (New York: Morrow, 1975).
85. "Track and bump" is a term coined by the author to describe this widely used patterning technique of oscillating one's attention between observing a pattern and doing something actively to change it. The gentle bump by the practitioner nudges the system to change while leaving the system enough room to remain the same if it is not ready for change.

Chapter 5

86. B. Cohen, *The Evolutionary Origins of Movement* (Amherst, Mass.: Self-published, 1990).
87. N. Smith and S. Simon, "The Action of Perceiving," an interview with Bonnie Bainbridge Cohen published in *Contact Quarterly* 12, no. 3 (Fall 1987).
88. Ibid.
89. F. Jones, *The Alexander Technique: Body Awareness in Action* (New York: Schocken Books, 1976).
90. F. Shapiro and M. Forrest, *Eye Movement Desensitization and Reprocessing* (New York: Basic Books, 1997).

Chapter 6

91. J. Barral and P. Mercier, *Visceral Manipulation* (Seattle: Eastland Press, 1989).
92. G. Tortora and S. Grabowski, *Principles of Anatomy.*
93. B. Cohen, *The Evolutionary Origins.*
94. E. Marieb, *Human Anatomy and Physiology* (Redwood, Calif.: Benjamin/Cummings, 1989).
95. Tortora and Grabowski, *Principles of Anatomy.*
96. Ibid.
97. Cohen, *Sensing, Feeling, and Action.*
98. I. Asimov, *On the Human Body and the Human Brain* (New York: Bonanza Books, 1985).
99. American Heart Association, "Heart and Stroke Statistics," American Heart Association Website (28 October 2002): <www.americanheart.org>.
100. J. Armour and J. Ardell, eds., *Neurocardiology* (New York: Oxford University Press, 1984); H. Gardener, *Frames of Mind* (New York: Basic Books, 1985).
101. C. Childre and H. Martin, *The Heartmath Solution* (San Francisco: Harper, 1999).
102. V. Hunt, *Infinite Mind: The Science of Human Vibrations* (Malibu, Calif.: Malibu Publishing, 1995), 13.
103. C. Norkin and P. Levangie, *Joint Structure and Functions: A Comprehensive Analysis*, 2nd ed. (Philadelphia: F. A. Davis, 1992).
104. R. Cailliet, *Knee Pain and Disability,* 3rd ed. (Philadelphia: F. A. Davis, 1992).

Chapter 7

105. B. Bobath, *Abnormal Postural Reflex Activity Caused by Brain Lesions,* 3rd ed. (Oxford, England: Butterworth-Heinemann, 1985).
106. B. Cohen, *The Evolutionary Origins.*
107. Ibid., 15–20.
108. B. Lipton, "The Biology of Consciousness," transcript of lecture presented at the University of British Columbia, 7 May 1995, 2–3.
109. P. Emerson, "Myofascial Manipulation," course outline (Denver, Colo.: Self-published, 2000).
110. A. Steindler, *Kinesiology of the Human Body* (Springfield, Ill.: Charles C. Thomas, 1955).
111. Ibid.

Chapter 8

112. M. Feldenkrais, *Awareness Through Movement*.
113. L. E. Sweigard, *Human Movement Potential: Its Ideokinetic Facilitation* (New York: Harper and Row, 1974).
114. Ibid.
115. D. Ingber, "The Architecture of Life," *Scientific American,* January 1998, 48–57.
116. A. Steindler, *Kinesiology.*
117. K. Luttgens, H. Deutsch and N. Hamilton, *Kinesiology.*
118. Ibid., 349.
119. G. Tortora and S. Grabowski, *Principles of Anatomy.*
120. Ibid.
121. R. Cailliet, *Knee Pain*.
122. A. Steindler, *Kinesiology.*
123. C. Sherrington, *The Integrative Action. of the Nervous System*.
124. I. A. Kapandji, *The Physiology of Joints, vol. 3: The Trunk and Vertebral Column* (Edinburgh: Churchill Livingstone, 1974; reprint, 1988).
125. M. Alter, *Science of Flexibility,* 2nd ed. (Champaign, Ill.: Human Kinetics, 1996), 78.

Chapter 9

126. M. Comerford, "The Psoas Is Not a Hip Flexor," public presentation at the Manual Therapies Seminars in Denver, Colorado, January 1999.
127. See S. Sahrmann, *Diagnosis and Treatment of Movement Impairment Syndromes* (St. Louis: Mosby, 2002); C. Richardson et al., *Therapeutic Exercises for Spinal Stabilization: Scientific Basis and Practical Techniques* (London: Churchill Livingstone, 1998); Kinetic Control Seminars at www.kinetic.control.com; and C. Norris, *Back Stability* (Champaign, Ill.: Human Kinetics, 2000).
128. I. A. Kapandji, *The Physiology of the Joints*.
129. R. McKenzie, *Treat Your Own Back,* 7th ed. (New Zealand: Spinal Publications, 1998).
130. C. Richardson, et al., *Therapeutic Exercises*.
131. Ibid.
132. J. Basmajian and C. DeLuca, *Muscles Alive*.
133. Ibid.
134. N. Bogduk, M. Pearcy, and G. Hadfield, "Anatomy and Biomechanics of the Psoas Major," *Clinical Biomechanics* 7 (1992): 109–119.
135. M. Comerford, "Dynamic Stability and Muscle Balance of the Lower Quadrant: Kinetic Control Movement Dysfunction Course," class tutor (Southamptom, U.K.: Self-published, 2001).
136. S. Gibbons, "Anatomy, Physiology, and Function of Psoas Major: A New Model of Stability." From proceedings of The Tragic Hip: Trouble in the Lower Quadrant, 11th Annual National Orthopeadic Conference, Halifax, Canada, 1999.
137. J. Travell and D. Simons, *Myofascial Pain and Dysfunction: The Trigger Point Manual,* vol. 2 (Baltimore: Williams and Wilkins, 1983), 89.
138. M. Comerford, "Dynamic Stability and Muscle Balance of the Upper Quadrant: Kinetic Control Movement Dysfunction Course," class tutor (Southamptom, U.K.: Self-published, 2001).
139. J. Upledger and J. Vredevoogd, *Cranialsacral Therapy* (Chicago: Eastland Press, 1983).

Chapter 10

140. I. A. Kapandji, *The Physiology of Joints*.
141. F. Kendall, E. McCreary, and P. Provance, *Muscles: Testing and Function with Posture and Pain,* 4th ed. (Baltimore: Williams and Wilkins, 1993).
142. R. Cailliet, *Low Back Pain Syndrome,* 4th ed. (Philadelphia: F. A. Davis, 1988).
143. F. Jones, *The Alexander Technique*.
144. R. Cailliet, *Understand Your Backache* (Philadelphia: F. A. Davis, 1984).
145. I. Bartenieff, *Body Movement: Coping with the Environment* (New York: Gordon and Breach, 1980), 246–47.
146. F. Kendall, E. McCreary, and P. Provance, *Muscles*.
147. R. Cailliet, *Shoulder Pain,* 3rd ed. (Philadelphia: F. A. Davis, 1991), 42–46.
148. R. Cailliet, *Low Back Pain Syndrome*, 5th ed. (Philadelphia: F. A. Davis, 1995).
149. H. Gray, *Gray's Anatomy,* 15th ed. (New York: Bounty Books, 1977), 558.
150. A. Steindler, *Kinesiology,* 436.
151. A. Michele, *Orthotherapy* (Philadelphia: M. Evans and Co. with Lippincott, 1971), 26.
152. I. A. Kapandji, *The Physiology of Joints*.
153. Ibid.
154. Cailliet, *Low Back Pain,* 5th ed.

Chapter 11

155. The International Somatic Movement Education and Therapy Association (ISMETA) was founded in 1988, at which time the International Movement Therapists Association-Registered Movement Therapist (IMTA-RMT) designation was established "as a registered mark with the U.S. Department of Labor, 'Movement Therapy' as a classification of instructional programs with the U.S. Department of Education, and 'Movement Therapist' as an occupational title with the U.S. Department of Labor." (*ISMETA Newsletter,* Summer 1999). For more information, write to ISMETA, 162 W. 21st St., #3S, NY, NY 10011.
156. From the ISMETA 1999 membership information publication.
157. F. Jones, *The Alexander*.
158. Ibid.
159. Ibid., 2.
160. F. M. Alexander, *Knowing How to Stop* (London: Chaterson, 1946).
161. After Laban's death, his followers split into various schools, which present the effort elements in slightly different combinations. This presentation comes out of the old Bartenieff lineage, which has since been revised to include four elements: space, time, weight, and flow.
162. R. Laban, *A Life for Dance: Reminiscences* (New York: Theater Arts Books, 1975).
163. J. Hodgson and V. Preston Dunlop, *Rudolph Laban: An Introduction to His Work and Influence* (Plymouth, England: Northcote House, 1990).
164. W. Lamb, *Posture and Gesture* (London: Duckworth, 1965).
165. Ibid.
166. C. Dell, *A Primer for Movement Description Using Effort-Shape Concepts* (New York: Dance Notation Bureau Press, 1977).
167. See M. North, *Personality Assessment through Movement* (London: MacDonald and Evans, 1970). See also J. Kestenberg, "The Role of Movement Patterns in Development: I, II, and III," *Psychoanalytic Quarterly* 14, no. 1 (1965); 14, no. 4 (1965); 16, no. 3 (1967).
168. From "What Are the Bartenieff Fundamentals?" LIMS Online Home Page (13 June 2002): <http://www.limsonline.org/about lims_bf.html>.
169. I. Bartenieff and D. Lewis, *Body Movement: Coping with the Environment* (New York: Gordon & Breach, 1980), 230.
170. Ibid., 3.
171. M. Feldenkrais, "Moshe on the Martial Arts," interview by D. Leri, *Feldenkrais Journal* no. 2 (1986).
172. M. Feldenkrais, *Awareness Through Movement*.
173. M. Feldenkrais and W. Schutz, "Movement and the Mind," from *The New Healers* (Berkeley, Calif.: New Dimensions, 1980).
174. M. Feldenkrais, "The Forebrain: Sleep, Consciousness, Awareness and Learning," interview by E. Rosenfeld, *Interface Journal* nos. 3–4 (1976): 1–4.
175. Ibid., 4.
176. M. E. Todd, *The Thinking Body* (Princeton, N.J.: Dance Horizons Books, 1937).
177. Ibid., 1–2.
178. L. E. Sweigard, *The Human Movement Potential: Ideokinetic Facilitation* (New York: Harper & Row, 1974).
179. Ibid.
180. E. Franklin, *Dynamic Alignment through Imagery* (Champaign, Ill.: Human Kinetics, 1996).
181. C. Brooks, *Sensory Awareness: The Rediscovery of Experiencing* (New York: Viking, 1974), 16.
182. B. Cohen, *Sensing, Feeling, and Action*.
183. Cohen was a student of the Bobaths, a husband-wife team of neurodevelopmental therapists in England. In her book *Abnormal Postural Reflex Activity Caused by Brain Lesions*, 3rd ed. (London: Butterworth Heinemann, 1985), Berta Bobath discusses these three divisions.
184. Ibid., 122.
185. Ibid., 159.
186. C. Shaffer, "Dancing in the Dark," *Yoga Journal* 77 (November/December 1987): 51.
187. V. Hunt, *Infinite Mind: The Science of Human Vibrations* (Malibu, Calif.: Malibu Publishing, 1995), 13–14.
188. L. Nelson and N. Smith, eds., *Contact Improvisation Sourcebook* (Northampton, Mass.: Contact Editions, 1997).

Chapter 12

189. E. Prosser, *Manual of Massage and Movement* (London: Lippincott, 1951).
190. I. Rolf, *Rolfing: The Integration of Human Structures* (New York: Harper & Row, 1977).
191. J. Oschman, *Readings on the Scientific Basis of Bodywork* (Dover, N.H.: Self-published, 1986).
192. J. Oschman, *Energy Medicine: The Scientific Basis* (London: Churchhill Livingstone, 2000), 131.
193. R. Schleip, from a presentation given at the Rolf Institute Annual Conference (Denver, 1987).

194. Judith Aston's approach has been compared to one developed by osteopath Lawrence Jones, described in *Strain, Counterstrain* (Colorado Springs, Colo.: The American Academy of Osteopathy, 1981). Jones's technique is based on the idea of taking a person into a "position of comfort" to release pain, holding it for 90 seconds, and then slowly bringing the client out of that position. This technique is classified as "indirect technique." In its opposite "direct technique," a practitioner moves the tissues directly toward their optimal functioning position. Although the mechanism of release is not well understood, it has been hypothesized that the passive placement of the body affects the mechanoreceptors and the proprioceptors in such a way that muscles find a new resting length. Strain-counterstrain is analogous to moving a gate with a spring closure so that the spring is no longer under tension. Once the spring has had a chance to relax in its new position, the gate will slowly close.
195. L. Low, "The Modern Body Therapies: A First-Hand Look at Leading Bodywork Therapies," *Massage Magazine* 16 (October/November 1988): 12–19, 48–55.
196. Judith Aston, telephone conversation with author, 15 June 1998.
197. W. Sutherland, *The Cranial Bowl* (Mankato, Minn.: Free Press Company, 1939).
198. J. Upledger and J. Vredevoogd, *Cranialsacral Therapy*.
199. J. Upledger, "Somato-Emotional Release" class handout, West Palm Beach, Fla., Upledger Institute, 1990.
200. J. Upledger and J. Vredevoogd, *Cranialsacral Therapy.*
201. D. Voss, M. Ionta, and B. Myers, *Proprioceptive Neuromuscular Facilitation.*
202. Ibid.
203. The nine PNF techniques are maximal resistance, rhythmic stabilization, quick reversal, contract-relax, holding, stretching, slow reversal, slow reversal-hold, and hold-relax-active. *Proprioceptive Neuromuscular Facilitation* offers an extensive discussion of these techniques.
204. M. Panjabi, *Clinical Biomechanics of the Spine* (Philadelphia: J. B. Lippincott Co., 1990), 88.
205. C. Richardson et al., *Therapeutic Exercises for Spinal Stabilisation: Scientific Basis and Practical Techniques* (London: Churchill Livingstone, 1998).
206. C. Richardson, G. Jull, and B. Richardson, "A Dysfunction of the Deep Abdominal Muscles Exists in Low Back Pain Patients," in *Proceedings of the World Confederation of Physical Therapists,* Washington, D.C., 1995, 932.
207. M. Comerford, "Movement Dysfunction: Dynamic Stability Rehabilitation of the Local and Global Muscles System for Sacro-Iliac Dysfunction" course tutor (Harrow, U.K.: Self-published, 2000).
208. A. Bergmark, "Stability of the Lumbar Spine: A Study in Mechanical Engineering," *Acta Orthopaedica: Scandinavica* 230 (supplemental): 20–24.

Chapter 13

209. G. Everly, *A Clinical Guide to the Treatment of Human Stress Response* (New York: Plenum, 1989).
210. L. Dossey, *Healing Words: The Power of Prayer and the Practice of Medicine* (New York: HarperCollins, 1993).
211. H. Selye, *The Stress of Life* (New York: McGraw-Hill, 1956), 1.
212. J. LeDoux, *Synaptic Self: How Our Brains Become Who We Are* (New York: Viking, 2002).
213. P. Levine, "Hakomi Bodywork Training."
214. C. Stroebel, *QR: The Quieting Reflex* (New York: Putnam, 1982).
215. H. Selye, "On the Real Benefits of Eustress," interview by L. Cherry, *Psychology Today,* March 1978, 60–70.
216. Selye, *Stress,* 1.
217. Ibid., 80.
218. J. Schultz and W. Luthe, *Autogenic Training* (New York: Grune & Stratton, 1959).
219. E. Charlesnorth, *The Relaxation and Stress Management Program: Autogenic Relaxation* (Houston: Stress Management Research Associates, 1981), audiotape.
220. T. Holmes and R. Rahe, "The Social Readjustment Scale," *Journal of Psychosomatic Research* 11 (1967): 213–18.
221. R. Stern and W. Ray, *Biofeedback: Potentials and Limits* (Lincoln: University of Nebraska Press, 1977) 5–6.
222. From the Biofeedback Certification Institute of America (BCIA) brochure titled "Guide to the Biofeedback Certification Program." For information about BCIA go to www.bcia.org.
223. W. Cannon, *The Wisdom of the Body* (New York: Norton, 1932).
224. E. Green and A. Green, *Biofeedback to Mind-Body Self-Regulation: Healing and Creativity* (New York: Delcorte Press, 1977), 26.
225. G. Engel, "The Need for a New Medical Model: A Challenge for Biomedicine," *Science* 196 (1977): 129–36.
226. G. Schrodt and A. Tasman, "Behavioral Medicine," from chapter 26 of *Essentials of Complimentary Alternative Medicine,* ed. W. B. Jonan and J. S. Levin (Baltimore: Lippincott, Williams, and Wilkins, 1999), 445.
227. R. Shellenberger and J. Green, *From the Ghost in the Box to Successful Biofeedback Training* (Greeley, Colo.: Health Psychology Publications, 1996).
228. Stern and Ray, *Biofeedback.*
229. C. Tart, ed. *Altered States of Consciousness* (New York: Doubleday Anchor Books, 1969).

230. J. Kamiya, "Operant Control of the EEG Alpha Rhythm and Some of Its Reported Effects on Consciousness," in *Altered States of Consciousness,* ed. C. Tart (New York: Doubleday Anchor Books, 1969), 519–29.
231. B. K. Bagchi and A. Wenger, "Electrophysiological Correlates of Some Yogi Exercises," *EEG Clinical Neurophysiology* Supplement 7 (1957): 132–49.
232. A. Kasmata and T. Hirai, "Science of Zazan," *Psychologia* 6 (1963): 86–91.
233. B. K. Anand, G. S. Chhina, and B. Singh, "Some Aspects of Electrocephalographic Studies in Yogis," *Electrocephalograph Clinical Neurophysiology* 13 (1961): 452–56.
234. C. M. Cade and N. Coxhead, *The Awakened Mind: Biofeedback and the Development of Higher States of Awareness* (Shaftesbury, Eng.: Element Books, 1989).
235. Ibid.
236. E. Jacobson, *Progressive Relaxation* (Chicago: University of Chicago Press, 1938).
237. Ibid., 1–17.
238. E. Jacobson, *The Biology of Emotions: New Understanding Derived form Biological Multidisciplinary Investigation: First Electrophysiological Measurements* (Springfield, Ill.: Charles C. Thomas, 1967), 7.
239. J. Basmajian, *Biofeedback: Principles and Practice for Clinicians* (Baltimore: Williams & Wilkins, 1979).
240. T. Budzynski, J. Stoyva, and C. Adler, "Feedback-Induced Muscle Relaxation: Application to Tension Headaches," *Journal of Behavior Therapy and Experimental Psychiatry* no. 1 (1970).
241. Green and Green, *Beyond Biofeedback.*
242. Ibid.
243. Ibid., 231.
244. Ibid.
245. Ibid.
246. R. K. Wallace, *The Physiological Effects of Transcendental Meditation* (Los Angeles: MUIPRESS, 1970).
247. H. Benson, *The Relaxation Response* (New York: Morrow, 1975).
248. H. Benson, *Timeless Healing* (New York: Simon and Schuster, 1996).
249. Ibid., 134.
250. J. Kaye, J. Morton, and M. Bowcutt, "Stress, Depression, and Psychoneuroimmunology," *Journal of Neuroscience and Nursing* 3, no. 2 (2000): 93–100.
251. J. Kiecolt-Glaser et al., "Psychological Influences on Surgical Recovery," *American Psychologist* 53, no. 11 (1998): 1209–18.
252. M. Biondi and A. Picardi, "Clinical and Biological Aspects of Bereavement and Loss-Induced Depression: A Reappraisal," *Psychotherapy and Psychosomatics* 65, no. 5 (1996): 229–45.
253. G. Miller et. al., "Psychosocial Predictors of Natural Killer Cell Mobilization during Marital Conflict," *Health Psychology* 18, no. 3 (1999): 262–71.
254. B. Moyers, *Healing and the Mind* (New York: Doubleday, 1993).
255. C. Pert, *Molecules of Emotion: Why You Feel the Way You Feel* (New York: Simon and Schuster, 1999).
256. S. Hall, "A Molecular Code Links Emotions, Mind, and Health," *Smithsonian,* June 1989, 69–71.
257. C. Pert, "The Wisdom of the Receptors: Neuropeptides, the Emotions, and the Bodymind," *Advances* 3 (Summer 1986): 8–16.
258. R. Ader and N. Cohen, "Behavior and the Immune System," in *Handbook of Behavioral Medicine* (New York: Guilford, 1984), 117–73.
259. S. Hall, "A Molecular Code."
260. R. Ader, D. Felton, and N. Cohen, *Psychoneuroimmunology*, 2nd ed. (New York: Academic Press, 1991).
261. B. Siegal, *Love, Medicine, and Miracles* (New York: Harper & Row, 1986).
262. C. Simonton, *Getting Well Again* (Los Angeles: Tarcher, 1978).
263. N. Cousins, *Anatomy of an Illness* (New York: Norton, 1979).

Chapter 14

264. B. F. Skinner, *Walden Two* (New York: Macmillan, 1948).
265. A. Beck, *Cognitive Therapy and Emotional Disorders* (New York: New American Library, 1976).
266. See M. McKay, M. Davis, and P. Fanning, *Thoughts and Feelings: The Art of Cognitive Stress Intervention* (Oakland, Calif.: New Harbinger Publications, 1994); and G. Martin and J. Pear, *Behavior Modification: What It Is and How to Do It* (Manitoba, Canada: Prentice Hall, 1996).
267. S. Maier and M. E. P. Seligman, "Learned Helplessness: Theory and Evidence," *Journal of Experimental Psychology: General* no. 105 (1976), 3–46.
268. M. E. P. Seligman, *Learned Optimism: How to Change Your Mind and Your Life* (New York: Pocket Books, 1990).
269. S. Andreas and C. Faulkner, eds., *NLP: The New Technology of Achievement* (New York: Quill William Morrow, 1994).
270. Ibid., 49.

271. R. Bandler and J. Grinder, *Frogs into Princes* (Moab, Utah: Real People Press, 1979), 61.
272. R. Bandler, *Using Your Brain—for a Change* (Moab, Utah: Real People Press, 1985).
273. S. Andreas and C. Andreas, eds., *Change Your Mind and Keep the Change* (Moab, Utah: Real People Press, 1987), 28–29.
274. Bandler, *Using Your Brain.*
275. Ibid., 85.

Chapter 15

276. This is not to imply that body-based psychotherapists touch their clients. It should be noted that it is usually considered unethical for psychotherapists to touch their clients, with the exceptions being a friendly handshake or a pat on the shoulder.
277. W. Reich, *Character Analysis,* 3rd ed. (New York: Noonday Press, 1949), 374.
278. Ibid., 384.
279. See A. Lowen, *Bioenergetics: The Revolutionary Therapy That Uses the Language of the Body to Heal the Problems of the Mind* (New York: Penguin, 1975), and J. Pierrakos, *Core Energetics* (Mendocino, Calif.: LifeRhythm, 1987).
280. Lowen, *Bioenergetics.*
281. R. Kurtz, *Body-Centered Psychotherapy: The Hakomi Method* (Mendocino, Calif.: LifeRhythm, 1990).
282. S. Keleman, *Your Body Speaks Its Mind* (Berkeley, Calif.: Center Press, 1975), 123.
283. S. Keleman, *Emotional Anatomy: The Structure of Experience* (Berkeley, Calif.: Center Press, 1985).
284. S. Keleman, *Your Body Speaks,* 30.
285. Ibid., 49.
286. S. Keleman, *Patterns of Distress: Emotional Insults and Human Form* (Berkeley, Calif.: Center Press, 1987).
287. S. Keleman, *Emotional Anatomy.*
288. S. Keleman, *Embodying Experience: Forming a Personal Life* (Berkeley, Calif.: Center Press, 1987).
289. Ibid., 23.
290. Ibid.
291. Ibid.
292. I. Chodorow, *Dance Therapy and Depth Psychology* (New York: Routledge, 1991), 27–28.
293. O. Rank, *The Trauma of Birth* (New York: Dover, 1993).
294. See, for example, W. Emerson, "What Is Birth Trauma?" Petaluma, Calif., 1996, photocopy; and A. Janov, *Imprints: The Lifelong Effects of the Birth Experience* (New York: Coward-McCann, 1983).
295. C. Caldwell, *Getting Our Bodies Back: Recovery, Healing and Transformation through Body-Centered Psychotherapy* (Boston: Shambhala, 1996).
296. F. Perls, *Gestalt Therapy Verbatim* (Moab, Utah: Real People Press, 1969), 4.
297. Ibid., 7.
298. Ibid., 21.
299. E. Gendlin, *Focusing,* 2nd ed. (New York: Bantam Books, 1978), 76.
300. Ibid.

GLOSSARY

abduction Moving away from the midline of the body, for example, lifting the leg or arm out to the side, or spreading the fingers or toes apart. *See also* **adduction**.

adaptation The structural and functional changes that occur in a species over a period of time to ensure survival. Darwin first identified this concept in his theory of how a specific species evolves.

adaptive pattern A movement pattern that develops to adapt to the chronic contraction of a number of muscles working to splint an injured or held area. Examples of adaptive patterns are a limp or the postural compensations a person makes to pain. *See also* **compensatory pattern** and **substitution pattern**.

adduction Moving toward the midline of the body, for example, lowering the leg or arm from an abducted position. *See also* **abduction**.

agonist The prime mover in an action: a contracting muscle. *See also* **antagonist**.

Alexander Technique An educational movement process developed by Mathias Alexander, based on establishing balance in the head-neck relationship through a three-step process: awareness, inhibition of habitual patterns, and primary control. The last step involves eliciting the head righting reflex to create a natural length, balance, and coordination between the head and the body.

anal rooting reflex Described by developmental specialist Bonnie Cohen as a reflex similar to mouthing or oral rooting reflexes in which an infant moves the anus toward tactile stimulation. This reflex underlies extension of the coccyx and reach patterns with the tail.

antagonist A muscle that lengthens on the opposite side of a contracting agonist muscle. *See also* **agonist**.

anterior tilt In reference to the movement of the pelvic girdle, when the top of the girdle tips in front of the bottom. *See also* **posterior tilt**.

approximation A technique of bringing two parts of the body together or into proximity, usually in reference to bones or ligaments. Approximation can be either sustained or rhythmic.

arc A C-shaped curve created by movement that is balanced on both ends of the moving part; in the spine, arcs have a continuity of tone between the head and the tail.

arcing A patterning exercise in which a person moves into spinal flexion, then extension, to a neutral position. Also, a type of joint movement in which both articulating bones move with even forces, which creates a balanced counter-rotation in the joint.

association A connection to, and awareness of, one's experience. In the context of neurolinguistic programming, going back and reliving an experience, seeing it through one's own eyes. *See also* **dissociation**.

asymmetrical tonic neck reflex (ATNR) A reflex that takes the head into diagonal extension with rotation.

Aston Patterning A collective term for the work of Judith Aston; which includes *Aston bodywork* and *myokinetics, arthrokinetics,* and *Aston Movement Education.*

authentic movement A therapeutic process developed by dance therapist Mary Whitehouse in which a psychotherapist observes, or "witnesses," the improvisational movement that a client explores as a physical form of free association and a vehicle for psychological processing. *See also* **witness**.

autogenics Developed by Johannes Schultz, a therapy in which people learn to put themselves into a mild state of self-induced hypnosis that is incompatible with states of tension.

autonomic flexibility The ability to move between stress reactions and relaxation, or between sympathetic tone and parasympathetic tone.

automatic movement Bonnie Cohen's version of *katsugen undo* (a movement practice created by a sect of Buddhist monks in Japan) that she teaches in Body-Mind Centering training, in which a person follows internal impulses to move, allowing a spontaneous movement improvisation to unfold and evolve in order to release tension in the autonomic nervous system.

autonomic nervous system (ANS) The part of the nervous system that controls automatic functions, including organ and glandular function. The ANS has two divisions: the parasympathetic, which slows down activity, and the sympathetic system, which initiates or speeds up activity.

autonomic patterning Any process of actively changing and improving patterns of tone in the autonomic nervous system.

autonomic proprioceptive facilitation (APF) Any method applied to change autonomic tone through the stimulation of self-awareness of a psychophysiological state. Includes techniques that use a sensory awareness of physiological tone—such as the heart beat, breath rate, and skin temperature—to realize therapeutic goals such as relaxation, stress management, and trauma resolution.

Awareness Through Movement The movement education part of the Feldenkrais Method.

axial compression In terms of the human body, the vertical loading of the joints due to weight bearing.

Babkin reflex A primitive reflex that is stimulated in an infant lying supine by putting quick, simultaneous pressure on the palms of both hands, which will cause the infant to rotate its head to midline, flex the neck, and open the mouth.

backward rotation In reference to pelvic motion, when the pelvis turns in the horizontal plane so that one hip moves backward, twisting the pelvis and lumbar spine. *See also* **forward rotation** and **lateral rotation**.

backward shift A term coined by Irmgaard Bartenieff to describe a backward movement of the pelvis. *See also* **forward shift**.

ballistic stretch Taking a limb or joint to its end of range and then stretching with repetitive bouncing.

Bartenieff Fundamentals A series of six basic movement exercises—thigh lift, pelvic shift, lateral shift, body half, arm circle, and condensation—delineated by Irmgaard Bartenieff, a student of Rudolph Laban, and taught with varying effort elements and spatial intentions. Used in movement education to coordinate effortless and balanced patterns. *See also* **Laban Movement Analysis**.

behaviorism A theory of psychology developed in the early twentieth century based on the notion that behavior is the result of conditioned reflexes that occur independent of an act of will.

bioenergetics A psychotherapeutic system developed by Alexander Lowen and John Pierrakos for resolving psychological issues as they relate to energetic body processes.

biofeedback (BF) therapy A therapeutic modality that teaches people how to regulate physiological patterns of stress and tension through mental control influenced by physiological feedback.

biopsychosocial medicine A term coined by psychologist George Engel that emphasizes the importance of understanding the interactions of biological, psychological, and social influences on an individual's presenting health problem.

body awareness The kinesthetic knowledge a person has about herself or himself from feeling physical sensations.

body image The mental image a person forms about his or her body. It may or may not be congruent with what the body actually looks like. Congruency reflects a healthy body image.

body-mind awareness Includes a sensory awareness of the bodily sensations generated by physiological processes, and of the changing tensions and positions caused by movement through space. Also includes cognitive awareness of thoughts, emotions, and the act of perceiving. Synonymous with **somatic awareness**.

Body-Mind Centering (BMC) A system of movement education plus touch-and-repatterning developed by Bonnie Cohen that is based on developmental movement education and the study of experiential anatomy.

body righting on body (BOB) reaction An equilibrium response that occurs when the pelvis is rotated and the chest and head follow the rotation. See also **neck righting on body (NOB) reaction**.

bound flow The quality of control in an ongoing movement sequence. A completely bound flow movement can be stopped at any point along its pathway; therefore, bound flow can be used to control a movement.

braced Indicates that a structure is supported by being buttressed or wedged between two elements; for example, the sacrum is braced between the hips and the legs.

braced arch An architectural structure supported by compression members buttressed evenly against a keystone member in between to support it. In terms of the skeletal structure, the pelvis is comparable to a braced arch; the two femurs buttress into two pelvic bones, which in turn buttress against the sacrum, the keystone of the arch.

bracing A holding pattern in which a person locks an area of the body with chronic muscular contractions as though protecting an existing injury or to prevent an injury.

breath cycle One round of inhalation and exhalation.

breath support An underlying support for the body created by alternating cycles of respiration, which fill and empty the ribcage and sinuses, alternating between a state of levity, which lifts and expands the body into a minor physiological extension, and gravity, which allows the body to rest and settle into a minor physiological flexion.

buoyancy The upward force of water that floats a body.

carving *See* **shaping**.

"cellular brain" The primitive communication network that exists within the cellular milieu; a level of consciousness and information processing that occurs on a cellular level. *See also* **cellular consciousness**.

cellular breathing *See* **cellular respiration**.

cellular consciousness A level of awareness that exists within a single cell and is associated with communication that occurs among a community of cells. *See also* **"cellular brain".**

cellular holding A Body-Mind Centering technique of hands-on touch and repatterning in which a practitioner holds another person and focuses attention on cellular fluids with an intention of establishing somatic contact and presence.

cellular respiration The exchange of oxygen and waste products (carbon dioxide) across cell membranes; associated with cellular breathing.

center of gravity (COG) The point in each body mass around which all parts are exactly balanced.

central initiation Movement that begins in the core of the body. *See also* **peripheral initiation**.

central nervous system (CNS) The brain and spinal cord, plus all the end organs that control all voluntary and involuntary behaviors and functions. The CNS has two divisions: the *autonomic* controls involuntary functions; the *skeletal* controls voluntary functions.

centrally mediated pain Pain caused by a breakdown of the central nervous system's ability to process pain, usually associated with an imbalance in neurotransmitters.

cerebral cortex The surface area of gray matter covering the cerebrum in the brain, which functions to coordinate higher nervous system activities, such as creative thought, planning, reflective thinking, and volitional movement.

cerebrospinal fluid (CSF) Fluid produced in the ventricles of the brain that circulates around the brain and spinal cord; CSF may also be found in the fascial network. *See also* **CSF pump** and **CR rhythm**.

character structure A term coined by Wilhelm Reich referring to the personality type, or structure, demonstrated by muscular armor. *See also* **character type** and **muscular armor**.

character types First described by Wilheim Reich, then developed in the context of bioenergetics by Alexander Lowen and John Pierrakos, a defensive position unconsciously assumed in the body, reflecting the personality. The five character types are schizoid, oral, psychopathic, masochistic, and rigid. *See also* **character structure** and **muscular armor**.

charge The buildup of energy in the body, usually associated with stress or distressing psychological issues.

circumduction The circular movement of a limb or finger that combines flexion, extension, abduction, adduction, and rotation.

closed kinematic chain A term to describe an action done with the active limb or part of the body moving against something, as in a push pattern. *See also* **open kinematic chain**.

close-packed position The position of a joint when the articulating surfaces of the bones are compressed together.

cognitive learning A change in behavior that is learned through mental or intellectual channels. *See also* **experiential learning**.

cognitive restructuring A therapeutic process in which a person learns to change patterns of thought in order to alleviate a psychological or physical problem and improve behavior and function.

cognitive skills Using mental abilities to change patterns, such as directing one's attention and intention toward a desired result, restructuring thoughts, or using visualization.

cognitive therapy A form of cognitive patterning in which a person learns to listen to subconscious thoughts and change them by replacing negative thoughts with positive ones.

compensatory holding pattern A holding pattern that develops as a result of pain caused by another holding pattern. *See also* **adaptive pattern** and **substitution pattern**.

complimentary alternative medicine (CAM) A term coined by the Office of Alternative Medicine (OAM) at the National Institutes of Health (NIH) to identify a large number of body-mind therapies, including yoga and martial arts, energy and spiritual healing, hypnosis, music therapy, aromatherapy, cognitive and behavioral therapy, biofeedback, acupuncture, and psychoneuroimmunology.

compression In the context of biomechanics, the compressive loading that occurs in joints as the result of weight bearing in both posture and movement. In the context of bodywork, hands-on pressure on the body.

compression member A structure that transfers weight to the ground. Compression members in the body are the bones.

compressive forces Any of the forces that increase compressive loading of the tissues, such as weight, gravity, and the forces generated by movement.

concentric contraction A contraction in which a muscle shortens. *See also* **eccentric contraction**, **isometric contraction**, and **isotonic contraction**.

connective tissue The most abundant tissue in the body, made up of ground substance (a base of intercellular fluid) and collagen fibers; functions to support, bind, protect, or transport substances within the body; examples are blood, bone, and cartilage.

concrete operations The third stage of Piaget's learning theory that lasts from about age seven to 11, in which a child begins to understand how one thing can change into another, and can describe how this change affects reality. *See also* **formal operations**, **preoperational stage**, and **sensorimotor learning**.

connective tissue adhesion A buildup of collagen fibers that forms knots in tissues and blocks motion.

constructive rest position (CRP) A position developed by Mabel Todd in which a person lies on her back with knees bent and arms folded across the chest or resting above the head; used for rest, recuperation, and improving alignment. *See also* **hooklying position**.

Contact Improvisation A dance form developed by Steve Paxton that is based on the spontaneous responses that two bodies have when they unexpectedly touch. Practiced by dancers using movement explorations with improvisational body contact.

continuity of tone An even quality of tone throughout the body or within one body system such as the muscular system. *See also* **tone**.

Continuum Movement An improvisational movement practice developed by Emilie Conrad in which a person combines breath, sound, and organic movement explorations to loosen and dissolve the boundaries of the ego on the body and awaken the fluid nature innate in living beings.

contractility The ability of a muscle to shorten.

contract-relax-antagonist-contract technique (CRAC) An inhibitory method to release and lengthen a tight muscle by first contracting it, then relaxing it, then stretching it, and during the stretch actively contracting its antagonist, which is thought to trigger an inhibitory response in the agonist and allow it to stretch more effectively.

contract-relax technique The facilitory method to release and lengthen a tight muscle by first contracting it against resistance, and then stretching it. The rationale behind this method is that the contraction triggers a reflex that causes the muscle to relax, thus allowing it to stretch more effectively directly after a contraction.

contralateral Movement that sequences from one arm to the opposite leg, or from one leg to the opposite arm. Crawling and walking are based on contralateral movements.

core issues Deeply rooted psychological issues that color all of a person's behaviors, attitudes, and somatic patterns.

core movement On a physical level, movement that initiates in and is supported by the center of the body. On a psychological level, movement that initiates as a result of one's own volition and effort.

core support Support that exists when weight and movement are as close to the center of the core of the body as possible.

cortical patterning Changing somatic patterns with mental control, using attention and intention, feedback, imagery, and cognitive restructuring.

coupling When two seemingly disparate elements become associated with each other, and the presence of one element brings up the image or memory of the other.

coupled pairs In terms of muscle physiology, agonist/antagonist pairs of muscles that work in opposition to each other due to spinal cord reflexes that facilitate the contraction of one while inhibiting the contraction of its pair.

cranialsacral (CS) therapy A gentle system of hands-on work based on freeing up the CS rhythm to release tension and tissue restrictions in the cranium and the entire body; derived from osteopathic principles and techniques.

CSF pump The fluid pump generated by the rhythmic motion of the ventricles in the brain as they fill with cerebrospinal fluid. *See also* **cerebrospinal fluid** and **CS rhythm**.

CS rhythm Body rhythms caused by the filling of cerebrospinal fluid within the ventricles of the brain. *See also* **cerebrospinal fluid** and **CSF pump**.

dance movement therapy A branch of psychotherapy based on the healing powers of creative expression through dance and movement.

depression A psychological state in which a person lacks emotion, marked by a heavy, lethargic affect. In reference to kinesiology, a return of the scapula from an elevated position to a normal position. *See also* **elevation**.

dermatomes A map of the areas innervated by each spinal nerve.

developmental movement patterns The basic neurological patterns established during early motor development that create the sensorimotor foundation of the nervous system. These patterns include yield, push, reach, and pull patterns through spinal, homologous, homolateral, and contralateral pathways.

developmental patterning Neuromuscular education and patterning based on the series of movement patterns that are first learned during early motor development.

developmental process A therapeutic process in which a person moves progressively to the next stage of his or her development.

differentiation of flexor/extensor tone Tone that develops from movement in a single joint. In the spine, differentiation starts at the head and gradually builds in a sequential manner down the spine.

dimensional cross In terms of the body, the cross made by the horizontal orientation of the shoulders and the vertical orientation of the spine and legs.

direct technique A hands-on technique of manual therapy in which a practitioner applies force to move the tissues out of a fixed, misaligned, or compressed position.

discharge The release of energy in the body.

diseases of adaptation The diseases that result from accumulative degeneration arising from prolonged exposure to factors that induce stress responses, including metabolic disorders or diseases such as obesity, diabetes, and hyperthyroidism; liver disease, gout, heart disease, cancer, ulcers, and immune dysfunction; and inflammatory diseases such as arthritis and rheumatism.

dissociation Loss of the awareness of an experience, or disconnecting from experience. In the context of neurolinguistic programming, seeing an experience from any viewpoint but one's own. In the context of skeletal patterning, a skill of isolating movement in a single joint or area, and then moving this area within it full range in order to gain control of its range. *See also* **association** and **dissociation of movement**.

dissociation of movement A basic patterning skill in which the movement of one joint or group of joints is isolated from the movement of another in order to gain control over the moving area.

dorsiflexion Flexing the ankle from an extended position. *See also* **plantar flexion**.

drag A force on bodies produced by a flow meeting direct pressure, resulting in turbulence and resistance, such as resistance a person experiences when walking into the wind.

dynamic system A system in which there is a two-way flow of information or energy. A system that lacks static properties, exists only through movement, and involves a feedback loop.

eccentric contraction A contraction in which a muscle slowly lengthens in response to an external force. *See also* **concentric contraction, isometric contraction,** and **isotonic contraction**.

edema An abnormal accumulation of interstitial fluid in the body that results in the swelling of tissues.

effort The amount of energy a person expends to carry out a movement.

effort elements In the context of Labanalysis, the qualities of effort one uses during movement: quick or sustained *time*, free or bound *flow*, direct or indirect attention to *space*, and strong or light *weight*.

elasticity The ability of a tissue to stretch; one of the properties inherent in muscle tissue.

electrodermal resistance (EDR) Instrumentation used in biofeedback training that provides feedback of sweat gland activity, measured from fingers. Used to build self-regulation skills of the autonomic nervous system.

electroencephalograph (EEG) Instrumentation used in biofeedback training that provides feedback of brain-wave activity, measured in different locations on the scalp. Used to induce relaxation and altered states of consciousness, and to control such conditions as epilepsy and migraines.

electromyograph (EMG) Instrumentation used to measure activity in muscles, used in biofeedback training to provide feedback about muscular activity, to teach relaxation skills, and to reduce pain caused by chronically contracted or dysfunctional muscles.

elevation In reference to kinesiology, the upward motion of the scapula. *See also* **depression**.

embody To make perceptible through energetic or physical movement; to become aware of and/or move through more of the body than a person is habituated to; to express through the body.

emotional intelligence A term coined by Daniel Goleman to describe the behavioral qualities that the average person with a thriving life seems to have. These qualities include self-awareness, self-control, empathy, the art of listening, conflict resolution skills, and the ability to cooperate.

emotional tone The overall emotional quality that influences the characteristics of a person's posture and movement.

emphasis In the context of Labanalysis, the elements that are emphasized in a movement sequence.

endpoints A term denoting the hands, feet, head, and tail.

energy Vigorous action, effort; the capacity for performing work; usable power and the resources for producing such power, strength, might, and vigor.

equilibrium responses The complex responses that reestablish balance in the body when either the center of gravity or the base of support shifts; usually coordinated at the level of the forebrain. Examples are protective stepping or spatial reaching with the limbs, both of which occur automatically when falling.

eustress Healthy stress that builds resistance, results in a healthy adaptive response, builds strength in the body and mind, and fortifies the body. *See also* **stress**.

eversion A movement of the foot in which the inner (lateral) arch is lifted. *See also* **inversion**.

excitability The ability of a muscle to receive and respond to nerve impulses.

exhalation fixation A holding pattern in which the person becomes stuck during the expiration phase of breathing. This pattern is usually marked by depression of the ribcage and an inability to take a full inhalation. *See also* **inhalation fixation**.

experiential learning A change in behavior that is learned as a result of how a person is affected by an experience; learning based on physical activity and sensorimotor perception. *See also* **cognitive learning**.

extensibility The ability of a muscle to be extended by a peripheral pull.

extension A movement that returns a joint from flexion.

extensor tone Tone in the muscles along the back of the body that takes the spine and limbs into extension with slight external rotation of the limbs. *See also* **flexor tone**.

external respiration The movement of air between the body and the outside environment; respiration in which the diaphragm and rib cage expand the lungs to pull in air. *See also* **internal respiration**.

extrinsic movement Movement that occurs in the outer layers of the body, usually involving the larger muscles that produce obvious, observable actions. *See also* **intrinsic movement**.

facilitate To induce an action. In terms of muscle function, to get a muscle to contract.

facilitation The process of eliciting movement. When used in reference to muscles, any method that elicits a muscular contraction, such as the PNF technique of pushing against resistance.

facilitory stretch A method of releasing tension in tight muscles by contracting the muscle prior to the stretch to elicit a stretch reflex, then stretching it. *See also* **contract-relax technique**.

fall and recovery In terms of kinesiology, the process of losing one's balance and regaining it in an instant. Also, a component of a normal gait pattern.

fascia A specialized form of connective tissue that wraps and binds every tissue in the body, creating a supportive, three-dimensional web, or fascial network, throughout the entire body. *See also* **fascial network**.

fascial adhesion A knot in the fascial network resulting in distorted body posture and movement caused by a buildup or bunching of collagen fibers and a decrease in fluid content; similar to scar tissue.

fascial network A matrix of connective tissue that supports other tissues throughout the body; the white, glistening sheaths around muscles and organs that collectively function as a support network.

Feldenkrais Method A method of movement education developed by Moshe Feldenkrais that is built upon the principle of changing movement by increasing an awareness of it.

felt sense A term coined by Eugene Gendlin to describe the vague experience, or "gut feeling," a person has during psychological processes; includes physical, emotional, and mental aspects. Is used to get to the core of an emotional issue and often leads to a deep yet relaxing physical and emotional shift. *See also* **focusing**.

fibromyalgia A chronic pain condition affecting the muscles and joints, diagnosed by tenderness in 11 or more of 18 specified spots. *See also* **myofascial pain syndrome (MFS)**.

fight-or-flight response A term coined by Walter Cannon to describe the body's generalized response to a stressful, or emergency, situation; involves stimulation of the sympathetic nervous system and adrenal glands, accompanied by increases in heart rate, breathing rate, blood flow, and blood pressure. *See also* **freeze response**.

flexion A movement that closes the angle of a joint; a movement that returns a joint from extension.

flexor tone The tone of the muscles and organs along the front of the body from the lower abdomen up, which takes the body into flexion with slight internal rotation of the limbs. *See also* **extensor tone**.

fluid forces Movement forces on the body that are generated by the currents or resistance to the currents of air or water; the forces that create buoyancy, lift, and drag on a body. *See also* **buoyancy, lift, drag**.

fluid support The fullness and volume of the fluids as they fill their surrounding containers, such as cells or circulatory tubes.

focusing A therapy developed by Eugene Gendlin based on the idea of "thinking with the body," using the felt sense as a primary tool. *See also* **felt sense**.

forebrain The part of the embryological brain from which the cerebrum and cerebral cortex arise. These parts of the brain are associated with advanced cognitive functions and self-awareness.

formal operations The final stage of Piaget's developmental learning theory, which begins around age 11 or 12, in which a child becomes aware of abstract thought. *See also* **concrete operations**, **preoperational stage**, and **sensorimotor learning**.

formative principle A concept developed by Stanley Keleman to describe the notion that a person is constantly shaping and reshaping, forming and reforming his or her body shape around that his or her psychological makeup. *See also* **formative process**.

formative process Stanley Keleman's theory of how a person forms the shape of the body in relationship to psychological processes; includes three phases: expansion, containment, and expression. *See also* **formative principle**.

forward rotation In reference to pelvic motion, when the pelvis turns in the horizontal plane so that one hip moves forward, twisting the pelvis and lumbar spine. *See also* **backward rotation** and **lateral rotation.**

forward shift A term coined by Irmgaard Bartenieff to describe a forward movement of the pelvis. *See also* **backward shift**.

framing Stopping and highlighting an event, experience, or phenomenon to give it emphasis. *See also* **reframing**.

free flow An ongoing quality of movement that is free, loose, and abandoned. For example, a swinging movement has a free flow quality.

freeze response A maladaptive reaction in which a person is physically immobilized by fear during a fight-or-flight response. *See also* **tonic immobility**.

frontal plane An imaginary plane made up of the longitudinal and the lateral dimensions, for example, the plane of a door frame. Also referred to as the coronal plane.

fundamental movement patterns Basic patterns of motion that involve flexion, extension, rotation of the limbs and trunk, circumduction of the limbs, and simultaneous condensation and extension of the entire body.

functional holding patterns Restrictions and limitations in body movement; the physiological and emotional patterns that limit the body's biological functions, including homeostasis and responses to stress.

Functional Integration The hands-on component of the Feldenkrais Method.

gate theory of pain A hypothesis developed by neuroscientists Ronald Melzack and Patrick Wall in the 1960s stating that painful stimuli from the smaller, deeper sensory nerve fibers may be blocked from reaching the central nervous system by applying sensory stimuli to larger, peripheral sensory nerves located in the skin.

general adaptation syndrome (GAS) A model developed by Hans Selye to describe the three stages of the stress response: the alarm reaction, the resistance stage, and exhaustion.

gestalt A pattern so fully integrated as a functional unit that it has properties that far exceed the sum of its parts.

Gestalt therapy An existential approach to psychotherapy developed by Fritz Perls that focuses on immediate behavior; helps people become aware of the fragmented aspects of their thoughts, emotions, and body awarenesses in order to reintegrate into a unified whole, or Gestalt.

gestural pattern In the context of Labanalysis, a pattern that sequences through a single body part; a gesture.

global stabilizers In terms of postural stabilization, the muscles that control a movement through its range.

glueing The adhering of fascial layers to each other.

goal orientation A focus on the end result of a modality rather than on the process.

gradation with rotation A concept developed by Irmgaard Bartenieff to describe how the gradual supination and pronation of the hand is gradated over the circumference of the motion of arm circumduction, which she refers to as an "arm circle."

gravity A constant force that pulls all bodies towards the center of the earth and gives them weight. *See also* **levity**.

ground reaction force The counterforce or resistance generated by the weight and friction of bodies against the ground. For example, the downward push of the toes accelerates the body forward in walking.

grounding In the context of bioenergetics, a concept developed by Alexander Lowen and John Pierrakos to describe the psychophysical process of getting in touch with reality through a physical and energetic connection with the ground upon which one is standing.

ground substance The fluid in fascia.

gyroscopic In reference to body movement, a three-dimensional twisting movement in which the three masses of the body each rotate around their own axis while rotating the whole spine around another axis in a coordinated, contralateral pattern.

habituation Learning that results from repetition of a behavior. The process of becoming a habit.

hand-eye coordination A coordination of movement between the hand and eyes, supported by numerous underlying reflexes that include the oral rooting and asymmetrical tonic neck reflexes.

hand-mouth coordination A coordination of movement between the hand and mouth, supported by oral rooting reflexes.

head righting reaction A reflex coordinated in the midbrain that bring the head to vertical from a non-vertical position.

hindbrain The part of the embryonic brain from which the pons, cerebellum, medulla oblongata, and brain stem arise. These parts of the brain coordinate reflexive movement and autonomic functions such as breathing, digestion, and metabolism.

hinging Extreme flexion or extension in one joint of the spine that bends the spine into an angle and exaggerates the spinal curves; common in the neck.

holding patterns Chronic muscular contractions that form as defense mechanisms. A blockage between two conflicting forces; in the body, holding patterns are evident in areas that are held in place and do not move.

holism The theory that all living beings are far more than the sum of their parts and that patterns of posture and movement reflect emotional, mental, and spiritual as well as physical aspects of a person. An approach to working with health patterns reflecting the function of the whole person rather than limiting the focus to one part.

homeostasis A state of physiological equilibrium maintained by internal feedback loops that regulate a stable yet dynamic internal environment.

homolateral Movement in which flexion of the arm and leg on one side sequences into extension on the other side.

homologous Simultaneous movement of either both arms or both legs.

hooklying position A supine position (lying on the back) with both knees bent, feet flat and parallel. Also referred to as "crooklying." *See also* **constructive rest position**.

horizontal plane An imaginary plane made up of the side-side and front-back dimensions. The four corners of the horizontal plane are akin to the four corners of a square table.

horizontal scanning A rotational movement of the head from side to side to scan the surrounding environment. *See also* **hand-eye coordination**.

hyperextension The extension of a joint past its neutral position in a direction that increases the angle of the joint past 180 degrees.

hyperventilation An imbalance in the exchange of gas in the body, in which the level of oxygen coming in exceeds the level of carbon dioxide going out; signs include dizziness, light-headedness, tingling in the extremities, tetany, and fainting.

hypnagogic Associated with the state of drowsiness preceding sleep.

hypnagogic images The images or visions that people tend to have when they are falling asleep. These images are thought to be a projection of impulses from the unconscious mind; they seem to pop out of nowhere, although they have been found beneficial in the process of psychoanalysis.

ideokinesis Using ideation, or imagery, to change movement.

ideokinetic facilitation A term coined by Lulu Sweigard to describe a method of changing movement through the use of mental imagery; also known as *ideokinesis*. *See also* **lines of movement**.

imprinting Discovered by ethnologist Konrad Lorenz, a behavior pattern rapidly established early in life when an infant or small child recognizes and mimics the innate characteristics of a parent or caretaker.

indirect technique A manual therapy technique in which the practitioner follows the client's tissues in and out of a pattern until the client's system spontaneously releases tension and rebalances.

inhalation fixation A holding pattern in which the person becomes stuck during the inspiration phase of breathing. A rigid, overly inflated ribcage and the inability to make a full exhalation usually mark this pattern. *See also* **exhalation fixation**.

inhibited In terms of muscle function, an inhibited muscle is one that is either not contracting or contracting too late. *See also* **over-facilitated**.

inhibition Something that stops movement. In the context of somatic patterning, inhibition is used to suspend a habitual body response in order to have time to choose a more efficient response.

inhibitory stretch A method of lengthening a tight muscle by contracting its antagonist to trigger a reflex that inhibits the agonist to release tension in it and improve the effectiveness of the stretch. *See also* **contract-relax-antagonist-contract (CRAC) technique**.

inversion A movement of the foot in which the outside edge (lateral arch) is lifted. *See also* **eversion**.

integration The synergistic functioning of all parts of a body or system. *See also* **movement integration**.

internal respiration The movement of oxygen from the lungs via the bloodstream to the cells of the body. *See also* **external respiration**.

interstitial fluid Fluid that is present in intercellular spaces, the spaces between cells in the body.

intra-abdominal pressure (IAP) An increase in pressure created in the abdominal cavity by the simultaneous contraction of the muscles of the abdominal wall, pelvic floor, and the respiratory diaphragm, resulting in an increased stiffness of trunk and lumbar spine.

intrapsychic processes Internal psychological processes. Therapy is referred to as *intrapsychic* when it focuses on a client's internal processes rather than on the interaction between client and psychotherapist, which is known as *interpersonal* therapy.

intrinsic movement Subtle internal movement that occurs through deep intrinsic muscles, particularly along the front of the spine, close to the long bones, and through the organs. *See also* **extrinsic movement**.

intuition A direct perception of truth; a keen and quick insight not based on cognitive processes and independent of any conscious reasoning process.

inward rotation Turning the leg or arm so that the knee or the crease of the elbow faces toward the body. *See also* **outward rotation**.

inversion A movement of the foot in which the inner (medial) arch is lifted. *See also* **eversion**.

ischemia Localized tissue anemia and lack of vitality caused by a stagnation in blood supply to that area.

isometric contraction A contraction in which the tension of a muscle remains the same; therefore, this type of contraction does not generate joint movement. *See also* **concentric contraction**, **eccentric contraction,** and **isotonic contraction**.

isotonic contraction A contraction in which the tension of a muscle remains even throughout the range of motion. Both eccentric and concentric contractions are isotonic. *See also* **concentric contraction**, **eccentric contraction,** and **isometric contraction**.

kinematic chain A series of joints linked together so that movement in one joint will produce movement in the other joints along the chain in a predictable manner.

kinesiology The study of the principles of mechanics and anatomy in relation to human movement.

kinesphere The area of space into which a person can reach while maintaining a stable base of support.

kinesthesia A bodily sense stimulated by changes in positions and tensions.

Kinetic Control A progressive, research-based method of stability training developed by physical therapist Mark Comerford and his colleagues.

kyphosis A backward curvature of the spine, found in the thorax spine. When abnormal and exaggerated, it is often called a "hunchback" curve. *See also* **lordosis**.

kyphotic curve A spinal curve that is concave toward the front, as in the normal sacral, thoracic, and cranial curves when viewed from the side. *See also* **lordotic curve**.

Labanalysis A system of movement analysis developed by Rudolph Laban that focuses on four areas of study: space, shape, effort, and body fundamentals. Used extensively in dance training and neuromuscular reeducation.

Laban Movement Analysis *See* **Labanalysis**.

Labanotation A system of shorthand to record dance movement developed by Rudoph Laban.

lack of continuity Discontinuity of movement or tone, or an incongruity between self-image and body awareness.

Landau reflex A midbrain reflex apparent in infants from three to six months of age who, when suspended in a horizontal position, extend the whole body, beginning with the head. Once the extension phase of the reflex is established, when the head is placed in passive flexion, the whole body flexes. The Landau extension pattern is also referred to as the "flying position."

lateral line In relation to human body, an imaginary line on the side of the body that bisects the body front to back, which travels through the middle of the ear, shoulder, hip, knee, and ankle. The lateral line might and might not be along the line of gravity, depending upon the posture of an individual.

lateral rotation In reference to pelvic motion, when the pelvis turns in the frontal plane so that one hip rises while the other lowers, taking the lumbar spine into a side-bending motion. *See also* **backward rotation** and **forward rotation**.

lateral shift A shift of the pelvis and trunk through space from one side to the other. See also **backward shift** and **forward shift**.

laws of motion Created by seventeenth-century physicist and mathematician Sir Isaac Newton, the three laws of motion govern the movement of physical bodies and demonstrate the relationship between force and matter generated by the gravitational pull. The *law of reaction* states that for every action there is an equal and opposite reaction; the *law of inertia* states that a body remains in a state of rest or of uniform motion until an unbalancing force acts upon it; and the *law of acceleration* states that the acceleration of any object is directly proportional to the force causing its acceleration.

learned helplessness Discovered by psychologist Martin Seligman, the state people sink into when they perceive that there are no adequate coping mechanisms to deal with or remove a source of stress. A person in a state of learned helplessness usually gives up fighting or trying to cope and sinks into depression.

learned optimism A cognitive therapeutic technique created by psychologist Martin Seligman in which a person learns how to work with dualistic thoughts by replacing negative thoughts with positive ones.

levity The opposite of gravity; a lightness that lifts and expands, seen in the body when the breath fills and lifts the lungs, and when air filling the sinuses lightens the skull. *See also* **gravity**.

lift A force produced by the flow of a current on one side of the body that is faster than the flow of the current on the other side.

limbic system A group of subcortical structures in the brain associated with emotion and motivation; includes the hypothalamus and amygdala. *See also* **forebrain, midbrain**.

line of force In the body, the direction taken by a force, such as weight or a push, as it travels from one joint to the next.

line of gravity An imaginary vertical line that passes through the center of gravity and changes with each shift in the position of the body.

lines of movement Identified by Lulu Sweigard as "the location and direction of a movement between specific skeletal parts, each beginning and ending in bone" (from *Human Movement Potential*, 193). *See also* **ideokinetic facilitation**.

local stabilizer In terms of postural stabilization, a muscle that controls the neutral position of a joint (usually used in reference to the intervertebral joints) within its neutral zone independent of the range or direction of movement.

lordosis A forward curvature of the spine, usually found in the lower back or neck. *See also* **kyphosis**.

lordotic curve A spinal curve that is convex toward the front, as in the normal neck and lower back curves when viewed from the side. *See also* **kyphotic curve**.

lumbar-pelvic rhythm The coordinated activity of spinal flexion, anterior pelvic tilting, and hip flexion, in the open-chain movements of forward bending or hip flexion, which increases the overall range of motion by distributing movement among these segments. *See also* **scapulohumeral rhythm**.

matching In the context of neurolinguistic programming, mirroring another person's qualities, such as breathing rate, tone of voice, representational system, or posture, in order to achieve rapport. *See also* **rapport** and **representational system**.

mechanical movement In terms of somatic patterning, an approach to movement education that focuses on the mechanical aspects of muscle and joint function.

mechanical stresses Five primary forces that act on the body: *tensile stresses, compression from gravity, shearing, torsion,* and *bending.*

micromovement A small, subtle movement that takes place internally. Often so small that an untrained observer cannot see them, micromovements are used to release tension and activate intrinsic muscles.

midbrain The part of the embryonic brain from which the thalamus and hypothalamus, an area generally called the limbic system, arise. These parts of the brain are associated with emotional responses and are a conduit through which information passes between the forebrain and hindbrain.

midline In terms of the body, the center of the body between the right and left sides.

mobility The motion of the body as it changes position and moves through space.

mobilizers In terms of postural stability, muscles that have phasic function, which generate fast, strong contractions to flex, extend, or rotate a joint or series of joints. *See also* **phasic function** and **stabilizers**.

modulate dualities A somatic patterning concept in which opposing elements in the body are balanced or brought into balance by the dual energies that they generate.

motility The internal movements of the body; often the unseen movements of organs and fluids, or movements initiated by physiological processes such as breathing or circulation.

motor processes The neurological sequences that involve the relay of information from the brain or spinal cord to the muscles, usually resulting in a movement response or the inhibition of a response. *See also* **sensory processes**.

motor planning The stage that precedes the initiation of a movement in which a person mentally prepares for the action.

motor unit A neuron plus all the muscle fibers it innervates.

mouthing *n.* A movement pattern that initiate in the lips and moves the mouth and throat; mouthing first appears during the stage of early development in which the infant roots, i.e., searches for the mother's nipple with his or her lips. *v.* Moving the lips and mouth in a gnawing, chewing, and gumming manner. *See also* **oral rooting reflex**.

movement Primarily the kinesiological motion of the body that can be observed in motion generated by the neuromuscular system; also, the intrinsic physiological motions of metabolic processes such as respiration, circulation, and digestion, as well as the motility of bodily fluids and tissues. In the context of this text, the sequence of physical, physiological, emotional, and mental motion through the body.

movement sequence A series of stages in a movement consisting of motor planning, initiation, action, completion, and recuperation.

muscle bracing First described by Edmund Jacobson, a chronic holding of inactive muscles in a state of flexion.

muscle tone The amount of contraction that occurs in a muscle at rest.

muscular armor A term coined by Wilhelm Reich to describe patterns of chronic muscular tension that block the flow of biological energy from the core of the body to the periphery, thereby repressing unmanageable and uncomfortable emotions, particularly those that cause anxiety. *See also* **character structure** and **character type**.

myofascia A single muscle or group of muscles plus all its related fascia.

myofascial pain syndrome (MFS) A chronic pain condition characterized by general tenderness in the muscles and specifically in trigger points. *See also* **fibromyalgia**.

navel radiation A developmental movement pattern marked by either flexion or extension of all limbs in a movement that either radiates in toward or out from the navel.

neck righting on the body (NOB) reaction An equilibrium response that occurs when the head is rotated and the chest and pelvis follow the rotation. *See also* **body righting on body (BOB) reaction**.

neoteny The retention of immature characteristics into adulthood, which allows humans to continue to learn and change throughout life.

neurolinguistic programming (NLP) A method of changing behavior by consciously reordering thought patterns and representational systems.

neurological actions As used in a developmental patterning context, the four most basic patterns of movement: yield, push, reach, and pull.

neuromuscular patterning Any methods used to reorganize and improve muscular control and coordination.

neuropeptide A neurotransmitter produced in the brain or in various locations outside the central nervous system; these regulate many of the body's states and functions. *See also* **neurotransmitter**.

neurotransmitter A chemical messenger produced within the brain and present at junctions between nerve cells to stimulate responses.

neutral position The position of a joint in which it is not flexed, extended, or rotated.

neutral position of the spine The position in which the joints of the spine are neither flexed nor hyperextended; extension of the spine.

neutral zone Defined by orthopedist Manohar Panajabi to describe the range in which a joint can move from its neutral position without resistance from its joint capsule or the surrounding ligaments, tendons, or muscles. *See also* **neutral position**.

nociceptors The small peripheral nerve endings found in the skin and throughout the body that relay sensations that are usually interpreted as pain to the brain for processing.

open kinematic chain A term to describe an action done with the active limb or part of the body moving freely in space, as in a reach pattern. *See also* **closed kinematic chain.**

opening pain Pain that occurs as tissues release holding patterns and begin to regain circulation and motion.

opposable thumbs Thumbs that move in opposition to the other fingers, allowing for the broad range of articulate and manipulative movement capacities of the human hands.

optical righting reaction A reflex stimulated by visual cues that brings the head to vertical and maintains it in this position. *See also* **head righting reaction**.

oral rooting reflex A primitive reflex stimulated by touch and smell that causes a newborn's mouth to search for the mother's nipple.

organic movement Movement having the characteristics of an organism; movement derived from the processes within a living organism, having a systematic coordination of parts.

organic movement practice A process-oriented, improvisational movement that a person uses to increase fluid circulation and relaxation, and to unwind both physical and psychological tension. This practice is carried out by focusing on releasing the body into the movement of the fluid rhythms inherent to any or all of the bodily systems.

organ support The fullness and volume of the organs and the space they occupy in the trunk.

orgasm reflex A term coined by Wilhelm Reich to describe the pulsation, or streaming, of energy and movement that occurs along the longitudinal axis of the body and is reflected in strong pulsating cycles of spinal flexion and extension; movement that occurs in the body when an orgasm fully sequences between the head and the pelvis.

orgone energy A term coined by Wilhelm Reich to describe biological energy that flows through the body; a concept developed as the physical counterpart to what Freud referred to as *libido*.

orienting response A movement made to orient oneself in the environment; usually involves head movement in a horizontal scanning that enables a person to look for danger.

oscillation between dualities A patterning technique in which a person volleys his or her focus between two elements that lack integration, such as tension and relaxation, or flexion and extension, to integrate them.

outward rotation Turning the leg or arm so that the knee or the crease of the elbow faces away from the body. *See also* **inward rotation**.

over-facilitated In terms of muscle function, a muscle that is working too hard, and thus is firing too often. *See also* **inhibited**.

paradoxical breathing A breathing pattern in which the diaphragm lifts up during contraction, moving in the opposite direction than it should, thereby decreasing lung volume; a pattern commonly seen when a person is in a state of fear or panic.

parasympathetic The branch of the autonomic nervous system that slows down the autonomic system and regulates vegetative metabolic functions such as digestion; usually associated with the relaxation response. *See also* **sympathetic.**

passive volition An attitude or use of will in which one sets an intention, then allows the body to realize the intention without the involvement of any conscious effort.

patterning *n.* Any physiotherapy designed to improve a malfunctioning nervous system by means of feedback from muscular activity. *v.* The process of changing patterns.

perception The brain's interpretation of bodily sensations such as what part of the body is moving, where it is moving, and how fast it is moving. Consciousness based on sensory information, such as tactile sensations, sound, color, taste, light. Also, a point of view, a mental image.

perceptual shift A general feeling of change in such aspects as tone, position, well-being, or even in a person's state of mind. A perceptual shift always accompanies changes in somatic patterns.

peripheral initiation Movement that begins in the body's periphery: the hands, feet, head, or tail. *See also* **central initiation**.

peripheral nervous system (PNS) The part of the nervous system that lies outside the brain, made up of the peripheral nerves and ganglia.

phasic A term used to describe the rate of a muscle contraction. A fast contraction.

phasic function The function of muscles that work to generate quick, strong movements, such as sprinting; these muscles, also called spurt muscles, operate in cycles of contraction and relaxation rather than sustained contractions. *See also* **mobilizers**.

physiological extension A subtle extension of the spine initiated by the inhalation cycle of respiration. In terms of developmental movement, a pattern in which the entire body extends in a single action that initiates in the feet, coccyx, and lower abdominal organs; a pattern strongest during a normal vaginal birth in which the infant pushes out from the feet.

physiological flexion A subtle flexion of the spine initiated by the exhalation cycle of respiration. In terms of developmental movement, a pattern in which the entire body flexes in a single action that initiates in the feet, coccyx, and lower abdominal organs.

physiological rhythm A body rhythm that is generated by a physiological process; examples are the breathing cycle, heartbeat, CSF pump, and the tissue pump of the muscles going through cycles of flexion and extension.

Pilates Method A system of conditioning developed by Joseph Pilates that is based on controlling the core of the body while one practices strengthening exercises.

plantar flexion Extending the ankle, such as by standing on the tip-toes or pointing the toes. *See also* **dorsiflexion**.

position of mechanical advantage A posture that is mechanically sound in which one body mass is aligned over another in a vertical posture, and each one stays vertically aligned with the others during movement.

posterior tilt In reference to the movement of the pelvic girdle, when the top of the girdle tips behind the bottom. *See also* **anterior tilt.**

postural stabilization *See* **stability training**.

postural stabilizers *See* **stabilizers**.

postural sway The subtle rocking motion that occurs when sitting or standing in a still, upright position, caused by the intermittent contractions of the tonic muscles.

postural tone The overall body tone that is used to maintain a specific posture.

posture *n.* A temperament or disposition in an observable stance. The position of the body. *v.* To posture is to pose, to assume a position, to take a conscious stand.

prenatal and paranatal psychology A new and as yet not broadly accepted branch of somatic psychology based on the premise that body and behavior patterns develop as a response to events and conditions that occur before, during, and shortly after birth.

preoperational stage A precognitive stage of learning identified by the learning theorist Jean Piaget in which a child starts to think in symbols and to use symbolic language to describe sensations and feelings. This stage begins when a child is around three years old and lasts until about age seven. *See also* **concrete operations**, **formal operations**, and **sensorimotor learning**.

prespinal movement Spinal movement that appears as if there were no bones around the spinal cord, having an undulating, snakelike quality; characteristic of invertebrate organisms such as the jellyfish and lancelet. *See also* **spinal movement**.

prevertebral patterns Patterns of movement that reflect the patterns of prevertebrate species, the primary patterns being cellular breathing, navel radiation, mouthing, and prespinal movements. *See also* **vertebral patterns**.

prime mover The agonist muscle, the muscle that initiates an action.

primitive reflexes Simple reflexes such as the tonic labyrinthine reflex, oral rooting reflex, and flexor withdrawal reflex, coordinated at a spinal cord and brain stem level, that appear between birth and approximately four months of age and disappear as they are integrated into more complex patterns.

process orientation A focus on the process of a modality rather than on the end result or goal.

progressive relaxation (PR) A therapeutic technique developed by Edmund Jacobson in which a person learns to relax by progressively tightening and releasing each muscle in the body.

propping Using a locked, hyperextended joint, usually the elbow or knee, to brace the body to hold it up.

pronation A movement of the forearm in which the palm of the hand is turned from a position that faces up to a position that faces down. *See also* **supination**.

protraction A lateral movement of the scapula away from the spine.

proprioception The sensations stimuli generate within the body. Proprioception comes from sensory receptors in the muscle spindles, joint proprioceptors, or golgi tendon organs.

proprioceptive feedback Information coming from the proprioceptors in the muscles, tendons, and joints that register movement, changes in position, and changes in muscle length and tendon tension.

proprioceptive neuromuscular facilitation (PNF) A method to activate the functional (neuromuscular) mechanisms by stimulating an awareness of movement.

proprioceptive neuromuscular facilitation (PNF) patterns A series of three-dimensional rotational patterns developed by Herman Kabat, designed to take the body, specifically the joints, through a full range of physiological motion.

protraction In reference to kinesiology, a lateral movement or abduction of the scapula away from the spine. *See also* retraction.

psychoneuroimmunology (PNI) A relatively new field of study, research, and therapy based on biochemical relationships between thoughts, emotions, and immune functions.

psychophysical education A style of movement education developed by Mabel Todd that focuses on an understanding of the body and posture, and the role of awareness and attitude in shaping movement.

psychosomatic Involving both the body and the mind; relating to or involving the bodily symptoms caused by mental or emotional states or disturbances.

pull The fourth of the four neurological actions, a movement that occurs after a reach and grasp, drawing a limb or the body through space.

push The second of the four neurological actions, a movement that separates the body from a supporting surface when a supporting limb or body part presses into the surface to push away from it.

rapport In the context of neurolinguistic programming, a connection that is established with another person from sharing or matching experiences, such as similar body rhythms, posture, body movements, or speech patterns. *See also* **matching**.

reach The third of the four neurological actions, an outwardly focused movement that causes the extension of a limb, the head, or the body into space.

reciprocal inhibition A principle described by physiologist Lord Sherrington describing muscle reflexes stating that when a muscle within a coupled pair is contracted, the contraction of its antagonist will be inhibited. *See also* **reciprocal innervation**.

reciprocal innervation A principle described by physiologist Lord Sherrington describing a reflex between coupled muscles in which the agonist muscles are connected to the antagonist muscles through neural synapses in the spinal cord that control basic reflexes such as the flexor withdrawal and extensor thrust. *See also* **reciprocal inhibition**.

recruitment order The order in which motor units within a muscle contract; the order in which muscles contract within a neuromuscular sequence.

reflective thinking In the context of somatic patterning, thoughts that reflect on the past or speculate about the future. Also, the cortical ability of humans to be aware of awareness.

reflex Specific automatic patterns of movement coordinated at spinal cord and hindbrain level that underlie all basic coordination.

reflexive movement Automatic movement.

reflexive sympathetic dystrophy (RSD) A chronic pain syndrome of unknown cause whose main symptom is that pain escalates rather than diminishes over time. RSD often begins with a minor bump or bruise.

reframing A technique in neurolinguistic programming used to separate a behavior from the secondary gain, or the intention of the behavior.

relaxation response A term coined by Dr. Herbert Benson to describe a response that can be elicited when four environmental conditions are met: a passive attitude, a quiet environment without interference, a word or phrase repeated over and over again, and a comfortable position. Relaxation skills require the ability to track autonomic tone and initiate a relaxation response during both rest and movement.

repetitive stress injury (RSI) An overuse injury to the tissues caused by the repetition of the same movement pattern.

representational system The perceptual channel (visual, auditory, kinesthetic, or a combination of these three) that a person uses to represent his or her reality.

resistance In terms of proprioceptive neuromuscular facilitation (PNF) techniques, resistance is the force applied by a practitioner that a client can move against to stimulate muscular responses and to organize an integrated chain of muscular contractions. Sustained resistance uses a constant force. Rhythmic resistance uses a force applied to intermittently give a client moments of rest between applications of force, used at the weakest point during a motion to increase strength; also called *intermittent resistance*.

responsiveness The ability to respond to a movement impulse and let it sequence through the entire body.

retraction In reference to kinesiology, a medial movement or adduction of the scapula toward the spine, "pinching the shoulder blades together." *See also* protraction.

reverie The state of consciousness between waking and sleeping; also called a "twilight state." This state is thought to be of therapeutic value when a person is able to stay awake during it, giving him or her access to subconscious processes. Also, this state is associated with the alpha-theta brain wave threshold and has been associated with states of deep relaxation and tissue regeneration.

righting reactions The complex, automatic movement patterns coordinated at a midbrain level that bring the head and torso into alignment, such as the head righting and optical righting reactions.

Rolfing A slang term to denote the somatic therapy developed by Ida P. Rolf called Structural Integration. *See also* **Rolfing Movement Education** and **structural integration**.

Rolfing Movement Education An adjunct method of movement education used in Rolfing that focuses on helping a client sense the effects of alignment of the body in the gravitational field on the structural integrity of the body.

rooting *See* **mouthing**.

sagittal plane An imaginary plane made up of the four corners of the longitudinal dimension and the front-back dimension. The plane in which a wheel turns.

scapula neutral The ideal position of the scapula in which it is most stable, marked by the balanced span of numerous muscles connecting the scapula to the arm and trunk. When in neutral, the medial border of the scapula rests about two and one-half inches from and parallel to the spine, the acromium is slightly higher than the superior medial angle of the scapula, and the scapula rests flat against the ribs and lies 15 to 30 degrees forward of the frontal plane.

scapulohumeral rhythm The ratio of movement between the scapula and humerus. Ideally, the scapula remains stable as a base of support during the first 45 to 60 degrees of respective arm abduction and flexion, after which the scapula and humerus move in an approximate one-to-two ratio. This ratio maximizes stability in the glenohumeral joint to prevent excessive shearing and ensure that the shoulder muscles function in an ideal range. *See also* **lumbar-pelvic rhythm.**

scoliosis An abnormal, lateral curvature of the spine, which has a number of causes: poor postural habits, asymmetry in bilateral muscle-use patterns, bone deformity, paralysis of muscles, visual defects that cause the head to tilt, hip disease, and congenital or neurological disorders.

secondary gain The benefits a person receives from a painful condition or illness.

self-image The mental picture a person forms of his or her personality as it is expressed through the body.

sensorimotor amnesia A term coined by somatic philosopher Thomas Hannah to describe a condition in which a person has a lack of body awareness and therefore is unable to sense movement in the body and lacks control over movement.

sensorimotor learning The first stage of cognitive development in Piaget's theory of learning, in which thinking is limited to immediate sensory input and motor responses. *See also* **formal operations**, **concrete operations**, and **preoperational stage**.

sensorimotor loop The cycle of sensory information that is processed and results in a motor response.

sensory awareness The perception of sensations in the body received through the sensory receptors of the skin, ears, eyes, nose, and musculoskeletal receptors. A meditative practice of tracking bodily sensation in order to expand perception and connect awareness with experience. Also, the process of tracking physical sensations to increase awareness and sensitivity in the body, which is widely used in somatic patterning.

Sensory Awareness A process and practice developed by Charlotte Selver used to become more fully aware of sensory perceptions and to refine this awareness.

sensory processes Neurological sequences that involve the relaying of information from the sensory nerves to the brain or spinal cord. *See also* **motor processes**.

shaping The process of carving a shape, either within the body or in space, with movement.

side load A structure hanging from the side, suspended by tensional pulleys. The arms hang as side loads from the tensional pull of the muscles and ligaments of the shoulder girdle.

skeletal nervous system (SNS) Also called the "somatic nervous system," the part of the peripheral nervous system that controls the voluntary functions of the skeletal muscles.

soma The living, breathing body in its all its wholeness. On a biological level, all of an organism except the germ cells.

somatic awareness Includes a sensory awareness of the bodily sensations generated by physiological processes, and of the changing tensions and positions caused by movement through space. Also includes cognitive awareness of thoughts, emotions, and the act of perceiving. Synonymous with body-mind awareness.

somatic patterning (SP) A therapeutic modality that works to change harmful or inefficient body-use patterns using awareness and movement as primary tools; an educational modality that works to improve posture and movement efficiency by focusing on the functional interrelationships of the parts of the body.

somatic resonance A physical connection between two or more people when their bodies vibrate and move at the same or similar frequencies. A positive physical rapport that occurs when people move in synchrony, and match or complement one another's patterns of movement, breath, speech, thought, and energetic somatic patterns.

somatic From the Greek root "soma" meaning the living organism in all its aspects, mental, physical and emotional. *See* **soma**.

somatics The field of study of the thinking body that expresses its intelligence in behavior and movement.

somato-emotional release A therapeutic hands-on method developed by John Upledger that is used to clear the body of energy blockages incurred during injury or trauma and incorporates unwinding.

spatial tension A tensional support of the body created by a directionally clear image coupled with a reach through the arm, leg, or spine. For example, a tightrope walker uses spatial tension to balance by reaching out through both arms.

spinal movement Movement characterized by patterns of flexion, extension, and side-bending through the spinal column. *See also* **prespinal movement**.

splinting A protective muscle spasm, or splint, that immobilizes an injured area during healing to prevent further injury.

stability dysfunction The failure of the body while moving because of unstable joints. The inability to control joint play during movement.

stability training A series of progressive exercises that build tonic function in the muscles that stabilize joints (particularly of the spine). The progression begins with precise, isometric contractions of stabilizer muscles with the spine in a neutral position, then co-contractions of groups of stabilizers, and culminates in stabilization that coordinates tonic control during phasic movements.

stabilizers In terms of postural stability, muscles that have tonic function, meaning that they generate slow, sustained contractions to stiffen the joints they span in order to hold these joints in a stable neutral position. *Local stabilizers* control the neutral position of a joint, and *global stabilizers* control a movement through its range. *See also* **mobilizers.**

stance phase In terms of gait patterns, the phase of movement in which the leg is bearing weight and the foot is in contact with the ground. *See also* **swing phase**.

startle reflex A defensive reflex in response to a loud noise or sudden threat, graded between a small contraction and a full-body response.

stillpoint The stopping of the cerebrospinal fluid (CSF) pump, either on its own or as a result of cranialsacral (CS) manipulation, which increases fluid pressure in the CS system. Stillpoints are induced by CSF practitioners to increase the strength of the CS pump.

stress The body's nonspecific response to external or internal demands, both positive and negative; wear and tear on the body.

stressor Any factor—environmental, cognitive, emotional, or physiological—that causes stress.

stress response The physiological response that the body automatically makes to a stressor.

stretch reflex A reflex that causes a skeletal muscle to contract after stretching; regulated by the muscle spindle.

stretch weakness A weakness that develops in a muscle under constant tension from being held in an elongated position, usually by a chronic contracture in the opposing muscle group.

Structural Integration A ten-step series of somatic education and manipulation techniques developed by Ida Rolf that results in the natural alignment of the body; also known as Rolfing.

substitution pattern When another muscle contracts to take over the job of a dysfunctional muscle.*See also* and **adaptivc pattern** *and* **compensatory pattern**.

supination A movement of the forearm in which the palm of the hand is turned from an position that faces down to a position that faces up. *See also* **pronation**.

support before movement A patterning concept stating that the more underlying support the body has prior to action, the more efficient the subsequent action will be.

sustained stretch A steady stretch that is held for 20 seconds or more.

swing phase In terms of gait patterns, the phase of movement in which the leg is swing freely and the foot is not in contact with the ground. *See also* **stance phase**.

sympathetic The branch of the autonomic nervous system that regulates arousal and speeds up metabolic functions required for fight, flight, or freeze. *See also* **parasympathetic.**

tender point A small, localized area of pain within a muscle, usually a nodule. *See also* **trigger point**.

tensegrity structure A structure supported by a balance between tensional forces, distributed along guylines, and compression support, distributed through rigid members, such as a tent.

tensile forces The forces in tensile elements or guylines that support weight, such as a rope that holds up a tent. In the body, tensional forces are especially evident in the span of myofascial tissues.

thermal feedback Biofeedback from thermisters (small apparatuses that attach to the fingers) to monitor peripheral blood flow by reading skin temperature, used in relaxation training. An easy biofeedback method because thermisters are inexpensive and easy to use.

thixotropy The property of a substance to change fluid states from a liquid or sol to a gel and back again, a process that is initiated by the heating or cooling of a substance. A property of fascia.

timeline A continuum of past-present-future; a cycle that occurs in time, such as birth, life, and death. In the context of neurolinguistic programming, a concept that teaches people how to link past, present, and future in healthy ways.

tissue pump The mechanical pump of body fluids, particularly interstitial and lymph, generated by the rhythmic contractions of muscles during movement.

tone The neural excitability of the tissues, particularly in the muscular system.

tonic A term used to describe the rate of a muscle contraction. A slow contraction.

tonic function The combined roles of the postural muscles to work in light, isometric contractions to maintain a neutral position of a joint and a neutral position of the spine.

tonic immobility Synonymous with the freeze response. Thought to be a response to physiological trauma. Described by trauma specialist Peter Levine as the natural response of animals to "play dead" when under attack; problematic in humans when this physiological state continues long after the attack or trauma is over.

tonic labyrinthine reflex A reflex stimulated by the tactile receptors in the skin and the movement of the otoliths in the inner ear that increases tone on the supporting surface of the body: flexor tone on the anterior side and extensor tone on the posterior side.

top load A supported structure that transfers weight to the structure below it; the head on the body.

track and bump A patterning technique in which a person oscillates between observing the shape of a posture or the direction of a movement, and giving the posture or movement direction and guidance with the nudge of intention. When done by a practitioner, he or she observes the movement visually or tactilely with touch, then bumps the client gently with tactile nudges to direct the motion.

transference Imagining that an experience coming from within is being caused by someone else.

trigger point (TP) An area of irritation in a tissue that is tender and hypersensitive when touched; can cause referred pain and tenderness, and sometimes involves autonomic responses and distorted proprioception. *See also* **tender point.**

unwinding In the context of cranialsacral therapy, the rhythmic unraveling of connective tissues that is initiated by physiological rhythms. Also, a gentle technique used in cranialsacral therapy in which the practitioner gently holds a client and passively unravels myofascial tension, following both the cranial sacral rhythm fueled by the movement of cerebrospinal fluid and the spiral pathways of the tissues as they unwind.

upright posture The vertical posture of humans in which the major body masses—head, thorax, and pelvis—are aligned and balanced over each other.

vertebral patterns The patterns of movement found in vertebrate species. *See also* **prevertebral patterns**.

volitional movement Movement that is directed by the will; voluntary movement. *See also* **reflexive movement**.

witness In dance therapy, a healing role passively taken on by an objective, nonjudgmental observer, the psychotherapist. *See also* **authentic movement**.

yield The first of the four basic neurological actions, a motor pattern involving deep relaxation and releasing into the supporting surface.

BIBLIOGRAPHY

Ader, R., and N. Cohen. "Behavior and the Immune System." From *Handbook of Behavioral Medicine.* New York: Guilford (1984):117–173.

Ader, R., D. Felton, and N. Cohen. *Psychoneuroimmunology.* 2nd ed. New York: Academic Press, 1991.

Alexander, F. M. *Knowing How to Stop*. London: Chaterson, 1946.

Alter, M. *Science of Flexibility.* 2nd ed. Champaign, Ill.: Human Kinetics, 1996.

American Heart Association. "Heart and Stroke Statistics." American Heart Association Website (28 October 2002): <www.americanheart.org>.

Anand, B. K., G. S. Cchina, and B. Singh. "Some Aspects of Electrocephalographic Studies in Yogis." *Electrocephalograph Clinical Neurophysiology* 13 (1961): 452–56.

Andrade, C., and P. Clifford. *Outcome-Based Massage.* Philadelphia: Lippincott Williams and Wilkins, 2001.

Andreas, S., and C. Faulkner, eds. *NLP: The New Technology of Achievement.* New York: Quill William Morrow, 1994.

———. *Change Your Mind and Keep the Change.* Moab, Utah: Real People Press,1987.

Armour, J., and J. Ardell, eds. *Neurocardiology*. New York: Oxford University Press, 1984.

Asimov, I. *On the Human Body and the Human Brain.* New York: Bonanza Books, 1985.

Ayres, J. *Sensory Integration and the Child.* Los Angeles: Western Psychological Services, 1972.

Bagchi, B. K., and A. Wenger. "Electrophysiological Correlates of Some Yogi Exercises." *EEG Clinical Neurophysiology* Supplement 7 (1957): 132–49.

Bandler, R. *Using Your Brain—for a Change*. Moab, Utah: Real People Press, 1985.

Bandler, R., and J. Grinder. *Frogs into Princes.* Moab, Utah: Real People Press, 1979.

Barasch, M. "Welcome to the Body-Mind Revolution." *Psychology Today* 24 (July/August 1993):58.

Barral, J., and P. Mercier. *Visceral Manipulation.* Seattle: Eastland Press, 1989.

Bartenieff, I., and D. Lewis. *Body Movement: Coping with the Environment*. New York: Gordon & Breach, 1980.

Basmajian, J. V. *Muscles Alive: Their Functions Revealed by Electromyography.* Baltimore: Williams and Wilkins, 1985.

———. *Biofeedback: Principles and Practice for Clinicians.* Baltimore: Williams and Wilkins, 1979.

Beck, A. *Cognitive Therapy and Emotional Disorders.* New York: New American Library, 1976.

Benson, H. *The Relaxation Response*. New York: Morrow, 1975.
———. *Timeless Healing*. New York: Simon and Schuster, 1996.
Bergmark, A. "Stability of the Lumbar Spine: A Study in Mechanical Engineering." *Acta Orthopaedica: Scandinavica* 230 Supplemental (1989): 20–24.
Biondi, M., and A. Picardi. "Clinical and Biological Aspects of Bereavement and Loss-Induced Depression: a Reappraisal." *Psychotherapy and Psychosomatics* 65, no. 5 (1996): 229–45.
Bobath, B. *Abnormal Postural Reflex Activity Caused by Brain Lesions*. 3rd ed. Oxford, England: Butterworth-Heinemann, 1985.
Bogduk, N., M. Pearcy, and G. Hadfield. "Anatomy and Biomechanics of the Psoas Major." *Clinical Biomechanics* 7 (1992): 109–19.
Brooks, C. *Sensory Awareness: The Rediscovery of Experiencing*. New York: Viking, 1974.
Budzynski, T., J. Stoyva, and C. Adler. "Feedback-Induced Muscle Relaxation: Application to Tension Headaches." *Journal of Behavior Therapy and Experimental Psychiatry* no. 1 (1970).
Cade, C., and N. Coxhead. *The Awakened Mind: Biofeedback and the Development of Higher States of Awareness*. Shaftesbury, Eng.: Element Books, 1989.
Cailliett, R. *Soft Tissue Pain and Disability*. 3rd ed. Philadelphia: F. A. Davis Company, 1996.
———. *Low Back Pain Syndrome*. 5th ed. Philadelphia: F. A. Davis Company, 1995.
———. *Pain: Mechanisms and Management*. Philadelphia: F. A. Davis Company, 1993.
———. *Knee Pain and Disability*. 3rd ed. Philadelphia: F. A. Davis Company, 1992.
———. *Shoulder Pain*. 3rd ed. Philadelphia: F. A. Davis Company, 1991.
———. *Low Back Pain Syndrome*. 4th ed. Philadelphia: F. A. Davis Company, 1988.
———. *Understand Your Backache*. Philadelphia: F. A. Davis Company, 1984.
Caldwell, C. *Getting Our Bodies Back: Recovery, Healing and Transformation Through Body-Centered Psychotherapy*. Boston: Shambhala, 1996.
Cannon, W. B. *The Wisdom of the Body*. New York: Norton, 1932.
Charlesnorth, E. "The Relaxation and Stress Management Program: Autogenic Relaxation." *Home Practice Audio Tapes*. Houston, Tex.: Stress Management Research Associates, 1981.
Childre, C., and H. Martin. *The Heartmath Solution*. San Francisco: Harper, 1999.
Chodorow, I. *Dance Therapy and Depth Psychology*. New York: Routledge, 1991.
Cohen, B. *Sensing, Feeling, and Action*. Northampton, Mass.: Contact Editions, 1993.
———. *The Evolutionary Origins of Movement*. Amherst, Mass.: Self-published, 1990.
———. *The Nervous System Manual*. Amherst, Mass.: Self-published, 1982.
Comerford, M. "Dynamic Stability and Muscle Balance of the Lower Quadrant: Kinetic Control Movement Dysfunction Course." Course tutor. Southamptom, U.K.: Self-published, 2001.
———. "Dynamic Stability and Muscle Balance of the Upper Quadrant: Kinetic Control Movement Dysfunction Course." Course tutor. Southamptom, U.K.: Self-published, 2001.
———. "Movement Dysfunction: Dynamic Stability Rehabilitation of the Local and Global Muscles System for Sacro-Iliac Dysfunction." Course tutor. Harrow, U.K.: Self-published, 2000.
Cousins, N. *Anatomy of an Illness*. New York: Norton, 1979.
Cowley, G. "Generation XXL." *Newsweek*, July 2000, 40–44.
Dacher, E. *Psychoneuroimmunology: The New Mind/Body Healing Program*. New York: Paragon House, 1991.
Darwin, C. *The Descent of Man*. Norwalk, Conn.: Easton Press, 1979.
Dell, C. *A Primer for Movement Description Using Effort-Shape Concepts*. New York: Dance Notation Bureau Press, 1977.
Dennis, R. J. "Functional Reach Improvement in Normal Older Women after Alexander Instruction." *Journal of Gerontology and Biological Sciences and Medical Sciences* 54, no. 1 (January 1999): M8–11.
Diamong, W., and S. Coniam. *The Management of Chronic Pain*. Oxford: Oxford University Press, 1997.
Dossey, L. *Healing Words: The Power of Prayer and the Practice of Medicine*. New York: HarperCollins, 1993.
Dusenbery, D. *Life at a Small Scale: The Behavior of Microbes*. New York: Scientific American Library, 1966.
Eisenberg, D. M., et al. "Trends in Alternative Medicine Use in the United States, 1990–1997: Results of a Follow-Up National Survey." *Journal of the American Medical Association* 11 (November 1998): 1569–75.
Emerson, P. "Myofascial Manipulation." Course outline. Denver, Colo.: Self-published, 2000.
Emerson, W. "What Is Birth Trauma?" Petaluma, Calif.: 1996.
Engel, G. "The Need for a New Medical Model: A Challenge for Biomedicine." *Science* 196 (1977): 129–36.
Everly, G. *A Clinical Guide to the Treatment of Human Stress Response*. New York: Plenum, 1989.

Feldenkrais, M. "Moshe on the Martial Arts." Interview by D. Leri. *Feldenkrais Journal* no. 2 (1986).
———. *The Master Moves.* Capitola, Calif.: Meta Publications, 1984.
———. *The Case of Nora: Body-Awareness as Healing Therapy*. New York: Harper and Row, 1977.
———. "The Forebrain: Sleep, Consciousness, Awareness and Learning." Interview by E. Rosenfeld. *Interface Journal* nos. 3–4 (1976): 1–4.
———. *Awareness Through Movement*. New York: Harper and Row, 1972.
Feldenkrais, M., and W. Schutz. "Movement and the Mind." From *The New Healers.* Berkeley, Calif.: New Dimensions, l980.
Foreign Language Press. *An Outline of Chinese Acupuncture: The Academy of Traditional Chinese Medicine.* Peking, 1975.
Franklin, E. *Dynamic Alignment Through Imagery*. Champaign, Ill.: Human Kinetics, 1996.
Gardener, H. *Frames of Mind.* New York: Basic Books, 1985.
Gazzaniga, M. *The Mind's Past*. Berkeley, Calif.: University of California Press, 1998.
Gendlin, E. *Focusing.* 2nd ed. New York: Bantam Books, 1978.
Gerber, R. *Vibrational Medicine: New Choices for Healing Ourselves.* Sante Fe, N. Mex.: Bear and Company, 1996.
Gibbons, S. G. "Anatomy, Physiology, and Function of Psoas Major: A New Model of Stability." The Tragic Hip: Trouble in the Lower Quadrant, 11th Annual National Orthopeadic Conference, Halifax, Canada, 1999.
Goleman, D. *Emotional Intelligence.* New York: Bantam, 1995.
Gray, H. *Gray's Anatomy.* 15th ed. New York: Bounty Books, 1977.
Green, E., and A. Green. *Biofeedback to Mind-Body Self-Regulation: Healing and Creativity.* New York: Delacorte Press, 1977.
Green, E. *The Ozawkie Book of the Dead: Alzheimer's Isn't What Your Think It Is.* Los Angeles: Philosophical Research Society, 2001.
Green, E., et al. "Anomalous Electrostatic Phenomena in Exceptional Subjects." *Subtle Energies* 2, no. 3 (1991): 69–97.
Greene, E., and B. Goodrich-Dunn. *The Psychology of the Body.* Baltimore: Lippincott Williams and Wilkins, 2004.
Greenspan, S. *The Growth of the Mind: The Endangered Origins of Intelligence.* Reading, Mass.: Addison-Wesley, 1997.
Hall, S. "A Molecular Code Links Emotions, Mind, and Health." *Smithsonian,* June 1989, 69–71.
Hanna, T. *Somatics: Reawakening the Mind's Control of Movement, Flexibility, and Health.* Reading. Mass.: Addison-Wesley, 1988.
———. *The Body of Life*. New York: Knopf, 1979.
Hodgson, J., and V. Preston-Dunlop. *Rudolph Laban: An Introduction to His Work and Influence*. Plymouth, Eng.: Northcote House, 1990.
Holmes, T., and R. Rahe. "The Social Readjustment Scale." *Journal of Psychosomatic Research* 11 (1967): 213–18.
Hunt, V. V. *Infinite Mind: The Science of Human Vibrations*. Malibu, Calif.: Malibu Publishing, 1989.
Ingber, D. "The Architecture of Life." *Scientific American,* January 1998, 48 57.
Jacobson, E. *The Biology of Emotions: New Understanding Derived from Biological Multidisciplinary Investigation: First Electrophysiological Measurements*. Springfield, Ill.: Charles C. Thomas, 1967.
———. *Progressive Relaxation*. Chicago: University of Chicago Press, 1938.
Janov, A. *Imprints: The Lifelong Effects of the Birth Experience*. New York: Coward-McCann, 1983.
Jonas, W., and J. Levin, eds. *Essentials of Complimentary Alternative Medicine.* Baltimore: Lippincott Williams and Wilkins, 2000.
Jones, F. P. *The Alexander Technique: Body Awareness in Action*. New York: Schocken, 1976.
Jones, L. *Strain and Counterstrain.* Colorado Springs, Colo.: American Academy of Osteopathy, 1981.
Kamiya, J. "Operant Control of the EEG Alpha Rhythm and Some of Its Reported Effects on Consciousness." In *Altered States of Consciousness.* Edited by C. Tart. New York: Wiley, 1969.
Kapandji, I. A. *The Physiology of Joints.* 2nd ed., vol. 2. London: Churchill Livingstone, 1982.
———. *The Physiology of Joints: The Trunk and Vertebral Column.* 2nd ed., vol. 3. Edinburgh: Churchill Livingstone, 1974.
Kasmata, A., and T. Hirai. "Science of Zazan." *Psychologia* 6 (1963): 86–91.
Kaye, J. Morton, and M. Bowcutt. "Stress, Depression, and Psychonueroimmunology." *Journal of Neuroscience and Nursing* 3, no. 2 (2000): 93–100.

Kein, H. A. *Clinical Symposia: Scoliosis* (vol. 30, no. 1). Summit, N. J.: CIBA, 1978.

Keleman, S. *Embodying Experience: Forming a Personal Life.* Berkeley, Calif.: Center Press, 1987.

———. *Patterns of Distress: Emotional Insults and Human Form.* Berkeley, Calif.: Center Press, 1987.

———. *Emotional Anatomy: The Structure of Experience.* Berkeley, Calif.: Center Press, 1985.

———. *Your Body Speaks Its Mind.* Berkeley, Calif.: Center Press, 1975.

Kendall, F., E. McCreary, and P. Provance. *Muscles: Testing and Function with Posture and Pain.* 4th ed. Baltimore: Williams and Wilkins, 1993.

Kestenberg, J. "The Role of Movement Patterns in Development: I, II, and III." *Psychoanalytic Quarterly* vol. 14, no.1 (1965); vol. 14, no. 4 (1965); vol. 16, no. 3 (1967).

Kiecolt-Glaser, J., et al. "Psychological Influences on Surgical Recovery." *American Psychologist* 53, no. 11 (November 1998): 1209–18.

Krieger, D. *Accepting Your Power to Heal: The Personal Practice of Therapeutic Touch.* Sante Fe, N. Mex.: Bear Books, 1993.

Kurtz, R. *Body-Centered Psychotherapy: The Hakomi Method.* Mendocino, Calif.: LifeRhythm, 1990.

Laban, R. *A Life for Dance: Reminiscences.* New York: Theater Arts Books, 1975.

Lamb, W. *Posture and Gesture.* London: Duckworth, 1965.

Laumer, U., M. Bauer, M. Fichter, and H. Milz. "Therapeutic Effects of the Feldenkrais Method of Awareness Through Movement in Patients with Eating Disorders." *Psychotherapy, Psychosomatic Medical Psychology Journal* 47, no. 5 (May 1997): 70–80.

LeDeoux, J. *The Synaptic Self: How Our Brains Become Who We Are.* New York: Viking, 2002.

———. *The Emotional Brain: The Mysterious Underpinnings of Emotional Life.* New York: Simon and Schuster, 1996.

Levine, P. A. *Waking the Tiger: Healing Trauma.* Berkeley, Calif.: North Atlantic Books, 1997.

Lipton, B. "The Biology of Consciousness." Transcript of lecture presented at the University of British Columbia, May 1995.

Lorenz, K. *King Soloman's Ring.* New York: Cromwell, 1952.

Low, L. "The Modern Body Therapies: A First-Hand Look at Leading Bodywork Therapies." *Massage Magazine* 16 (October/November 1988): 12–19, 48–55.

Lowen, A. *Narcissism: Denial of the True Self.* New York: Collier Books, Macmillan Publishing Co., 1985.

———. *Bioenergetics: The Revolutionary Therapy That Uses the Language of the Body to Heal the Problems of the Mind.* New York: Penguin, 1975.

———. *Betrayal of the Body.* New York: Macmillan, 1967.

Luskin, F. M., et al. "A Review of Mind-Body Therapies in the Treatment of Cardiovascular Disease." *Alternative Therapies in Health and Medicine* 4, no. 3 (May 1998): 46–61.

Luttgens, K., H. Deutsch, and N. Hamilton. *Kinesiology: Scientific Basis of Human Motion.* 8th ed. Dubuque, Iowa: Brown and Benchmark, 1992.

Maier, H. *Theories of Child Development.* New York: Harper and Row, 1969.

Maier, S., and M. E. P. Seligman. "Learned Helplessness: Theory and Evidence." *Journal of Experimental Psychology: General* 105 (1976): 3–46.

Marieb, E. N. *Human Anatomy and Physiology.* 4th ed. Redwood City, Calif.: Benjamin/Cummings, 1998.

Martin, G., and J. Pear. *Behavior Modification: What It Is and How to Do It.* University of Manitoba: Prentice Hall, 1996.

McKay, M., M. Davis, and P. Fanning. *Thoughts and Feelings: The Art of Cognitive Stress Intervention.* Oakland, Calif.: New Harbinger Publications, 1994.

McKenzie, R. *Treat Your Own Back.* 7th ed. New Zealand: Spinal Publications, 1998.

Melzack, R., and P. Wall. *The Challenge of Pain.* Rev. ed. New York: Basic Books, 1982.

Michele, A. *Orthotherapy.* Philadelphia: M. Evans and Co. with Lippincott, 1971.

Miller, G., et. al. "Psychosocial Predictors of Natural Killer Cell Mobilization during Marital Conflict." *Health Psychology* 18, no. 3 (1999): 262–71.

Montagu, A. *Touching: The Human Significance of Skin.* 3rd ed. New York: Harper and Row, 1986.

Moore, N. "A Review of Alternative Medicine Courses Taught at U.S. Medical Schools." *Alternative Therapies in Health and Medicine* 4, no. 3 (May 1998): 90–101.

Moyers, B. *Healing and the Mind.* New York: Doubleday, 1993.

Nelson, L., and N. Smith, eds. *Contact Improvisation Sourcebook.* Northampton, Mass.: Contact Editions, 1997.

Norkin, C., and P. Levangie. *Joint Structure and Functions: A Comprehensive Analysis.* 2nd ed. Philadelphia: F. A. Davis Company, 1992.
North, M. *Personality Assessment through Movement*. London: MacDonald and Evans, 1970.
Norris, C. *Back Stability.* Champaign, Ill.: Human Kinetics, 2000.
Oschman, J. *Energy Medicine: The Scientific Basis.* London: Churchhill Livingstone, 2000.
———. *Readings on the Scientific Basis of Bodywork*. Dover, N.H.: Self-published, l986.
Pagels, H. *Cosmic Code*. New York: Bantam, 1982.
Panjabi, M. "The Stabilizing System of the Spine, Part 2: Neutral Zone and Instability Hypothesis." *Journal of Spinal Disorders* 5 (1992):90–97.
———. *Clinical Biomechanics of the Spine.* Philadelphia: J.B. Lippincott Co., 1990.
Panjabi, M., K. Abumi, J. Duranceau, and T. Oxland. "Spinal Stability and Intersegmental Forces. A Biomechanical Model." *Spine* 14 (1989): 94–200.
Pearce, J. *Evolution's End: Claiming the Potential of Our Intelligence*. San Francisco: Harper Collins, 1992.
Perls, F. *Gestalt Therapy Verbatim*. Moab, Utah: Real People Press, 1969.
Pert, C. *Molecules of Emotion: Why You Feel the Way You Feel.* New York: Simon and Schuster, 1999.
———. "The Wisdom of the Receptors: Neuropeptides, the Emotions, and the Bodymind." *Advances* 3 (Summer 1986): 8–16.
Pierrakos, J. *Core Energetics*. Mendocino, Calif.: Life Rhythms, 1987.
Prosser, E. *Manual of Massage and Movements.* London: Lippincott, 1951.
Rank, O. *The Trauma of Birth.* New York: Dover, 1993.
Reich, W. *The Function of the Orgasm.* Vol. 1. New York: Farrar, Straus and Giroux, 1973.
———. *Character Analysis.* 3rd ed. New York: Noonday Press, 1949.
Richardson, C., G. Jull, J. Hides, and P. Hodges. *Therapeutic Exercises for Spinal Segmental Stabilization: Scientific Basis and Clinical Approach*. London: Churchill Livingstone, 1999.
Richardson, C., G. Jull, and B. Richardson. "A Dysfunction of the Deep Abdominal Muscles Exists in Low Back Pain Patients." In *Proceedings: World Confederation of Physical Therapists,* Washington, D. C., 1995.
Rolf, I. P. *Rolfing: The Integration of Human Structures*. New York: Harper and Row, 1977.
Sahrmann, S. *Diagnosis and Treatment of Movement Impairment Syndromes.* St. Louis: Mosby, 2002.
Schacklock, M. "The Chronic Back: An Evidence-Based Approach to Prevention and Treatment of Persistent Back Pain." Class handout. Self-published, 2002.
Schrodt, G., and A. Tasman. "Behavioral Medicine." From chapter 26 of *Essentials of Complimentary Alternative Medicine,* edited by W. B. Jonan and J. S. Levin, 445. Baltimore: Lippincott Williams and Wilkins, 1999.
Schultz, J., and W. Luthe. *Autogenic Training.* New York: Grune and Stratton, 1959.
Schulz, M. L. *Awakening Intuition: Using Your Mind-Body Network for Insight and Healing.* New York: Three Rivers Press, 1998.
Schutz, W. "Movement and the Mind." Interview with Moshe Feldenkrais published in *The New Healers.* Berkeley, Calif.: New Dimensions, 1980.
Seligman, M. E. P. *Learned Optimism: How to Change Your Mind and Your Life.* New York: Pocket Books, 1990.
Selye, H. "On the Real Benefits of Eustress," interview by L. Cherry. *Psychology Today,* March 1978, 60–70.
———. *The Stress of Life.* New York: McGraw-Hill, 1956.
Shaffer, C. "Dancing in the Dark." *Yoga Journal* 77 (November/December 1987): 48–55, 94, 98.
Shapiro, F., and M. Forrest. *Eye Movement Desensitization and Reprocessing.* New York: Basic Books, 1997.
Shellenberger, R., and J. Green. *From the Ghost in the Box to Successful Biofeedback Training.* Greeley, Colo.: Health Psychology Publications, 1996.
Sherrington, C. *The Integrative Action of the Nervous System.* London: Cambridge University Press, 1952.
Siegal, B. *Love, Medicine, and Miracles.* New York: Harper & Row, 1986.
Siegfried, M., and D. Simons. *Muscle Pain: Understanding Its Nature, Diagnosis, and Treatment.* Baltimore: Lippincott Williams and Wilkins, 2001.
Simonton, C. *Getting Well Again.* Los Angeles: Tarcher, 1978.
Skinner, B. F. *Walden Two.* New York: Macmillan, 1948.
Spalding, B. T. *The Life and Teachings of the Masters of the Far East*. Vol. 2. Marina del Ray, Calif.: DeVorss and Co., 1972.
Spencer J., and J. Jacobs. eds. *Complimentary and Alternative Medicine: An Evidence Based Approach.* St. Louis: Mosby, 1999.

Spencer, J., and J. Jacobs. eds. *Complimentary and Alternative Medicine: An Evidence-Based Approach.* St. Louis: Mosby, 1999.

Stallibrass, C. "An Evaluation of the Alexander Technique for the Management of Disability in Parkinson's Disease: A Preliminary Study." *Clinical Rehabilitation* 11, no. 1 (February 1997): 8–12.

Steindler, A. *Kinesiology of the Human Body*. Springfield, Ill.: Charles C. Thomas, 1955.

Stern, D. *The Interpersonal World of the Infant.* New York: Basic Books, Inc., 1985.

Stern, R. M., and W. Ray. *Biofeedback: Potentials and Limits.* Lincoln: University of Nebraska Press, 1977.

Stroebel, C. *QR: The Quieting Reflex.* New York: Putnam, 1982.

Sutherland, W. *The Cranial Bowl.* Mankato, Minn.: Free Press Company, 1939.

Sweigard, L. E. *The Human Movement Potential: Ideokinetic Facilitation*. New York: Harper & Row, 1974.

Taber's Cyclopedic Medical Dictionary. 17th ed. Philadelphia: F. A. Davis, 1993.

Tart, C., ed. *Altered States of Consciousness.* New York: Doubleday Anchor Books, 1969.

Todd, M. E. *The Thinking Body*. Princeton, N.J.: Dance Horizons Books, 1937.

Tortora, G. J., and S. R. Grabowski. *Principles of Anatomy and Physiology.* 8th ed. Menlo Park, Calif.: Addison Wesley Longman Co., 1996.

Travell, J., and D. G. Simons. *Myofascial Pain and Dysfunction: The Trigger Point Manual.* Vol. 1. Baltimore: Williams and Wilkins, 1983.

Upledger, J. E. "Somato-Emotional Release." Class handout. West Palm Beach, Fla.: Upledger Institute, 1990.

Upledger, J. E., and J. D. Vredevoogd. *Cranialsacral Therapy*. Chicago: Eastland Press, 1983.

U.S. Department of Health and Human Services. *Healthy People 2010: Understanding and Improving Health*. Washington, D.C.: Health and Human Services, 2000.

Voss, D. E., M. K. Ionta, and B. J. Myer. *Proprioceptive Neuromuscular Facilitation: Patterns and Techniques.* 3rd ed. New York: Harper and Row, 1985.

Wallace, R. K. *The Physiological Effects of Transcendental Meditation.* Los Angeles: MUIPRESS, 1970.

Watts, A. *This Is It: And Other Essays on Zen and Spiritual Experience*. New York: Vintage Books, 1958.

Wetzel, M., D. Eisenberg, and T. Kaptchuk. "Courses Involving Complementary and Alternative Medicine at U.S. Medical Schools." *Journal of the American Medical Association* 280, no. 9 (September 1998): 784–87.

Whitehouse, M. "Reflections on a Metamorphosis." Paper presented at the Developmental Conference on Dance, University of California, Los Angeles, 1968.

Wilson, E., and C. Schneider. *Human Activity: A Primer in Psychobiology*. Boulder, Colo.: Self-published, 1988.

———. *The Challenge of Chronic Muscle Pain.* Boulder, Colo.: Self-published, 1988.

INDEX

A

B

C

D

E

F

G

H

I

J

K

L

M

N

O

P

Q

R

S

T

U

V

W

Y

PATTERNING EXERCISE APPENDIX

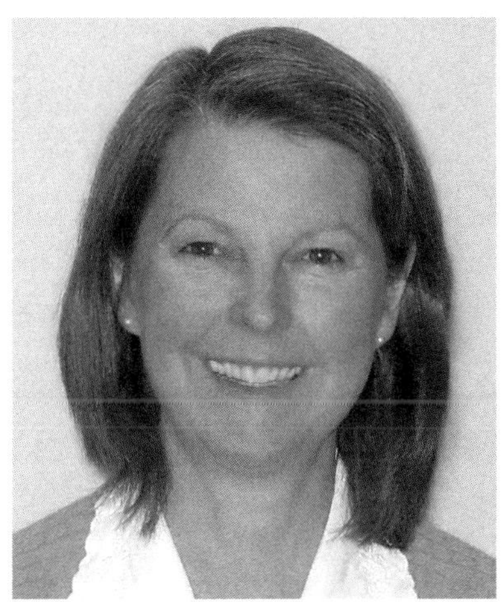

About the Author

Mary Ann Foster BA, CMT, is a certified massage therapist who has been in private practice in the Denver/Boulder area since 1981. She has a B.A. in Body-Mind Therapies and specializes in movement instruction for health care professionals with an emphasis on postural muscle training, body mechanics, self-care, and client education.

An avid researcher and writer, Mary Ann is also author of *Therapeutic Kinesiology: Musculoskeletal Systems, Palpation, and Body Mechanics* (Pearson, 2012), was a contributor to *Teaching Massage* (LWW and ABMP, 2008), and has written regularly for *Massage and Bodywork Magazine.* She developed Somatic Patterning out of diverse studies in therapeutic massage, Laban movement analysis, Rolfing® movement integration, Body-Mind Centering®, cranialsacral therapy, Hakomi Body-Centered Therapy, and graduate studies in somatic psychology.

Mary Ann has taught movement and kinesiology classes at a number of colleges and massage schools for over 25 years, including the Boulder College of Massage Therapy and Naropa, and has worked with diverse populations, including nurses, dancers, and yoga and Pilates teachers, as well as physical and occupational therapists. She has taught seminars on a national level and teaches master classes in neuromuscular patterning for manual therapists and professional movement teachers.

Mary Ann's students describe her as a clear and enthusiastic instructor with an innovative and knowledgeable presentation. In her seminars, she encourages students to cultivate body awareness and efficient movement through therapeutic and experiential exercises. She runs NCBTMB-approved professional courses for manual therapists, providing students with cutting-edge tools for neuromuscular patterning.